Fatty Liver Disease: NASH and Related Disorders

Fatty Liver Disease: NASH and Related Disorders

Edited by

Geoffrey C. Farrell
Director, Storr Liver Unit, Westmead Hospital, Department of Medicine,
University of Sydney, Sydney, NSW 2006, Australia

Jacob George
Director, Clinical Hepatology, Storr Liver Unit, Westmead Hospital,
Department of Medicine, University of Sydney, Sydney, NSW 2006, Australia

Pauline de la M. Hall
University of Cape Town, Department of Anatomical Pathology, Faculty of Medicine,
Observatory, Cape Town 7925, South Africa

Arthur J. McCullough
Division of Gastroenterology, MetroHealth Medical Center and
Schwartz Center for Metabolism and Nutrition, Cleveland, OH 44102-1998, USA

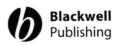

Blackwell
Publishing

© 2005 Blackwell Publishing Ltd
Blackwell Science, Inc., 350 Main Street, Malden, Massachusetts 02148-5020, USA
Blackwell Publishing Ltd, 9600 Garsington Road, Oxford OX4 2DQ, UK
Blackwell Science Asia Pty Ltd, 550 Swanston Street, Carlton, Victoria 3053, Australia

First published 2005

Library of Congress Cataloging-in-Publication Data

Fatty liver disease : NASH and related disorders / edited by Geoffrey C. Farrell . . .
[et al.].
        p.   ;   cm.
   Includes bibliographical references and index.
   ISBN 1-4051-1292-1 (alk. paper)
1. Fatty liver.
   [DNLM: 1. Fatty Liver. WI 700 F252 2004] I. Farrell, Geoffrey C.

RC848.F3F38 2004
616.3′62—dc22

                                                          2004009034

ISBN 1–4051–1292–1

A catalogue record for this title is available from the British Library

Set in 9/11.5pt Sabon by Graphicraft Limited, Hong Kong
Printed and bound in Great Britain at CPI Bath, Bath

Commissioning Editor: Alison Brown
Managing Editor: Rupal Malde
Production Editor: Nick Morgan
Project Manager: Sue Hadden
Production Controller: Kate Charman

For further information on Blackwell Publishing, visit our website:
http://www.blackwellpublishing.com

The publisher's policy is to use permanent paper from mills that operate a sustainable
forestry policy, and which has been manufactured from pulp processed using
acid-free and elementary chlorine-free practices. Furthermore, the publisher ensures
that the text paper and cover board used have met acceptable environmental
accreditation standards.

Contents

Contributors

Paul Angulo
Associate Professor of Medicine, Mayo Medical
School, and Senior Associate Consultant, Division of
Gastroenterology and Hepatology, Mayo Clinic and
Foundation, 200 First Street SW, Rochester,
MN 55905, USA

Nathan M. Bass
Professor of Medicine and Medical Director,
UCSF Liver Transplant Program, Division of
Gastroenterology, PO Box 0538, University of
California, San Francisco, CA 94143-0538, USA

Christiane Bode
Chief, Section of Physiology of Nutrition, Hohenheim
University, Garbenstrasse 28, D-70599 Stuttgart,
Germany

J. Christian Bode
Professor of Medicine (retired), Honoldweg 18,
D-70193 Stuttgart, Germany

Elisabetta Bugianesi
Gastroenterology Department, University of Turin,
Turin, Italy

Anne Burke
Assistant Professor of Medicine, University of
Pennsylvania School of Medicine, Division of
Gastroenterology, 3 Ravdin, 3400 Spruce Street,
Philadelphia, PA 19104-4283, USA

Stephen H. Caldwell
University of Virginia, Hospital West,
PO Box 800708, Charlottesville, VA 22042-3399,
USA

Vikas Chandhoke
Center for Liver Diseases, Inova Fairfax Hospital,
Department of Medicine, 3300 Gallows Road, Falls
Church, VA 22042-3300, USA

Shivakumar Chitturi
Block AG 45, Anna Nagar, Chennai, India 600 040

Andrew D. Clouston
Department of Pathology, University of Queensland,
The Princess Alexandra Hospital, Ipswich Road,
Woolloongabba, Brisbane, Queensland 4102,
Australia

Ann K. Daly
Centre for Liver Research, The Medical School,
University of Newcastle, Framlington Place,
Newcastle Upon Tyne NE2 4HH, UK

Christopher P. Day
Professor of Liver Medicine, Centre for Liver
Research, The Medical School, University of
Newcastle, Framlington Place, Newcastle Upon Tyne
NE2 4HH, UK

Anna-Mae Diehl
Director, Duke Liver Center, and Chief, Division of
Gastroenterology, Duke University Medical Center,
Genome Science Research Building #1, Suite 1073,
595 LaSalle Street, Durham, NC 27710

Geoffrey C. Farrell
Director, Storr Liver Unit, Westmead Hospital,
Department of Medicine, University of Sydney,
Sydney, NSW 2006, Australia

Bernard Fromenty
INSERM U-481, Hôpital Beaujon, 100 Boulevard du
Général Leclerc, 92118 Clichy Cedex, France

Jacob George
Head, Clinical Hepatology, Storr Liver Unit,
Westmead Hospital, Department of Medicine,
University of Sydney, Sydney, NSW 2006,
Australia

Geraldine M. Grant
Center for Liver Diseases, Inova Fairfax Hospital,
Department of Medicine, 3300 Gallows Road,
Falls Church, VA 22042-3300, USA

Pauline de la M. Hall
Professor of Pathology, University of Cape Town,
Department of Anatomical Pathology, Faculty
of Medicine, Observatory, Cape Town 7925,
South Africa

Stephen A. Harrison
Assistant Professor of Medicine, University of Texas,
Brooke Army Medical Center, 3851 Roger Brooke
Drive, Fort Sam Houston, TX 7823, USA

Yves Horsmans
Service de Gastro-enterologie, Cliniques
Universitaires Saint Luc, Université Catholique de
Louvain, Brussels, Belgium

Anita Impagliazzo Hylton
Division of Gastroenterology and Hepatology,
Box 800708, University of Virginia Health
Sciences Center, Charlottesville, VA 22908, USA

Richard Kirsch
Registrar, University of Cape Town, Department of
Anatomical Pathology, Faculty of Health Sciences,
Observatory, Cape Town 7925, South Africa

Joel E. Lavine
Professor and Vice Chair, Department of Pediatrics,
University of California San Diego Medical Center,
200 West Arbor Drive, MC 8450, San Diego,
CA 92103-8450, USA

Isabelle A. Leclercq
Collaborateur Scientifique du FNRS, Université
Catholique de Louvain, Laboratoire de Gastro-
entérologie, Avenue E. Mounier 53, B 1200
Brussels, Belgium

Zhiping Li
Assistant Professor, Department of Medicine,
Division of Gastroenterology, Johns Hopkins
University, 720 Rutland Avenue, Baltimore,
MD 21205, USA

Keith D. Lindor
Professor of Medicine, Mayo Medical School, and
Head and Consultant, Division of Gastroenterology
and Hepatology, Mayo Clinic Foundation,
200 First Street SW, Rochester,
MN 55905-0002, USA

Michael R. Lucey
Professor of Medicine and Chief, Section of
Gastroenterology and Hepatology, University of
Wisconsin-Madison Medical School,
600 Highland Avenue, Madison,
WI 53792-5124, USA

Giulio Marchesini
Associate Professor of Metabolic Disease, University
of Bologna, Department of Internal Medicine,
Unit for Metabolic Diseases, Policlinico S. Orsola,
Via Massarenti 9, I-40138 Bologna, Italy

Arthur J. McCullough
Director, Division of Gastroenterology, MetroHealth
Medical Center, 2500 Metrohealth Drive, Cleveland,
OH 44102-1998, USA

Raphael B. Merriman
Division of Gastroenterology, University of California,
PO Box 0538, San Francisco, CA 94143-0538, USA

Brent Neuschwander-Tetri
Associate Professor of Internal Medicine,
Saint Louis University School of Medicine,
Division of Gastroenterology and Hepatology,
3635 Vista Avenue, PO Box 15250, St Louis,
MO 63110-0250, USA

Dominique Pessayre
Institut National de la Santé et de la Recherche,
Unit 481, Hôpital Beaujon, 100 Boulevard du
General Leclerc, 92118 Clichy Cedex, France

Elizabeth E. Powell
Department of Gastroenterology and Hepatology,
The Princess Alexandra Hospital, Ipswich Road,
Woolloongabba, Queensland 4102, Australia

Thierry Poynard
Service d'hépatogastroentérologie, Hôpital Pitié
Salpêtrière, 47–83 Boulevard de l'Hôpital,
Paris 75013, Fance

Vlad Ratziu
Service d'hépatogastroentérologie, Hôpital Pitié
Salpêtrière, 47–83 Boulevard de l'Hôpital,
Paris 75013, France

Varman T. Samuel
Yale University School of Medicine, S269 TAC,
300 Cedar Street, New Haven, CT 06520, USA

Arun J. Sanyal
Medical College of Virginia, Internal Medicine/
Gastroenterology, MCV Station Box 980711,
Richmond, VA 23298-0711, USA

Jeffrey B. Schwimmer
Division of Gastroenterology, Hepatology and
Nutrition, Department of Pediatrics, University of
California, San Diego, and Children's Hospital and
Health Center, 200 West Arbor Drive, San Diego,
CA 92103-8450, USA

Gerald I. Shulman
Investigator, Howard Hughes Medical Institute,
295 Congress Avenue, BCMM, New Haven,
CT 06510, USA

Zobair M. Younossi
Director, Center for Liver Diseases, Inova
Fairfax Hospital, Department of Medicine,
3300 Gallows Road, Falls Church, VA 22042-3300,
USA

Preface

Non-alcoholic fatty liver disease (NAFLD), like hepatitis C and HIV, is a disease of our generation. Mostly unrecognized prior to 1980 and seldom taken seriously until the past few years, NAFLD has seemingly been thrust upon us unexpectantly like an orphaned child left at our clinical bedside. In fact, NAFLD was conceived during the industrial revolution, which caused food to be processed differently, provided that food more abundantly and made physical work less demanding. In the 1980's, information technology and virtual reality have enhanced sedentary lifestyles and the decline of physical activity, key factors in exacerbating lifestyle disorders. NAFLD shares these roots with its older siblings—obesity and diabetes mellitus—but is only now being accepted into the full family of the metabolic syndrome.

The clinical importance of this disease is introduced in the first chapter of this book, which is the first devoted exclusively to NAFLD and its more serious form—non-alcoholic steatohepatitis (NASH). In Chapter 1, the editors have introduced the seminal issues related to NAFLD; its definition, epidemiology, pathophysiology and treatment. The nascent yet expanding knowledge of these issues served not only as the basis for developing this book, but also for the selection of its topics and contributing authors.

This disease currently impacts virtually all fields of clinical medicine and will continue to do so with increasing prevalence and adversity to patients. The misconception that NAFLD is benign is fading, but there remain some lingering doubts. This book should dispel those doubts, convince the reader that NAFLD and especially NASH is important, and clarify which affected persons are the ones we need to worry most about. NAFLD/NASH is common, expensive to society, adversely affects quality of life and causes liver-related death in a significant, but still imprecisely known percentage of patients. Certainly important questions remain. Why does only a subset of NAFLD patients develop NASH? What is the interaction between genetic and environmental factors in NAFLD? Is our current knowledge of the natural history and pathophysiology of NAFLD sufficient to recommend management algorithms (including the indications for liver biopsy) or treatments that are cost effective with an acceptable risk benefit ratio? Hopefully, this book will serve as a platform from which these questions can be answered and from which clinicians can gain some confidence in the management of this disease that remains a mosaic of evolving complex issues. Interactions between the determinants of metabolic disease and other disorders, especially hepatitis C and alcoholic liver disease, is one very important advance in understanding with practical implications for patient care.

The editors would like to thank each of the authors for their efforts in this work. We also want to acknowledge the pathologists who have contributed such high quality histologic micrographs. We appreciate the authors' patience and gracious tolerance to the timelines, deadlines and urgent e-mails that are inevitably associated with this type of work. Their expertise and ability to share their knowledge have made this book a very informative and readable text. Our colleagues at Blackwell Publishing have been extremely helpful in guiding us through the editorial process and we appreciate their professional input. Finally, we wish to thank both the patients with NAFLD and the clinicians who care for them. These are the people for whom this book was written and without whom it would not have been achieved.

The Editors

1

Overview: an introduction to NASH and related fatty liver disorders

Geoffrey C. Farrell, Jacob George, Pauline de la M. Hall &
Arthur J. McCullough

Key learning points

1 Non-alcoholic steatohepatitis (NASH) is a form of metabolic liver disease in which fatty change (steatosis) is associated with lobular inflammation, hepatocyte injury, polymorphs and/or hepatic fibrosis.
2 NASH comprises a pathogenic link in the chain of non-alcoholic fatty liver diseases (NAFLD) that extends from bland steatosis to some cases of 'cryptogenic cirrhosis'.
3 NAFLD and NASH are usually hepatic manifestations of the insulin resistance syndrome, but the factors that transform steatosis to NASH remain unclear.
4 In 20–25% of cases, NASH may progress to advanced stages of hepatic fibrosis and cirrhosis; liver failure then becomes the most common cause of death.
5 Clinicians should consider NAFLD/NASH as a primary diagnosis by its metabolic associations with obesity, insulin resistance and type 2 diabetes, rather than simply as a disease of exclusion.
6 Correction of insulin resistance by lifestyle modification (dietary measures and increased physical activity) is a logical approach to prevent or reverse NAFLD/NASH.

Abstract

This chapter introduces the history, definitional and semantic issues, spectrum and general importance of non-alcoholic fatty liver diseases (NAFLD). Non-alcoholic steatohepatitis (NASH) is a form of metabolic liver disease in which fatty change (steatosis) is associated with lobular inflammation, hepatocyte injury and/or hepatic fibrosis. It comprises a pathogenic link in the chain of NAFLD that extends from bland steatosis to some cases of 'cryptogenic cirrhosis'. NAFLD and NASH are usually hepatic manifestations of the insulin resistance (or metabolic) syndrome (syndrome X), but the factors that transform steatosis to NASH remain unclear. NAFLD/NASH is the most common type of liver disease in affluent societies, affecting between 2 and 8% of the population. NASH typically causes no symptoms. When present, clinical features such as fatigue, hepatomegaly and aching hepatic discomfort are non-specific. In 20–25% of cases, NASH may progress to advanced stages of hepatic fibrosis and cirrhosis; liver failure then becomes the most common cause of death, and hepatocellular carcinoma (HCC) may occasionally occur. Correction of insulin resistance by dietary measures and increased physical activity (lifestyle intervention) is a logical approach to prevent or reverse early NASH, and modest weight reduction can normalize liver test abnormalities. Drug therapy aimed at reversing insulin resistance, correcting diabetes and lipid disorders, or providing 'hepatocellular protection' has been shown to improve liver tests in short-term small studies, but larger randomized controlled trials are needed to establish whether any of these approaches arrest progression of hepatic fibrosis and prevent liver complications, and at what stage interventions are cost-effective.

History of NASH

In 1980, Ludwig *et al.* [1] described a series of patients who lacked a history of 'significant' alcohol intake but in whom the liver histology resembled that of alcoholic liver disease. They were the first to use the term 'non-alcoholic steatohepatitis' for this condition, the principal features of which were hepatic steatosis (fatty change), inflammation and exclusion of alcohol as an aetiological factor. Further small case series were published during the next 15 years [2–10]. After much debate, the entity of NASH became accepted, but it is only in the last 10 years that NASH and other forms of metabolic (non-alcoholic) fatty liver diseases (NAFLD) have been widely recognized and diagnosed in clinical practice. The pace of research into the pathogenesis, natural history and treatment of NAFLD/NASH has acclerated in the last 5 years (Fig. 1.1). Thus, Marchesini and Forlani [11] were able to locate only 161 articles which addressed this topic between 1980 and 1999 (approximately 8/year) but 122 in 2000–01 (approx-

imately 60/year). These advances have been reviewed elsewhere [11–19].

What is NASH?

Terminology and definitions

The spectrum of fatty liver disease associated with metabolic determinants and not resulting from alcohol (NAFLD) extends from hepatic steatosis through steatohepatitis to cirrhosis (Table 1.1). As described in Chapter 2, NASH can be defined pathologically as significant steatohepatitis not resulting from alcohol, drugs, toxins, infectious agents or other identifiable exogenous causes (Table 1.2). However, standardized definitions are lacking, particularly of what pathology is encompassed by 'significant steatohepatitis' (such as types 3 or 4 NAFLD; see Table 1.1). Outstanding challenges confronting pathological definition include the following.

1 Agreement on the importance, validity and concordance between observers of histological features of hepatocellular injury, especially ballooning degeneration.
2 Categorizing the grade and diagnostic reliability of patterns of hepatic fibrosis.
3 Interpretation of what cases of 'cryptogenic cirrhosis' can be attributed to NASH.

This book adopts general recommendations on nomenclature for what comprises NASH that are similar to those suggested by Brunt *et al.* [20] and

1950	• Cirrhosis noted in diabetics
1970s	• Jejuno-ileal bypass liver disease resembles alcoholic hepatitis
1979/80	• Ludwig *et al.* [1] Coined term NASH for steatohepatitis in non-drinkers
	• ~8 papers/year
	• Small series
	• NASH is benign (Powell *et al.* 1990 [8])
1994	• Expanded scope of NASH (Bacon *et al.* 1994 [10])
1996	• CYP2E1 induced in rodent dietary model
	• Endotoxin induces inflammation in steatotic liver
1998	• CYP2E1 induced in human NASH
	• First NIH conference on NASH
	• Pivotal importance of insulin resistance
1999	• Several animal models
	• First clinical trials
2002	• ~60 papers/year
	• AASLD single topic conference
	• First European and Japanese single topic conferences
	• NASH established as part of insulin resistance syndrome
2004	• Release of first book on NAFLD/NASH

Fig. 1.1 Chronology of the pace of research into pathogenesis, natural history and treatment of NAFLD/NASH.

Table 1.1 Categories of non-alcoholic fatty liver diseases (NAFLD): relationship to NASH. (After Matteoni *et al.* [15].)

Category	Pathology	Clinicopathological correlation
Type 1	Simple steatosis	Known to be non-progressive
Type 2	Steatosis plus lobular inflammation	Probably benign (not regarded as NASH)
Type 3	Steatosis, lobular inflammation and ballooning degeneration	NASH without fibrosis—may progress to cirrhosis
Type 4	Steatosis, ballooning degeneration and Mallory bodies, and/or fibrosis	NASH with fibrosis—may progress to cirrhosis and liver failure

Table 1.2 Causes of secondary steatohepatitis.

Alcohol (alcoholic hepatitis)
Drugs (tamoxifen, amiodarone, methotrexate)
Copper toxicity (Wilson's disease, Indian childhood cirrhosis)
Jejuno-ileal bypass (see Chapter 20)
Other causes of rapid profound weight loss (massive intestinal resection, cachexia, bulimia, starvation)
Hypernutrition in adults (parenteral nutrition, intravenous glucose)
A-betalipoproteinaemia
Jejunal diverticulosis (contaminated bowel syndrome)
Insulin resistance syndromes (familial and acquired lipodystrophies, polycystic ovary syndrome)

discussed at a single topic conference of the American Association for Study of Liver Diseases (AASLD), September 2002, Atlanta, Georgia (see Chapter 2) [19,20].

When one particular cause of steatohepatitis is evident, the term steatohepatitis is qualified (e.g. alcoholic steatohepatitis, drug-induced steatohepatitis, experimental [dietary] steatohepatitis). Such cases are often referred to as 'secondary NASH' (Table 2.2; see Chapters 13, 20 and 21). Because of its strong association with 'metabolic' determinants (obesity, insulin resistance, type 2 diabetes, hyperlipidaemia), the acronym 'MeSH' has been been suggested as an alternative for 'idiopathic' (or 'primary') NASH, but seems unlikely to gain widespread acceptance.

Non-alcoholic fatty liver diseases

The term NAFLD is gaining acceptance and is useful because it is more comprehensive than NASH (Table 1.1) [15–17]. NAFLD includes less significant forms of steatosis either alone (type 1 NAFLD) or with inflammation but no hepatocyte ballooning or fibrosis

(type 2). The term NAFLD will be used here when the pathology of metabolic liver disease is not known, or when specifically referring to the fuller spectrum. This now includes some cases of cryptogenic cirrhosis in which steatohepatitis and steatosis are no longer conspicuous.

Primary and secondary steatohepatitis: the importance of alcohol

A key definitional issue is potential overlap between 'primary' (metabolic) NAFLD/NASH and pathologically similar fatty liver diseases associated with a single causative factor (Table 1.2). The most important consideration is the level of alcohol consumption considered unlikely to have any causal role in liver disease. Early publications describing 'alcoholic hepatitis-like lesions' were in non-drinkers or those with minimal intake (less than one drink a week in the Ludwig series). Since then, reports of NAFLD/NASH have used a variety of thresholds for alcohol intake. Some have required rigorous alcohol restriction, particularly for cases of 'cryptogenic cirrhosis' attributable to

NASH (e.g. none, or less than 40 g/week) [21,22]. Conversely, other authors have allowed alcohol intake to be as high as 210 g/week [23].

It is noted that 30 g/day is close to the level of 40 g/day associated with an increased risk of cirrhosis in women [24]. Safe levels of alcohol intake have also been difficult to define for other liver diseases, such as hepatitis C for which less than 10 g/day was recommended by the first National Institutes of Health (NIH) Consensus Conference in 1997 [25], but up to 30 g/day for men and 20 g/day for women by the second NIH Consensus Conference [26]. In this book, the definition of NASH requires alcohol intake to have never been greater than 140 g/week (ideally, ≤ 20 g/day for men and ≤ 10 g/day for women). However, it is acknowledged that there may be potential for even these low levels of alcohol intake levels to contribute to cell injury, fibrogenesis and hepatocarcinogenesis in steatohepatitis. Conversely, it remains possible that low levels of alcohol intake confer health benefits in obese persons with liver disease [27]. The implications for recommending optimal levels of alcohol intake

for people with NAFLD/NASH are considered in Chapter 15.

Interaction between steatohepatitis and other liver disorders

Another challenge is when the metabolic determinants of NASH (Table 1.3) coexist with known causes of liver disease. The latter include 'moderate' levels of alcohol intake (30–60 g/day in men, 20–40 g/day in women), hepatitis C and potentially hepatotoxic drugs (methotrexate, tamoxifen, calcium-channel blockers, highly active antiretroviral therapy) [28]. The likelihood that steatosis or the metabolic determinants that result in NASH contribute to liver injury and fibrotic severity of other liver diseases is canvassed in Chapter 23.

Importance of NASH

Reasons why NASH is an important form of liver disease are summarized in Table 1.4.

Table 1.3 Metabolic associations of NASH.

Type 2 diabetes mellitus
Family history of type 2 diabetes
Insulin resistance, with or without glucose intolerance
Central obesity (waist : hip ≥ 0.85 in women, ≥ 0.90 in men; waist > 85 cm in women, > 97 cm in men*)
Obesity (BMI ≥ 30 kg/m^2 in white people, ≥ 27 kg/m^2 in Asians)
Hypertriglyceridaemia
Rapid and massive weight loss in overweight subjects

* Values vary between countries; 90 cm for women and 102 cm for men often used in USA.

Table 1.4 Reasons why NAFLD/NASH is important.

High prevalence of fatty liver disorders in urbanized communities with affluent ('Western') economies throughout the world
Most common cause of abnormal liver tests in community—?2–8% of population have NAFLD
NASH now rivals alcoholic liver disease and chronic hepatitis C as reason for referral to gastroenterologist or liver clinic
NASH is a potential cause of cirrhosis, which may be 'cryptogenic', and lead to end-stage liver disease
Liver failure is most common cause of death in patients with cirrhosis resulting from NASH
Standardized mortality of liver disease in type 2 diabetes greatly exceeds vascular disease
NASH recurs after liver transplantation
Hepatic steatosis as a cause of primary graft non-function after liver transplantation
Role of metabolic determinants of NASH in pathogenesis of other liver diseases, particularly hepatitis C and alcoholic cirrhosis
Possible role of NASH/hepatic steatosis in hepatocarcinogenesis

The NASH epidemic

In much of the world, abnormal liver tests attributable to hepatic steatosis or NASH have become the most common liver disease in the community. Depending on how an abnormal value for aminotransferase is defined in studies, such as the Third National Health and Nutritional Examination Survey (NHANES III), between 3 and 23% of the adult population may have NAFLD/NASH [29–31]. In studies that have employed hepatic imaging, autopsy or biopsy approaches, approximately 70% of obese people have hepatic steatosis and/or raised alanine aminotransferase (ALT) [12,21, 27,31–37]; NASH is present in approximately 20% of these [7,27]. In old autopsy studies, ~ 10% of diabetics had cirrhosis, but other factors (hepatitis B and C) were possible confounding variables. In more recent studies, both the prevalence and severity of NASH appear to be increased considerably in patients with type 2 diabetes [11,21,36,38–40].

The epidemiology of NAFLD/NASH is discussed in Chapter 3. Based on the continuing epidemic of obesity and type 2 diabetes through much of the world, it is likely that the prevalence of NASH will increase further during the next decade. In the USA and Australia, up to 60% of men and 45% of women are now overweight, and about one-third of these are obese [41, 42]. Similar increases have been noted in societies that until the last one or two generations were participating in physically active ('hunter gatherer') lifestyles (see Chapter 18). The prevalence of type 2 diabetes has doubled, trebled or increased 10- to 20-fold (as in Japanese youth) during the last decade, rates reaching 40% or more of the adult population in some communities [43–45]. Childhood cases of NASH are also clearly related to obesity and type 2 diabetes (see Chapter 19) [46,47]. Some possible reasons for high rates of obesity and type 2 diabetes in contemporary affluent societies ('east' and 'west', 'north' and 'south'), and the implications for prevention and interruption of NASH are discussed in Chapters 3–5 and 18.

NAFLD/NASH varies in severity and clinical outcome

Steatosis alone has an excellent prognosis. It seems probable that most cases of steatosis with lobular inflammation but without conspicuous hepatocyte injury or fibrosis (NAFLD type 2) behaves in the same way, with very low rates of fibrotic progression (see Chapter 3). However, 20–25% of cases with NASH have or will progress to cirrhosis [15,16,19,21,22,39]. There is mounting evidence that a proportion of cases of 'cryptogenic cirrrhosis' may be attributable to NASH, in which the histological features of steatohepatitis have resolved (see Chapter 14) [15,21,31,35,48]. Rare cases of subacute hepatic failure have also been attributed to possible NASH [49].

Earlier studies of NAFLD/NASH emphasized the good overall prognosis [8,10]. More recent studies that have defined cases according to fibrotic severity indicate that those with significant fibrosis may progress to liver failure [15,22,50]. Among cases of cirrhosis, the risk of death or liver transplantation may be as high as cirrhosis resulting from hepatitis C (both ~ 30% at 7 years) [15,16,22,50]. If this indolent progressive course is confirmed in larger prospective studies, NASH will cause a formidable disease burden in forthcoming decades.

A few well-documented cases of cirrhosis resulting from NASH have presented with, or less commonly have terminated in HCC [16,51]. HCC was recently noted to be a cause of death among obese patients with cryptogenic cirrhosis [52,53]. However, it is not clear that all such cases were caused by NASH [22], and several were diagnosed within 9 months of presentation. Others have suggested that steatosis could increase the risk of HCC associated with other liver diseases [54,55], but conflicting data have been noted (see Chapter 22).

Metabolic risk factors for NASH may worsen other liver diseases

As well as providing the setting for NASH, insulin resistance, obesity, type 2 diabetes and hepatic steatosis are now recognized as factors that favour fibrotic progression in hepatitis C [56,57]. Obesity is also an independent risk factor for alcoholic cirrhosis [58]. Thus, 'NASH determinants' may contribute to the overall burden of cirrhosis directly as the hepatic complication of obesity, insulin resistance and diabetes, and indirectly as factors that favour cirrhosis among people with chronic viral hepatitis or alcoholism (see Chapter 23).

When should the clinician think of NASH?

Clinicians need to consider that NAFLD/NASH is the most likely cause of liver test abnormalities in the

Table 1.5 Pointers to NAFLD/NASH in clinical practice.

Unexplained elevation of ALT and GGT, typically minor, in a person with metabolic risk factors (Table 1.3)

'Rubbery' hepatomegaly

Recent weight gain and expanding waistline

Lifestyle or medication changes favouring weight gain (marriage, retirement, unemployment, antidepressants)

Family history of type 2 diabetes, NAFLD, vascular disorders or hyperlipidaemia

Raised serum ferritin not attributable to iron storage disorder or alcohol

Abnormalities of hepatic imaging—diffuse echogenicity on ultrasonogram ('bright liver'), radiolucency on CT

Patient with chronic HCV infection and diabetes and/or obesity, 'rubbery' hepatomegaly or steatosis with HCV genotype 1 infections (see Chapter 23)

Patient with chronic HBV infection, raised ALT but non-detectable HBV DNA in presence of metabolic risk factors

---

ALT, alanine aminotransferase; CT, computerized tomography; GGT, gamma-glutamyl transpeptidase; HBV DNA, hepatitis B virus DNA; HCV, hepatitis C virus.

presence of metabolic risk factors (Table 1.3), and when other causes of liver disease have been excluded (see Chapter 13). The importance of considering NAFLD/NASH as a primary diagnosis, rather than purely as a disease of exclusion, is emphasized in this book (see Chapter 5).

NAFLD/NASH is usually suspected because of abnormal liver biochemical tests in an apparently healthy person with no symptoms (Table 1.5). However, fatigue, or vague discomfort over the liver with 'rubbery' hepatomegaly are common. Significant hepatic pain and tenderness are rare. The presence of a firm liver edge, or more rarely a palpable spleen, muscle wasting, ascites, jaundice or hepatic encephalopathy indicate possible cirrhosis, with or without complications of portal hypertension and hepatic decompensation (see Chapters 13 and 14).

In a person with abnormal liver biochemistry tests, a history of recent weight gain or an expanding waistline are often clues to the diagnosis of NASH. However, rapid and extensive weight loss in an obese person can lead to an initial diagnosis of NASH. Such weight loss may occur through intercurrent illness, older forms of obesity surgery (see Chapter 20) or drastic reductions in energy intake caused by fasting, bulimia or 'crash' dieting (Table 1.2). Cycles of rapid weight gain followed by precipitant *weight loss* have led to cirrhosis or hepatic decompensation [3].

The past medical and family history often provide clues to metabolic disorders that underlie NASH [59], particularly type 2 diabetes, and other features and complications of insulin resistance such as arterial hypertension and coronary heart disease [11]. Similarly,

laboratory tests, such as a raised serum urate, triglyceride, low-density lipoprotein (LDL) cholesterol and low levels of high-density lipoprotein (HDL) cholesterol are pointers to insulin resistance. The genetic factors that could predispose to NASH are considered in Chapter 6, and the insulin resistance syndrome is discussed in Chapter 5.

A raised serum ferritin level is a common 'confounder' in cases of NAFLD/NASH [60–62]. As in alcoholic liver disease, this most often reflects increased hepatic release of ferritin as an 'acute phase reactant', reflecting the hepatic inflammatory response and increased permeability of steatotic and injured hepatocytes. If a persistently raised serum transferrin saturation suggests increased body iron stores, haemochromatosis gene testing should be conducted in those with a northern European or Celtic background. The proposed role of hepatic iron in worsening fibrotic severity in NASH is controversial (see Chapter 7) [60–62].

Confirming the diagnosis is NASH

Liver biochemical function tests, serum lipids and other laboratory results

Abnormal biochemical results (liver function tests) typically comprise minor (1.5- to 5-fold) elevations of ALT and gamma-glutamyl transpeptidase (GGT). The following laboratory tests may provide clues to the presence of cirrhosis: low platelet count, raised aspartate aminotransferase (AST) that is higher than ALT, and subtle changes in serum albumin or bilirubin that are not attributable to other causes (see Chapter 14).

Fasting hypertriglyceridaemia is present in 25–40% of patients with NASH [8,9,10,16,39]. It may be associated with hypercholesterolaemia (increased LDL cholesterol, particularly with low levels of HDL and a high LDL : HDL ratio). This pattern of lipid disorders is a feature of the insulin resistance syndrome.

Anthropometric measurements

Because nearly all patients with NASH have central obesity, anthropometric measurements should be routinely recorded at liver clinic visits (see Chapter 15). Height and weight are used to calculate body mass index (BMI), while girth (circumference at umbilicus), or waist : hip ratio form simple pointers to central obesity (see Chapters 5 and 15 for details). Some nutritionists recommend waist circumference as more useful than body weight for monitoring benefits of lifestyle change in overweight people.

Determination of insulin resistance

The near universal association of NASH with insulin resistance means that tests to document this pathophysiological state should form part of the approach to diagnosis. Fasting serum insulin and blood glucose levels can be used to construct the relatively crude (but practically useful) homoeostasis model assessment of insulin resistance (HOMA-IR). Values for HOMA-IR differ between population subgroups. Thus, application of this method requires reference to a local group of normal age-matched controls.

As discussed in Chapter 4, diabetologists prefer an 'active' measure of insulin sensitivity as opposed to a fasting one; the latter will be misleading when there is secondary failure of insulin secretion by pancreatic β cells. A simplified 75-g oral glucose tolerance test with 1 and 2 h blood glucose and serum insulin levels can be very informative. Fasting serum C-peptide level is an excellent measure of insulin production. It therefore appears to be a sensitive indicator of insulin resistance that can be used in hepatological practice.

Hepatic imaging

Hepatic imaging performed as part of investigations into abdominal pain, abnormal liver tests or suspected hepatic malignancy may be the first clue to the presence of steatosis [63]. The sensitivity of hepatic ultra-sound for steatosis (increased echogenicity, or 'bright liver') appears fairly high, particularly when extensive steatosis (involving at least 33% hepatocytes) is present [63]. CT also appears to be relatively sensitive for hepatic steatosis, and has the advantage that nodularity resulting from cirrhosis may sometimes be appreciated. Careful attention should be given to features of portal hypertension (portal vein dilatation, splenomegaly, retroperitoneal varices). Otherwise, both ultrasonography and computerized tomography (CT) have low positive predictive value for detecting features of cirrhosis.

Neither ultrasonography nor CT is able to distinguish NASH from other forms of NAFLD (see Chapter 13). Thus, while hepatic imaging is useful for providing supportive evidence in favour of hepatic steatosis, it cannot substitute for liver biopsy for elucidating the fibrotic severity of NASH.

Newer imaging techniques (dual-energy X-ray absorptiometry [DEXA], magnetic resonance imaging [MRI]) are also valuable in determining body composition. Total body fat can be estimated accurately with DEXA, but greater interest will come from studies attempting to discern patterns of adipose tissue distribution (visceral versus subcutaneous or ectopic); these patterns are likely to correlate more closely with insulin resistance (see Chapter 4).

Liver biopsy

Clinical guidelines for when liver biopsy is indicated for suspected NASH are not yet standardized [16,18], with views ranging from the nihilistic to the enthusiastic! In considering whether a liver biopsy is indicated, one approach is to assess risk factors for fibrotic severity (obesity, diabetes, age over 45 years, and AST : ALT > 1) and to seek 'warning signs' of cirrhosis (see Chapter 14) [15,16,18]. One approach is not to recommend biopsy at first referral (see Chapter 15). If lifestyle intervention aimed at correcting insulin resistance and central obesity fails to normalize liver tests, and particularly if there are warning signs for cirrhosis or the patient expresses a strong desire to know the severity of their liver disease, the physician should proceed to liver biopsy (see Chapters 13 and 15). Liver biopsy interpretation is described in Chapter 2.

In following any paradigm for liver biopsy, it should be noted that liver test abnormalities in NASH are poorly related to fibrotic severity. Some patients with NASH cirrhosis may have normal ALT levels. A nihilistic approach to liver biopsy for NASH therefore raises the concern that some patients with advanced hepatic fibrosis and/or cirrhosis would not be counselled and monitored appropriately. Further, liver biopsy can sometimes produce unexpected findings indicative of another liver disease, thereby changing management.

Why does NASH happen?

The recurrence of NASH after orthotopic liver transplantation (see Chapter 17) is a dramatic demonstration of the importance of extrahepatic (metabolic) factors in its pathogenesis. Among these, genetic and acquired abnormalities of fatty acid turnover and oxidation are likely to be crucial in causing steatohepatitis [16,17,19,64]; some facilitate accumulation of free fatty acids (FFA), others favour the operation of oxidative stress. Factors that facilitate recruitment of an hepatic inflammatory (or innate immune) response, or determine the tissue response to liver injury are other potentially relevant variables.

Human and animal studies have started to address key issues in NASH pathogenesis, such as the nature of insulin resistance—why it occurs, whether it is responsible for inflammation and liver cell injury as well as FFA accumulation, the mechanisms for inflammatory recruitment and perpetuation, the biochemical basis and significance of oxidative stress, the cell biological basis of hepatocye injury and the pathogenesis of fibrosis (see Chapters 4, 7, 8 and 10–12). It seems likely that many such factors are genetically determined (see Chapter 6). In this way, NASH, like type 2 diabetes, atherosclerosis and some cancers, is the outcome of an interplay between several genetic and environmental factors.

Lipid accumulation also favours increased concentrations of FFA that may be directly toxic to hepatocytes. It has recently been proposed that such 'lipotoxicity' in NASH results from failure of leptin or other hormones that modulate insulin sensitivity to correct for insulin resistance [65]. The humoral and dietary modulation of insulin receptor signalling that underlies this new concept is discussed in Chapter 4. The fatty liver also provides an excess of unsaturated FFA, oxidation of which results in the autopropagative process of lipid peroxidation. It is now clear that the steatotic liver is more susceptible to oxidative stress, as well as to injury after injection of endotoxin [16,18,64].

The liver normally responds to the chronic presence of oxidants by increasing synthesis of protective antioxidant pathways, such as those based on reduced glutathione (GSH). If GSH levels are depleted (as with fasting, toxins such as alcohol, or consumption by pro-oxidants), the products of lipid peroxidation create and amplify oxidative stress. In turn, oxidative stress can cause liver injury (e.g. by triggering apoptosis and inciting inflammation). The mechanisms that may trigger and perpetuate inflammatory recruitment in NASH, and the importance of cytokines such as tumour necrosis factor-α (TNF-α) are discussed in Chapter 10.

Evidence has been deduced from human studies as well as in experimental models that cytochrome P450 2E1 (CYP2E1) is overexpressed in steatohepatitis [66–68], most likely because of impaired insulin receptor signalling. CYP2E1 is a potential source of reduced (reactive) oxygen species (ROS). In the absence of CYP2E1, CYP4A takes on the role as an alternative microsomal lipid oxidase, and it too may generate ROS [67]. CYP2E1 and CYP4A catalyze the ω and ω-1 hydroxylation of long-chain fatty acids. The products are dicarboxylic fatty acids, which cannot be subjected to mitochondrial β-oxidation and are so targeted to the peroxisome for further oxidation. In turn, this generates hydrogen peroxide (coupled to catalase) as an essential by-product [69].

The relative importance of metabolic sites of ROS generation in hepatocytes (mitochondria, endoplasmic reticulum, peroxisomes), and products of the inflammatory response in contributing to oxidative stress in steatohepatitis remains unclear; interactive processes are likely to operate [64]. However, mitochondria could be a critical source of ROS in fatty liver disorders (see Chapter 11) [38,70].

Hepatic inflammation and cellular injury to hepatocytes can induce and activate transforming growth factor-β (TGF-β), which has a key role in activating stellate cells to elaborate extracellular matrix as part of the wound healing process. It is now apparent that leptin has a key role in hepatic fibrogenesis, and leptin also appears to be necessary for appropriate liver regeneration as part of the 'wound healing' response to chronic steatohepatitis and other forms of liver injury (see Chapter 12). Thus, leptin, originally characterized as an anti-obesity hormone acting on the central nervous system to regulate appetite, could have multiple roles in the pathogenesis of NASH by modulating fat deposition in hepatocytes (anti-lipotoxicity), and regulating the hepatic fibrotic and regenerative response to steatohepatitis. A more detailed account of the cell biology of NASH is presented in Chapter 12.

Approaches to management of NASH

Lifestyle adjustments

Attempts to correct steatosis and liver injury in NASH can begin before the diagnostic process is complete (see Chapter 15). The aim is to correct insulin resistance and central obesity. Rapid and profound weight loss is potentially dangerous for the person with fatty liver disease [3]. It is prudent and more realistic to recommend slow reductions in body weight that are achievable and sustainable by permanent changes in lifestyle. It has been shown that such reductions improve liver tests [71], and there is mounting evidence that this is associated with removal of fat from the liver, decreased necroinflammatory change and even resolution of fibrosis [72,73].

In accordance with the results of recent type 2 diabetes intervention studies [74,75], physical activity should include at least 20 min of exercise each day (140 min/week), equivalent to rapid walking. The essentials of dietary modification are the same as for diabetes: reduce total fat to less than 30% of energy intake, decrease saturated fats, replace with complex carbohydrates containing at least 15 g fibre, and rich in fruit and vegetables. Consideration of low versus high glycaemic foods (e.g. brown or basmati rice versus conventional long or short-grain white rice); reduction of simple sugars and alcohol intake is also likely to be beneficial.

Some authors have advocated referral to a dietitian or 'personal case manager' to provide education and closer supervision of dietary regimens and lifestyle interventions [73–75]. Approaches to lifestyle modification and weight reduction are discussed in more detail in Chapter 15. The effectiveness and cost-efficacy of such approaches are important aspects that warrant further study.

Measures to control hyperlipidaemia and hyperglycaemia

Increased physical activity and low-fat diet improve insulin sensitivity and can, in some cases, reverse insulin resistance. The value of exercise in improving glycaemic control in diabetes is now generally accepted. In other respects, treatment of diabetes in patients with NASH should conform to conventional approaches, although this may change in future if drugs that help reverse insulin resistance live up to initial promise against NAFLD/NASH without causing unacceptable weight gain. These agents include metformin and the thiolazinediones (see Chapter 16). Drugs that correct lipid disorders, anti-oxidants (vitamin E, betaine) and other hepatoprotective agents (ursodeoxycholic acid) are also under study in NASH (see Chapter 16).

Concluding remarks: can NAFLD/NASH be prevented or reversed?

Because liver failure does not occur in NAFLD/NASH unless cirrhosis has developed, reducing or reversing fibrotic progression must be the ultimate objective of treatment. While several agents improve liver tests over the short term in patients with NAFLD/NASH (see Chapter 16), none have yet (June 2003) been shown to have long-term efficacy and to impact on fibrotic progression (but see Chapter 24). In the absence of evidence of such efficacy, patients should currently only receive drug therapy directed at NASH within the context of a clinical trial, particularly as some of the compounds presently under study carry toxic potential or other unwanted effects (see Chapters 16 and 24).

There is now compelling evidence that type 2 diabetes can be prevented (or at least delayed in onset) by lifestyle interventions [74,75]. Both the Finnish and US Diabetes Intervention Projects showed a 58% reduction in incidence of type 2 diabetes among those at high risk could be achieved with only modest reductions in body weight [74,75]. NASH, another consequence of insulin resistance (see Chapter 5), should also be preventable by changes in diet and physical activity. There is now evidence that weight reduction and lifestyle changes nearly always improve liver tests in NAFLD, and also have potential to improve liver histology in obese patients with hepatitis C or fatty liver disorders [71–73] (Chapter 24). Whether this approach would be a cost-effective way to reduce the number of patients progressing to cirrhosis and liver failure is clearly worthy of study.

References

1 Ludwig J, Viaggiano TR, McGill DB, Oh BJ. Non-alcoholic steatohepatitis: Mayo Clinic experience with an hitherto unnamed disease. *Mayo Clin Proc* 1980; **55**: 434–8.

2 Adler M, Schaffner F. Fatty liver hepatitis and cirrhosis in obese patients. *Am J Med* 1979; **67**: 811–6.

3 Capron J-P, Delamarre J, Dupas J-L *et al.* Fasting in obesity: another cause of liver injury with alcoholic hyaline? *Dig Dis Sci* 1982; **27**: 265–8.

4 Itoh S, Yougel T, Kawagoe K. Comparison between non-alcoholic steatohepatitis and alcoholic hepatitis. *Am J Gastroenterol* 1987; **82**: 650–4.

5 Diehl AM, Goodman Z, Ishak KG. Alcohol-like liver disease in non-alcoholics: a clinical and histologic comparison with alcohol-induced liver disease. *Gastroenterology* 1988; **95**: 1056–62.

6 Lee RG. Non-alcoholic steatohepatitis: a study of 49 patients. *Hum Pathol* 1989; **20**: 594–8.

7 Wanless IR, Lentz JS. Fatty liver hepatitis (steatohepatitis) and obesity: an autopsy study with analysis of risk factors. *Hepatology* 1990; **12**: 1106–10.

8 Powell EE, Cooksley WGE, Hanson R *et al.* The natural history of non-alcoholic steatohepatitis: a follow-up study of 42 patients for up to 21 years. *Hepatology* 1990; **11**: 74–80.

9 Fiatarone JR, Coverdale SA, Batey RG, Farrell GC. Non-alcoholic steatohepatitis: impaired antipyrine metabolism and hypertriglyceridaemia may be clues to its pathogenesis. *J Gastroenterol Hepatol* 1991; **6**: 585–90.

10 Bacon BR, Farahvash MJ, Janney CG, Neuschwander-Tetri BA. Non-alcoholic steatohepatitis: an expanded clinical entity. *Gastroenterology* 1994; **107**: 1103–9.

11 Marchesini G, Forlani G. NASH: From liver diseases to metabolic disorders and back to clinical hepatology. *Hepatology* 2002; **35**: 497–9.

12 Seth SG, Gordon FD, Chopra S. Non-alcoholic steatohepatitis. *Ann Intern Med* 1997; **126**: 137–45.

13 Ludwig J, McGill DB, Lindor KD. Non-alcoholic steatohepatitis. *J Gastroenterol Hepatol* 1997; **12**: 398–403.

14 James OFW, Day CP. Non-alcoholic steatohepatitis (NASH): a disease of emerging identity and importance. *J Hepatol* 1998; **29**: 495–501.

15 Matteoni CA, Younossi ZM, Gramlich T *et al.* Non-alcoholic fatty liver disease: a spectrum of clinical and pathological severity. *Gastroenterology* 1999; **116**: 1413–9.

16 Angulo P. Non-alcoholic fatty liver disease. *N Engl J Med* 2002; **16**: 1221–31.

17 Younossi ZM, Diehl AM, Ong JP. Non-alcoholic fatty liver disease: an agenda for clinical research. *Hepatology* 2002; **35**: 746–52.

18 Farrell GC. Okuda Lecture. Non-alcoholic steatohepatitis: what is it, and why is it important in the Asia-Pacific region. *J Gastroenterol Hepatol* 2003; **18**: 124–38.

19 Neuschwander-Tetri BA, Caldwell SH. Non-alcoholic steatohepatitis: summary of an AASLD single topic conference. *Hepatology* 2003; **37**: 1202–19.

20 Brunt EM, Janney CG, Di Bisceglie AM, Neuschwander-Tetri BA, Bacon BR. Non-alcoholic steatohepatitis: a proposal for grading and staging the histological lesions. *Am J Gastroenterol* 1999; **94**: 2467–74.

21 Angulo P, Keach JC, Batts KP, Lindor KD. Independent predictors of liver fibrosis in patients with non-alcoholic steatohepatitis. *Hepatology* 1999; **30**: 1356–62.

22 Hui JM, Kench JG, Chitturi S *et al.* Long-term outcomes of cirrhosis in NASH compared to hepatitis C: same mortality, less cancer. *Hepatology* 2003; **38**: 420–7.

23 Mulhall BP, Ong JP, Younossi Z. Non-alcoholic fatty liver disease: an overview. *J Gastroenterol Hepatol* 2002; **17**: 1136–43.

24 Norton R, Batey R, Dwyer T, MacMahon S. Alcohol consumption and the risk of alcohol related cirrhosis in women. *Br Med J* 1987; **295**: 80–2.

25 Consensus Development Panel. National Institutes of Health Consensus Development Conference Panel Statement. Management of hepatitis C. *Hepatology* 1997; **26** (Suppl. 1): 2S–10S.

26 National Institutes of Health Consensus Development Conference Statement. Management of Hepatitis C, June 10–12, 2002. *Hepatology* 2002; **36** (Suppl. 1): S3–S21.

27 Dixon JB, Bhathal PS, O'Brien PE. Non-alcoholic fatty liver disease: predictors of non-alcoholic steatohepatitis and liver fibrosis in the severely obese. *Gastroenterology* 2001; **121**: 91–100.

28 Farrell GC. Drugs and steatohepatitis. *Semin Liver Dis* 2002; **22**: 185–94.

29 Erby JR, Silberman C, Lydick E. Prevalence of abnormal serum alanine aminotransferase levels in obese patients and patients with type 2 diabetes. *Am J Med* 2000; **109**: 588–90.

30 Clark JM, Brancati FL, Diehl AM. Non-alcoholic fatty liver disease. *Gastroenterology* 2002; **122**: 1649–57.

31 Ruhl CE, Everhardt JE. Determinants of the association of overweight with elevated serum alanine aminotransferase activity in the United States. *Gastroenterology* 2003; **124**: 71–9.

32 Bellentani S, Sacoccio G, Masutti F *et al.* Prevalence and risk factors for hepatic steatosis in northern Italy. *Ann Intern Med* 2000; **132**: 112–7.

33 Hasan I, Gani RA, Machmud R *et al.* Prevalence and risk factors for non-alcoholic fatty liver in Indonesia. *J Gastroenterol Hepatol* 2002; **17** (Suppl): A154.

34 Caldwell SH, Oelsner DH, Iezzoni JC *et al.* Cryptogenic cirrhosis: clinical characterization and risk factors for underlying disease. *Hepatology* 1999; **29**: 664–9.

35 Ratziu V, Giral P, Charlotte F *et al.* Liver fibrosis in overweight patients. *Gastroenterology* 2000; **118**: 1117–23.

36 Marchesini G, Brizi M, Morselli-Labate AM *et al.* Association of non-alcoholic fatty liver disease with insulin resistance. *Am J Med* 1999; **107**: 450–5.

37 Marceau P, Biron S, Hould FS *et al.* Liver pathology and the metabolic syndrome X in severe obesity. *J Clin Endocrinol Metab* 1999; **84**: 1513–7.

38 Sanyal AJ, Campbell-Sargent C, Mirshahi F *et al.* Non-alcoholic steatohepatitis: association of insulin resistance and mitochondrial abnormalities. *Gastroenterology* 2001; **120**: 1183–92.

39 Chitturi S, Abeygunasekera S, Farrell GC *et al.* NASH and insulin resistance: insulin hypersecretion and specific association with the insulin resistance syndrome. *Hepatology* 2002; **35**: 373–8.

40 Pagano G, Pacini G, Musso G *et al.* Non-alcoholic steatohepatitis, insulin resistance and metabolic syndrome: further evidence for an etiologic association. *Hepatology* 2002; **35**: 367–72.

41 www.cdc.gov/nccdphp/dnpa/obesity/trends/maps/index.htm

42 Dunstan DW, Zimmet PZ, Welborn TA *et al.* The rising prevalence of diabetes and impaired glucose tolerance: the Australian Diabetes, Obesity and Lifestyle Study. *Diabetes Care* 2002; **25**: 829–34.

43 Daniel M, Rowley KG, McDermott R, O'Dea K. Diabetes and impaired glucose tolerance in Aboriginal Australians: prevalence and risk. *Diabetes Res Clin Pract* 2002; **57**: 23–33.

44 Zimmet P, Alberti KG, Shaw J. Global and societal implications of the diabetes epidemic. *Nature* 2001; **414**: 782–7.

45 Omagari KH, Kadokawa Y, Masuda J *et al.* Fatty liver in non-alcoholic non-overweight Japanese adults: incidence and clinical characteristics. *J Gastroenterol Hepatol* 2002; **17**: 1089–105.

46 Rashid M, Roberts E. Non-alcoholic steatohepatitis in children. *J Paediatr Gastroenterol Nutr* 2000; **30**: 48–53.

47 Manton ND, Lipsett J, Moore DJ *et al.* Non-alcoholic steatohepatitis in children and adolescents. *Med J Aust* 2000; **173**: 476–9.

48 Poonawala A, Nair SP, Thuluvath PJ. Prevalence of obesity and diabetes in patients with cryptogenic cirrhosis: a case study. *Hepatology* 2000; **32**: 689–92.

49 Caldwell SH, Hespenheide EE. Subacute liver failure in obese women. *Am J Gastroenterol* 2002; **97**: 2058–62.

50 Falck-Ytter Y, Younossi ZM, Marchesini G, McCullough AJ. Clinical features and natural history of non-alcoholic steatosis syndromes. *Semin Liver Dis* 2001; **21**: 17–26.

51 Shimada M, Hashimoto E, Taniai M *et al.* Hepatocellular carcinoma in patients with non-alcoholic steatohepatitis. *J Hepatol* 2002; **37**: 154–60.

52 Ratziu V, Bonhay L, Di Martino V *et al.* Survival, liver failure, and hepatocellular carcinoma in obesity-related cryptogenic cirrhosis. *Hepatology* 2002; **35**: 1485–93.

53 Bugianesi E, Leone N, Vanni E *et al.* Expanding the natural history of non-alcoholic steatohepatitis: from cryptogenic cirrhosis to hepatocellular carcinoma. *Gastroenterology* 2002; **123**: 134–40.

54 Marrero JA, Fontana RJ, Su GL *et al.* NAFLD may be a common underlying liver disease in patients with hepatocellular carcinoma in the United States. *Hepatology* 2002; **36**: 1349–54.

55 Garcia-Monzon C, Martin-Perez E, Iacono OL *et al.* Characterization of pathogenic and prognostic factors of non-alcoholic steatohepatitis associated with obesity. *J Hepatol* 2000; **33**: 716–24.

56 Hourigan LF, Macdonald GA, Purdie D *et al.* Fibrosis in chronic hepatitis C correlates with body mass index and steatosis. *Hepatology* 1999; **29**: 1215–9.

57 Hwang SJ, Luo JC, Chu CW *et al.* Hepatic steatosis in chronic hepatitis C virus infection: prevalence and clinical correlation. *J Gastroenterol Hepatol* 2001; **16**: 190–5.

58 Naveau S, Giraud V, Borotto E *et al.* Excess weight risk factor for alcoholic liver disease. *Hepatology* 1997; **25**: 108–11.

59 Struben VMD, Hespenheide EE, Caldwell SH. Non-alcoholic steatohepatitis and cryptogenic cirrhosis within kindreds. *Am J Med* 2000; **108**: 9–13.

60 George DK, Goldwurm S, MacDonald GA *et al.* Increased hepatic iron concentration in non-alcoholic steatohepatitis is associated with increased fibrosis. *Gastroenterology* 1998; **114**: 311–8.

61 Younossi ZM, Gramlich T, Bacon BR *et al.* Hepatic iron and non-alcoholic fatty liver disease. *Hepatology* 1999; **30**: 847–50.

62 Chitturi C, Weltman M, Farrell GC *et al.* HFE mutations, hepatic iron, and fibrosis: ethnic-specific associations of NASH with C282Y but not with fibrotic severity. *Hepatology* 2002; **36**: 142–8.

63 Saadeh S, Younossi ZM, Remer EM *et al.* The utility of radiological imaging in non-alcoholic fatty liver disease. *Gastroenterology* 2002; **123**: 745–50.

64 Chitturi S, Farrell GC. Etiopathogenesis of non-alcoholic steatohepatitis. *Semin Liver Dis* 2001; **21**: 27–41.

65 Chitturi S, Farrell GC, Frost L *et al*. Serum leptin in NASH correlates with hepatic steatosis but not fibrosis: a manifestation of lipotoxicity? *Hepatology* 2002; **36**: 403–9.

66 Weltman MD, Farrell GC, Ingelman-Sundberg M, Liddle C. Hepatic cytochrome P4502E1 is increased in patients with non-alcoholic steatohepatitis. *Hepatology* 1998; **27**: 128–33.

67 Leclercq IA, Farrell GC, Field J, Robertson G. CYP2E1 and CYP4A as microsomal catalysts of lipid peroxides in murine non-alcoholic steatohepatitis. *J Clin Invest* 2000; **105**: 1067–75.

68 Chalasani N, Gorski C, Asghar MS *et al*. Hepatic cytochrome P450 2E1 activity in non-diabetic patients with non-alcoholic steatohepatitis. *Hepatology* 2003; **37**: 544–50.

69 Reddy JK. Non-alcoholic steatosis and steatohepatitis III: peroxisomal β-oxidation, PPARα, and steatohepatitis. *Am J Physiol Gastrointest Liver Physiol* 2001; **281**: G1333–9.

70 Caldwell SH, Swerdlow RH, Khan EM *et al*. Mitochondrial abnormalities in non-alcoholic steatohepatitis. *J Hepatol* 1999; **31**: 430–4.

71 Palmer M, Schaffner F. Effect of weight reduction on hepatic abnormalities in overweight patients. *Gastroenterology* 1990; **99**: 1408–13.

72 Ueno T, Sugawara H, Sujaku K *et al*. Therapeutic effects of restricted diet and exercise in obese patients with fatty liver. *J Hepatol* 1997; **27**: 103–7.

73 Hickman IJ, Clouston AD, MacDonald GA *et al*. Effect of weight reduction on liver histology and biochemistry in patients with chronic hepatitis C. *Gut* 2002; **51**: 89–94.

74 Diabetes Prevention Program Research Group. Reduction in the incidence of type 2 diabetes with lifestyle intervention or metformin. *N Engl J Med* 2002; **346**: 393–403.

75 Tuomilehto J, Lindstrom J, Eriksson J G *et al*. Prevention of type 2 diabetes mellitus by changes in lifestyle among subjects with impaired glucose tolerance. *N Engl J Med* 2001; **344**: 1343–50.

2

Pathology of hepatic steatosis, NASH and related conditions

Pauline de la M. Hall & Richard Kirsch

Key learning points

1 Non-alcoholic steatohepatitis (NASH) is the term used to describe liver injury that occurs with little or no alcohol consumption, but which closely resembles alcoholic hepatitis, and is characterized by steatosis, hepatocyte injury (ballooning degeneration and/or necrosis), a mixed inflammatory infiltrate that includes neutrophils, with or without pericellular fibrosis.
2 Non-alcoholic fatty liver disease (NAFLD) is a preferable term because it refers to a spectrum of liver injury that includes simple steatosis, non-specific steatohepatitis and NASH.
3 Reports of liver biopsies showing NAFLD/NASH should include the grade and stage in words, with or without a numerical score.
4 Some cases of cryptogenic cirrhosis are likely to be the result of 'burnt-out' NASH, which can recur after liver transplant.
5 Hepatocellular carcinoma is now recognized as a rare complication of cirrhosis likely due to NASH.

Abstract

This chapter provides general background information on the pathology of NAFLD/NASH for non-pathologists, as well as practical help for anatomical pathologists who report liver biopsies. The main emphasis is on the definition and illustration of the various patterns of liver injury that form the broad spectrum of injury encompassed by the terms non-alcoholic fatty liver disease (NAFLD) and non-alcoholic steatohepatitis (NASH). Difficult concepts, such as the essential requirements and minimal requirements for a diagnosis of NASH, are addressed. Currently, the broader term NAFLD is probably preferable because it embraces simple steatosis and non-specific steatohepatitis than does the more narrow term NASH, in which the pathology is virtually identical to that seen in alcoholic hepatitis and which is usually complicated by fibrosis. An approach is suggested for the diagnosis of cirrhosis associated with NASH and 'cryptogenic' cirrhosis seen in people with clinical risk factors for NASH. Finally, the relatively new concept that hepatocellular carcinoma (HCC) forms part of the spectrum of NASH complicated by cirrhosis is discussed briefly.

Introduction

In a landmark study in 1980, Ludwig *et al.* [1] described a series of patients who lacked a history of 'significant' alcohol intake but in whom the liver histology resembled that of alcoholic liver disease. They coined the term NASH to describe the principal features of this condition; namely, hepatic steatosis and inflammation and an aetiology that was 'non-alcoholic'. During the next two decades it became apparent that the histopathological definition of NASH was subject to a wide range of interpretations. In many studies, the presence of mild focal macrovesicular steatosis and lobular inflammation, mainly or exclusively composed of mononuclear cells, was regarded as sufficient for the histological diagnosis of NASH, while some insisted on the presence of ballooning degeneration, and still others required neutrophils and/or fibrosis. There is still no international consensus regarding the histopathological criteria for the diagnosis of NASH. Some have proposed that in addition to steatosis and lobular inflammation, either ballooning degeneration or perivenular or pericellular fibrosis should be present [2,3] (see also Chapter 24).

In their first paper on grading and staging NASH, Brunt *et al.* [4] stated that in grade 1 injury one 'may see occasional ballooned zone 3 hepatocytes', but in a subsequent review article Brunt *et al.* [5] required hepatocellular ballooning to be present for the diagnosis of NASH. Burt *et al.* [6] used the term steatohepatitis when steatosis, ballooning of hepatocytes and any degree of centrilobular fibrosis was present, while Diehl *et al.* [7] regarded centilobular fat accumulation, and Mallory bodies or zone 3 perivenular and pericellular fibrosis as cardinal features of NASH. Some pathologists occasionally make a diagnosis of 'NASH' even in the absence of steatosis (B. Brunt, personal communication, see also Chapter 24). Presumably, this is when the clinical setting is appropriate for NASH and the biopsy shows all the features required for a diagnosis of NASH apart from steatosis. However, it seems counter-intuitive to use a diagnostic term that includes steatosis in cases where there is no steatosis.

Clinicopathological studies have been vexed by these inconsistencies, leading to considerable confusion amongst pathologists, clinicians and patients. In an attempt to 'tighten the screws', Lee [2] suggested that the diagnosis of NASH should be reserved for liver biopsies in which the pathology closely resembles that of alcoholic steatohepatitis. Sheth *et al.* [3], Brunt *et al.* [4], Brunt [5] and Burt *et al.* [6], amongst others, have supported this suggestion. The features in liver biopsies diagnosed as NASH should fulfil the criteria for alcoholic hepatitis laid down by the International Hepatopathology Study Group: hepatocyte necrosis and the presence of neutrophils amongst

the inflammatory cells, with or without Mallory bodies [8]. Although liver injury diagnosed as NASH should be indistinguishable from alcoholic hepatitis, the liver injury is generally less severe, with fewer or no Mallory bodies [6,8–11]. In addition, some of the patterns of injury (e.g. sclerosing hyaline necrosis) seen in alcoholic hepatitis are not usually evident in NASH [9].

According to such rigid criteria, milder forms of steatohepatitis, which bear little resemblance to alcoholic hepatitis, are effectively excluded from being designated as NASH, leading to the apparent paradox that 'steatosis + inflammation + insignificant alcohol intake' do not necessarily equal 'non-alcoholic steatohepatitis'. In addition, many hepatopathologists, who work with animal models for alcohol-induced liver injury, point out that alcohol-related liver injury in humans is also frequently non-specific-without Mallory bodies and with few or no polymorphs, rather than 'classic' steatohepatitis with ballooning, neutrophil polymorphs and Mallory bodies, to support the validity of their models [12]. Again, it is parodoxical that the same non-specific pattern of steatohepatitis in human non-drinkers, which is identical to that seen experimentally in association with alcohol, should not be designated by the words 'non-alcoholic steatohepatitis'.

To overcome some of the problems outlined above, Matteoni *et al.* [13] suggested the term 'non-alcoholic fatty liver diseases' (NAFLD), which they divided into four categories:
* *Type 1:* steatosis alone
* *Type 2:* steatosis plus lobular inflammation
* *Type 3:* steatosis, lobular inflammation and ballooning degeneration of hepatocytes
* *Type 4:* steatosis, ballooning degeneration and Mallory bodies and/or fibrosis

NAFLD is a useful 'umbrella' term that covers a broad spectrum of liver injury and encompasses steatosis (type 1), a pattern of non-specific steatohepatitis that does not resemble alcoholic hepatitis (type 2) and NASH (types 3 and 4). The finding that NAFLD types 3 and 4 are associated with the worst clinical outcomes provides support for such a classification [13].

Ludwig *et al.* [1], in the initial paper on NASH, used the term 'insignificant amounts of alcohol' and reported that 'most patients had less than one drink a week'. However, there is a lack of consensus as to what constitutes 'insignificant' or 'negligible' alcohol intake. A recent review on NASH reports on studies that have allowed from 40 to 210 g/week ethanol [14]. It is possible that the alcohol, particularly the higher doses, is contributing to liver injury, in at least some if not all of these patients.

Liver pathology

Light microscopy

Steatosis

Steatosis (fatty liver) is characterized by the accumulation of fat droplets in hepatocytes. In NAFLD the fat is seen mainly as large single macrovesicular droplets that displace the nucleus to the periphery of the cell (Plate 1, facing p. 22); a lesser amount of microvesicular fat may be seen as large numbers of smaller droplets surrounding a central nucleus (Plate 2). In early or mild NAFLD, the fat is seen in zone 3 hepatocytes. Simple steatosis is reversible in a matter of days to weeks.

Biochemically, steatosis is defined as an accumulation of lipid in the liver exceeding 5% of the liver weight [15]. We, and others, consider the presence of fat droplets in up to 5% of hepatocytes as within normal limits [16], while others regard the presence of any steatosis as abnormal and allocate a score of 1 for even the mildest forms (Table 2.1) [4,5]. When the steatosis is entirely microvesicular in type, other aetiologies including alcohol and drugs and, where appropriate, acute fatty liver of pregnancy should be considered. Steatotic livers may also contain 'fat cysts,' and lipogranulomas that are mainly located in zone 3, and are composed of aggregates of lipid-laden macrophages that stain positively with an antibody to CD 68.

There is uncertainty about the minimum criteria for the diagnosis of any type of hepatitis in fatty livers. The presence of one or two focal collections of mononuclear cells in the parenchyma (Plate 1) or occasional mononuclear cells in the portal tracts is not sufficient to warrant a diagnosis of NAFLD/NASH types 2–4. Nor does the existence of one or more clinical risk factors for NASH justify the designation of simple fatty

liver as NASH in the absence of hepatocyte injury and a mixed inflammatory infiltrate. However, a diagnosis of NAFLD type 1 would be appropriate in such livers.

Alcoholic hepatitis

The essential features are steatosis, hepatocyte necrosis and a neutrophil polymorph infiltrate. Ballooned hepatocytes and Mallory bodies are frequently seen but are not obligatory for the diagnosis of alcoholic hepatitis [7,17].

Steatohepatitis

This is a term that implies the presence of both fatty change and hepatocyte injury accompanied by inflammation. Ludwig *et al.* [1] made the selection criteria for inclusion in their study 'moderate to severe macrovesicular fatty change and lobular inflammation'. They further described the features in liver biopsies as focal necrosis and a mixed inflammatory infiltrate. Most of their cases contained Mallory bodies and showed varying degrees of fibrosis. Thus, the originally described features of NASH (Plates 3–6) clearly resemble those of alcoholic hepatitis.

Hepatocyte injury can be in the form of ballooning degeneration that is reversible, or hepatocyte necrosis or apoptosis that is irreversible. Some [4,5,16], but not all authors [7,18], consider the presence of ballooning degeneration as an absolute requirement for a diagnosis of NASH. Ballooned hepatocytes are enlarged and have pale cytoplasm as a result of fluid retention (Plates 3, 4). The problem is that small fat droplets can give the cytoplasm a 'cobweb-like' appearance that closely resembles that of mildly hydropic cells. Further, in end-stage cirrhosis, bile stasis, particularly in hepatocytes at the periphery of the regeneration nodules, results in hydropic change that gives the cells a ballooned appearance.

Fat stains (oil red O on frozen tissue, or post-fixation in osmium tetroxide), which are not routinely performed, are required to reliably distinguish between fluid and fat. Apoptotic hepatocytes, seen as shrunken eosinophilic cells with pyknotic nuclei, can be seen in NASH but are never as prominent as in viral hepatitis. Necrotic hepatocytes are not usually prominent, but a mixed inflammatory infiltrate comprising neutrophils, lymphocytes and ceroid-laden Kupffer cells can be seen at the sites where necrotic hepatocytes have disappeared. Again, some authors [4,5], but not others [7,18], require neutrophils for a diagnosis of NASH.

Table 2.1 Grading of steatosis. (After Brunt [5], with permission of the author.)

Grade 1	Fat droplets in < 33% hepatocytes
Grade 2	Fat droplets in 33–66% hepatocytes
Grade 3	Fat droplets in > 66% hepatocytes

Table 2.2 Grading of necroinflammation. (After Brunt [5], with permission of the author.)

Grade	Ballooning	Lobular inflammation	Portal inflammation
Grade 1 Mild	Occasional, zone 3 hepatocytes	Polymorphs and mononuclear cells, mild and scattered	None or mild
Grade 2 Moderate	Obvious, present in zone 3	Polymorphs associated with ballooned hepatocytes, +/− mild mononuclear cells	None, mild or moderate
Grade 3 Severe	Marked, predominantly zone 3	Polymorphs concentrated in areas of ballooning Inflammation more than in grade 2	Mild or moderate, *not* marked

Mallory bodies are seen in hepatocytes, particularly in zone 3 and especially in those cells showing ballooning degeneration. They appear as irregularly shaped, deeply eosinophilic masses in the cytoplasm (Plate 3). Mallory bodies are composed of cytokeratin polypeptides, which stain with an antibody to ubiquitin [19]. They are often seen in NASH but, as the case in alcoholic hepatitis [8], the presence of Mallory bodies is not obligatory for a diagnosis of NASH.

Another unresolved problem is how much necroinflammation is required for a diagnosis of NASH; to some extent this can be overcome by using a grading system either as words (mild, moderate, marked) or a numerical grade (1–3) (Table 2.2).

Fibrosis and cirrhosis
In both alcoholic hepatitis and NASH, fibrosis is first seen in zone 3 (centrilobular region). The fibrosis is characteristically pericellular in distribution (Plate 4), but perivenular fibrosis may also be present. Some authors advocate the presence of early fibrosis as an essential feature for the diagnosis of NASH [6,18]. In children with NASH (see Chapter 19 for a more detailed discussion) the fibrosis tends to be in the portal tracts rather than in zone 3 (Plate 5A, B).

In clinical series, approximately 20% of patients with NASH progress to cirrhosis [2,7,13]. In the staging of NASH, the fibrosis can progress, albeit slowly, to cirrhosis (Plate 6). In established cirrhosis, there is complete loss of the normal lobular architecture and replacement by regenerative nodules of hepatocytes that are completely surrounded by bands of fibrous tissue [7]. Marked fibrosis can be seen in haematoxylin and eosin (H&E) stained sections, but special stains such as Sirius red (Plate 7), van Gieson or Masson

Table 2.3 Staging of fibrosis*

Stage 1	Zone 3 pericellular fibrosis (focal or extensive)
Stage 2	Zone 3 pericellular fibrosis (focal or extensive) plus portal fibrosis (focal or extensive)
Stage 3	Bridging fibrosis (focal or extensive)
Stage 4	Cirrhosis, +/− foci of residual pericellular fibrosis

trichrome are needed for a more accurate estimate of the severity of fibrosis. The Sirius red stain is preferred for morphometric analysis because, unlike the Masson trichrome stain, it reacts specifically with collagen and does not stain other matrix proteins [20].

Brunt [5] has developed and refined a staging system for fibrosis in NASH (Table 2.3). Cirrhotic livers usually show active steatohepatitis (personal observation of the editors). However, in end-stage liver disease coming to transplantation, the hepatic steatosis and necroinflammation may no longer be apparent. In this situation, the cirrhosis is described as 'inactive' (cryptogenic cirrhosis) and NASH is sometimes designated as 'burnt-out' [21].

Glycogenated nuclei
The presence of pseudo-inclusions of glycogen in hepatocyte nuclei is non-specific, but they are frequently seen in diabetes mellitus [22] and are therefore a frequent finding in NASH.

Electronmicroscopy

Megamitochondria (giant mitochondria)
Enlarged mitochondria, often containing paracrystalline inclusions, are a frequent ultrastructural finding in

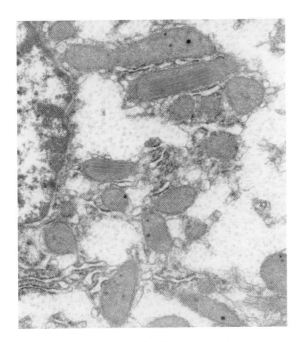

Fig. 2.1 Electron micrograph of liver from obese patient with NAFLD showing giant mitochondria with paracrystalline inclusions. Magnification ×48 000. Image courtesy of Dr S. Caldwell, University of Virginia, Charlottesville, USA.

NASH (Fig. 2.1) (Plate 5(b)) [23]. Megamitochondria are well recognized in alcoholic liver disease, even in the early stages, and occasionally they can even be recognized by light microscopy as eosinophilic intracytoplasmic globules in H&E-stained sections of liver. However, because giant mitochondria are now becoming increasingly recognized in NASH in both humans [23] and animal models [24], their presence in liver biopsies showing steatohepatitis does not necessarily point to an alcoholic aetiology. The causes and effects of mitochondrial injury in NASH are discussed in Chapter 11.

Clinicopathological correlation

Histopathologists cannot make a diagnosis of NASH purely on morphological grounds; clinicopathological correlation is essential. Problems for the histopathologist include the following:

• Whether or not to use the term NASH when the steatosis is mild, hepatocyte injury minimal, without ballooning, and the inflammatory infiltrate is composed purely of mononuclear cells. This is a particular problem when the patient does not drink alcohol but has one or more risk factors for NAFLD/ NASH. Currently, many pathologists prefer to term this pattern of injury NAFLD type 2 because the features do not meet the strict criteria for a diagnosis of NASH.

• What terminology to use when the alcohol history is not known or has not been stated on the request form. It is unwise to use the term 'non-alcoholic' in the diagnosis under these circumstances; rather, a diagnosis of 'steatohepatitis of uncertain aetiology' is suggested, along with a recommendation for clinicopathological correlation.

During the last decade, clinicians and pathologists have moved from an era of incorrectly diagnosing alcoholic hepatitis in people who were non-drinkers to overdiagnosing NASH, sometimes in excessive alcohol drinkers. At this stage, the significance of this milder form of non-specific hepatitis, especially in patients with risk factors for NASH, is uncertain. A small study of serial liver biopsies from patients with psoriasis receiving low-dose methotrexate showed a subset with risk factors for NASH. These patients all had non-specific steatohepatitis, not 'classic' NASH, yet showed progressive liver fibrosis while on methotrexate unlike those who had no risk factors for NASH [18].

Pathologists are frequently asked for advice about the need for liver biopsy in patients in whom NASH is suspected on clinical grounds. The results of a study by Angulo *et al.* [25] enable the pathologist to provide some guidance to clinicians. The only correlate for steatosis was the body mass index (BMI), while for steatohepatitis a high correlation was found between the severity of fibrosis and the following:

• BMI
• Older age
• Type 2 diabetes mellitus (insulin resistance)
• Aspartate aminotransferase : alanine aminotransferase (AST : ALT) ratio > 1
• Female gender [26].

Studies are currently in progress to determine whether female gender is indeed a risk factor for progressive liver injury (J. George, personal communication). This type of information has enabled better selection of patients in whom a liver biopsy is likely to yield significant pathology (NASH or NAFLD types 3 and 4) (see also Chapter 24).

Differential diagnosis

From the pathologist's perspective, the main differential diagnosis is between alcoholic hepatitis and NASH [10,11]. It is not possible to differentiate between the two conditions purely on morphological grounds; however, the more severe the hepatitis in terms of the amount of necroinflammation, the greater the number of Mallory bodies and the higher the stage of fibrosis, the more likely the injury is caused by alcohol rather than metabolic factors [7].

Increasingly, drugs are being reported as a cause of liver injury that is identical to alcoholic hepatitis and often of equal or greater severity. As discussed in Chapter 1, the editors recommend that this be called drug-induced steatohepatitis rather than NASH, particularly because different pathogenic mechanisms may be involved.

Coexistent liver disease

NAFLD/NASH may coexist with a number of other liver diseases including hepatitis C, hepatic iron overload (both primary in association with HFE mutations, and secondary overload resulting from a range of causes), primary biliary cirrhosis and α_1-antitrypsin deficiency (for a detailed discussion see Chapter 23) [27].

Chronic hepatitis C

Steatosis has long been recognized as a frequent morphological finding in liver biopsies from patients with hepatitis C [28]. The steatosis in hepatitis C may be related to the direct ability of the virus, in particular genotype 3, to induce steatosis [29,30], and/or to alcohol or to the presence of risk factors for NASH (see also Chapter 24).

Steatosis in hepatitis C, when associated with risk factors for NASH, is an independent predictor of fibrosis [29] and has been shown to accelerate the progression of liver damage [31].

From a histological perspective, steatosis associated with hepatitis C *per se* differs from that of NAFLD in that it is usually focal, without a zonal distribution, and is not associated with ballooning degeneration, Mallory bodies or pericellular or perivenular fibrosis [28]. The presence of these features in a biopsy from a patient with hepatitis C is strongly suggestive of coexistent NASH.

Hepatic siderosis

Increased stainable iron, usually mild (grade 1–2), has been documented in liver biopsies from patients with NASH; the frequency varies from 18 to 65% (Plate 8) [4,31].

Several studies have reported an increased prevalence of *HFE* gene mutations in patients with NASH [32–34]. One study suggested a correlation between increased hepatic iron and fibrosis [32], but this has not been confirmed by later studies [26,35]. Hepatic iron overload has been documented in liver biopsies from patients with the insulin resistance syndrome [36].

It has been suggested that iron may serve as a 'second hit' in steatotic livers, leading to the development of NASH [37]. This suggestion is supported by a study using an animal model of NASH in which excess dietary iron increased the amount of necroinflammation in steatotic livers (see Chapters 7 and 8) [38].

A Perls' Prussian blue stain for iron should be performed on liver biopsies showing NASH; the report should include a comment about the absence or presence of excess iron, and the grade of iron 1–4 (the iron grading relates to the percentage of hepatocytes that contain stainable iron: grade 1, up to 25%; grade 2, 25 to 50%; grade 3, 50 to 75%; and grade 4, iron in 75 to 100% of hepatocytes).

NAFLD/NASH in children

NAFLD is increasingly recognized in the paediatric population, particularly in obese children in the peripubertal years [39–42]. Although the full spectrum of morphological changes seen in adult NAFLD can be seen in children [40,41], it is noteworthy that in paediatric NAFLD the tendency is for inflammation and fibrosis to be predominantly in the portal tracts (Plate 5A–D) [39,40,42]. In particular, Baldridge et al. [39] drew attention to the invariable presence of a mixed inflammatory infiltrate in portal tracts, and portal fibrosis with only rare foci of lobular inflammation in some cases, and only one case with Mallory bodies. Hepatic fibrosis is usual and tends to occur early, but cirrhosis is not regarded as a frequent component of paediatric NASH [39,43]. Nevertheless, there have been recent case reports of children developing cirrhosis within 1–3 years of presentation with NASH [41]. Other causes of steatohepatitis, such as metabolic diseases, drugs and toxins (especially Wilson's disease), including alcohol in older children and adolescents, malnutrition, short gut syndrome and cystic fibrosis, must be excluded before diagnosing NAFLD in children (for a more detailed account see Chapter 19) [43].

Effects of treatment

The reversibility of steatosis is well recognized in both alcoholic and non-alcoholic steatohepatitis and usually occurs quite rapidly once the underlying cause has been removed or modified. Of much greater importance is the potential reversibility of hepatic fibrosis as a result of either modification in lifestyle or drug therapy, in particular drugs that improve insulin sensitivity. Pathologists are frequently asked to evaluate serial liver biopsies in individual patients or as part of clinical research projects. Grading of hepatic fibrosis in sections stained for collagen (e.g. Sirius red or Masson trichrome) is essential—and can be subjective or objective (Table 2.2). Up to one-third of patients with NASH progress to cirrhosis, but there are also case reports of serial liver biopsies describing a decrease in necroinflammation and fibrosis with time [44]. Recent reports of reversal of liver pathology by life style modification or drug treatment (rosiglitazone, piaglitazone) of NASH are summarized in Chapter 24.

Sampling variability and inter-observer variability

Concern has been expressed about sampling error in studies of serial liver biopsies. This is likely to be less than in diseases of bile ducts (e.g. primary biliary cirrhosis where the bile duct injury is known to be patchy) and frequently affects medium-sized bile ducts that may not be included in the biopsy. An autopsy study of NASH to document regional variation in grades of liver injury and stage of fibrosis could answer concerns about sampling variability.

The other potential problem with multicentre trials to evaluate drug therapy, where the 'gold standard' is evaluation of serial liver biopsies, is inter-observer variability. A study of liver biopsies showing NASH that addressed this problem showed that there was 'significant, substantial or moderate concordance' for the extent of steatosis, ballooning degeneration, perivenular fibrosis, grade of fibrosis and glycogenated nuclei, but less agreement about other features.

These included the location, degree and type of inflammation [45].

NASH-associated cirrhosis, 'cryptogenic' cirrhosis and recurrence of NAFLD/NASH after liver transplantation

Cirrhosis is a well-documented complication of NASH, the reported incidence varying from 7 to 26% (Plates 6,7) [2,7,13]. Several studies have addressed the predictive value of the initial liver biopsy findings in terms of which features correlate with 'aggressive outcomes'. Ratziu et al. [46] described significant steatosis (more than 40% of hepatocytes) and 'early' necroinflammatory activity in fatty livers as predictors of subsequent fibrosis.

There is a growing recognition that 'cryptogenic' cirrhosis may, in some cases, represent 'burnt-out' NASH. This suggestion is supported by the following:
• The prevalence of obesity and diabetes in patients with cryptogenic cirrhosis is reported to be similar to that in NASH and far exceeds that seen in patients with cirrhosis resulting from other causes [47].
• There have been several reports of patients with NASH, followed with serial liver biopsies, which showed disappearance of steatosis and inflammation with development of cirrhosis [21,48].
• Rashid and Roberts [43] suggested that at least some adults who have cryptogenic cirrhosis in adulthood may have had NASH since childhood.
• Extensive histopathological examination of explanted livers from patients transplanted for cryptogenic cirrhosis has revealed steatosis, with or without inflammation (often focal), in many cases where no such changes were apparent before transplantation [49].
• The frequent recurrence of non-alcoholic steatosis or steatohepatitis in patients receiving liver transplants for cryptogenic cirrhosis provides further evidence that NASH is an important cause of cryptogenic cirrhosis (Plate 9) [49–53].

In patients with NASH who develop cirrhosis, the strict morphological criteria for the diagnosis of NASH may no longer be apparent. Currently, there are no defined criteria for the diagnosis of NASH in cirrhosis [54]. Some authors regard the presence of steatosis (with or without inflammation) in a cirrhotic liver as diagnostic of NASH once other causes have been excluded by appropriate serological, biochemical and histological means, in patients who do not consume alcohol [49].

Hui *et al.* [54] have suggested the following working classification for cirrhosis in liver biopsies, explanted or autopsy livers, from patients with the clinical risk factors for NASH and no or minimal alcohol intake.

1 *Definite NASH-associated cirrhosis:* liver pathology characteristic of NASH

2 *Probable NASH-associated cirrhosis:* steatosis and non-specific steatohepatitis (NAFLD type 2)

3 *Possible NASH-associated cirrhosis*

   (a) No steatosis but necroinflammation suggestive of NASH

   (b) Steatosis but no necroinflammation

4 *Cryptogenic cirrhosis:* inactive cirrhosis without evidence of steatohepatitis, even after extensive sampling of the liver.

Clearly, previous liver biopsies showing features of NASH would support a diagnosis of NASH as the cause of cirrhosis even if steatohepatitis were no longer apparent. However, such biopsies are seldom available because patients with 'early' NASH tend to be asymptomatic. If these patients come to liver transplant, the diagnosis may be made retrospectively following extensive sampling of the explanted liver or recurrence of NASH in the allograft. Ayata *et al.* [49] examined nine explanted livers with cirrhosis attributed to NASH. The features of NASH were usually only present focally, involving just a few regenerative nodules. The findings were steatosis (78%), grade 2–3 inflammation (67%), Mallory hyaline (56%) and glycogenated nuclei (44%). Interestingly, large-cell dysplasia was present in 78% of these livers, compared to 17% in livers from patients with cirrhosis resulting from other causes.

Hepatocellular carcinoma: a complication of NAFLD/NASH?

Hepatocellular carcinoma (Plate 10) has become an increasingly recognized complication of NASH. Thus, a number of reports have appeared of tumours developing in patients with NASH, some of whom were followed over several years, and in others presenting *de novo* with cirrhosis associated with NASH [13,44, 55–59]. Two recently published series of HCC from Italy [58] and the USA [57] indicated that underlying liver disease may be NAFLD/NASH in 4% (23 of 641) and 13% (14 of 105) of patients with HCC, respectively. These conclusions were based on the presence of either histological features of NASH or clinical features associated with NAFLD, including obesity, diabetes and hyperlipidaemia. Moreover, the authors suggested that this might be an underestimate of the true prevalence of NAFLD in this group because the histological features of steatosis and inflammation often decrease as NASH progresses. It is essential for past history of alcohol ingestion and previous hepatitis B to be excluded in such cases (see also Chapter 24), particularly because other studies have not shown an association between NASH and HCC [54]. However, larger prospective studies of patients with NAFLD/NASH are required to confirm the proposed aetiological association with HCC, and to evaluate the risk of HCC in this group of patients.

The morphology of HCC developing in NASH cirrhosis is indistinguishable from that of HCC occurring in cirrhosis resulting from other aetiologies (Plate 10); trabecular, solid and pseudoglandular patterns have been described [58].

Careful surveillance of patients with NASH has enabled early detection of these tumours and successful treatment in several cases [58]. It has been suggested that obesity-related cell proliferation and altered apoptosis may have a role in the development of HCC in these patients (see Chapter 12). Interestingly, large-cell dysplasia was seen in 7 of 9 explanted livers (78%) from NASH patients undergoing liver transplantation, compared to only 3 of 18 (17%) of cirrhotic livers resulting from other causes [49]. Two such foci contained HCC. Clearly, mention of the presence or absence of dysplastic foci should be included in reports of liver biopsies showing NASH.

Conclusions

Although there is still a lack of general agreement about the nomenclature and diagnostic criteria for the spectrum of liver injury encompassed by the terms NAFLD/NASH, there is no doubt about the increasing prevalence and growing importance of this type of liver pathology. There is an urgent need for a standardized approach, based on internationally accepted criteria, to the reporting of liver biopsies showing 'fatty liver disease'.

References

1 Ludwig J, Viggiano TR, McGill DB, Ott BJ. Non-alcoholic steatohepatitis: Mayo Clinic experiences with a hithero unnamed disease. *Mayo Clin Proc* 1980; **55**: 434–5.

2 Lee RG. Non-alcoholic steatohepatitis: tightening the morphological screws on a hepatic rambler. *Hum Pathol* 1989; **20**: 594–8.

3 Sheth SG, Gordon FD, Chopra S. Non-alcoholic steatohepatitis. *Ann Intern Med* 1997; **126**: 137–45.

4 Brunt EM, Janney CG, Di Bisceglie AM, Neuschwander-Tetri BA, Bacon BR. Non-alcoholic steatohepatitis: a proposal for grading and staging the histological lesions. *Am J Gastroenterol* 1999: **94**: 2462–74.

5 Brunt EM. Non-alcoholic steatohepatitis: definition and pathology. *Semin Liver Dis* 2001; **21**: 3–16.

6 Burt AD, Mutton A, Day CP. Diagnosis and interpretation of steatosis and steatohepatitis. *Semin Diagn Pathol* 1998; **15**: 246–58.

7 Diehl AM, Goodman Z, Ishak KG. Alcohol-like liver disease in non-alcoholics. *Gastroenterology* 1988; **95**: 1056–62.

8 Anthony PP, Ishak KG, Nayak NC, *et al.* Alcoholic liver disease: morphological manifestations. *Lancet* 1981; **1**: 707–11.

9 Brunt EM. Alcoholic and non-alcoholic steatohepatitis. *Clin Liver Dis* 2002; **6**: 399–420.

10 Pinto HC, Baptista A, Camilo ME *et al.* Non-alcoholic steatohepatitis: clinicopathological comparison with alcoholic hepatitis in ambulatory and hospitalized patients. *Dig Dis Sci* 1996; **41**: 224–9.

11 Itoh S, Yougel T, Kawagoe K. Comparison between non-alcoholic steatohepatitis and alcoholic hepatitis. *Am J Gastroenterol* 1987; **82**: 650–4.

12 Hall P de la M, Lieber CS, DeCarli LM, *et al.* Animal models for alcoholic liver disease: a critical review. *J Alcohol Clin Exp Res* 2001; **25**: 254–61S.

13 Matteoni CA, Younossi ZM, Gramlich T *et al.* Non-alcoholic fatty liver disease: a spectrum of clinical and pathological severity. *Gastroenterology* 1999; **116**: 1413–9.

14 Mulhall BP, Ong JP, Younossi Z. Non-alcoholic fatty liver disease: an overview. *J Gastroenterol Hepatol* 2002; **17**: 1136–43.

15 Cairns SR, Peters T. Biochemical analysis of hepatic lipid in alcoholic and diabetic and control subjects. *Clin Sci (Lond)* 1983; **65**: 645–2.

16 Wanless IR, Lentz JS. Fatty liver hepatitis (steatohepatitis) and obesity: an autopsy study with analysis of risk factors. *Hepatology* 1990; **12**: 1106–10.

17 Beckett AG, Livingstone AV, Hill KR. Acute alcoholic hepatitis. *Br Med J* 1961; **ii**: 1113–9.

18 Langman G, Hall P de la M, Todd G. The role of non-alcoholic steatohepatitis in methotrexate-induced liver injury. *J Gastroenterol Hepatol* 2001; **16**: 1395–401.

19 French SW. Mechanisms of alcoholic liver injury. *Can J Gastroenterol* 2000; **14**: 327–32.

20 Plummer JL, Ossowicz CJ, Whibley C, Ilsley AH, Hall PD. Influence of intestinal flora on the development of fibrosis and cirrhosis in a rat model. *J Gastroenterol Hepatol* 2000; **15**: 1307–11.

21 Caldwell SH, Oelsner DH, Iezzoni JC *et al.* Cryptogenic cirrhosis: clinical characterization and risk factors for underlying disease. *Hepatology* 1999; **29**: 664–9.

22 Nagore N, Scheuer PJ. The pathology of diabetes mellitus. *J Pathol* 1988; **156**: 155–60.

23 Caldwell SH, Swerdlow RH, Khan EM *et al.* Mitochondrial abnormalities in non-alcoholic steatohepatitis. *J Hepatol* 1999; **31**: 430–4.

24 Kirsch R, Clarkson V, Shephard EG *et al.* A rodent nutritional model of non-alcoholic steatohepatitis: species, strain and sex difference studies. *J Gastroenterol Hepatol* 2003; **18**: 1272–82.

25 Angulo P, Keach JC, Batts KP, Lindor KD. Independent predictors of liver fibrosis in patients with non-alcoholic steatohepatitis. *Hepatology* 1999; **30**: 1356–62.

26 Chitturi S, Weltman M, Farrell GC *et al.* HFE mutations, hepatic iron, and fibrosis: ethnic-specific association of NASH with C282Y but not with fibrotic activity. *Hepatology* 2002; **36**: 142–9.

27 Brunt EM, Ramrakhiani S, Cordes BG *et al.* Concurrence of histologic features of steatohepatitis with other forms of liver disease. *Mod Pathol* 2003; **16**: 49–56.

28 Lefkowitch JH, Scåhiff ER, Davis GL *et al.* Pathological diagnosis of chronic hepatitis C: a multicentre comparative study with chronic hepatitis B. *Gastroenterology* 1993; **104**: 595–603.

29 Monto A, Alonzo J, Watson JJ, Grunfeld C, Wright TL. Steatosis in chronic hepatitis C: relative contributions of obesity, diabetes mellitus, and alcohol. *Hepatology* 2002; **36**: 729–36.

30 Negro F. Hepatitis C and liver steatosis: is it the virus? Yes it is, but not always. *Hepatology* 2002; **36**: 1050–2.

31 Adinolfi LE, Gambardella M, Andreana A *et al.* Steatosis accelerates the progression of liver damage of chronic hepatitis C patients and correlates with specific HCV genotype and visceral obesity. *Hepatology* 2001; **33**: 1358–64.

32 Bacon BR, Farahvash MJ, Janney CG, Neuschwander-Tetri BA. Non-alcoholic steatohepatitis: an expanded clinical entity. *Gastroenterology* 1994; **107**: 1103–9.

33 George DK, Goldwurm S, MacDonald GA *et al.* Increased hepatic iron concentration in non-alcoholic steatohepatitis is associated with increased fibrosis. *Gastroenterology* 1998; **114**: 311–8.

34 Bonkowsky HL, Jawaid T, Bacon BR *et al*. Non-alcoholic steatohepatitis and iron: increased prevalence of mutations of the HFE gene in non-alcoholic steatohepatitis. *J Hepatol* 1999; **31**: 421–9.

35 Younossi ZM, Gramlich T, Bacon B *et al*. Hepatic iron and fatty liver disease. *Hepatology* 1999; **30**: 847–50.

36 Turlin B, Mendler MH, Moirand R *et al*. Histological feature of the liver in insulin resistance-associated iron overload. *Am J Clin Pathol* 2001; **116**: 263–70.

37 Day CP, James OFW. Steatohepatitis: a tale of two hits? *Gastroenterology* 1998; **114**: 842–5.

38 Kirsch R, Verdonk RC, Twala M *et al*. Iron potentiates liver injury in the rat nutritional model of non-alcoholic steatohepatitis (NASH). *J Hepatol* 2002; **36** (Suppl. 1): 148, 534A.

39 Baldridge AD, Perez-Atayde AR, Graeme-Cook F, Higgins L, Lavine JE. Idiopathic steatohepatitis in childhood: a multicentre retrospective study. *J Paediatr* 1995; **127**: 700–4.

40 Manton ND, Lipsett J, Moore DJ *et al*. Non-alcoholic steatohepatitis in children and adolescents. *Med J Aust* 2000; **173**: 476–9.

41 Molleston JP, White F, Teckman J, Fitzgerald JF. Obese children with steatohepatitis can develop cirrhosis in childhood. *Am J Gastroenterol* 2002; **97**: 2460–2.

42 Moran JR, Ghishan FK, Halter SA, Green HL. Steatohepatitis in obese children: a cause of chronic liver dysfunction. *Am J Gastroenterol* 1983; **78**: 374–7.

43 Rashid M, Roberts EA. Non-alcoholic steatohepatitis in children. *J Pediatr Gastroenterol Nutr* 2000; **30**: 48–53.

44 Powell EE, Cooksley GE, Hanson R *et al*. The natural history of non-alcoholic steatosis: a follow-up study of 42 patients for up to 21 years. *Hepatology* 1990; **11**: 74–80.

45 Younossi ZM, Gramlich T, Liu YC *et al*. Non-alcoholic fatty liver disease: assessment of variability in pathological interpretations. *Mod Pathol* 1998; **11**: 560–5.

46 Ratziu V, Giral P, Charlotte F *et al*. Liver fibrosis in overweight patients. *Gastroenterology* 2000; **118**: 1117–23.

47 Poonawala A, Nair SP, Thuluvath PJ. Prevalence of obesity and diabetes in patients with cryptogenic cirrhosis: a case–control study. *Hepatology* 2000; **32**: 689–92.

48 Abdelmalek M, Ludwig J, Lindor KD. Two cases from the spectrum of non-alcoholic steatohepatitis. *J Clin Gastroenterol* 1995; **20**: 127–30.

49 Ayata G, Gordon FD, Lewis WD *et al*. Cryptogenic cirrhosis: clinicopathologic findings at and after liver transplantation. *Hum Pathol* 2002; **33**: 1098–104.

50 Kim WR, Poterucha JJ, Porayko MK *et al*. Recurrence of non-alcoholic steatohepatitis following liver transplantation. *Transplantation* 1996; **62**: 1802–5.

51 Carson K, Washington MK, Treem WR *et al*. Recurrence of non-alcoholic steatohepatitis in a liver transplant recipient. *Liver Transplant Surg* 1997; **3**: 174–6.

52 Molloy RM, Komorowski R, Varma RR. Reccurent non-alcoholic steatohepatitis and cirrhosis after liver transplantation. *Liver Transplant Surg* 1997; **3**: 177–8.

53 Ong J, Younossi ZM, Reddy V *et al*. Cryptogenic cirrhosis and posttransplantation non-alcoholic fatty liver disease. *Liver Transpl* 2001; **7**: 797–801.

54 Hui JM, Kench JG, Chitturi S *et al*. Long-term outcomes of cirrhosis in non-alcoholic steatohepatitis compared with hepatitis C. *Hepatology* 2003; **38**: 420–7.

55 Cotrim HP, Parana R, Braga E, Lyra L. Non-alcoholic steatohepatitis and hepatocellular carcinoma: natural history? *Am J Gastroenterol* 2000; **95**: 3018–9.

56 Zen Y, Katayanagi K, Tsuneyama K *et al*. Hepatocellular carcinoma arising in non-alcoholic steatohepatitis. *Pathol Int* 2001; **51**: 127–31.

57 Marrero JA, Fontana RJ, Su GL *et al*. NAFLD may be a common underlying liver disease in patients with hepatocellular carcinoma in the United States. *Hepatology* 2002; **36**: 1349–54.

58 Buguianesi E, Leone N, Vanni E *et al*. Expanding the natural history of non-alcoholic steatohepatitis: from cryptogenic cirrhosis to hepatocellular carcinoma. *Gastroenterology* 2002; **123**: 134–40.

59 Shimada M, Hashimoto E, Taniai M *et al*. Hepatocellular carcinoma in patients with non-alcoholic steatohepatitis. *J Hepatol* 2002; **37**: 154–60.

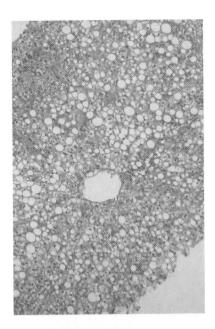

Plate 1 Steatosis/NAFLD type 1. Liver showing macrovesicular steatosis with minor inflammatory changes that are insufficient to be diagnosed as necroinflammation. Haematoxylin and eosin, objective × 10.

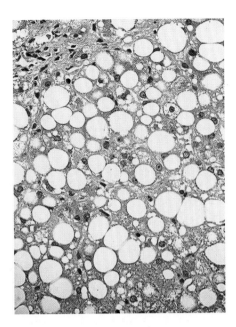

Plate 2 Steatosis/NAFLD type 1. Liver showing simple steatosis, mainly macrovesicular, but with some microvesicular fat droplets. Haematoxylin and eosin, objective × 20.

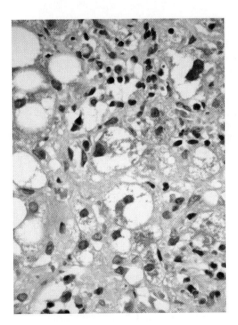

Plate 3 NASH. The hepatocytes show ballooning degeneration with Mallory bodies and an inflammatory infiltrate. Haematoxylin and eosin, objective × 40.

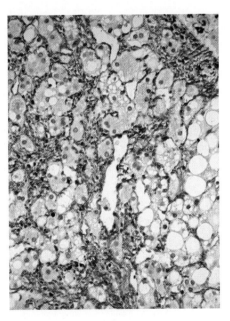

Plate 4 Macrovesicular steatosis and pericellular fibrosis in zone 3. Sirius red, objective × 20.

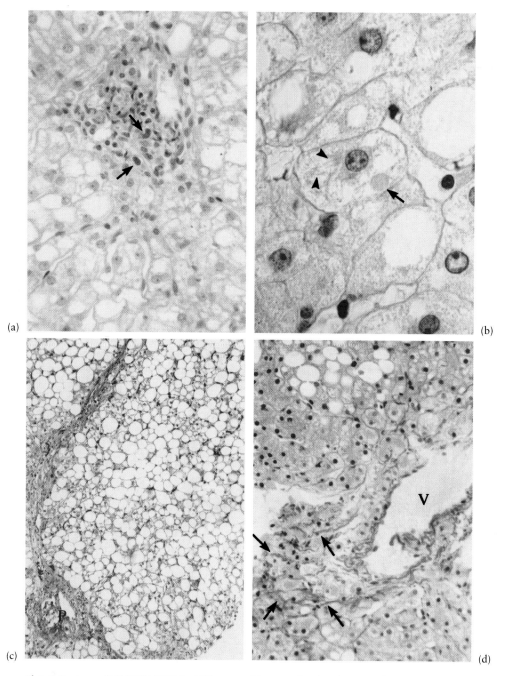

(a)

(b)

(c)

(d)

Plate 5 Features of NASH/NAFLD in children. (a) Mild portal mixed inflammatory infiltrate including occasional eosinophils (arrows). Haematoxylin and eosin, objective × 20. (b) Megamitochondria are observed in the cytoplasm of a hepatocyte. The round cytoplasmic hyaline inclusion (arrow) represents a megamitochondrion slightly smaller than the nucleus of the hepatocyte. The arrowheads indicate needle-shaped megamitochondria. Haematoxylin and eosin, objective × 40. (c) Trichrome stain to highlight collagen (blue) reveals portal fibrosis with portal to portal bridging. Objective × 4. (d) Mild sclerosis of terminal hepatic vein and radiating pericellular (Disse space) fibrosis. Trichrome stain, objective × 10.

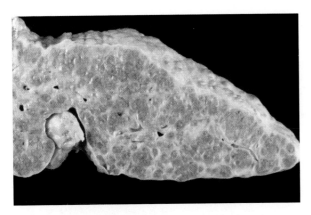

Plate 6 Explanted cirrhotic liver from a patient with NASH.

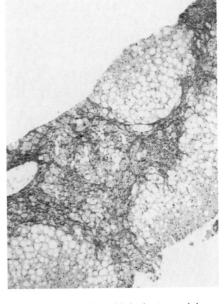

Plate 7 NASH with established micronodular cirrhosis. Regenerative nodules are surrounded by bands of fibrous tissue. The hepatocytes show macrovesicular fatty change. Sirius red, objective × 10.

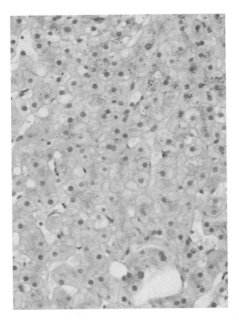

Plate 8 Mild hepatic siderosis and steatosis. Small amounts of iron are present within hepatocytes in a non-zonal distribution. Perls' Prussian blue stain, objective × 20.

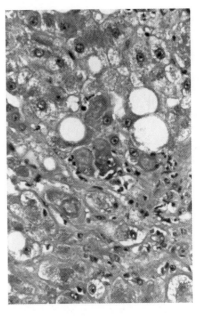

Plate 9 Recurrent NASH post-transplant. The liver shows steatosis and severe necroinflammation with Mallory bodies. Haematoxylin and eosin, objective × 40. Image courtesy of Dr T. Gramlich, Cleveland, USA.

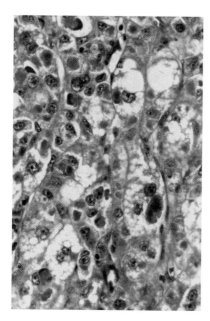

Plate 10 Hepatocellular carcinoma occurring in NASH/cirrhosis. Haematoxylin and eosin, objective × 40. Image courtesy of Dr T. Gramlich, Cleveland, USA.

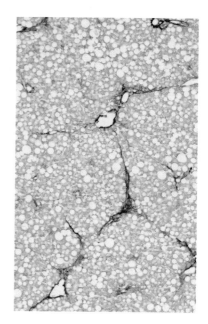

Plate 11 Hepatic fibrosis in rats fed a methionine- and choline-deficient diet for 12 weeks. Portal–portal and central portal bridging fibrosis is evident. Sirius red, objective × 10.

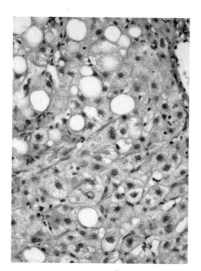

Plate 12 Perisinusoidal and perivenular fibrosis in chronic hepatitis C with steatosis. The collagen deposition is seen as fine fibres staining red. The classical features of coexistent NASH were not present in this biopsy. Haematoxylin-van Gieson, objective × 20.

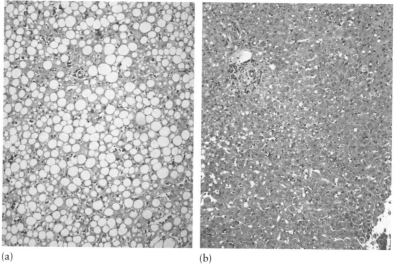

(a)   (b)

Plate 13 Effect of weight loss on steatosis in chronic hepatitis C. In the original biopsy (a), severe steatosis was present. Following weight loss there was a significant improvement in steatosis (b) despite persisting viral infection. This patient also had a reduced fibrosis score after weight loss. Haematoxylin and eosin, objective × 10.

The epidemiology and risk factors of NASH

Arthur J. McCullough

Key learning points

1 Non-alcoholic steatohepatitis (NASH), the most severe form of non-alcoholic fatty liver disease (NAFLD), is emerging as a common, clinically important type of chronic liver disease in industrialized countries, and rates are increasing in many developing countries.

2 Available data indicate that the prevalence rates for NAFLD and NASH have increased from previous estimates, and are now in the range 17–33% for NAFLD and 5.7–17% for NASH.

3 This increase and high prevalence is related to societal changes in obesity and genetic factors.

4 In some population-based surveys, hepatic steatosis is more strongly associated with obesity than heavy alcohol use.

5 NASH is a progressive fibrotic disease, in which cirrhosis and liver-related death occur in up to 20% and 12%, respectively, over a 10-year period.

6 NASH-associated cirrhosis can also decompensate into subacute liver failure, progress to hepatocellular carcinoma and recur post-transplantation. In contrast, steatosis alone has a more benign clinical course, although progression to cirrhosis appears to have occurred in 3% of these patients.

7 The strong link between obesity and type 2 diabetes and NAFLD/NASH is of particular concern given the increasing recognition of NASH in children.

8 The major risk factors for advanced fibrosis include diabetes or obesity, aspartate aminotransferase : alanine aminotransferase ratio > 1, patients older than 50 years and hepatic histology (presence of hepatocellular injury and fibrosis).

9 A number of important unresolved issues must be clarified before the true epidemiology and natural history of NAFLD and NASH can be fully understood.

Abstract

Non-alcoholic steatohepatitis (NASH)—the most severe form of non-alcoholic fatty liver disease (NAFLD)—is emerging as a common clinically important type of chronic liver disease in industrialized countries. The available data, which are based on screening population studies using the diagnostic modalities of ultrasound and liver function tests, now indicate the prevalence rates for both NAFLD and NASH have increased from previous estimates. They are now estimated to be in the range 17–33% for NAFLD and 5.7–16.5% for NASH. Because NAFLD and NASH are associated with insulin resistance and obesity, these prevalence rates are expected to increase worldwide, concurrent with the pandemic epidemic of obesity and type 2 diabetes. The importance of these observations stems from the fact that NASH is a progressive fibrotic disease, in which cirrhosis and liver-related death occur in up to 20% and 12% of these patients, respectively, over a 10-year period. This is of particular concern given the increasing recognition of NASH in children. The major risk factors for advanced fibrosis include the presence of diabetes or obesity, an aspartate aminotransferase : alanine aminotransferase (AST : ALT) ratio > 1, patients older than 50 years and hepatic histology. However, a number of important unresolved issues must be clarified before the true epidemiology and natural history of this disease can be fully understood.

Introduction

Epidemiology evaluates the incidence, prevalence, distribution and control of a disease in a specific or selected population. Unfortunately, our knowledge of the epidemiology of NAFLD and its more severe form NASH must be considered wanting in all of these areas. There are no incidence data and the prevalence data are conflicting, while our understanding of the population(s) most affected is only nascent [1].

Disagreement exists regarding patient demographics and which patients are most likely to be affected [2–4]. The distribution is worldwide [1]. However, while most of the available data have been obtained from the adult populations in the USA, Australia and western Europe [5,6], there is great concern over the emergence of NASH in children [7,8] and among the large populations of non-Western countries [9,10,11], as well as its emergence in developing countries (see Chapter 18) [12].

Our imprecise knowledge of NAFLD/NASH epidemiology results from a number of factors:

1 The relative recent recognition of NAFLD/NASH as an important disease.

2 The silent, often indolent nature of NAFLD/NASH.

3 Published trials that have used indirect surrogate serum markers or radiological tests to diagnose NAFLD/NASH.

4 Lack of consensus regarding the histological diagnosis of NAFLD/NASH (see Chapter 2), as well as the quantity of alcohol ingestion consistent with the diagnosis [1,13].

Regardless of these limitations, the available data indicate that NAFLD/NASH is the most common form of liver disease [1,14] and its prevalence is expected to

increase concurrent with the worldwide epidemic of obesity and type 2 diabetes mellitus [15].

NASH is an increasingly common problem worldwide and has been reported in Australia [16,17], India [9,18], Japan [10,19], the Middle East [11], New Zealand [20], North America [3,21–24], South America [25], northern Europe [26,27] southern Europe [28,29] and South East Asia [30]. The international impact of NAFLD/NASH is discussed in more detail in Chapter 18. However, despite its emergence as an important clinical entity, the true prevalence remains unknown. The reasons for this are predominantly related to vagaries in the histological definition, limitations in the diagnostic methods and the selected patient populations studied thus far.

Definition of NASH

Histology

The histopathology of NAFLD/NASH is discussed in Chapter 2. However, when reviewing the prevalence data, it is important to emphasize that NASH should be considered as the most severe form of a larger spectrum of NAFLD, with histological findings ranging from fat alone to fat plus inflammation and fat plus hepatocyte injury (ballooning degeneration) with or without fibrosis, polymorphonuclear (PMN) leukocytes or Mallory hyaline. Only fat plus hepatocyte injury with or without fibrosis should be considered to be NASH (NAFLD type 3 or 4; see Chapter 1). The significance of these histological categories rests not only on the fact that the prevalence varies by histology, with steatosis alone with or without inflammation being more common than NASH (Table 3.1), but clinical outcomes also vary by histological category (see Chapter 14).

As shown in Fig. 3.1, cirrhosis develops in 15–25% of NASH patients [3,16,21,22]. Once developed,

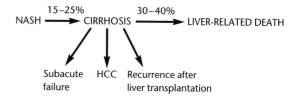

Fig. 3.1 Natural history of NASH. HCC, hepatocellular carcinoma.

Table 3.1 Prevalence of NAFLD and NASH.

Study population	Prevalence (%)
SELECTED STUDY POPULATIONS	
Liver biopsy	
Nonomara *et al.* [82]	(1.2)
Propst *et al.* [81]	15 (4.8)
Hultcrantz *et al.* [27]	54
Skelly *et al.* [66]	66 (34)
Daniel *et al.* [67]	84
Mathieson *et al.* [64]	42
Ratziu *et al.* [83]	79 (49)
CT scan	
El-Hassan *et al.* [11]	10
Postmortem analysis	
Random deaths	
Hilden *et al.* [84]	24
Ground [85]	16 (2.1)
Hospitalized deaths	
Wanless & Lenz [23]	
Lean	3
Obese	19
Surgical patients	
Adult living liver donors	
Marcos *et al.* [86]	20
Bariatric surgery	
Marceau *et al.* [87]	86 (14)
Del Gaudio *et al.* [88]	78 (21)
Luyek *et al.* [89]	74
Dixon *et al.* [48]	71 (25)
Klain *et al.* [90]	56 (29)
Silverman *et al.* [91]	78 (21)
GENERAL POPULATION SCREENING	
Ultrasound	
Nomura *et al.* [10]	23
Lonardo *et al.* [94]	22
Bellentani *et al.* [28]	
Lean	16
Obese	76
Liver enzyme screening	
Patt *et al.* [72]	14–21
NHANES III	3–23
Clark *et al.* [69]	23
Clark *et al.* [71]	23
Ruhl & Everhart [70]	3
Lean	1
Obese	6

Numbers in square brackets indicate the reference number for the specific study cited. Numbers in parentheses indicate the percentage of patients with hepatic histology consistent with NASH in studies that differentiated NASH from less severe forms of NAFLD.

30–40% of these patients may succumb to liver-related death over a 10-year period [22], the mortality rate being similar to [31] or worse than [32] cirrhosis associated with hepatitis C. NASH is also now considered the major cause of cryptogenic cirrhosis [33]. NASH-associated cirrhosis can also decompensate into subacute liver failure [34], progress to hepatocellular carcinoma (HCC) [35–39] and re-occur post-transplantation [40,41]. In contrast, steatosis alone is reported to have a more benign clinical course [22,26], although progression of fibrosis to cirrhosis has occurred in 3% of patients with steatosis alone in the author's series [22].

Definition of non-alcoholic

By definition, excessive alcohol consumption excludes the diagnosis of NAFLD. However, the definition of 'excessive' has been elusive and a wide range of alcohol has been allowed in previous reports [1,13]. Early studies allowed no alcohol use [2,21,42] while more recent studies have allowed 40 g/week [16,43] or up to 140 and 210 g/week for women and men, respectively [2,22,26,28,44,45]. Confounding this issue is a recent study describing endogenous alcohol production in NASH patients related to the degree of obesity [46], as well as the protective effect of moderate alcohol intake in the prevention of diabetes [47], and the development of NASH in morbidly obese patients undergoing bariatric surgery [48]. Although there is no consensus regarding the definition of 'non-alcoholic' in NAFLD patients, it seems reasonable to exclude patients from this diagnosis if current or past (within 5 years) alcohol intake has exceeded more than 20 g/day in women and 30 g/day in men. Life time total may be important (see Chapter 24). Because there is no clinical feature or laboratory test sufficiently sensitive to detect small amounts of alcohol intake, a careful history from the patient, the patient's family and other health care providers involved in the patient's management is paramount [49].

Diagnosis of NASH

The diagnosis of NASH is reviewed in detail in Chapter 12. However, a brief discussion is warranted here because the prevalence of NASH is very much dependent on the accuracy of the diagnosis. Liver biopsy is considered the gold standard for diagnosis and is the only method for differentiating NASH from steatosis with or without inflammation [50,51]. However, performing liver biopsies as a screening test in population-based studies to determine prevalence rates of NASH is not feasible. Consequently, radiological and serum liver function tests (LFTs) have been used as indirect or surrogate tests to estimate the prevalence of NAFLD and NASH. However, both have limitations, as displayed in Table 3.2.

Hepatic imaging

Ultrasound, computerized tomography (CT) scan, magnetic resonance imaging (MRI), and proton magnetic resonance spectroscopy (^{1}H MRS) have all been used to assess hepatic fat deposition in the liver [51–60]. While some studies have described superiority of a particular modality [52,54,56,59], a recent study [51] demonstrated ultrasound, CT scan and MRI have similar diagnostic accuracy for quantitating the severity of steatosis when fat deposition is more than 33% of the liver volume. ^{1}H MRS has greater sensitivity than the other three modalities and has been shown to detect as little as 5% fat deposition in the liver [52]. MRI is useful for confirming the nature of hepatic steatosis when it occurs focally rather than its usual diffuse pattern [61], while calibrated CT scans may be useful in monitoring hepatic fat content over time [53]. However, differences between NASH and steatosis are not apparent with any of the radiological modalities [51,57]. Even though two studies [62,63] have evaluated test characteristics for ultrasound and found that ultrasound leads to an incorrect diagnosis of fatty liver in 15–33% of patients, the most recent data, as well as cost considerations [14], have made ultrasound the most common imaging modality used for evaluating hepatic steatosis.

Liver function tests

A number of studies have reported that NAFLD is the most common cause of chronically elevated serum enzymes (ALT, AST, gamma-glutamyl transpeptidase [GGT]) of unexplained aetiology. With histology as the gold standard, NAFLD is found in 42–84% of such cases [64–67], while 85% of those with indicative ultrasonographical appearances have NAFLD [68].

These results provided the rationale for using LFT abnormalities to estimate the prevalence of NAFLD in screening population studies [69–72]. The limitations of this approach have been discussed elsewhere [14,73–75] and include the following:

1 Lack of specificity; this results in an overestimation of prevalence.

2 Although LFTs are usually mildly elevated in NAFLD (see Chapters 13 and 15) [1,76,77], values can be normal [78,79].

3 Serum LFT abnormalities do not correlate with the degree of steatosis or fibrosis [78,79].

4 The normal limits for ALT in population studies have been revised downward with values individualized by gender and for individuals with obesity or the metabolic syndrome [68].

These limitations indicate that earlier reports of NAFLD prevalence rates based on serum LFTs may be either overestimates because of lack of specificity, or underestimates because of lack of sensitivity of the values used for normal cut-off.

Prevalence

Table 3.1 provides estimates of the prevalence of NAFLD obtained from studies that evaluated different patient populations using various methodologies [1,5,80]. These studies can be separated into two

Table 3.2 Limitations to current screening methods to diagnose NAFLD.

Liver function tests	Ultrasound
Upper limit for normal values being revised	Operator dependent
Levels decrease with freezing	Logistically difficult for large screening studies
May be normal in an unknown percentage of patients	May be inaccurate in up to 33% of patients
Which LFT(s) to use is not clear	Does not detect steatosis if < 33% of liver volume

general categories: highly selected population studies and general screening population studies. The studies that used highly selected patient populations suffer from ascertainment bias. However, they have high specificity because histology was used in the large majority of these studies to diagnose not only the presence, but the type of NAFLD. The general population screening studies provide more representative prevalence rates, but also suffer from the limitations of their diagnostic techniques: hepatic imaging methods and LFTs (see above). Furthermore, without histology these general screening studies cannot identify the type of NAFLD.

Selected study populations

In patients undergoing liver biopsy, the prevalence has ranged between 15% and 84% for NAFLD and between 1.2% and 49% for NASH [27,64–67,81–83]. This wide range is related to differences in case ascertainment. One study [68] performed biopsies on patients found to have NAFLD on ultrasound, while others [27,64,66,67] performed biopsies only on patients with chronically elevated LFTs.

While this information is helpful, better estimates of prevalence can be obtained from studies investigating patients who had random deaths. Analyses of livers from individuals who died randomly from automobile [84] or airplane [85] crashes showed prevalence rates for NAFLD of 24% and 16%, respectively, while the prevalence of NASH was 2.4 and 2.1%. However, all these studies used selected populations and therefore these data do not reflect the true prevalence of either NAFLD or NASH in the general population [1].

In healthy young adults being evaluated as donors for living-related orthotopic liver transplantation, fatty liver disease was found in 20%, despite normal ALT levels [86].

An autopsy study found NAFLD in 19% of obese patients and 3% of normal weight patients [23]. Although the histological description provided did not allow for distinguishing NASH from other types of NAFLD reliably, the study emphasizes the close association between obesity and fatty liver. It further found that the presence of diabetes mellitus was a more important risk factor for fibrosis than obesity.

In morbidly obese patients undergoing bariatric surgery [48,87–91], NAFLD was present in 56–78% of patients while NASH occurred in 21–39%.

NAFLD also occurs in children. Consistent with results in adults, approximately 3% of overweight children have steatosis [8,92]. This proportion increases to 53% in obese children [93].

General population studies

As shown in Table 3.1, the general population studies have used either ultrasound or LFTs to make the diagnosis of NAFLD.

Ultrasound
In Japanese and Italian studies that performed hepatic ultrasonography prospectively in general population studies [10,28,94], NAFLD was observed in 16–23% of individuals. Among these studies perhaps the most representative is the Dionysos study. This was performed in 1990–92 and screened almost 7000 patients in two towns in northern Italy in order to determine the spectrum and prevalence of liver disease in the general population [28,95,96]. Fat was found in 16% and 76% of normal weight and obese individuals, respectively. In the normal weight subjects who consumed more than 30 g/day alcohol, the prevalence of steatosis increased to 46%, a rate that increased to 95% in obese heavy drinkers.

The Dionysos study indicates that fatty liver disease is frequently present in healthy subjects and is essentially always present in obese subjects consuming more than 30 g/day alcohol. Of interest was the observation that hepatic steatosis is more strongly associated with obesity than heavy alcohol use [28].

Liver function tests
Although NAFLD has been reported to be a common cause of liver disease in physicians' offices [97,98], only recently has the prevalence of NAFLD, based on population studies, been reported. In the USA, the Third National and Nutritional Examination Survey (NHANES III) has provided the most extensive evaluation of NAFLD prevalence. NHANES III was performed between 1988 and 1994. It was sponsored by the United States (US) Centers for Disease Control (CDC) and included over 12 000 adults from the general US population. NAFLD was diagnosed when there was an elevation in ALT, AST or GGT without any other identifiable liver disease as the cause. As shown in Table 3.3, there have been three different studies from the NHANES database, with prevalences

	NHANES III		
	Clark [69]	Ruhl [70]	Clark [71]
Prevalence (%)	23	2.8	7.9
LFTs (U/L)	AST, ALT, GGT (> 30)	ALT (> 43)	AST, ALT F(> 31), (> 31) M(> 37), (> 40)
Exclusions	Appropriate	Diabetics	Appropriate

Table 3.3 Prevalence of NAFLD.

Numbers in brackets indicate the reference number for the specific study cited.
F, female; M, male.

ranging from 2.8% to 23% [69–71]. This wide discordance in prevalence rates for NAFLD in the NHANES study is caused by a number of differences in inclusion criteria for the three studies [14,73,74]:
1 Whether or not diabetic patients were excluded
2 What liver function tests were used
3 The level of elevation in the liver function tests that were considered abnormal
4 Whether the abnormal cut-off level for liver function tests should be adjusted for gender.

The initial analysis [69] had the highest prevalence of 23%; this analysis did not exclude diabetic patients and used any increment above 30 U/L in any of three tests (ALT, AST or GGT). In a subsequent analysis by the same authors [71], the prevalence decreased to 7.9% because GGT was excluded from the analysis and the cut-off levels for ALT and AST were increased for male subjects. The third analysis [70] reported only a 2.8% prevalence rate when only ALT was used, the normal cut-off level was increased to 43 U/L and diabetic patients were not included. In this study, the prevalence rate was 1% in normal weight patients and 6% for combined overweight and obese patients.

This variation in prevalence among the three separate analyses for the same data set can be related to the issues discussed above. However, the essence of the uncertainty in the prevalence rates for NAFLD resides in the problem of defining NAFLD in epidemiological studies based on non-invasive tests without a liver biopsy. There are a number of pertinent questions that need to be answered for future studies. If liver function tests are used, should ALT be used alone or with other biochemical tests [14,73,74,99]? What level of eleva-

tion should be considered abnormal [68]? Should different cut-off levels for normal values differ between men and women [68]?

Regardless of these issues, it is clear from the NHANES III data set that NAFLD is extremely common, occurs in both men and women, and there is a positive correlation between the prevalence of NAFLD and obesity as estimated from body mass index (BMI).

In all likelihood, the 23% prevalence rate for NAFLD obtained in the first analysis [69] is most accurate for a number of reasons. First, there is little reason to use ALT alone rather than ALT, AST and GGT [14,73, 74,99]. Secondly, there is no reason to exclude diabetics. Not only do diabetics now account for 7% of the US population, but diabetes is also a risk factor for both steatosis and NASH. Thirdly, the upper limit of normal for ALT levels used in this analysis are closest to the newly suggested values that have been revised downward [68]. Finally, a 23% prevalence is most consistent with the ultrasound screening studies, which reported rates between 16% and 23% [10,28].

Current estimates of prevalence

Because of the imprecision of both the imaging methods and liver function tests discussed above and displayed in Table 3.2, the prevalence of NAFLD can be at best an estimate. However, the available data provide sufficient information to allow reasonable estimates, at least for populations in North America, Australia/New Zealand and western Europe. Based on all the studies discussed above and listed in Table 3.1, the prevalence of NAFLD ranges between 1% and 24% in normal weight individuals [70,84], with the best studies reporting 16–20% [28,86]. In obesity the range is 6–86% [70,87], with the best estimates having prevalence rates between 19% and 76% [23,28]. Using the rates from the best studies and assuming 23% of the population is obese, the over-all prevalence of NAFLD rests between 17% and 33%.

Estimating the prevalence of NASH is more problematic because no general population screening study has obtained liver histology; this makes the distinction between NASH and the less severe forms of NAFLD (steatosis with or without inflammation) impossible. However, in a variety of the selected population studies discussed above and in Table 3.1, the ratio of NASH : NAFLD was one-third to half. Therefore, using a conservative estimate, the prevalence of NASH should be 5.7% (one-third of 17%) but could be as high as 17% (half of 33%) using liberal estimates.

Risk factors

Insulin resistance

Metabolic syndrome
The metabolic syndrome (also known as the insulin resistance syndrome) comprises five major features [100,101]: hypertension, central obesity, elevated fasting blood sugar, high triglycerides and low high-density lipoproteins, which are associated with insulin resistance. The presence of any three of the five components allows the diagnosis of metabolic syndrome to be made [100]. It is now recognized that insulin resistance syndrome is important in the pathophysiology of NAFLD and is present even in NAFLD patients who are normal weight and have normal carbohydrate tolerance [102,103]. Although the initial site and cause of insulin resistance is unknown, a large number of studies indicate that fatty liver is the hepatic component of the insulin resistance syndrome [17,24,29,102–105].

In a recent large cross-sectional study of severely obese subjects [106], the risk of hepatic steatosis increased exponentially with each addition of the components of the insulin resistance syndrome. In addition, the presence of the metabolic syndrome makes it more likely that a patient will have NASH rather than steatosis [29,107 and see Chapter 24]. These data are not surprising and are consistent with earlier demographic studies that found NAFLD in 25–90%, 21–55% and 3–92% in patients with obesity, diabetes and dyslipidaemias (three of the more important components of the metabolic syndrome), respectively [2,3,16,17,21,22,29,42,105–108].

Obesity and type 2 diabetes mellitus are being particularly recognized for their importance in NAFLD, both as clinical associations and as pathophysiological factors.

Obesity
Although NAFLD and its more severe form—NASH—may develop in non-obese patients, the majority of NAFLD occurs in obese or overweight individuals. Three studies have reported that less than 50% of their patients with NAFLD were obese [3,107,109]. In the other studies, the median prevalence rate of obesity in NAFLD patients was 71%, with the range of 57–93% [2,16,21,22,29,42,43,105,107,108]. Virtually all children with NAFLD are obese [7,8] (see Chapter 19).

The high prevalence rate of obesity in NAFLD may be explained by its association with hepatic steatosis [110]. A number of studies [43,83,90,111–118] have established obesity as a risk factor for hepatic steatosis and fibrotic liver disease. It has been proposed that lipid-laden hepatocytes then act as a reservoir for hepatotoxic agents that are more susceptible to a 'second hit' injury by components such as endotoxins and cytokines [119,120] in the production of reactive oxygen species (ROS) [121]. These ROS then cause lipid peroxidation and activation of cytokines, processes that stimulate fibrogenesis [121–124] and cause cell death [121].

This increased fat mass assumes greater significance with recent information that the adipocyte is now recognized to be an endocrine tissue capable of secreting a number of potential toxic substances [125,126] that may induce insulin resistance. Of these adipocyte residing substances, tumour necrosis factor (TNF) [127,128], resistin [129], leptin [130] and free fatty acids [130,131] correlate with insulin resistance and may be particularly relevant to the development of type 2 diabetes [131,132].

Adiponectin is a recently recognized peptide that is secreted from the adipocyte [133] and is decreased in obesity. This is important because adiponectin increases insulin sensitivity and has been demonstrated to decrease hepatic steatosis in animal models [134]. The potential importance of declining adiponectin levels in NASH pathogenesis is discussed in Chapter 24.

It should be emphasized that the distribution of fat may be more important than the total fat mass. Visceral fat, rather than total fat mass, has been shown to be a predictor of hepatic steatosis [135–138] as well as hyperinsulinaemia, decreased hepatic insulin extraction and peripheral insulin resistance [139]. Furthermore, lipolysis in visceral adipose tissue is more resistant to insulin [140], thereby providing a source of hepatoxic fatty acids in hyperinsulinaemic states. Decreasing visceral fat has also been shown to decrease hepatic insulin resistance [141,142]. Of note, lean NASH patients may have central adiposity [107]. This may explain the subgroup of non-obese patients [3] that have been suggested to represent the lean part of a spectrum of insulin resistance subjects (frequently of Asian origin) in which genes may play a part [143].

Diabetes

In addition to obesity, diabetes may be a particularly important risk factor. A number of studies have shown that hepatic fibrosis is more common in obese patients with diabetes [22,23,48,144]. A recent study has confirmed that in NAFLD patients, diabetes is an independent predictor for cirrhosis and liver-related deaths [145]. The reason for this is unclear but may be caused by additional oxidative stress [146,147].

Predictors for advanced fibrotic disease

In addition to histology (the presence or absence of NASH), a number of risk factors have been identified as predictors for the development of progressive fibrosis and cirrhosis: obesity [23,43,83], diabetes [22,23,43], age [43,83,148], arterial hypertension [48,105], AST : ALT ratio [43,149,150], triglycerides [83], elevated ALT [48,83], iron [44], extent of steatosis [83, 105] and the grade of hepatic inflammation [23,43,83].

Table 3.4 displays a combination of the strongest predictive factors along with their acronyms that have been used by different investigators to predict fibrosis in patients with fatty liver [43,48,83,149]. The presence of either obesity and/or type 2 diabetes are the most robust predictors of fibrosis [22,23,43,83,105, 149]. Age (over 45 or 50 years) is a strong predictive factor for cirrhosis [22,23,43,149], which probably reflects the duration of time that steatosis is at risk for a subsequent second hit. An elevated ALT level [48, 83], an AST : ALT ratio > 0.8 [43,149], arterial hypertension [48,105], triglycerides [84] and a high insulin resistance index [48] are also all strong predictors.

Data from the BARD or BARG acronyms, for example, would predict a patient with fatty liver on ultrasound who is less than 45 years old, has neither obesity nor diabetes and an AST : ALT ratio < 0.8, has

	BARD [43]	BARG [149]	BAAT [83]	HAIR [48]
BMI	×	×	×	
Age	×		×	
AST : ALT	×	×		
ALT			×	×
Diabetes	×			
HgbA1c		×		
Triglycerides			×	
Hypertension				×
Insulin resistance index				×

Table 3.4 Prediction acronyms for advanced fibrosis in NAFLD.

Numbers in brackets indicate reference numbers. Hgb, haemoglobin.
BARD: BMI ≥ 30; age ≥ 45 years; ratio of AST : ALT ≥ 1 and diabetes.
BARG: BMI ≥ 28; ratio of AST : ALT ≥ 0.8 and HgbA1c ≥ 5.2. This predicts NASH, not necessarily advanced fibrosis.
BAAT: BMI ≥ 28; age ≥ 50 years; ALT ≥ twice normal and triglycerides ≥ 1.7 mmol/L.
HAIR: hypertension; ALT > 40 and insulin resistance ≥ 5.0 defined by Quicki.

only a minimal risk for developing significant fibrosis. In contrast, almost two-thirds of patients with diabetes or obesity, age over 45 years and an AST : ALT ratio > 0.8 will have significant fibrosis.

This information can be used to determine the usefulness of performing a liver biopsy in patients with fatty liver by targeting a population with a high likelihood for having NASH (for implications in clinical management, see Chapter 15).

Implications for the future

Although the current prevalence rates of NAFLD and NASH are a major health care problem, additional concern arises from the fact that the prevalence can be expected to increase in concert with the rapidly growing prevalence of obesity and type 2 diabetes. In the USA, the prevalence of obesity in adults has increased from 15% to 25% in women and from 10% to 20% in men over the 30-year epoch between 1961 and 1991 [151], such that 22.5% of the population of the USA is now obese [152,153]. In children, however, the prevalence has more than doubled. Data from the US National Longitudinal Survey of Youth between 1986 and 1998 showed that the prevalence of overweight increased steadily and significantly [154]. Thus, by 1998, overweight prevalence increased to 22% among African Americans, 22% among Hispanics and 12% among non-Hispanic whites [154]. If the current rate continues, the prevalence of obesity could reach 40% by 2025 [155].

As would be expected, the prevalence of insulin resistance and type 2 diabetes has also increased [156] along with this increase in obesity. A dramatic increase in obesity during the past decade has been accompanied by a 25% increase in the prevalence of type 2 diabetes such that 7–10% of the US population now have type 2 diabetes. Data from NHANES III indicate that among those in whom type 2 diabetes has been diagnosed, 67% have a BMI of at least 27, and 46% have a BMI of at least 30. Both BMI and weight gain are major factors for diabetes, and BMI is one of the strongest predictors of diabetes. The previous studies showing changes in BMI at the population level foreshadow similar changes in diabetes [157–160]. Recent data have also shown that the prevalence of a self-report of diagnosed diabetes increased from 4.9% to 9.7% in 2000 [156]. Therefore, approximately 15 million US adults aged 18 years or older have

diagnosed diabetes (6.3 million men and 8.7 million women). If undiagnosed cases are considered, it is likely that almost 10% of the adult population have diabetes [161].

The importance of these societal changes is emphasized by a population study of patients with type 2 diabetes, in which the standardized mortality rates from liver disease exceeded those from cardiovascular disease [162]. There is also an emerging epidemic of type 2 diabetes among children, especially among minorities whose proportion in the USA is increasing [163]. There are already increasing reports of NASH in children [43,44,164] (see Chapter 19). Therefore, the full impact of NAFLD and NASH will not be felt until these children become adults and develop the long-term effects of diabetes and obesity.

Conclusions

The available data indicate that the prevalence rates for NAFLD and NASH have increased from previous estimates [1]. They are now estimated to be in the range 17–33% for NAFLD and 5.7–17% for NASH. Such high prevalence rates are a result of the worldwide epidemic of obesity [15,165–167], which has resulted from a combination of societal lifestyle changes [15,165–172] and genetic susceptibility [132, 173–175]. From an epidemiological prospective, the obesity epidemic has major economic and psychological implications [176]. The direct costs of obesity and its comorbidities represent 5.7% of the national health expenditure in the USA [177] and, perhaps more importantly, adversely affects quality of life [178]. This obesity and the consequently NAFLD epidemic is yet another disease of affluence [179] and shows no signs of abating. Although many therapeutic interventions are discussed subsequently in the book, the epidemiological data suggest a change in behaviour that would affect energy balance by as little as 420 kJ/day would prevent weight gain and arrest the epidemics of both obesity and NAFLD [180].

References

1 Falck-Ytter Y, Younossi ZM, Marchesini G, McCullough AJ. Clinical features and natural history of non-alcoholic steatosis syndromes. *Semin Liver Dis* 2001; **21**: 17–26.

2 Ludwig J, Viggiano TR, McGill DB, Ott BJ. Non-alcoholic steatohepatitis: Mayo Clinic experience with a hither to unnamed disease. *Mayo Clin Proc* 1980; **55**: 434–8.

3 Bacon BR, Farahvash MJ, Janney CG, Neuschwander-Tetri BA. Non-alcoholic steatohepatitis: an expanded clinical entity. *Gastroenterology* 1994; **107**: 1103–9.

4 Youssef WI, McCullough AJ. Steatohepatitis in obese individuals. *Best Pract Res Clin Gastroenterol* 2002; **16**: 733–47.

5 AGA technical review on non-alcoholic fatty liver disease. *Gastroenterology* 2002; **23**: 1705–25.

6 Harrison SA, Kadakia S, Lang KA, Schenker S. Non-alcoholic steatohepatitis: what we know in the new millennium. *Am J Gastroenterol* 2002; **97**: 2714–24.

7 Baldridge AD, Perez-Atayde AR, Graeme-Cook F, Higgins L, Lavine JE. Idiopathic steatohepatitis in childhood: a multicenter retrospective study. *J Pediatr* 1994; **127**: 700–4.

8 Rashid M, Roberts E. Non-alcoholic steatohepatitis in children. *J Pediatric Gastroenterol Nutr* 2000; **30**: 48–53.

9 Agarawal SR, Maihotra V, Sakhuja P, Sarin SK. Clinical biochemical and histological profile of non-alcoholic steatohepatitis. *Indian J Gastroenterol* 2001; **20**: 183–6.

10 Nomura H, Kashiwagi S, Hayashi J *et al*. Prevalence of fatty liver in a general population of Okinawa, Japan. *Jpn J Med* 1988; **27**: 142–9.

11 El-Hassan AY, Ibrahim EM, Al-Mulhim FA, Nabhan AA, Chammas MY. Fatty infiltration of the liver: analysis of prevalence, radiological and clinical feature and influence on patient management. *Br J Radiol* 1992; **65**: 774–8.

12 Zimmet B, Albert KG, Shaw J. Global and societal implications of the diabetes epidemic *Nature* 2001; **414**: 782–7.

13 Youssef W, McCullough AJ. Diabetes mellitus, obesity and hepatic steatosis. *Semin Gastrointest Dis* 2002; **13**: 7–30.

14 Clark JM, Diehl AM. Defining non-alcoholic fatty liver disease: implications or epidemiologic studies. *Gastroenterology* 2003; **124**: 248–50.

15 Seidell JC. Obesity, insulin resistance and diabetes: a world wide epidemic. *Br J Nutr* 2000; 83 (Suppl. 1): 55–8.

16 Powell EE, Cooksley WGE, Hanson R *et al*. The natural history of non-alcoholic steatohepatitis: a follow-up study of 42 patients for up to 21 years. *Hepatology* 1990; **11**: 74–80.

17 Chitturi S, Abeygunasekera S, Farrell GC *et al*. NASH and insulin resistance: insulin secretion and specific association with the insulin resistance syndrome. *Hepatology* 2002; **35**: 373–8.

18 Amarapurkar DN, Amarapurkar AD. Non-alcoholic steatohepatitis: clinicopathology profile. *J Assoc Physicians India* 2000; **48**: 311–3.

19 Ikai E, Ishizaki M, Suzuki Y *et al*. Association between hepatic steatosis, insulin resistance and hyperinsulinaemia as related to hypertension in alcohol consumers and obese people. *J Hum Hypertens* 1995; **9**: 101–5.

20 Samarasinghe D, Tasman-Jones C. The clinical associations with hepatic steatosis: a retrospective study. *N Z Med J* 1992; **105**: 57–8.

21 Lee RG. Non-alcoholic steatohepatitis: a study of 49 patients. *Hum Pathol* 1988; **20**: 594–8.

22 Matteoni CA, Younossi ZM, Gramlich T *et al*. Non-alcoholic fatty liver disease: a spectrum of clinical and pathological severity. *Gastroenterology* 1999; **116**: 1413–9.

23 Wanless IR, Lentz JS. Fatty liver hepatitis (steatohepatitis) and obesity: an autopsy study with analysis of risk factors. *Hepatology* 1990; **12**: 1106–10.

24 Chalasani N, Deeg MA, Persohn S, Crabb DN. Metabolic and anthropometric evaluation of insulin resistance in non-diabetic patients with non-alcoholic steatohepatitis. *Am J Gastroenterol* 2003; **98**: 1849–55.

25 Araujo LM, DeOliveira DA, Nunes DS. Liver and biliary ultrasonography in diabetic and non-diabetic obese women. *Diabetes Metab* 1998; **24**: 455–62.

26 Teli MR, James OFW, Burt AD, Bennett MK, Day CP. The natural history of non-alcoholic fatty liver: a follow-up study. *Hepatology* 1995; **22**: 1714–9.

27 Hultcrantz R, Glaumann H, Lindberg, Nilsson LH. Liver investigation in 149 asymptomatic patients with moderately elevated activities of serum transaminases. *Scand J Gastroenterol* 1986; **21**: 109–13.

28 Bellentani S, Saccoccio G, Masatti F *et al*. Prevalence of and risk factors for hepatic steatosis in Northern Italy. *Ann Intern Med* 2000; **132**: 112–7.

29 Cortez-Pinto H, Camilu ME, Baptista A, DeOliveira AG, DeMoura MC. Non-alcoholic fatty liver: another feature of the metabolic syndrome? *Clin Nutr* 199; **18**: 353–8.

30 Hasan I, Gani RA, Machmud R, Prevalence and risk factors for non-alcoholic fatty liver in Indonesia. *J Gastroenterol Hepatol* 2002; **17** (Suppl. A): 30.

31 Hui JM, Kench JG, Chitturi S *et al*. Long-term outcomes of cirrhosis in non-alcoholic steatohepatitis compared with hepatitis C. *Hepatology* 2003; **38**: 420–7.

32 Ratziu V, Bonyhay L, DiMartino V *et al*. Survival, liver failure, and hepatocellular carcinoma in obesity related cryptogenic cirrhosis. *Hepatology* 2002; **35**: 1485–93.

33 Caldwell SH, Oelsner DH, Iezzoni JC *et al*. Cryptogenic cirrhosis: clinical characterization and risk factors for underlying disease. *Hepatology* 1999; **32**: 689–92.

34 Caldwell SH, Hespenheide EE. Subacute liver failure in obese women. *Am J Gastroenterol* 2002; **97**: 2058–67.

35 Bugianesi E, Leone A, Vanni E *et al.* Expanding the natural history of non-alcoholic steatohepatitis: from cryptogenic cirrhosis to hepatocellular carcinoma. *Gastroenterology* 2002; **123**: 134–40.

36 Shimada M, Hashimoto E, Taniai M *et al.* Hepatocellular carcinoma in patients with non-alcoholic steatohepatitis. *J Hepatol* 2002; **37**: 154–60.

37 Cotrim HP, Parana R, Brago E, Lyra L. Non-alcoholic steatohepatitis and hepatocellular carcinoma: natural history? *Am J Gastroenterol* 2000; **95**: 3018–9.

38 Zen Y, Katayanagi K, Tsuneyama K *et al.* Hepatocellular carcinoma arising in non-alcoholic steatohepatitis. *Pathol Int* 2001; **51**: 127–31.

39 Nair S, Mason A, Eason J, Loss G, Perillo RP. Is obesity an independent risk factor for hepatocellular carcinoma in cirrhosis? *Hepatology* 2002; **76**: 150–5.

40 Ong J, Younossi ZM, Reddy V *et al.* Cryptogenic cirrhosis and post-transplantation non-alcoholic fatty liver disease. *Liver Transpl* 2001; **7**: 707–801.

41 Contos MJ, Cales W, Sterling RK *et al.* Development of non-alcoholic fatty liver disease after liver transplantation for cryptogenic cirrhosis. *Liver Transpl* 2001; **7**: 363–73.

42 Diehl AM, Goodman Z, Ishak KG. Alcohol-like liver disease in non-alcoholics: a clinical and histologic comparison with alcohol-induced liver injury. *Gastroenterology* 1998; **44**: 311–8.

43 Angulo P, Keach JC, Batts KP, Lindor KD. Independent predictors of liver fibrosis in patients with non-alcoholic steatohepatitis. *Hepatology* 1999; **30**: 1356–62.

44 George DK, Goldwurm S, MacDonald GA *et al.* Increased hepatic iron concentration in non-alcoholic steatohepatitis is associated with increased fibrosis. *Gastroenterology* 1998; **114**: 311–8.

45 Bonkovsky HL, Jawhid Q, Tortorelli K *et al.* Non-alcoholic steatohepatitis and iron: increased prevalence of mutations of the HFE gene in non-alcoholic steatohepatitis. *J Hepatol* 1999; **31**: 421–9.

46 Nair S, Cope K, Terrence RH. Obesity and female gender increase breath ethanol concentration and potential implications for the pathogenesis of non-alcoholic steatohepatitis. *Am J Gastroenterol* 2001; **96**: 1200–4.

47 Hu FB, Manson JE, Stampfer MJ. Diet, lifestyle and the risk of type 2 diabetes in women. *N Engl J Med* 2001; **345**: 790–7.

48 Dixon JR, Bathol PS, O'Brien PE. Non-alcoholic fatty liver disease: predictors of non-alcoholic steatohepatitis and liver fibrosis in the severely obese. *Gastroenterology* 2001; **12**: 91–100.

49 Dasarthy S, McCullough AJ. Alcohol induced liver injury. In: Schiff ER, Sorrell MF, Maddrey WC, eds. *Schiff's Diseases of the Liver*, 9th edn, Philadelphia: Lippincott Raven, 2002: 1019–57.

50 Bianchi L. Liver biopsy in elevated liver function tests? An old question revisited. *J Hepatol* 2001; **35**: 290–4.

51 Saadeh S, Younossi ZM, Remer EM *et al.* The utility of radiological imaging in non-alcoholic fatty liver disease. *Gastroenterology* 2002; **123**: 745–50.

52 Szezepaniak LS, Babcock EE, Schick F *et al.* Measurement of intracellular triglyceride stores by 'H spectroscopy: validation *in vivo*. *Am J Physiol* 1999; **276**: E977–89.

53 Ricci C, Lungo R, Gioulis E *et al.* Non-invasive *in vivo* quantitative assessment of fat content in human liver. *J Hepatol* 1997; **27**: 108–13.

54 Fishbein MH, Gardner KG, Potter CJ, Schmalbrock P, Smith MA. Introduction of fast MR imaging in the assessment of hepatic steatosis. *Magn Reson Imaging* 1997; **15**: 287–93.

55 Levenson H, Greensite F, Hoefs J *et al.* Fatty infiltration of the liver: quantification with phase-contrast MR imaging at 1.5 T vs biopsy. *Am J Roentgenol* 1991; **156**: 307–12.

56 Mendler MH, Bouillet P, LeSidaner A *et al.* Dual energy CT in the diagnosis and quantification of fatty liver-limited clinical value in comparison to ultrasound and single-energy CT, with special reference to iron overload. *J Hepatol* 1998; **28**: 785–94.

57 Siegelman ES, Rosen MA. Imaging of hepatic steatosis. *Semin Liver Dis* 2001; **21**: 71–80.

58 Longo R, Pollesello P, Ricci C, Masutti F, Kvam BJ. Proton MR spectroscopy in quantitative *in vivo* determination of fat content in human liver steatosis. *J Magn Reson Imaging* 1995; **4**: 281–5.

59 Jacobs JE, Birnbaum BA, Shapira MA *et al.* Diagnostic criteria for fatty infiltration of the liver on contrast enhanced helical CT. *Am J Roentgenol* 1998;171-659-664.

60 Hulcrantz R, Gabrielson N. Patients with persistent elevation of aminotransferases: investigation with ultrasonography, radionuclide imaging and liver biopsy. *J Intern Med* 1993; **233**: 7–12.

61 Mitchell DG. Focal manifestations of diffuse liver disease at MR Imaging. *Radiology* 1992; **185**: 1–11.

62 Joseph A, Saverymuttu S, Al-Sam S *et al.* Comparison of liver histology with ultrasonography in assessing diffuse parenchymal liver disease. *Clin Radiol* 1991; **43**: 26–31.

63 Graif M, Yanuka M, Baraz M. Quantitative estimation of attenuation in ultrasound video images: correlation with histology in diffuse liver disease. *Invest Radiol* 2000; **35**: 319–24.

64 Mathieson NL, Franzen LE, Fryden A, Fuberg U, Bodenar G. The clinical significances of slightly to moderately increased liver transaminase values in asymptomatic patients *Scand J Gastroenterol* 1999; **34**: 55–91.

65 AGA Technical review on the evaluation of liver chemistry tests. *Gastroenterology* 2002; **123**: 1367–84.

66 Skelly MM, James PD, Ryder SD. Findings on liver biopsy to investigate abnormal liver function tests in the absence of diagnostic serology. *J Hepatol* 2001; **35**: 195–9.

67 Daniel S, Ben-Menachem T, Vasudevan G, Ma CK, Blumenkehl M. Prospective evaluation of unexplained chronic liver transaminases abnormalities in asymptomatic patients. *Am J Gastroenterol* 1999; **94**: 3010–4.

68 Prati D, Taioli E, Zanella A *et al.* Updated definitions of health ranges for serum amino transferase levels. *Ann Intern Med* 2002; **137**: 1–9

69 Clark JM, Brancati FL, Diehl AM. Non-alcoholic fatty liver disease. *Gastroenterology* 2002; **122**: 1649–57.

70 Ruhl CE, Everhart JE, Determinants of the association of overweight with elevated serum alanine aminotransferase activity in the United States. *Gastroenterology* 2003; **124**: 71–9.

71 Clark JM, Brancat FL, Diehl AM. The prevalence and etiology of elevated aminotransferase levels in the United States. *Am J Gastroenterol* 2003; **98**: 960–7.

72 Patt CH, Yoo HY, Dibadji K, Flynn J, Thuluvath PJ. Prevalence of transaminases abnormalities in asymptomatic health subjects. *Dig Dis Sci* 2003; **48**: 797–801.

73 Yu AS, Keefe EB. Elevated AST or ALT to non-alcoholic fatty liver disease: accurate predictor of disease prevalence? *Am J Gastroenterol* 2003; **98**: 955–6.

74 Yu AS, Keefe EB. Non-alcoholic fatty liver disease. *Rev Gastroenterol Disord* 2002; **2**: 11–9.

75 Berasain C, Betes M, Panizo A *et al.* Pathological and virological findings in patients with persistent hypertransaminemia of unknown etiology. *Gut* 2000; **47**: 429–35.

76 Pratt DS, Kaplan MM. Evaluation of abnormal liver enzyme results in asymptomatic patients. *N Engl J Med* 2000; **342**: 1266–71.

77 Alba LM, Lindor K. Non-alcoholic fatty liver disease. *Aliment Pharmacol Ther* 2003; **17**: 977–86.

78 Mofrad P, Contos M, Haque M *et al.* Clinical and histologic spectrum of non-alcoholic fatty liver disease with normal ALT values. *Hepatology* 2003; **37**: 1286–92.

79 Noaguchi H, Tazawa Y, Nishinomiya F, Takada G. The relationship between serum transaminases activities and fatty liver in children with simple obesity. *Acta Paediatr Jpn* 1995; **37**: 621–5.

80 Neuschwander-Tetri BA, Caldwell SH. Non-alcoholic steatohepatitis: summary of an AASLD single topic conference. *Hepatology* 2003; **37**: 1202–19.

81 Propst A, Propst T, Judmaier G, Vogel W. Prognosis in non-alcoholic steatohepatitis [Letter]. *Gastroenterol* 1995; **108**: 1607.

82 Nonomura A, Mizukami Y, Unoura M. Clinico-pathologic study of alcoholic-like liver disease in non-alcoholics; non-alcoholic steatohepatitis and fibrosis. *Gastroenterol Jpn* 1992; **27**: 521–8.

83 Ratziu V, Giral P, Charlotte F *et al.* Liver fibrosis in overweight patients. *Gastroenterology* 2000; **118**: 1117–23.

84 Hilden M, Christoffersen P, Juhl E *et al.* Liver histology in a 'normal' population: examinations of 503 consecutive fatal traffic casualties. *Scand J Gastroenterol* 1977; **12**; 593–9.

85 Ground KE. Liver pathology in review. *Aviat Space Environ Med* 1982; **53**: 14–8.

86 Marcos A, Fisher RA, Jam JM *et al.* Selection and outcome of living donors for adult right lobe. *Transplantation* 2000; **69**: 2410–5.

87 Marceau P, Biron S, Hould FS *et al.* Liver pathology and the metabolic syndrome X in severe obesity. *J Clin Endocrinol Metab* 1999; **84**: 1513–7.

88 DelGaudio A, Boschi L, DelGaudio GA, Mastrangel L, Munars D. Liver damage in obese patients. *Obes Surg* 2001; **11**: 254–7.

89 Lucyckx FA, Desaive C, Tiry A *et al.* Liver abnormalities in severely obese subjects: effect of drastic weight loss after gastroplasty. *Int J Obes* 1998; **22**: 222–6.

90 Klain J, Fraser D, Goldstein J *et al.* Liver histology in the morbidly obese. *Hepatology* 1989; **10**: 873–6.

91 Silverman EM, Sapala JA, Appelman HD. Regression of hepatic steatosis in morbidly obese persons after gastric bypass. *Am J Clin Path* 1995; **104**: 23–31.

92 Franzese A, Vasjro P, Argenziano A *et al.* Liver involvement in obese children: ultrasound and liver enzyme levels at diagnosis and during follow-up in an Italian population. *Dig Dis Sci* 1997; **42**: 1428–32.

93 Tuminaga K, Kurata JH, Chen YK *et al.* Prevalence of fatty liver in Japanese children and relationship to obesity: an epidemiological ultrasonography survey. *Dig Dis Sci* 1995; **40**: 2002–9.

94 Lonardo A, Bellini M, Tartoni P *et al.* The bright liver syndrome: prevalence and determinants of a 'bright' liver echo pattern. *Ital J Gastroenterol Hepatol* 1997; **29**: 351–6.

95 Bellentani S, Tiribelli C, Saccoccio G *et al.* Prevalence of chronic liver disease in the general population of northern Italy: the Dionysos study. *Hepatology* 1994; **20**: 1442–9.

96 Bellentani S, Tiribelli C. The spectrum of liver disease in the general population: lesson from the Dionysos study. *J Hepatol* 2001; **35**: 531–7.

97 Navarro VJ, St. Louis T, Bell BZ, Sofair AN. Chronic liver disease in the primary care practices of Waterbury, Connecticut [Letter]. *Hepatology* 2003; **38**: 1062.

98 Byron D, Minuk G. Clinical hepatology: profile of an urban, hospital-based practice. *Hepatology* 1996; **24**: 813–5.

99 Yokoyama H, Morriya S, Homma Y, Ogawa T. Association between α-glutamyltranspeptidase activity and status of disorder constituting insulin resistance syndrome. *Alcohol Clin Exp Res* 2003; **27** (Suppl.): 225–55.

100 National Institutes of Health. *The Third Report of the National Cholesterol Education Program Expert Panel on Detection Evaluation, and Treatment of High Blood Cholesterol in adults (Adult Treatment Panel III).* Bethesda, MD: National Institutes of Health, 2001: NIH Publication 01-2610.

101 Ford ES, Giles WH, Dietz WH. Prevalence of the metabolic syndrome among US adults. *J Am Med Assoc* 2002; **287**: 356–9.

102 Marchesini G, Brizi M, Morselli-Labate AM *et al.* Association of non-alcoholic fatty liver disease with insulin resistance. *Am J Med* 1999; **107**: 450–6.

103 Marchesini G, Brizi M, Bianchi G *et al.* Non-alcoholic fatty liver disease: a feature of the metabolic syndrome. *Diabetes* 2001; **40**: 1844–50.

104 Sanyal AJ, Campbell-Sargent C, Mirshahi F *et al.* Non-alcoholic steatohepatitis: association of insulin resistance and mitochondrial abnormalities. *Gastroenterology* 2001; **120**: 1183–92.

105 Willner IR, Waters B, Patil SR *et al.* Ninety patients with non-alcoholic steatohepatitis: insulin resistance, familial tendency, and severity of disease. *Am J Gastroenterol* 2001; **96**: 2957–61.

106 Knobler H, Schattner A, Zhornick T *et al.* Fatty liver: an additional and treatable feature of the insulin re-existence syndrome. *Q J Med* 1999; **92**: 73–9.

107 Marchesini G, Bugianessi E, Forlani G *et al.* Non-alcoholic fatty liver, steatohepatitis and the metabolic syndrome. *Hepatology* 2003; **37**: 917–23.

108 Laurin J, Lindor KD, Crippin J *et al.* Ursodeoxycholic acid or clobifrate in the treatment of non-alcohol induced steotohepatitis: a pilot study. *Hepatology* 1996; **23**: 1464–7.

109 Cortez-Pinto H, Baptista A, Camilo E *et al.* Non-alcoholic steatohepatitis in ambulatory and hospitalized patients. *Dig Dis Sci* 1996; **41**: 172–9.

110 McCullough AJ, Falck-Ytter Y. Body composition and hepatic steatosis as precursors for fibrotic liver disease. *Hepatology* 1999; **29**: 1328–39.

111 Anderson T, Gluud C. Liver morphology in morbid obesity: a literature study. *Int J Obes* 1984; **8**: 97–106.

112 Kern WH, Heger AH, Payne JH DeWind LT. Fatty metamorphosis of the liver in morbid obesity. *Arch Pathol* 1973; **96**: 342–6.

113 Nasrallah SM, Wills CE, Gallambos JT. Hepatic morphology in obesity. *Dig Dis Sci* 1981; **26**: 325–7.

114 Ioannou GN, Weiss NS, Kowdley KV, Dominitz J. Is obesity a risk factor for cirrhosis related death or hospitalization? A population-based cohort study. *Gastroenterology* 2003; **125**: 1053–9.

115 Braillon A, Capron JP, Herve MA, Degott C, Quenum C. Liver in obesity. *Gut* 1985; **26**: 133–9.

116 Nomura F, Ohnishi K, Satomura T. Liver function on moderate obesity: a study in 534 moderately obese subjects among 4613 male company employees. *Int J Obes* 1986; **10**: 349–54.

117 Angulo P. Non-alcoholic fatty liver disease. *N Eng J Med* 2002; **346**: 1221–31.

118 Das UN. Is obesity an inflammatory condition. *Nutrition* 2001; **17**: 953–966.

119 Day CP, James OF. Hepatic steatosis: innocent bystander or guilty party? *Hepatology* 1998; **27**: 1463–6.

120 Day CP, James OFW. Steatohepatitis: a tale of two 'hits'? *Gastroenterology* 1998; **114**: 842–5.

121 Pessayre D, Berson A, Fromenty B, Mansouri A. Mitochondria in steatohepatitis. *Semin Liver Dis* 2001; **21**: 57–69.

122 Parola M, Pinzani M, Casini A *et al.* Stimulation of lipid peroxidation or 4-hydroxynonenal treatment increases procollagen α1 (1) gene expression in human liver fat-storing cells. *Biochem Biophys Res Commun* 1993; **194**: 1044–50.

123 Lee KS, Buck M, Houghlum K, Chojkier M. Activation of hepatic stellate cells by TGF-β and collagen type 1 is mediated by oxidative stress through c-myo expression. *J Clin Invest* 1995; **96**: 2461–8.

124 Bedossa P, Houghlum K, Trautwein C, Holstege A, Chojkier M. Stimulation of collagen α1 (1) gene expression is associated with lipid peroxidation in hepatocellular injury: a link to tissue fibrosis. *Hepatology* 1994; **19**: 1262–71.

125 Shuldiner AR, Yang R, Gong DW. Resistin, obesity and insulin resistance: the emerging role of the adipocyte as an endocrine organ. *N Engl J Med* 2001; **345**: 1345–6.

126 Ahima RS, Filer JS. Adipose tissue as an endocrine organ. *Trends Endocrinol Metab* 2000; **11**: 327–32.

127 Katsuki A, Sumida T, Murashima S *et al.* Serum levels of tumor necrosis factor α are increased in obese patients with non-insulin-dependent diabetes mellitus. *J Clin Endocrinol Metab* 1998; **83**: 859–62.

128 Hotamisligil GS, Peraldi P, Budavaria D *et al.* IRS-1 mediated inhibition of insulin receptor kinase activity in INF-α and obesity-induced insulin resistance. *Science* 1996; **271**: 665–8.

129 Steppan CM, Bailey St, Bhat S. The hormone resistin links obesity to diabetes. *Nature* 2001; **409**: 307–12.

130 Lomquist F, Arner P, Nordfors L *et al*. Overexpression of the obese (OB) gene in adipose tissue of human obese subjects. *Nat Med* 1995; **1**: 950–3.

131 Bergman RN, Ader M. Free fatty acids and pathogenesis of type 2 diabetes mellitus. *Trends Endocrinol Metab* 2000; **11**: 351–6.

132 Nadler ST, Attie AD. Please pass the chips: genomic insights into obesity and diabetes. *J Nutr* 2001; **131**: 2078–81.

133 Berg AH, Combs TP, Scherer PE. ACRP30/adiponectin: an adipokine regulating glucose and lipid metabolism. *Trends Endocrinol Metab* 2002; **13**: 84–9.

134 Xu A, Wang Y, Keshaw H *et al*. The fat deprived hormone adiponectin alleviates alcoholic and non-alcoholic fatty liver diseases in mice. *J Clin Invest* 2003; **112**: 91–100.

135 Kral JG, Schaffner F, Pierson RN, Wang J. Body fat topography as an independent prediction of fatty liver. *Metabolism* 1993; **42**: 548–51.

136 Banerji MA, Buckley MC, Chalken RL *et al*. Liver fat, serum triglycerides and visceral adipose tissue in insulin-sensitive and insulin-resistant black men with NIDDM. *Int J Obes Relat Metab Disord* 1995; **19**: 846–50.

137 Tominga K, Kurara JH, Chen YK *et al*. Prevalence of fatty liver in Japanese children and relationship to obesity: an epidemiological ultrasonography survey. *Dig Dis Sci* 1995; **40**: 2002–9.

138 Omagari K, Kadokawa Y, Masuda J *et al*. Fatty liver in non-alcoholic non-overweight Japanese adults: incidence and clinical characteristics. *J Gastroenterol Hepatol* 2002; **17**: 1098–105.

139 Peiris AN, Mueller RA, Smith GA, Struve MF, Kissebah AH. Splanchnic insulin metabolism in obesity: influence of body for distribution. *J Clin Invest* 1986; **78**: 1648–57.

140 Meek SE, Nair KS, Jensen MD. Insulin regulation of regional free fatty acid metabolism. *Diabetes* 1999; **48**: 10–4.

141 Barzilai N, Banerjee S, Hawkins M, Chen W, Rossetti L. Calorie restriction reverses hepatic insulin resistance in aging by decreasing visceral fat. *J Clin Invest* 1986; **78**: 1648–57.

142 Barzilai N, She L, Liu BQ *et al*. Surgical removal of visceral fat reverses hepatic insulin resistance. *Diabetes* 1999; **48**: 94–8.

143 Marchesini G, Orlani G. NASH: from liver disease to metabolic disorders and back to clinical hepatology. *Hepatology* 2002; **35**: 497–99.

144 Falchuk KR, Fiske SC, Haggitt RC. Pericentral hepatic fibrosis and intracellular hyalin in diabetes mellitus. *Gastroenterology* 1980; **78**: 535–41.

145 Younossi ZM, Gramlich T, Matteoni CA, Boparai N, McCullough AJ. Non-alcoholic fatty liver disease in patients with type II diabetes. *Clin Gastroenterol Hepatol* 2004; **2**: 262–5.

146 Evan JL, Goldfine ID, Maddux BA, Grudsky GM. Oxidative stress and stress activated signaling pathways: a unifying hypothesis of type 2 diabetes. *Endocr Rev* 2002; **23**: 599–622.

147 Davis G, Ciabottni G, Congoli A *et al*. *In vivo* formation of 8-ISO-prostaglandin F22 and platelet activation in diabetes mellitus. *Circulation* 1999; **99**: 224–9.

148 Garcia-Monzon C, Martin-Perez E, Iacono OL. Characterization of pathogenic and prognostic factors of non-alcoholic steatohepatitis associated with obesity. *J Hepatol* 2000; **33**: 716–24.

149 Harrison SA, Oliver DA, Torgerson S, Paul H, Neuschwander BA. NASH: clinical assessment of 501 patients from two separate academic medical centers with validation of a clinical scoring system for advanced hepatic fibrosis. *Hepatology* 2003; **34** (Suppl.): 511A.

150 Sorbi D, Boynton J, Lindor KD. The ratio of aspartate amino transferase to alanine amino transferase: potential value in differentiating nonalcoholic steatohepatitis from alcoholic liver disease. *Am J Gastroenterol* 1999; **94**: 1018–22.

151 Fiegal KM. Trends in body weight and overweight in the US population. *Nutr Rev* 1996; **54**: S97–S100.

152 Kuczmarski RJ, Carroll MD, Fiegal KM, Troiano RP. Varying body mass index cut-off points to describe overweight prevalence among US adults: NHANES III (1988–94). *Obes Res* 1997; **5**: 542–58.

153 Centers for Disease Control and Prevention. Update: prevalense of overweight among children, adolescents, and adults. *Arch Pediatr Adolesc Med* 1995; **149**: 1085–91.

154 Strauss RS, Pollock HA. Epidemic increase in childhood overweight, 1986–98. *J Am Med Assoc* 2001; **286**: 2845–8.

155 Kopelman PG. Obesity as a medical problem. *Nature* 2000; **404**: 635–43.

156 Harris MI, Fiegal KM, Vowle CC *et al*. Prevalence of diabetes, impaired fasting glucose, and impaired glucose tolerance in US adults: the Third National Health and Nutrition Examination Survey, 1998–94. *Diabetes Care* 1998; **21**: 518–24.

157 Holbrook TL, Barrett-Conor E, Wingard DL. The association of lifetime weight and weight control patterns with diabetes among and women in an adult community. *Int J Obes* 1989; **13**: 723–9.

158 Chan JM, Stampfer MJ, Rimm EB *et al*. Obesity, fat distribution, and weight gain as risk factors for clinical diabetes in men. *Diabetes Care* 1994; **17**: 961–9.

159 Colditz GA, Willett WC, Rotnitzky A, Mansour JE. Weight gain as a risk factor for clinical diabetes in women. *Ann Intern Med* 1995; **122**: 481–6.

160 Hanson RL, Narayan KM, McCance DR *et al*. Rate of weight gain, weight fluctuation, and incidence of NIDDM. *Diabetes* 1995; **43**: 261–2.

161 Mokdad A, Ford E, Bowman B *et al*. Diabetes trends in the United States, 1990–98. *Diabetes Care* 2000; **23**: 1278–83.

162 deMarco R, Locatelli F, Zoppini G *et al*. Cause-specific mortality in type 2 diabetes: the Verona Diabetes Study. *Diabetes Care* 1999; **22**: 756–61.

163 Rosenbloom AL, Young RS, Joe JR, Winter NE. Emerging epidemic of type 2 diabetes in youth. *Diabetes Care* 1999; **22**: 345–54.

164 Kocak N, Yuce A, Gurakan K. Obesity: a cause of steatohepatitis in children. *Am J Gastroenterol* 2000; **95**: 1099–100.

165 Yanovski S, Yanovski JA. Obesity. *N Engl J Med* 2002; **346**: 591–602.

166 Uauy R, Albala C, Kain J. Obesity trends in Latin America: transiting from under- to overweight. *J Nutr* 2002; **131**: 8935–95.

167 King H, Aubert RE, Herman WH. Global burden of diabetes 1995–2025: prevalence, numerical estimates, and projections. *Diabetes Care* 1998; **21**: 1414–31.

168 Hinsworth HP. Diet and the innocence of diabetes mellitus. *Clin Sci* 1935; **2**: 117–48.

169 Kimm SYS, Glynn NW, Kriska AM *et al*. Decline in physical activity in black girls and white girls during adolescence. *N Engl J Med* 2002; **347**: 709–15.

170 Kruger HS, Venter CS, Vorster HH, Margetts BM. Physical inactivity is the major determinant of obesity in black women in the northwest province, South Africa: the Thusa Study. *Nutrition* 2002; **18**: 422–7.

171 Van Dam RM, Rimm E, Willett WC *et al*. Dietary patterns and risks for type 2 diabetes mellitus in US men. *Ann Intern Med* 2002; **136**: 201–9.

172 Kawate R, Yanakido M, Nishimoto Y. Diabetes mellitus and its vascular complications in Japanese migrants on the island of Hawaii. *Diabetes Care* 1979; **2**: 161–70.

173 Pratley RE. Gene–environment interactions in the pathogenesis of type 2 diabetes mellitus, lessons learned from the Pima Indians. *Proc Nutr Soc* 1998; **57**: 175–81.

174 Ashrafi K, Chang FY, Watts JL *et al*. Genome-wide RNAi analysis of *Caenorhabditis elegans* fat regulatory genes. *Nature* 2003; **421**: 709–15.

175 Groop L. Genetics of the metabolic syndrome. *Br J Nutr* 2000; 83 (Suppl. 1): 539–48.

176 Kottke TE, Wu LA, Hoffman RS. Economic and psychological implications of the obesity epidemic. *Mayo Clin Proc* 2003; **78**: 92–4.

177 Wolf AM, Colditz GA. Current estimates of the economic cost of obesity in the United States. *Obes Res* 1998; **6**: 97.

178 Kushner RF, Foster GD. Obesity and quality of Life. *Nutrition* 2000; **16**: 947–52.

179 James OF, Day CP. Non-alcoholic steatohepatitis: another disease of affluence. *Lancet* 1995; **353**: 1634–6.

180 Hill JO, Wyatt HR, Reed GW, Peters JC. Obesity and the environment: where do we go from here? *Science* 2003; **299**: 853–5.

4 Insulin resistance in NAFLD: potential mechanisms and therapies

Varman T. Samuel & Gerald I. Shulman

Key learning points

1 Non-alcoholic fatty liver disease (NAFLD) is found in approximately two-thirds of obese individuals and half of patients with type 2 diabetes, but the exact nature of relationships between the metabolic disorders and NAFLD continues to be debated.

2 Peripheral insulin resistance refers to diminished insulin-mediated uptake while hepatic insulin resistance refers to the inability of insulin to suppress hepatic glucose production.

3 Glucose tracer experiments enable investigators to quantify glucose flux *in vivo*, specifically the rates of endogenous (primarily hepatic) glucose production and whole body glucose disposal.

4 The hyperinsulinaemic–euglycaemic clamp method remains the gold standard for measuring insulin responsiveness *in vivo*. For studies of hepatic insulin sensitivity, a low dose of insulin (10–20 $\mu m/m^2$) is typically used.

5 The rate of hepatic glucose production is the sum of net hepatic gylcogenolysis and the rate of gluconeogenesis; quantifying these two components is complex.

6 The current model of peripheral insulin resistance links intramyocellular fat accumulation to prevention of insulin-mediated activation of phosphatidylinositol-3 (PI3) kinase through impaired insulin receptor substrate-1 (IRS-1) tyrosine phosphorylation, thereby limiting the movement of the glucose transporter GLUT4 from its intracellular compartment to the plasma membrane.

7 Hepatic fat accumulation can lead specifically to hepatic insulin resistance through a block in the insulin signalling cascade at the level of IRS-2-associated PI3 kinase activity.

8 High-fat feeding appears to result in marked hepatic fat accumulation and hepatic insulin resistance prior to any alteration in peripheral insulin action.

Abstract

With the continued high prevalence of obesity and type 2 diabetes mellitus in the USA and elsewhere, clinicians and investigators have developed an appreciation for the link between non-alcoholic fatty liver disease (NAFLD) and hepatic insulin resistance. A number of techniques are now available for studying the mechanism of fat-induced hepatic insulin resistance in humans. The hyperinsulinaemic–euglycaemic clamp technique enables the quantification of hepatic glucose production and hepatic insulin responsiveness. ^{13}C magnetic resonance spectroscopy and the ^2H_2O method provide complementary techniques for determining the rates of glycogenolysis and gluconeogenesis, respectively. Accumulation of fat within the liver is clearly associated with decreased hepatic responsiveness to insulin and possibly with increased hepatic gluconeogenesis. The mechanism behind fat-induced hepatic insulin resistance is likely to be analogous to the mechanism of fat-induced skeletal muscle insulin resistance. Thus, accumulation of a fatty acid metabolite may activate a cascade of kinases involving protein kinase C (PKC), C-Jun N-terminal kinase (JNK)-1 and/or inhibitor of κB kinase β (IKK-β), thereby blocking the insulin signalling pathway via increased serine phosphorylation of insulin receptor substrates (IRS-1 in muscle, IRS-2 in liver). In turn, this limits the ability of insulin to increase peripheral glucose uptake, decrease hepatic glucose output and increase hepatic glycogen synthesis. Possible therapeutic agents for fat-induced hepatic insulin resistance include metformin, which acts by decreasing gluconeogenesis, and the thiazolidinediones, which shift fat away from the liver (hepatocytes) and into fat stores (adipocytes).

Introduction

The prevalence of obesity and type 2 diabetes mellitus continues to increase worldwide. As of 2001, approximately 1 in 5 US adults was categorized as obese, and 1 in 12 carried a diagnosis of type 2 diabetes mellitus (T2DM). This translates into over 40 million obese adults and 16 million patients with T2DM [1]. Similar trends are being observed in many countries around the world (see Chapters 3 and 18). NAFLD is found in approximately two-thirds of the obese patients and 50% of patients with diabetes mellitus (see Chapter 3). However, while obesity, diabetes and NAFLD are certainly linked, the nature of their relationship remains debated.

Insulin resistance, a cardinal feature of the metabolic syndrome and T2DM, can be classified as peripheral insulin resistance and/or hepatic insulin resistance. Peripheral insulin resistance primarily refers to diminished insulin-mediated uptake of glucose in skeletal muscle and adipocytes, while hepatic insulin resistance refers to the inability of insulin to decrease hepatic glucose production. There is a growing consensus that accumulation of fat within skeletal muscle is the key pathogenic event leading to peripheral insulin resistance. Briefly, accumulation of fatty acid metabolites within the muscle initiates a series of signalling reactions that increases the phosphorylation of specific serine residues (e.g. S307) on IRS-1, the major insulin receptor substrate in muscle. This block in the insulin signalling cascade limits the ability of insulin to stimulate glucose uptake by muscle. In contrast to this well-defined model for fat-induced peripheral insulin resistance, a paradigm for fat-induced hepatic insulin resistance is still emerging. A number of investigators have begun to focus on the mechanism of hepatic insulin resistance. This chapter reviews the methodology for studying hepatic glucose metabolism, the putative mechanisms for insulin resistance in NAFLD, and the impact of therapeutic agents on hepatic insulin resistance and hepatic fat content.

Methodologies for studying glucose metabolism *in vivo*

Principles of the glucose tracer experiment

Glucose tracer experiments enable investigators to quantify glucose flux *in vivo*, specifically the rates of endogenous (primarily hepatic) glucose production and whole body glucose disposal. This section provides the reader with an overview of the theories and practice of tracer experiments. For a more thorough and detailed description, the reader is referred to the excellent text by R. Wolfe, *Radioactive and Stable Isotope Tracers in Biomedicine* [2].

Most studies of glucose kinetics utilize Steele's steady state equations to determine glucose flux. Briefly, the measurements depend on attaining a steady state of tracer within the total body pool of the glucose that is being measured. At this point, the proportion of the labelled glucose to the unlabelled glucose is constant. Knowing the rate at which the glucose is being introduced into the system, and the relative concentration of the labelled glucose within the system, one can calculate the turnover of glucose within the pool.

Figure 4.1 shows a sample model for this process. In state A, a single pool of glucose is represented. There is production, or appearance, of this glucose by the body and use, or disappearance, of the metabolite by the body. The rates of appearance and disappearance are R_a and R_d, respectively. As steady state production and use are balanced, so $R_a = R_d$. A typical experiment will begin with the introduction of labelled glucose into the system (represented by I in Fig. 4.1). Initially, the proportion of labelled glucose to unlabelled glucose will be low (state B). However, with continuous infusion of

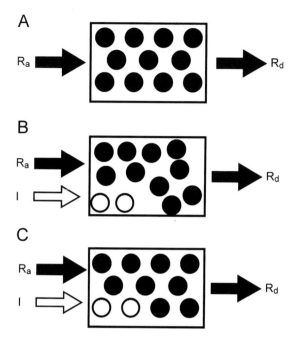

Fig. 4.1 Schematic representation of single metabolite pool. In state A, the pool exists in steady state. The introduction of a tracer (infusion I) in state B, perturbs this pool. With time, the pool reaches a new steady state (state C) at which point the ratio of the rate of appearance of glucose (R_a) to rate of tracer infusion (I) is equal to the relative amounts of metabolite to tracer. The filled circles represent unlabelled metabolite, and the open circles the labelled tracer. R_d, rate of disappearance or use of glucose.

the labelled glucose, this proportion will increase until a new steady state is achieved (state C).

In human subjects, a steady state of isotopic enrichment may not be achieved for 3–4 h. Ideally, the amount of tracer introduced should not perturb the system: it should neither change the concentration of the glucose within the pool nor alter the rates of appearance or disappearance. This is mostly a concern for experiments utilizing stable isotope tracers of glucose ($[1\text{-}^{13}C]$ glucose or $[6,6\text{-}^2H]$ glucose). Additionally, the body should use the tracer in the exact same manner as the unlabelled glucose. With these caveats, at steady state, the ratio of labelled tracer to unlabelled glucose will equal the ratio of R_a : I or:

$$\frac{[\text{labelled glucose}]}{[\text{unlabelled glucose}]} = \frac{R_a}{I}.$$

To solve for R_a:

$$R_a = \frac{I}{([\text{labelled glucose}]/[\text{unlabelled glucose}])}.$$

In the basal state, R_a will equal the rate of endogenous glucose production. In the insulin-stimulated state, one measures R_d, which will equal the rate of whole body glucose disposal.

Measuring insulin response: the clamp experiment

The hyperinsulinaemic–euglycaemic clamp method of DeFronzo *et al.* [3] remains the gold standard for assessing insulin responsiveness *in vivo*. The use of the term 'clamp' refers to the maintaining or clamping the plasma glucose at a constant level, usually 100 mg/dL, with a variable infusion of glucose. At the authors' laboratory, the clamp experiment starts with a basal infusion of tracer for 180 min to determine the basal endogenous rate of glucose production. The clamp begins with a primed and/or continuous infusion of insulin and a variable of glucose infusion (GINF). For studies of hepatic insulin sensitivity, typically a low dose of insulin (10–20 mU/m^2) is used. For studies of insulin-stimulated whole body glucose disposal, higher levels (40–120 mU/m^2) have been employed. The degree of insulin responsiveness is directly proportional to the GINF.

Once a steady state is achieved, the plasma samples are obtained in order to determine the isotopic enrichment. At steady state, the rate of appearance of glucose will equal the rate of disposal. The total flux of glucose into the body can only come from endogenous glucose production or the glucose infusion. Using the isotopic enrichment at the end of the clamp experiment, one can calculate R_d. Endogenous glucose production (EGP) is the sum total of all glucose released into the circulation by the body. During the clamp experiment, EGP is calculated as follows:

At steady state $\quad R_a = R_d$

During the clamp $\quad R_a = \text{EGP} + \text{GINF}$

therefore $\quad R_d = \text{EGP} + \text{GINF}$

or $\quad \text{EGP} = R_d - \text{GINF}$

In most studies, EGP is equated to hepatic glucose production (HGP). However, this may over-represent the contribution of the liver to total EGP. In basal conditions, renal gluconeogenesis contributes 10–15% of total EGP, although under some conditions this contribution may increase to as high as 45% [4]. In addition to the kidney, some recent evidence suggests that the small intestine also has gluconeogenic potential under insulinopenic conditions [5,6]. Thus, depending on the conditions under which EGP is measured, equating HGP to EGP may slightly overestimate the true rate of hepatic glucose production.

The rate of hepatic glucose production is the sum of the rate of net hepatic glycogenolysis and the rate of gluconeogenesis. Quantifying these two components of hepatic glucose production is complex. The following section discusses two of the prevailing methodologies.

Before the application of ^{13}C-magentic resonance spectroscopy (MRS) to the study of hepatic glucose metabolism, the available methods were either invasive (liver biopsy [7,8], hepatic venous catheterization [9]) or relied on indirect approaches using various substrate tracers [10–12]. ^{13}C-MRS enables the serial direct non-invasive measurement of hepatic glycogen *in vivo* [13]. ^{13}C has a natural abundance of 1.1% and thus permits for the measurement of carbon-containing compounds by MRS *in vivo*. By comparing the signal intensity of the C-1 of glycogen to a glycogen phantom of known concentration, it is possible to calculate the concentration of glycogen per volume of liver. Subsequently, the volume of the liver can be obtained from a three-dimensional reconstruction of the liver using serial MRS sections and used to calculate total liver glycogen. Thus, using serial measurements of hepatic glycogen concentration, one can measure the rate of net hepatic glycogenolysis. If the total rate of endogenous glucose production is measured simultaneously, using a tracer technique discussed above, it is possible to calculate the rate of gluconeogenesis by subtracting the rate of net hepatic glycogenolysis from the rate of glucose production.

Using such an approach, several key findings have been made regarding hepatic glucose metabolism in the fed and fasted states (Fig. 4.2). After a meal, liver glycogen concentration increases in a near linear fashion, peaking at approximately 5 h [14]. During this period of hepatic glycogen synthesis, where exogenous glucose is absorbed from the gut, endogenous glucose production is suppressed. Of the glucose ingested in a meal, approximately 20% is incorporated into hepatic glycogen [15]. About two-thirds of this glycogen is formed via the direct pathway of glycogen synthesis (glucose → G6P → G1P → UDP-glucose → glycogen) and the remainder via the indirect, or gluconeogenic, pathway (pyruvate → G6P →, etc.). Approximately 5 h after a meal, and hepatic glycogen begins to be broken down at a linear rate and up to approximately 22 h [13,16]. During this period, hepatic glycogen breakdown accounts for 40–50% of total EGP. Gluconeogenesis accounts for the remainding or 50–60% of EGP during the early part of a fast.

In contrast, previous studies had estimated that hepatic glycogenolysis accounted for approximately 70–80% and gluconeogenesis approximately 20–30% of EGP after 12–24 h fasting. However, prior to the application of ^{13}C-MRS to measure the rate of glycogen breakdown *in vivo* in fasting humans, it had not been possible to directly measure net hepatic glycogenolysis, and thus to calculate accurately rates of gluconeogenesis. Between 22 and 46 h, net hepatic glycogenolysis accounts for approximately 20% and gluconeogenesis approximately 80% of EGP. Between 46 and 64 h, net hepatic glycogenolysis accounts for less than 5% and gluconeogenesis for approximately 95% of EGP.

Magnusson *et al.* [17] applied the same techniques to determine the relative contributions of gluconeogenesis in patients with T2DM. They measured the rate of glycogenolysis and EGP in control and diabetic subjects fasted over 23 h. The rate of EGP was increased by approximately 25% in the diabetic subjects (8.9 ± 0.5 T_2DM versus 11 ± 0.6 µmol/kg/min in control). They found that this increase in EGP was largely accounted for by an approximate 20% increase in the percentage contribution of gluconeogenesis to EGP (88 ± 2% in T_2DM versus 70 ± 6% in controls).

Landau *et al.* [18,19] subsequently developed the use of ^2H_2O (D_2O) to determine the relative contributions of gluconeogenesis to EGP (Fig. 4.3). ^2H_2O is given orally to enrich the total body water pool with a final proportion of 0.5%. As shown in Fig. 4.3, glucose formed from gluconeogenesis obtains a hydrogen molecule from body water in two steps:

1 Isomerization of dihydroxyacetone phosphate with glyceraldehyde 3-phosphate labels C-5.

2 Isomerization of fructose 6-phosphate with glucose 6-phosphate labels C-2.

In contrast, glucose derived from glycogenolysis will obtain a hydrogen molecule from body water only at C-2 as the result of isomerization of glucose 6-phosphate with fructose 6-phosphate. Thus, the ratio of ^2H enrichment at C-5 to C-2 will equal the percentage

(a)

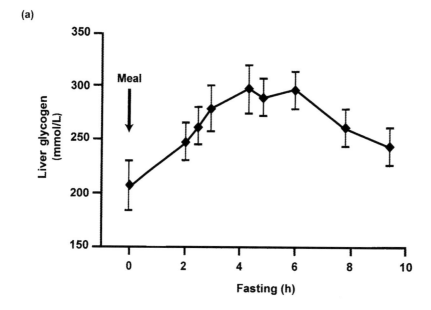

(b)

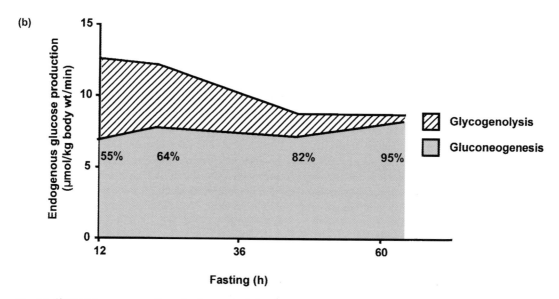

Fig. 4.2 ^{13}C-MRS assessment of hepatic glycogen in fed and fasted states. (a) Hepatic glycogen concentration after a meal. (Adapted from Taylor *et al.* [14].) (b) Contribution of gluconeogenesis and glycogenolysis to endogenous glucose production during a fast. Numbers indicate percentage contribution of gluconeogenesis. (Adapted from Rothman *et al.* [13] and Petersen *et al.* [16].)

contribution of gluconeogenesis to EGP. As an illustration, assume an equal contribution of glycogenolysis and gluconeogenesis to hepatic glucose production. ^{2}H at the C-2 position would arise equally from glycogenolysis and the other half from gluconeogenesis. Glucose produced from gluconeogenesis also has an equal chance of being labelled at C-5 as being labelled C-2. Thus, the ratio of ^{2}H enrichment at C-5 : C-2

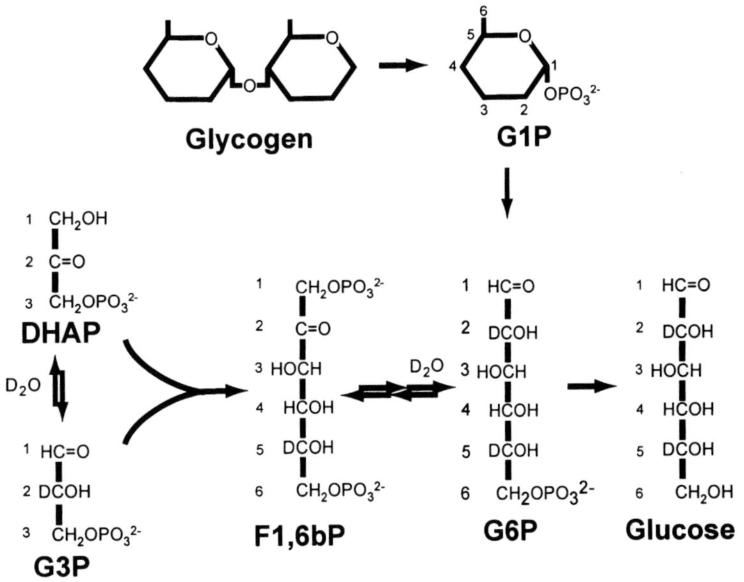

Fig. 4.3 Incorporation of deuterium (^{2}D) into glucose from body water. ^{2}D is incorporated into carbon 2 (C2) of glyceraldehyde 3-phosphate during the triose phosphate isomerase step. This will ultimately yield a ^{2}D label on C5 of glucose. ^{2}D is incorporated onto C2 during the isomerization of glucose 6-phosphate (G6P) with fructose 6-phosphate (F6P). All glucose obtained from glycogen will be labelled on C2. All glucose obtained from gluconeogenesis from glyceraldehyde 3-phosphate (GA3P) will be labelled at either C2 or C5.

would be 50%. If, on the other hand, gluconeogenesis accounted for 100% of glucose production, the ratio of ^{2}H at C-5 : C-2 would be equal. By multiplying the percentage contribution of gluconeogenesis by the rate of endogenous glucose production (determine using a tracer infusion), one can calculate the rate of gluconeogenesis. The rate of glycogenolysis is then estimated as the difference between total EGP and gluconeogenesis.

The challenge with this method lies in the determination of the isotopic ratios at C-5 and C-2. In order to determine the deuterium enrichment at C-5, glucose is first converted into xylose and the xylose into formaldehyde. The C-5 carbon is retained on formaldehyde, which is then converted into hexamethylenetetramine (HMT) for analysis by gas chromatography/mass spectroscopy (GC/MS). In order to determine the deuterium enrichment at C-2, glucose is first converted into ribitol phosphate and arabitol phosphate. Formaldehyde is formed from the C2 carbon of these polyol phosphates and converted into HMT.

Recently, a ^{2}H-^{13}C MRS method has been developed for determining the positional enrichments of deuterium on a glucose molecule [20,21]. This method enables the simultaneous determination of ^{2}H enrichment at carbon 2, 5 and 6, allowing for the determination of the relative contributions to EGP from glycogenolysis, and gluconeogenesis from both glyc-

erol and phosphoenolpyruvate. This ^{2}H-MRS method was recently compared to the GC/MS method of Landau with excellent correlation [22]. Using the ^{2}H$_2$O technique, gluconeogenesis was found to account for approximately 50% of EGP after an overnight fast and nearly 100% of EGP after 42 h of fasting [18]. These results confirmed the earlier results obtained using ^{13}C-MRS measures of the rate of glycogenolysis.

A recent study compared all three methods (^{13}C MRS, ^{2}H-MRS and the HMT-GC/MS method) in control and diabetic subjects [23]. In control subjects fasted for 14–18 h, the percentage contribution of gluconeogenesis determined by ^{13}C-MRS, ^{2}H-MRS and HMT-GC/MS were similar to each other and confirmed previous findings ($65 \pm 3\%$ versus $63 \pm 3\%$ versus $51 \pm 3\%$, respectively). By comparison, while all three methods demonstrated an increase in gluconeogenesis in subjects with T2DM, the two MRS methods yielded higher estimates than the HMT-GC/MS method, respectively ($85 \pm 2\%$ versus $75 \pm 2\%$ versus $63 \pm 3\%$). While the reason for this discrepancy remains unknown, one possibility could be the fact that the ^{2}H$_2$O method measures *total* glycogenolysis while the MRS method measures *net* glycogenolysis. The difference between these two rates may therefore reflect glycogen cycling (glycogen $\rightarrow$ G6P $\rightarrow$ glycogen) [24].

43

Mechanism of fat-induced skeletal muscle insulin resistance

Studies of skeletal muscle insulin resistance serve as an important reference point from which to proceed to a discussion of hepatic insulin resistance. In skeletal muscle, insulin increases glucose uptake. By binding to its receptor, insulin activates the insulin receptor tyrosine kinase activity, resulting in the phosphorylation of IRS-1 on specific tyrosine sites. IRS-1 binds to and activates phosphatidylinositol 3 kinase (PI3 kinase), which subsequently leads to the translocation of glucose transporter (GLUT4)-containing vesicles to the plasma membrane. The current model of peripheral insulin resistance links intramyocellular fatty acid metabolite accumulation with a blunting of insulin-mediated increases in glucose transport. Specifically, intramyocellular fat accumulation prevents insulin-mediated activation of IRS-1-associated PI3 kinase activity, ultimately limiting the movement of the glucose transporter GLUT4 from its intracellular compartment to the plasma membrane.

This model has evolved over several decades. In the 1960s, Randle et al. first formed a hypothesis linking obesity with insulin resistance. The essential tenets were that increased delivery of free fatty acids (FFA) promoted fatty acid oxidation and inhibited glucose oxidation. Fat oxidation increases intramitochondrial acetylCoA/CoA and NADH/NAD$^+$, which, in turn, would lead to the inactivation of pyruvate dehydrogenase (PDH), the enzyme responsible for the conversion of pyruvate into acetylCoA. Inactivation of PDH would lead to increases in intracellular citrate, which inhibit phosphofructokinase (PFK), a key glycolytic enzyme. The block in PFK would lead to accumulation of glucose 6-phosphate (G6P), which then blocks hexokinase 2. Inhibition of hexokinase 2 activity then leads to an increase in intracellular glucose, and subsequently a decrease in glucose uptake.

The link between fatty acids and insulin resistance was demonstrated in a cross-sectional study comparing lean normoglycaemic offspring of patients with T2DM with age- and BMI-matched controls. An inverse correlation was seen between plasma FFA and insulin sensitivity [25]. Using ^{1}H-MRS and the hyperinsulinaemic–euglycaemic clamp method, Krssak et al. [26] measured intramyocellular lipid (IMCL) content and insulin sensitivity in normal individuals. They, and others [27], found that IMCL was even a stronger predictor of insulin resistance. In order to better delineate the biochemical mechanisms of insulin resistance, Perseghin et al. [28] measured the changes in muscle glycogen and G6P in lean offspring of patients with T2DM against matched controls. In contrast to the control subjects, muscle glycogen synthesis was approximately 60% lower in the offspring. The impairment in glycogen synthesis was associated with an approximate 40% decrease in the accumulation of G6P under hyperinsulinaemic conditions. These data suggested that insulin resistance in the offspring of patients with T2DM was caused by an impairment in the ability of insulin to activate either transport or phosphorylation of glucose. To summarize, accumulation of fat with the muscle is associated with a decrease in insulin action, possibly because of a defect in either glucose transport or phosphorylation.

To strengthen the causal link between lipids and insulin resistance, Roden et al. [29] infused normal insulin-sensitive subjects with either glycerol or Intralipid/heparin. Infusion of Intralipid elevates plasma triglycerides, which are then hydrolyzed into fatty acids and glycerol by lipoprotein lipase released from the endothelium by heparin. Insulin action was then assessed with a euglycaemic–hyperinsulinaemic clamp. Using ^{13}C-MRS spectroscopy, they found that after 3 h of Intralipid/heparin infusion, the rate of insulin-mediated glycogen synthesis began to decrease. This decrease in glycogen synthesis was preceded by a drop in the concentration of G6P, as assessed by ^{31}P-MRS. This finding was in contrast to the Randle model, which would have predicted that increased fatty acids would lead to an accumulation of G6P. Instead, these data suggested that the increase in fatty acids resulted in insulin resistance through a block in either glucose transport or phosphorylation activity. In order to distinguish between these two possibilities, Dresner et al. [30] studied normal subjects with a similar glycerol versus Intralipid/heparin infusion protocol, in combination with ^{13}C-MRS to look specifically at intracellular glucose. They found that, compared to the glycerol infusion, the Intralipid/heparin infusion was associated with lower concentrations of intracellular glucose and a failure to increase G6P concentrations. This suggested that elevations in fatty acids led to insulin resistance through a defect in insulin-stimulated glucose transport activity. Furthermore, based on muscle biopsies obtained from these subjects, the apparent defect in insulin-stimulated glucose uptake was associated with impaired activation of IRS-1-associated PI3 kinase activity. Thus, elevations in fatty acids could lead to peripheral insulin resistance through a defect in the insulin signalling cascade, which limited the ability of insulin to increase muscle glucose transport activity.

How is fat accumulation linked to insulin resistance?

Animal studies have helped to elucidate the cellular mechanisms of peripheral insulin resistance. Several candidate kinases have emerged as possible mechanisms for fatty acid-induced insulin resistance. Accumulation of a fat metabolite within the muscle is associated with activation of the serine kinase, PKC-θ [31,32]. Increased intramyocellular fat metabolites have also been associated with activation of IKK-β [33]. This association has been strengthened by the finding that inhibition of IKK-β activity, either by salicylate treatment or gene knockout, protects against fat-induced insulin resistance [34,35]. Furthermore, IKK-β has been shown to increase serine phosphorylation of IRS-1 at key residues *in vitro* [36]. Once it is serine phosphorylated, IRS-1 cannot be tyrosine phosphorylated by the insulin receptor, and therefore cannot bind to and activate PI3 kinase.

The third candidate is the stress-activated protein kinase, JNK1 (also known as mitogen activated protein kinase 8). JNK1 activity is increased in both dietary and genetic models of obesity. Furthermore, knockout mice deficient in JNK1 appear to be protected from diet-induced insulin resistance [37]. Like IKK-β, JNK1 has also been shown to be capable of serine phosphorylating IRS-1 at the crucial S307 residue [38].

Current data also support a role for PKC and IKK activation in the pathogenesis of fat-induced insulin resistance in humans. Thus, increased activity of PKC-θ has been noted in the muscle of patients with T2DM [39]. Further, lipid infusion in normal volunteers increases total PKC activity. However, in these latter studies, lipid infusion was associated with activation of both PKC-β2 and δ, but not θ. Finally, analogous to the inhibition of IKK-β in rodents, the use of high-dose salicylates was shown to improve insulin responsiveness in patients with T2DM [40].

A model for fat-induced hepatic insulin resistance

The primary role of insulin in hepatic glucose metabolism is to promote glucose storage via activation of glycogen synthase and inhibition of hepatic glucose production. When insulin binds to its receptor, it activates a signalling cascade in hepatocytes that is similar to the cascade in myoctyes [41]. The insulin receptor tyrosine phosphorylates its substrates (IRS), which in turn activate PI3 kinase. In contrast to muscle, IRS-2—not IRS-1—is the predominant substrate for the insulin receptor in the liver [42,43]. This leads to the subsequent activation of protein kinase B (PKB/Akt2) [44]. Akt2 will phosphorylate and inactivate glycogen synthase kinase-3 (GSK3). Under basal conditions, GSK3 phosphorylates and inactivates glycogen synthase. Once removed from this tonic inhibition, glycogen synthase will promote the storage of glucose as glycogen. In addition, insulin may alter expression of key genes within the liver to promote glycolysis and fatty acid synthesis and inhibit gluconeogenesis. The key question then is how fat accumulation within the liver leads to hepatic insulin resistance.

Liver-lipoprotein lipase overexpressing mouse

One model in which to study the mechanism for hepatic insulin resistance is the liver-lipoprotein lipase (LPL) overexpressing mouse. LPL is the rate-limiting enzyme for the hydrolysis of triglyceride from triglyceride-rich lipoproteins, such as chylomicrons and very-low-density lipoproteins (VLDL). By crossing a transgenic mouse expressing human LPL under the control of apo A-1 (A-1 LPL) promoter with an heterozygote LPL knockout (het ko) mouse, it was possible to generate a mouse in which LPL was expressed primarily in the liver [45]. The resulting liver LPL/het ko has accumulation of triglyceride within the liver (Fig. 4.4a). Using the hyperinsulinaemic–euglycaemic clamp technique, insulin sensitivity of this mouse was assessed [46]. While whole body glucose metabolism and muscle glucose uptake were normal, the ability of insulin to suppress endogenous glucose production was markedly diminished (Fig. 4.4b).

Alterations in the insulin signalling cascade were also assessed in this model (Fig. 4.5). Insulin-mediated increases in insulin receptor tyrosine phosphorylation were identical in the control and LPL0/A-1-LPL mice. However, the LPL0/A-1-LPL mice failed to demonstrate increases in IRS-2 tyrosine phosphorylation and IRS-2-associated PI3 kinase activity. This model illustrates how hepatic fat accumulation can lead

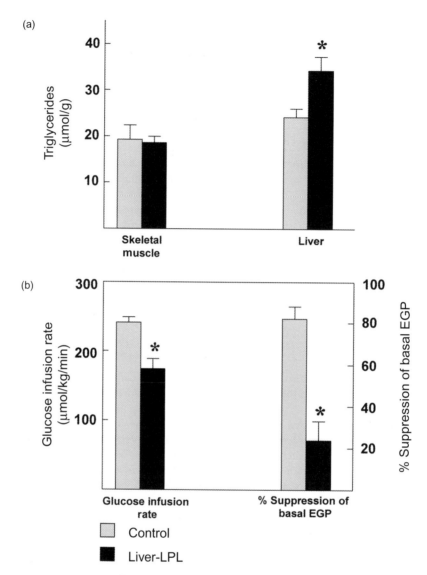

Fig. 4.4 Metabolic characterization of liver-lipoprotein lipase (L-LPL) overexpressing mouse. (a) Triglyceride content of tissues, as labelled. (b) Glucose infusion rate and suppression of basal endogenous glucose production (EGP) during a hyperinsulinaemic–euglycaemic clamp. The grey bars represent the wildtype control, and the black bars the L-LPL transgenic mice. (From Kim *et al*. [46].)

specifically to hepatic insulin resistance through a block in the insulin signalling cascade.

Fatless mouse

Another murine model of hepatic fat accumulation and hepatic insulin resistance is the fatless mouse. By expressing a dominant-negative protein A-ZIP/F under the control of the adipocyte specific AP-1 promoter, Moitra *et al*. [47] generated mice that are devoid of white adipose tissue. Without adipocytes, these mice develop fat accumulation in the muscle and the liver. When studied under the hyperinsulinaemic–euglycaemic clamp, these fatless mice displayed profound peri-

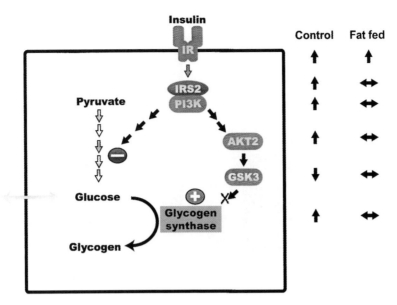

Control   Fat fed

Fig. 4.5 Schematic for hepatic insulin signalling. Insulin acts to activate glycogen synthesis and inhibit gluconeogenesis. To the right, the arrows summarize the normal (control) response to insulin compared to the changes incurred with hepatic fat accumulation (fat-fed). Upward arrows indicate an increase, horizontal arrows no change, and downward arrows a decrease. AKT2, protein kinase 13; GSK, glycogen synthase kinase; IR, insulin receptor; IRS-2, insulin receptor substrate 2; PI3K, phosphatidylinositol-3 kinase.

pheral and hepatic insulin resistance [48]. Analysis of insulin signalling in the liver showed that insulin failed to increase IRS-2-associated PI3 kinase activity. Remarkably, this phenotype can be rescued by transplantation of fat pads from wildtype littermates [48]. With restoration of adipocytes, tissue triglyceride levels normalize, as does muscle and hepatic insulin sensitivity. Furthermore, this is associated with improvements in insulin-stimulated PI3 kinase activity. Thus, these results in the fatless mouse model also support the hypothesis that hepatic fat accumulation leads to insulin resistance through a proximal block in the insulin signalling cascade at the level of IRS-2-associated PI3 kinase.

The development of hepatic insulin resistance before peripheral insulin resistance has also been documented in canine models of high-fat feeding [49]. Twelve weeks of isocaloric high-fat feeding in normal dogs resulted in marked impairments in hepatic insulin action at 6 and 12 weeks of the high-fat diet. In contrast, the ability of insulin to increase whole body glucose disposal and suppress plasma FFA concentration was unchanged, indicating that muscle or adipocyte insulin sensitivity remained unaltered. In conclusion, high-fat feeding appears to result in marked hepatic fat accumulation and hepatic insulin resistance prior to any alteration in peripheral insulin action. The mechanism of fat-induced hepatic insulin resistance may be similar to muscle, involving the activation of PKC-ε and a block in the insulin signalling pathway at the level of IRS-2.

Human studies of insulin resistance with lipodystrophy: the role of leptin in hepatic insulin sensitivity

Lipodystrophy is a collection of discrete genetic and acquired disorders that are marked by a failure of proper adipocyte formation (see Chapter 21). Affected individuals have markedly diminished subcutaneous fat. All forms are characterized by hypertriglyceridaemia, insulin resistance and visceral fat deposition. Hepatic steatosis is common. Shimomura et al. [50] found that in a mouse model of lipodystrophy, leptin therapy normalized insulin resistance beyond what could be accounted for by food restriction. On this basis, Oral

Effect of leptin on liver size

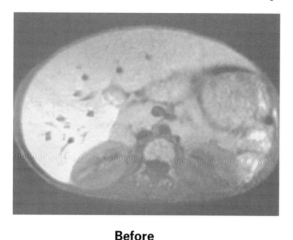
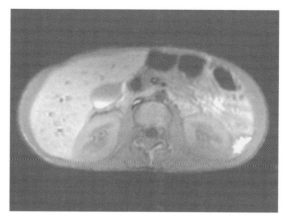

Before **After**

☐ Pretreatment
■ Post-treatment

Fig. 4.6 Effect of leptin on hepatic and intramyocellular fat content in patients with congenital lipodystrophy. The open bars are the pretreatment values, the filled bars are the post-treatment values. (From Oral *et al.* [51] and Petersen *et al.* [52].)

et al. [51] hypothesized that leptin therapy may be a novel therapeutic agent in human subjects with congenital lipodystrophy. They found that replacement of leptin to physiological levels markedly improved metabolic indices, as well as strikingly reduced fasting blood glucose, serum lipids and liver function test abnormalities.

To quantify the affects of leptin therapy on liver and muscle insulin resistance, Petersen *et al.* [52] performed hyperinsulinaemic–euglycaemic clamps with ^{1}H-MRS measures of hepatic triglyceride content on three subjects with lipodystrophy. When compared to age- and weight-matched controls, basal rates of glucose production were approximately doubled in the lipodystrophic patients (3.6 ± 0.8 versus 1.9 ± 0.1 mg/kg/min). In addition, the ability of insulin to suppress endogenous glucose production was markedly impaired. When compared to the pretreatment state, leptin therapy was associated with an approximate 90% reduction in hepatic triglyceride content and approximately 33% reduction in skeletal muscle triglyceride content (Fig. 4.6). Leptin therapy increased whole body glucose disposal from 3.5 ± 0.3 to 6.1 ± 1.0 mg/kg/min (Fig. 4.7a). Hepatic insulin respon-

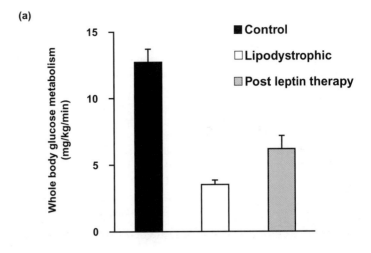

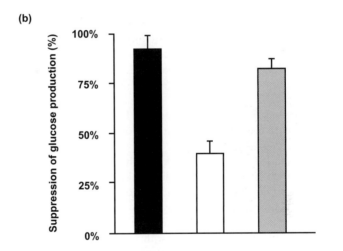

Fig. 4.7 Metabolic characterization of control subjects and patients with lipodystrophy before and after leptin treatment (From Petersen *et al.* [52]). (a) Insulin-stimulated whole body glucose disposal during hyperinsulinaemic–euglycaemic clamp. (b) Suppression of endogenous glucose production by insulin. The black bars are the control subjects, the open bars represent the lipodystrophic subjects before therapy, and the grey bars the lipodystrophic subjects after leptin therapy.

siveness improved dramatically, from 40% ± 6% to 82 ± 5%. Thus, leptin therapy reduced hepatic and intramyocellular lipid content and the reductions were associated with improvements in hepatic insulin responsiveness and whole body glucose disposal. Leptin therapy may have exerted this affect by a decrease in energy intake. In fact, in the only patient in whom intake was monitored, caloric intake decreased from approximately 8500 kJ/day to approximately 4000 kJ/day. In contrast, there was no change in energy expenditure as assessed by indirect calorimetery.

Lipodystrophy is a rare disorder that represents the very end of the spectrum of hepatic fat accumulation. The question therefore arises as to whether the more common variety of fatty liver seen in obese individuals is linked with hepatic insulin resistance? The author is aware of only a few studies that address this issue (but see Chapters 1, 5 and 24). Marchesini *et al.* [53] obtained metabolic variables in 46 patients with NAFLD and compared the results to 92 age- and sex-matched controls. They assessed insulin resistance using the homoeostasis model assessment method (HOMA), which generates a measure of insulin resistance based on plasma insulin and glucose (insulin/$22.5 \times e^{-\ln(glucose)}$). Their results indicated that patients with NAFLD are more insulin-resistant than controls. However, the interpretation of this result should be tempered by the discrepancy in weights between controls and patients (BMI 24.2 versus 28.2 kg/m^2). In addition, in some groups of patients, the HOMA method does not always correlate well with the degree of insulin resistance derived from the gold standard hyperinsulinaemic–euglycaemic clamp [54,55].

A subsequent study by the same group did employ the clamp technique [56]. In this study, they compared 30 patients with NAFLD with 10 control subjects and 10 subjects with T2DM. When compared to control subjects, insulin-stimulated whole body disposal was diminished in the subjects with T2DM and NAFLD (6.62 ± 1.4 versus 3.2 ± 0.7 versus 3.31 ± 1.1 mg/kg/min, control versus T2DM versus NAFLD, respectively). Suppression of hepatic glucose production was also diminished, compared with controls, in the patients with T2DM and NAFLD (82 ± 14% versus 65 ± 4% versus 63 ± 9%). Unfortunately, there was again a discrepancy in weight between the controls and the other groups (24 ± 2 versus 29 ± 4 versus 27 kg/m^2, respectively). In addition, the suppression of hepatic glucose production that these investigators achieved in normal subjects was somewhat less than that the authors typically achieve in normal insulin-sensitive individuals (more than 90%). One reason for this is that the length of the clamp was only 2 h, and this may not have been adequate to establish a steady state of the tracer used.

Sanyal et al. [57] used a two-step euglycemic–hyperinsulinemic clamp to assess insulin sensitivity in patients with fatty liver and those who had progressed to NASH, as confirmed by liver biopsy. They did not measure suppression of hepatic glucose production in their control subjects. In the subjects with fatty liver alone, a low dose of insulin (10 mU/m^2/min) suppressed hepatic glucose production by 76%, as compared to 54% in those with NASH. At the high insulin dose (40 mU/m^2/min), hepatic glucose production was completely suppressed in both groups. Given the small numbers, the apparent difference between the two groups was not statistically significant. As in the other studies, the subjects with fatty liver and NASH were significantly heavier than the controls (31 versus 33 versus 24 kg/m^2, NASH, fatty liver and control subjects, respectively).

Despite the design difficulties with these studies, the impression from existing data is that hepatic fat accumulation does seem to be associated with hepatic insulin resistance. However, drawing clear conclusions about the impact of hepatic fat accumulation on hepatic insulin resistance requires careful weight matching. If one group is heavier than the other, it will be difficult to separate any impact of increased peripheral insulin resistance on hepatic glucose metabolism. This will subsequently make it difficult to attribute the measured changes in hepatic insulin sensitivity purely to a pathological process within the liver.

Treatment options for hepatic insulin resistance

Metformin

Metformin, a biguanide, has been used to treat patients with T2DM for over 30 years. It improves liver function test abnormalities, at least temporarily, in some patients with NAFLD (see Chapter 16). Although metformin was known to lower fasting glucose, the exact mechanism by which it did so was unknown. Using [6,6-^{2}H] glucose measures of endogenous glucose production combined with ^{13}C-MRS measures of net hepatic glycogenolysis and ^{2}H$_2$O measures of gluconeogenesis, Hundal et al. [58] studied nine diabetic subjects before and after 3 months of metformin therapy; they compared the results with seven age-, sex- and weight-matched controls. At baseline, the diabetic subjects had increased rates of endogenous glucose production. Using ^{13}C-MRS measures of net hepatic glycogenolysis and ^{2}H$_2$O measures of gluconeogenesis, it was clear that increased hepatic gluconeogenesis accounted for the increase in EGP. After 3 months of metformin therapy, the EGP was lowered in the diabetic subjects, mainly as a result of decreasing the rate of hepatic gluconeogenesis. Although metformin has been shown to decrease hepatic steatosis and improve hepatic insulin sensitivity in ob/ob mice [59], as of the time of writing, there has not been any published report to link metformin therapy with improvements in hepatic fat content in humans.

Marchesini et al. [60] evaluated metformin therapy in non-diabetic subjects with NASH. Metformin therapy was associated with a modest decrease in BMI and waist circumference, normalization of serum aminotransferase elevations and reduction in liver volume in patients with NASH. While metformin may be a potential agent in the treatment of fat-induced hepatic insulin resistance and NASH, more studies are required.

Thiazolidinediones

The thiazolidinediones (TZDs) are peroxisome

proliferator-activated receptor γ (PPARγ) agonists that improve insulin sensitivity. They have therefore been used in the treatment of T2DM. In a study of troglitazone, 93 patients were randomly assigned to placebo or one of four regimens and were studied with hyperinsulinaemic–euglycaemic clamps before and after 6 months of therapy [61]. Troglitazone decreased basal hepatic glucose production but there was no difference in hepatic insulin sensitivity. However, the clamp for this protocol employed a high dose of insulin $(120\,mU/m^2)$ and may not have been able to detect modest changes in hepatic insulin sensitivity. Troglitazone did exert marked dose-responsive improvements in glucose disposal during a meal tolerance test and under the hyperinsulinaemic–euglycaemic clamp.

While it appears conclusive that TZDs do improve peripheral insulin responsiveness, the question remains as to how they do this. As PPARγ is mainly expressed in adipocytes with apparently weaker expression in the liver and skeletal muscle (there are species differences), the mechanism of their beneficial action is not yet understood. Given this discordance between the site of PPARγ expression and the site of drug effects, it was hypothesized that TZDs worked by redistributing fat from the liver and muscle into the adipocyte.

In a subsequent study, rosiglitazone was given to nine patients with T2DM in order to assess changes in insulin sensitivity (as assessed by the hyperinsulinaemic–euglycaemic clamp) and tissue fat content (as measured by ^{1}H-MRS) [62]. Insulin-mediated suppression

(a)

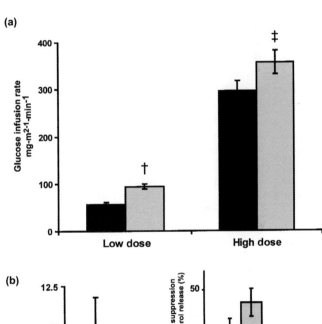

Fig. 4.8 Rosiglitazone therapy in patients with type 2 diabetes mellitus. (Adapted from Mayerson *et al.* [60].) (a) Glucose infusion rate during low- $(20\,mU/m^2)$ and high-dose $(120\,mU/m^2)$ hyperinsulinaemic–euglycaemic clamp. (b) Tissue triglyceride concentration before and after rosiglitazone therapy. Inset represents percentage suppression of subcutaneous adipocyte glycerol release assessed by microdialysis during low-dose insulin clamp. The black bars represent the pre-rosiglitazone values and the grey bars the post-rosiglitazone values.

(b)

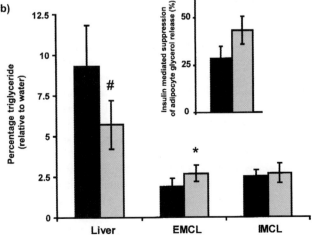

of lipolysis in subcutaneous fat was also assessed by measuring glycerol release by microdialysis. After 3 months of therapy, rosiglitazone was associated with an approximate 40% decrease in hepatic triglyceride content, an approximate 40% increase in extramyocellular triglyceride content, but no significant change in intramyocellular triglyceride content (Fig. 4.8b). Despite the lack of a measurable change in intramyocellular triglyceride content, rosiglitazone improved insulin-mediated whole body glucose disposal (Fig. 4.8a). This apparent disconnection between intramyocellular triglyceride and peripheral insulin action underscores the fact that intramyocellular triglyceride is only a crude marker for the active metabolite responsible for fat-induced insulin resistance [31].

These findings were associated with enhanced adipocyte insulin responsiveness as reflected by improved suppression of adipocyte lipolysis (Fig. 4.8b, inset). In summary, rosiglitazone seems to exert its beneficial effects by shifting intracellular lipid from resistant organs into the adipocytes, possibly through improving the insulin sensitivity of adipocytes.

These findings have been duplicated with pioglitazone treatment [63]. In patients with T2DM, pioglitazone improved both hepatic and peripheral insulin sensitivity. While this study did not measure hepatic or intramyocellular fat content, there appeared to be a redistribution of fat from visceral fat stores into subcutaneous fat.

Conclusions

Studies of the mechanisms of peripheral insulin resistance point to fat-induced activation of various inflammatory signalling kinases (PKCθ, IKK-β and JNK1) that may, in turn, serine phosphorylate IRS-1, thereby preventing its participation in the insulin signalling cascade. As a result, the ability of insulin to increase GLUT4 translocation is impaired. This is reflected by decreased whole body glucose disposal in various models of insulin resistance. The mechanisms of fat-induced hepatic insulin resistance are likely to be similar. Thus, accumulation of fat within the liver has been shown to result in a block in insulin signalling at IRS-2. This proximal block in the insulin signalling cascade may limit the ability of insulin to activate hepatic glycogen synthesis and suppress hepatic glucose production. However, a role for PKC, IKK-β and/or JNK1 in the pathogenesis of fat-induced hepatic insulin resistance, as opposed to peripheral insulin resistance, remains to be defined. In addition, based on studies in patients with diabetes, accumulation of fat within the liver may also be associated with increased hepatic gluconeogenesis; the exact mechanism accounting for this increase also needs to be established. Using the studies of peripheral insulin resistance as a guide, in combination with the available new MRS and isotopic techniques, the answers to many of these questions are likely to be answered in the next decade.

References

1 Mokdad AH, Ford ES, Bowman BA, *et al*. Prevalence of obesity, diabetes, and obesity-related health risk factors, 2001. *J Am Med Assoc* 2003; **289**: 76–9.

2 Wolfe RR. *Radioactive and Stable Isotope Tracers in Biomedicine: Principles and Practice of Kinetic Analysis*. New York: Wiley-Liss, 1992.

3 DeFronzo RA, Tobin JD, Andres R. Glucose clamp technique: a method for quantifying insulin secretion and resistance. *Am J Physiol* 1979; **237**: E214–23.

4 Stumvoll M, *et al*. Renal glucose production and utilization: new aspects in humans. *Diabetologia* 1997; **40**: 749–57.

5 Mithieux G, Bady I, Gautier A, *et al*. The induction of control genes in intestine gluconeogenesis is sequential during fasting and maximal in diabetes. *Am J Physiol Endocrinol Metab* 2004; **286**: E370–5.

6 Croset M, Rajas F, Zitoun C, *et al*. Rat small intestine is an insulin-sensitive gluconeogenic organ. *Diabetes* 2001; **50**: 740–6.

7 Beringer A, Thaler H. [Quantitative studies of glycogen content of the liver in normal and sick persons. II. The influence of fructose and glucose on glycogen storage.] *Wien Klin Wochenschr* 1964; **76**: 627–30.

8 Beringer A, Thaler H. [On quantitative studies of the glycogen content of the liver in healthy and diseased subjects. III. Action mechanism of glucagon.] *Wien Med Wochenschr* 1965; **115**: 105–7.

9 Wahren J, Felig P, Cerasi E, *et al*. Splanchnic and peripheral glucose and amino acid metabolism in diabetes mellitus. *J Clin Invest* 1972; **51**: 1870–8.

10 Landau BR. Limitations in the use of [U-13C6] glucose to estimate gluconeogenesis. *Am J Physiol* 1999; **277**: E408–13.

11 Landau BR. Quantifying the contribution of gluconeogenesis to glucose production in fasted human subjects using stable isotopes. *Proc Nutr Soc* 1999; **58**: 963–72.

12 Landau BR, Fernandez CA, Previs SF, *et al*. A limitation in the use of mass isotopomer distributions to measure gluconeogenesis in fasting humans. *Am J Physiol* 1995; **269**: E18–26.

13 Rothman DL, *et al*. Quantitation of hepatic glycogenolysis and gluconeogenesis in fasting humans with ^{13}C NMR. *Science* 1991; **254**: 573–6.

14 Taylor R, *et al*. Direct assessment of liver glycogen storage by ^{13}C nuclear magnetic resonance spectroscopy and regulation of glucose homeostasis after a mixed meal in normal subjects. *J Clin Invest* 1996; **97**: 126–32.

15 Petersen KF, *et al*. Contribution of net hepatic glycogen synthesis to disposal of an oral glucose load in humans. *Metabolism* 2001; **50**: 598–601.

16 Petersen KF, *et al*. Contribution of net hepatic glycogenolysis to glucose production during the early postprandial period. *Am J Physiol* 1996; **270**: E186–91.

17 Magnusson I, *et al*. Increased rate of gluconeogenesis in type II diabetes mellitus: a ^{13}C nuclear magnetic resonance study. *J Clin Invest* 1992; **90**: 1323–7.

18 Landau BR, *et al*. Contributions of gluconeogenesis to glucose production in the fasted state. *J Clin Invest* 1996; **98**: 378–85.

19 Chandramouli V, *et al*. Quantifying gluconeogenesis during fasting. *Am J Physiol* 1997; **273**: E1209–15.

20 Jones JG, *et al*. An integrated ^{2}H and ^{13}C NMR study of gluconeogenesis and TCA cycle flux in humans. *Am J Physiol Endocrinol Metab* 2001; **281**: E848–56.

21 Jones JG, *et al*. Quantitation of gluconeogenesis by ^{2}H nuclear magnetic resonance analysis of plasma glucose following ingestion of [2]H$_2$O. *Anal Biochem* 2000; **277**: 121–6.

22 Burgess SC, *et al*. Analysis of gluconeogenic pathways *in vivo* by distribution of ^{2}H in plasma glucose: comparison of nuclear magnetic resonance and mass spectrometry. *Anal Biochem* 2003; **318**: 321–4.

23 Kunert O, *et al*. Measurement of fractional whole-body gluconeogenesis in humans from blood samples using ^{2}H nuclear magnetic resonance spectroscopy. *Diabetes* 2003; **52**: 2475–82.

24 Petersen K, *et al*. Mechanism by which glucose and insulin inhibit net hepatic glycogenolysis in humans. *J Clin Invest* 1998; **101**: 1203–9.

25 Perseghin G, *et al*. Metabolic defects in lean non-diabetic offspring of NIDDM parents: a cross-sectional study. *Diabetes* 1997; **46**: 1001–9.

26 Krssak M, *et al*. Intramyocellular lipid concentrations are correlated with insulin sensitivity in humans: a ^{1}H NMR spectroscopy study. *Diabetologia* 1999; **42**: 113–6.

27 Perseghin G, *et al*. Intramyocellular triglyceride content is a determinant of *in vivo* insulin resistance in humans: a [1]H-^{13}C nuclear magnetic resonance spectroscopy assessment in offspring of type 2 diabetic parents. *Diabetes* 1999; **48**: 1600–6.

28 Perseghin G, *et al*. Increased glucose transport-phosphorylation and muscle glycogen synthesis after exercise training in insulin-resistant subjects. *N Engl J Med* 1996; **335**: 1357–62.

29 Roden M, *et al*. Mechanism of free fatty acid-induced insulin resistance in humans. *J Clin Invest* 1996; **97**: 2859–65.

30 Dresner A, *et al*. Effects of free fatty acids on glucose transport and IRS-1-associated phosphatidylinositol 3-kinase activity. *J Clin Invest* 1999; **103**: 253–9.

31 Yu C, *et al*. Mechanism by which fatty acids inhibit insulin activation of insulin receptor substrate-1 (IRS-1)-associated phosphatidylinositol 3-kinase activity in muscle. *J Biol Chem* 2002; **277**: 50230–6.

32 Griffin ME, *et al*. Free fatty acid-induced insulin resistance is associated with activation of protein kinase C theta and alterations in the insulin signaling cascade. *Diabetes* 1999; **48**: 1270–4.

33 Lin X, *et al*. Protein kinase C-theta participates in NF-κB activation induced by CD3-CD28 costimulation through selective activation of IκB kinase β. *Mol Cell Biol* 2000; **20**: 2933–40.

34 Yuan M, *et al*. Reversal of obesity- and diet-induced insulin resistance with salicylates or targeted disruption of IκKβ. *Science* 2001; **293**: 1673–7.

35 Kim JK, *et al*. Prevention of fat-induced insulin resistance by salicylate. *J Clin Invest* 2001; **108**: 437–46.

36 Gao Z, *et al*. Serine phosphorylation of insulin receptor substrate 1 by inhibitor κB kinase complex. *J Biol Chem* 2002; **277**: 48115–21.

37 Hirosumi J, *et al*. A central role for JNK in obesity and insulin resistance. *Nature* 2002; **420**: 333–6.

38 Aguirre V, *et al*. Phosphorylation of Ser307 in insulin receptor substrate-1 blocks interactions with the insulin receptor and inhibits insulin action. *J Biol Chem* 2002; **277**: 1531–7.

39 Itani SI, *et al*. Increased protein kinase C theta in skeletal muscle of diabetic patients. *Metabolism* 2001; **50**: 553–7.

40 Hundal RS, *et al*. Mechanism by which high-dose aspirin improves glucose metabolism in type 2 diabetes. *J Clin Invest* 2002; **109**: 1321–6.

41 Saltiel AR Kahn CR. Insulin signalling and the regulation of glucose and lipid metabolism. *Nature* 2001; **414**: 799–806.

42 Kido Y, *et al*. Tissue-specific insulin resistance in mice with mutations in the insulin receptor, IRS-1, and IRS-2. *J Clin Invest* 2000; **105**: 199–205.

43 Previs SF, *et al*. Contrasting effects of IRS-1 versus IRS-2 gene disruption on carbohydrate and lipid metabolism *in vivo*. *J Biol Chem* 2000; **275**: 38990–4.

44 Cross DA, *et al*. Inhibition of glycogen synthase kinase-3 by insulin mediated by protein kinase B. *Nature* 1995; **378**: 785–9.

45 Merkel M, *et al*. Lipoprotein lipase expression exclusively in liver: a mouse model for metabolism in the neonatal period and during cachexia. *J Clin Invest* 1998; **102**: 893–901.

46 Kim JK, Fillmore JJ, Chen Y, *et al*. Tissue-specific overexpression of lipoprotein lipase causes tissue-specific insulin resistance. *Proc Natl Acad Sci USA* 2001; **98**: 7522–7.

47 Moitra J, Mason MM, Olive M, *et al*. Life without white fat: a transgenic mouse. *Genes Dev* 1998; **12**: 3168–81.

48 Kim JK, Gavrilova O, Chen Y, *et al*. Mechanism of insulin resistance in A-ZIP/F-1 fatless mice. *J Biol Chem* 2000; **275**: 8456–60.

49 Kim SP, Ellmerer M, van Citters GW, *et al*. Primacy of hepatic insulin resistance in the development of the metabolic syndrome induced by an isocaloric moderate-fat diet in the dog. *Diabetes* 2003; **52**: 2453–60.

50 Shimomura I, Hammer RE, Ikemoto S, *et al*. Leptin reverses insulin resistance and diabetes mellitus in mice with congenital lipodystrophy. *Nature* 1999; **401**: 73–6.

51 Oral EA, Simha V, Ruiz E, *et al*. Leptin-replacement therapy for lipodystrophy. *N Engl J Med* 2002; **346**: 570–8.

52 Petersen KF, Oral EA, Dufour S, *et al*. Leptin reverses insulin resistance and hepatic steatosis in patients with severe lipodystrophy. *J Clin Invest* 2002; **109**: 1345–50.

53 Marchesini G, Brizi M, Morselli-Labate AM, *et al*. Association of nonalcoholic fatty liver disease with insulin resistance. *Am J Med* 1999; **107**: 450–5.

54 Katsuki A, Sumida Y, Urakawa H, *et al*. Neither homeostasis model assessment nor quantitative insulin sensitivity check index can predict insulin resistance in elderly patients with poorly controlled type 2 diabetes mellitus. *J Clin Endocrinol Metab* 2002; **87**: 5332–5.

55 Ferrara CM Goldberg AP. Limited value of the homeostasis model assessment to predict insulin resistance in older men with impaired glucose tolerance. *Diabetes Care* 2001; **24**: 245–9.

56 Marchesini G, Brizi M, Bianchi G, *et al*. Nonalcoholic fatty liver disease: a feature of the metabolic syndrome. *Diabetes* 2001; **50**: 1–7.

57 Sanyal A, Campbell-Sargent C, Clore J. Non-alcoholic steatohepatitis: association of insulin resistance and mitochondrial abnormalities. *Gastroenterology* 2001; **120**: 1183–92.

58 Hundal R, Krssak M, Dufour S, *et al*. Mechanism by which metformin reduces glucose production in type 2 diabetes. *Diabetes* 2000; **49**: 2063–9.

59 Lin HZ, Yang SQ, Chuckaree C, *et al*. Metformin reverses fatty liver disease in obese, leptin-deficient mice. *Nat Med* 2000; **6**: 998–1003.

60 Marchesini G, Brizi M, Bianchi G, *et al*. Metformin in non-alcoholic steatohepatitis. *Lancet* 2001; **358**: 893–4.

61 Maggs DG, Buchanan TA, Burant CF, *et al*. Metabolic effects of troglitazone monotherapy in type 2 diabetes mellitus: a randomized, double-blind, placebo-controlled trial. *Ann Intern Med* 1998; **128**: 176–85.

62 Mayerson AB, Hundal RS, Dufour S. *et al*. The effects of rosiglitazone on insulin sensitivity, lipolysis, and hepatic and skeletal muscle triglyceride content in patients with type 2 diabetes. *Diabetes* 2002; **51**: 797–802.

63 Miyazaki Y, Mahankali A, Matsuda M, *et al*. Effect of pioglitazone on abdominal fat distribution and insulin sensitivity in type 2 diabetic patients. *J Clin Endocrinol Metab* 2002; **87**: 2784–91.

5 NASH as part of the metabolic (insulin resistance) syndrome

Giulio Marchesini & Elisabetta Bugianesi

Key learning points

1 Insulin resistance is the common factor among the metabolic conditions now characterized as the insulin resistance syndrome or as more recently termed the metabolic syndrome.

2 The best working definition of the metabolic syndrome is the presence of at least 3 of the following conditions (defined using standardized criteria): central obesity, elevated fasting blood glucose, hypertension, hypertriglyceridemia, and decreased high density lipoproteins.

3 Non-alcoholic fatty liver disease (NAFLD) can now be considered the hepatic component of the metabolic syndrome.

4 The presence of the metabolic syndrome is associated with non-alcoholic steatohepatitis and advanced fibrosis among NAFLGD patients.

5 The same lifestyle interventions proven effective for the other diseases associated with the metabolic syndrome may also be effective for NAFLD/NASH.

Abstract

Non-alcoholic fatty liver disease (NAFLD) and its more serious form non-alcoholic steatohepatitis (NASH) are associated with several diseases (obesity, type 2 diabetes, dyslipidaemia and hypertension), with insulin resistance being the common factor. These conditions cluster to form the 'insulin resistance syndrome' or, according to a recent proposal, the 'metabolic syndrome', carrying a high risk for cardiovascular complications. NASH itself, as well as pure fatty liver, is an insulin-resistant state, not only in subjects with additional metabolic disorders, but also in lean normoglycaemic patients. The prevalence of the metabolic syndrome, according to well-defined criteria, is higher in NAFLD patients compared with the general population. NAFLD patients with the metabolic syndrome have a higher prevalence and severity of fibrosis and necroinflammatory activity, compared to subjects with pure fatty liver. The presence of the metabolic syndrome is associated with a high risk of NASH among NAFLD subjects, after correction for sex, age and body mass. In particular, it is associated with a high risk of severe fibrosis. The increasing prevalence of obesity, coupled with diabetes, dyslipidaemia, hypertension and the metabolic syndrome puts a very large population at risk for succumbing to liver failure in the next decades. Because treatment with lifestyle interventions have proven effective in the metabolic diseases associated with the metabolic syndrome, studies with similar lifestyle interventions in NASH are eagerly awaited.

Introduction

Since the first description of NASH was made in 1980, a close association with clinical and laboratory findings indicative of insulin resistance has been reported. The relevance of the metabolic disorders associated with NAFLD has changed from an occasional and incidental finding to the view that these disorders may be involved in the pathophysiology of NAFLD. In this chapter we review the evidence supporting a causative role for insulin resistance in the histological spectrum of NAFLD, ranging from isolated steatosis to NASH.

Association of fatty liver with metabolic disorders

Most cases of NAFLD occur in patients with obesity (60–95%), type 2 diabetes mellitus (28–55%) and hyperlipidaemia (27–92%). These metabolic conditions are well-known risk factors for 'primary NAFLD', occurring independently from other causes of fatty liver such as pharmacological treatment, intravenous infusions and surgical procedures.

The prevalence of NAFLD in obesity is particularly relevant. The spreading of obesity as a worldwide epidemic [1] puts millions of people at risk of developing progressive liver disease in the next few decades (see Chapter 3). Very recent data are dramatic. In 1 year (from 2000 to 2001), the prevalence of obesity (BMI $\geq$ 30 kg/m^2) increased in the USA by 5.6% (by more than 1% of the total population) [2]. In severe obesity, the prevalence of liver abnormalities is virtually the rule. In 551 patients undergoing bariatric surgery, the prevalence of fatty liver was 86%, fibrosis was observed in 74% and mild necroinflammation in 24% [3]. The risk of steatosis was higher in men, and increased exponentially with additional metabolic disorders (impaired glucose tolerance, hypertension, dyslipidaemia). In over-weight or obese patients with abnormal liver function tests and no evidence of overt liver disease, liver biopsy revealed septal fibrosis in 30%, including cirrhosis in 10% [4]. A score combining body mass index (BMI), age, alanine aminotransferase and triglyceride levels was predictive of septal fibrosis. Dixon *et al.* [5] confirmed the high prevalence of fibrosis in severe obesity, and found that a quantitative index of insulin resistance (homoeostasis model

assessment [HOMA]) was highly predictive of NASH. Obese women are also at risk of developing subacute liver failure, and there is evidence of a possible underlying NASH in a few cases [6].

The prevalence of diabetes also is increasing. In 1 year, the prevalence increased in the USA by 0.6% of the total population (from 7.3 to 7.9%), an increase of 8.2% [2], and projections for the next decades are dramatic. In older studies of patients with diabetes, fatty liver was present at histological examination in 50% of cases [7], but no recent data are available. Ultrasonographical evidence of 'bright' liver is virtually the rule, but the technique is not specific enough for epidemiological studies (see Chapter 3). No systematic study of liver biopsy has ever been performed in type 2 diabetic patients with abnormal liver function tests (elevated aminotransferase), although epidemiological studies suggest that liver disease may be an important cause of death in diabetes. In a cohort of patients with type 2 diabetes, the standardized mortality rates for liver cirrhosis were exceedingly high (odds ratio [OR], 2.52; 95% confidence interval [CI], 1.96–3.20), and significantly contributed to overall mortality [8].

Obesity and diabetes may exert an additive or, more probably, a synergistic effect on the risk of hyperlipidaemia, thereby increasing the prevalence of cardiovascular disease.

In most studies, NAFLD is not to limited to subjects with metabolic disorders, but a subset of apparently lean patients without evidence of diabetes or dyslipidaemia is invariably reported; in one study nearly all of these had central obesity [10]. This consideration underscores the possible existence of an inherited or acquired metabolic disturbance, which is probably amplified by high-risk lifestyle behaviours. These patients pose a particular challenge from both a diagnostic and therapeutic standpoint.

NAFLD and measurement of insulin resistance

Several methods are available for a quantitative assessment of insulin resistance, which prove that NAFLD is significantly associated with reduced biological effects of endogenous as well as exogenous insulin (Table 5.1).

In epidemiological studies, insulin resistance was quantified by the HOMA technique. The method, based

Table 5.1 Quantitative studies of insulin resistance in NAFLD.

Author	Reference	Method
Marchesini *et al.* (1999)	[9]	HOMA
Dixon *et al.* (2001)	[5]	HOMA
Chitturi *et al.* (2002)	[10]	HOMA
Facchini *et al.* (2002)	[29]	HOMA
Comert *et al.* (2001)	[13]	Euglycaemic clamp
Marchesini *et al.* (2001)	[14]	Euglycaemic clamp
Sanyal *et al.* (2001)	[15]	Two-step euglycaemic clamp
Vanni *et al.* (2001)	[16]	Two-step euglycaemic clamp (Abstract)
Pagano *et al.* (2002)	[11]	Frequently-sampled intravenous glucose tolerance test

HOMA, homoeostasis model assessment. Note that in a few studies HOMA was coupled with the quantitative insulin sensitivity check index (QUICKI) method, based on the log transformed insulin-glucose product.

on a complex theoretical concept, derives insulin resistance from the simple product of fasting glucose (in mmol/L) and insulin (in μU/mL). In 1999, Marchesini *et al.* [9] found that HOMA insulin resistance was nearly doubled in 46 NAFLD cases, compared to 92 matched controls. This difference was entirely a result of increased insulin concentration, with normal or near-normal glucose levels. Stepwise logistic regression analysis identified insulin resistance as the best predictive index for classifying patients with NAFLD. When coupled with fasting triglyceride concentrations, 180-min blood glucose and average insulin concentrations in response to oral glucose, HOMA contributed to a model correctly classifying 41 of 46 patients with NAFLD and 89 of 92 control subjects.

Because of the relatively greater importance of insulin concentrations over glucose levels, the sole measurement of insulin may also be indicative of insulin resistance in non-diabetic patients. These results were confirmed by Chitturi *et al.* [10], who examined 66 patients with biopsy-proven NASH. According to their study, insulin resistance (measured by HOMA) is an essential requirement of NASH, independent of the degree of obesity (but note the high frequency of central obesity). In addition, nearly all NASH patients fulfilled minimal criteria for the insulin resistance syndrome. When compared to a control group with chronic hepatitis C, matched for age, sex and severity of fibrosis, the measure of insulin resistance was significantly higher in NASH patients.

Pagano *et al.* [11] measured insulin sensitivity by means of the frequently-sampled intravenous glucose

tolerance test in 19 NASH patients without obesity or overt diabetes. Reduced insulin sensitivity was present in the majority of cases, and nearly half fulfilled two criteria for the diagnosis of the metabolic syndrome, according to the European Group for the Study of Insulin Resistance (see below) [12].

The euglycaemic clamp technique remains the gold standard for the quantitative measurement of insulin sensitivity (see Chapter 4). When coupled with stable isotopes, it gives clues to the site of insulin resistance (hepatic versus peripheral tissues). Four clamp studies confirmed that insulin resistance is the rule in NAFLD, with minor differences in the final message (Table 5.2) [13–16]. The amount of glucose infused to maintain euglycaemia during the clamp study, proportional to the insulin-mediated glucose disposal by muscle tissue, is reduced by nearly 50% in NAFLD patients, to an extent similar to that observed in patients with type 2 diabetes. Data do not change when studies are limited to NAFLD subjects with normal weight, glucose regulation and lipid levels (triglycerides and high-density lipoprotein [HDL] cholesterol), but total glucose disposal shows an inverse correlation with basal plasma insulin levels [16]. In addition, the insulin-mediated suppression of lipolysis also is less effective (−69% in NAFLD versus −84% in controls), to a degree similar for the insulin-mediated suppression of hepatic glucose production (−63% in NAFLD versus −84% in controls) [14]. The latter defect is not present in lean NAFLD subjects with normal lipid profile and glucose tolerance [16]; notably, these patients show a reduced suppression of C-peptide levels during the clamp,

Table 5.2 Comparison of clamp studies in NAFLD.

	Comert et al. [13]	Marchesini et al. [14]	Sanyal et al. [15]	Vanni et al. [16]
Total glucose disposal	−35%	−50%	−45% in NASH −33% in fatty liver	−45%
HGP	–	Normal	–	Normal
Glucose oxidation	–	–	Decreased in NASH vs. fatty liver	Decreased
Insulin-mediated suppression of HGP	–	Defective	–	Normal
Free fatty acid levels	–	+20%	Normal or elevated	Normal
Glycerol levels	–	–	↑50%	+40%
Lipolysis	–	–	Increased in NASH vs. fatty liver	+40%
Lipid oxidation	–	–	Increased in NASH vs. fatty liver	+20%
Insulin-mediated suppression of lipolysis	–	Defective	Defective	Defective
Additional results	–	1 Data similar to type 2 diabetes 2 Correlation with waist girth 3 Also present in lean subjects	1 NASH correlates with microcristalline inclusions	1 LDL-cholesterol particles more susceptible to oxidation

HGP, hepatic glucose production; LDL, low-density lipoprotein.
+ and − indicate differences versus controls, when not otherwise specified.

suggesting an initial impairment in the feedback regulation of the pancreatic β-cell insulin secretion.

When tracer glycerol is added to tracer glucose, the effects of insulin resistance on lipid metabolism can also be quantified. In the presence of insulin resistance, the antilipolytic effect of insulin on adipose tissue should be reduced, leading to an increased free fatty acid (FFA) flux. Remarkably, not only are FFA concentrations high after an overnight fast, but also they fail to suppress appropriately after meals, in spite of elevated or high-normal postprandial insulin levels. In addition to exacerbating the insulin resistance in muscle, this hyperlipidaemia can influence liver function and give rise to intrahepatic fat accumulation. This is particularly so when the FFA arise from expanded visceral fat stores, which pour large amounts of FFA in the portal circulation.

The rate of appearance of glycerol provides a quantitative reflection of lipolytic activity in adipose tissue, because glycerol is assumed to arise predominantly from adipose tissue lipolysis. FFA released in excess during lipolysis can be either oxidized or utilized in the liver. Their role is to provide hepatic energy needs and to serve as substrate for ketone body production. They are also used for re-esterification and delivery of triglycerides into the circulation as very-low-density lipoproteins (VLDL).

Sanyal et al. [15] found a progression in the severity of insulin resistance on glucose metabolism from the stage of pure fatty liver to NASH, whereas the effects on lipid metabolism were less clear. Both glucose oxidation and glycogen synthesis were found to be reduced in lean as well as obese NAFLD patients, compared to healthy subjects. Insulin-mediated suppression of fatty acid and glycerol levels were generally reduced, but lipid oxidation was increased only in NASH. β-Hydroxybutyrate levels increased stepwise with increasing insulin infusion rates, indicating that the hepatic fatty acid oxidation was also increased.

Table 5.3 Metabolic features of insulin resistance in various clinical disorders.

	NAFLD	Cirrhosis	Obesity	Type 2 diabetes
Total glucose disposal	↓	↓	↓	↓
Glucose oxidation	↓	↔	↓	↓
Non-oxidative glucose disposal	↓	↓	↓	↓
Suppression of hepatic glucose output	↓ ↔	↔	↓	↓
Suppression of lipolysis	↓	↔	↓	↓
Insulin secretion	↑	↑	↑	↓↑

The pattern of insulin resistance so far described in NAFLD patients is more like that observed in patients with type 2 diabetes or in their relatives, than in patients with cirrhosis. Non-diabetic patients with cirrhosis are characterized by hyperinsulinaemia, both in the fasting state and following glucose load, but basal endogenous glucose production is normal, and is normally suppressed by insulin. In contrast, both diabetic and NAFLD patients have a blunted insulin-mediated suppression of hepatic glucose production and decreased rates of both oxidative and non-oxidative (glycogen synthesis) glucose metabolism.

The derangement in lipid metabolism so far described is to be expected in NAFLD patients with obesity or hypertriglyceridaemia, but it is still present when these confounding factors are absent. In a selected population of lean NAFLD patients with normal glucose tolerance and lipid levels, lipolysis was increased by approximately 40% in the basal state and less efficiently inhibited after insulin administration. Although the percentage decrease of glycerol turnover was comparable to controls after insulin administration (−62%), its absolute value remained higher in NAFLD patients (Bugianesi et al., personal communication). Likewise, lipid oxidation was higher in the basal state and less efficiently inhibited by insulin. The pattern of metabolic defects in non-obese non-diabetic NAFLD patients is thus consistent with accelerated lipolysis —the immediate result of insulin resistance in adipose tissue—being responsible for the increased FFA supply and their oxidative use at the whole body level. The finding of a tight correlation between lipid oxidation and glucose production/disposal, may suggest that the hepatic and peripheral insulin resistance in these NAFLD patients was primarily the consequence of insulin resistance in fat tissues.

The main source of increased lipid turnover in NAFLD patients is not clear. However, an important role for visceral adiposity has been proposed. It is generally accepted that visceral adipose tissue is more insulin-resistant than subcutaneous adipose tissue [17], and people with increased visceral fat are characterized by a more severe deterioration of their lipid profile [18]. The association of NAFLD with central adiposity and increased lipolysis, as assessed by anthropometric measurements [10,14], needs to be confirmed by a quantitative nuclear magnetic resonance (NMR) assessment of visceral fat.

Finally, the role of insulin resistance in NAFLD is supported by pilot therapeutic studies. Troglitazone, an insulin-sensitizing drug, significantly reduces transaminase levels, with inconclusive results on liver histology [19] (but see Chapter 24). In an animal model of NASH in obese leptin-deficient mice [20] and in humans [21], metformin reduces transaminase levels, which return to normal in approximately 50% of cases. Metformin also improves other metabolic abnormalities associated with the insulin resistance syndrome [22].

In summary, a large body of evidence indicates that NAFLD may stem from a defect of insulin activity, involving both glucose and lipid metabolism, which explains the link with the associated metabolic disorders. In the scenario of metabolic and liver disease, NAFLD looks very much like type 2 diabetes and obesity, but also shares features common to more advanced liver disease (Table 5.3). However, the defects are not necessarily linked to the presence of obesity and diabetes. Lean subjects with normal fasting glucose and normal glucose tolerance may also present with NAFLD. These subjects are nevertheless characterized by enlarged waist girth, and possibly belong to the subgroup of normal-weight metabolically obese patients (usually with central obesity, see Chapter 18), a phenotype more frequently observed in subjects of Asian descent. Considering the importance of lifestyle behaviours in the pathogenesis of metabolic disorders, lean NAFLD patients might be subjects with a primary (genetic?) defect of insulin activity, where healthy lifestyles have not yet permitted the expression of the usual phenotype of the insulin resistance syndrome.

Iron and the insulin resistance syndrome

Iron deposition has long been known to cause clinical and laboratory findings similar to those observed in the insulin resistance syndrome. Moirand *et al.* [23] described a syndrome characterized by increased serum iron and liver iron deposition, associated with abnormal glucose tolerance, overweight or obesity, dyslipidaemia and insulin resistance. Patients were predominantly male and middle-aged, with a slightly increased prevalence of the compound heterozygote *HFE* mutation C282Y/H63D. Steatosis was present in 25% of patients and NASH in 27%. Portal fibrosis (grades 0–3) was present in 62% of patients (grade 2 or 3 in 12%) in association with steatosis, inflammation and increased age. This syndrome, insulin resistance-associated hepatic iron overload (IRHIO), occurs both in the absence and in the presence of increased transferrin saturation and serum ferritin and is frequently associated with NASH [24].

This association stimulated research on the possible role of iron in the pathogenesis of NASH. Iron is an ideal culprit for fatty liver disease. Iron deposition in genetic haemochromatosis is associated with insulin resistance and diabetes mellitus. Iron is a potent oxidative agent and might trigger oxidative stress with resultant liver injury. The relationship between hepatic iron overload and hyperinsulinaemia and/or insulin resistance may be twofold. Transferrin receptors, glucose transporters and insulin-like growth factor II receptors co-localize in cultured adipocytes, and are simultaneously regulated by insulin. Any genetic or acquired condition characterized by increased serum and liver iron is expected to downregulate glucose transporters, leading to hyperinsulinaemia and insulin resistance. Alternatively, if insulin resistance and hyperinsulinaemia were the primary defects, alterations in iron metabolism would be expected [25].

An increased peripheral iron burden has also been reported in other conditions characterized by insulin resistance. In males, hypertension is characterized by a higher prevalence of increased iron stores and metabolic abnormalities that are part of the IRHIO syndrome [26]. The prevalence of IRHIO among type 2 diabetic patients is as high as 40%, and can be associated with a higher prevalence of steatosis and inflammation [27]. Iron depletion improves metabolic control and insulin sensitivity [28]. A similar improvement in insulin sensitivity has been observed in obese subjects with impaired glucose tolerance [29].

The hypothesis that iron might be the cause of NASH has received much attention, but available data do not completely support this conclusion (Table 5.4). A large proportion of NAFLD patients have no evidence of hepatic iron overload, and no differences are present in clinical features in relation to iron status [30]. In addition, iron status does not classify patients according to the histological severity of their liver disease [31], and serum indices of iron overload do not correlate with measures of insulin sensitivity [14]. However, recent data do suggest that iron may have a role; iron depletion to a level of near-iron deficiency by quantitative phlebotomy produces a near normalization of alanine aminotransaminase and a marked reduction of fasting and glucose-stimulated insulin. Also, HOMA values were reduced in most cases, but did not return to normal values [29]. (The potential role of iron as a factor determining fibrotic severity of NASH is discussed in Chapters 1 and 7.)

Insulin resistance, oxidative stress and cytokines

The role of iron, if present, might be mediated by oxidative stress, which might also be generated by different conditions. Insulin resistance is an atherogenic state, characterized by oxidative changes of circulating low-density lipoprotein (LDL) cholesterol particles, induced by an excessive activity of free radicals [32], and a role for hyperinsulinaemia is suggested. Quinones-Galvan *et al.* [33] demonstrated that acute physiological hyperinsulinaemia enhances the oxidative susceptibility of LDL-cholesterol particles and reduces the vitamin E content in the LDL molecule. These changes are well characterized in type 2 diabetes, but they may also be present in hyperinsulinaemic

Table 5.4 Pros and cons for a role of iron in the insulin-resistance syndrome and NASH.

Pros	Cons
1 Iron overload is associated with insulin-resistance	1 A poor correlation exists between *HFE* mutations and iron stores
2 A link at subcellular level connects transferrin receptors and glucose transporters	2 In NASH, iron overload is not associated with a higher prevalence of features of the metabolic syndrome
3 Serum and liver iron are frequently increased in NASH patients	3 Iron status does not classify patients according to the severity of liver disease
4 Serum iron is increased in hypertension and diabetes	4 Indices of iron overload do not correlate with quantitative measures of insulin resistance
5 Iron depletion improves diabetes control	
6 Iron depletion reduces transaminase levels in obese subjects with impaired glucose tolerance	

normoglycaemic conditions, such as obesity, essential hypertension and dyslipidaemia. Human liver biopsy specimens, when assessed for lipid peroxidation by staining for 3-nitrotyrosine, showed higher levels of lipid peroxidation in NASH relative to fatty liver and controls [15]. The levels of thiobarbituric acid reactive substances (TBARS), a gross measure of lipid peroxidation, also are increased in NAFLD.

Finally, insulin resistance might stem from cytokine activation. In animal models, the chronic activation of IKKβ, the kinase that activates nuclear factor β, is associated with the presence of insulin resistance. Conversely, the administration of salicylate to inhibit IKKβ abolishes lipid-induced insulin resistance in the skeletal muscle of animals [34]. Cytokines might represent the link between insulin resistance and oxidative stress. Oxidant and inflammatory stresses are powerful activators of the IKKβ pathway, possibly via tumour necrosis factor α (TNF-α), suggesting a direct link between oxidative stress and insulin resistance. Whether treatment with antioxidants (e.g. vitamin E) might improve insulin sensitivity remains to be proven.

Definition of the metabolic syndrome

The clustering of metabolic disorders had been known for a long time before Avogaro *et al.* [35] first reported the association of obesity, hyperlipidaemia and diabetes in 1967. Hypertension is also frequently present.

These features are independently related to cardiovascular mortality, which has given rise to the name of 'deadly quartet' for this syndrome [36].

In 1988, Gerald Reaven proposed the term 'syndrome X' [37] to define the contemporary presence of diabetes and/or impaired glucose tolerance, hypertriglyceridaemia, low HDL-cholesterol and hypertension. He pointed out the role of hyperinsulinaemia and insulin resistance in the pathogenesis of the disease [37]. The metabolic disorder is probably much wider and other features might be added. Most subjects have evidence of additional metabolic disorders (elevated urate concentrations, impaired fibrinolysis and endothelial dysfunction).

The primary role of hyperinsulinaemia is supported by several cross-sectional and longitudinal studies [38]. Central obesity, type 2 diabetes, hyperlipidaemia and hypertension are all characterized by raised insulin concentrations, and elevated insulin levels predict the development of the metabolic disorder [39]. Accordingly, DeFronzo and Ferrannini [40] proposed the term 'insulin resistance syndrome' to define this clustering of diseases.

The borders of the syndrome remain difficult to define. The critical number of metabolic disorders to define the syndrome has not been specified; the disorders may progressively develop over the course of time, with obesity usually occurring first, followed by hyperlipidaemia and diabetes. Hypertension may frequently be present independently from other components. In addition, the 'normal' limits for the individual disorders have been repeatedly changed in the last few years, so as to prevent a clear-cut assessment.

The first attempt to define the metabolic syndrome came from the World Health Organization (WHO). The expert committee setting new criteria for the definition of diabetes proposed a classification based on the presence of one out of two necessary conditions (altered glucose regulation and insulin resistance), coupled with two additional features (Table 5.5) [41]. These criteria may be easily applied to diabetic populations, but are not useful in a general setting. The assessment of insulin resistance requires complex techniques. Surrogate markers (fasting insulin, HOMA values), although validated by correlation analysis [42], have no defined 'normal' limits.

New criteria were defined by the European Group for Insulin Resistance in 1999, limiting the syndrome to non-diabetic subjects [12], but the critical problem of insulin resistance was not set.

In 2001 a new proposal by the Third Report of the National Cholesterol Education Expert Panel on Detection, Evaluation, and Treatment of High Blood Cholesterol in Adults (Adult Treatment Panel III, ATPIII) [43] provided a working definition of the metabolic syndrome, based on a combination of five categorical and discrete risk factors, which can easily be measured in clinical practice, and are suitable for epidemiological purposes. The limits for individual components (central obesity, hypertension, hypertriglyceridaemia, low HDL-cholesterol and hyperglycaemia) are derived from the guidelines of the international societies or the statements of WHO [1,41,43,44]. It is important to note that the anthropometric criteria vary between ethnic groups, with values being substantially lower among Asians (see Chapter 18).

NASH as part of the metabolic syndrome

A very recent study with a large number of NAFLD patients was specifically aimed at assessing the prevalence of the metabolic syndrome in relation to liver histology. In 304 consecutive NAFLD patients without overt diabetes, Marchesini *et al.* [45] defined the metabolic syndrome according to the ATPIII proposal. The population had a mean age of 41 years and a BMI of 27.5, but nearly 80% were overweight or obese. Over 80% were males. At least one criterion for the metabolic syndrome was present in 96% of females

Table 5.5 Comparison of different diagnostic criteria for the metabolic syndrome.

WHO proposal (1998, revised 1999) [41]
Altered glucose regulation
or
insulin resistance
plus
two of the following:

1 Obesity (BMI ≥ 30 kg/m^2 or WHR > 1.0 [M] or > 0.9 [F])
2 High triglycerides (> 150 mg/dL) or low HDL-cholesterol (< 35 mg/dL [M] or < 39 mg/dL [F])
3 Hypertension (≥ 140/90 mmHg)
4 Microalbuminuria (> 30 μg/min)

EGIR proposal (1999) [12]
No diabetes
Hyperinsulinaemia
or
insulin resistance
plus
two of the following:

1 Impaired fasting glucose (glucose, 110–126 mg/dL)
2 Hypertension (≥ 140/90 mmHg)
3 High triglycerides (> 175 mg/dL) or low HDL-cholesterol (< 39 mg/dL), independently of gender
4 Central obesity (waist girth ≥ 94 cm [M] or ≥ 80 cm [F])

ATP III proposal (2001) [43]
Three of the following:

1 Waist girth (> 102 cm [M] or > 88 cm [F])
2 Arterial pressure (≥ 130/85 mmHg)
3 Triglycerides (≥ 150 mg/dL)
4 HDL-cholesterol (< 40 mg/dL [M] or < 50 mg/dL [F])
5 Glucose (≥ 110 mg/dL)

BMI, body mass index; F, female; HDL, high-density lipoprotein; M, male; WHR, waist : height ratio.

and 83% of males, and three criteria were fulfilled in 60% of females and 30% of males (Fig. 5.1). The prevalence of the metabolic syndrome increased with increasing BMI, from 18% in normal-weight subjects to 67% in obese subjects.

The presence of the metabolic syndrome was significantly associated with female gender (OR, 3.08; 95% CI, 1.57–6.02) and age (OR, 1.54; 1.23–1.93 per 10 years) after adjustment for BMI class. The presence of impaired fasting glucose (blood glucose ≥ 110 mg/dL)

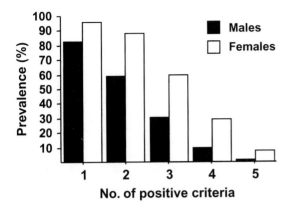

Fig. 5.1 Frequency of criteria for the metabolic syndrome (ATPIII proposal—Expert Panel on Detection, Evaluation and Treatment of High Blood Cholesterol in Adults [43]) in NAFLD patients according to gender. Note that the presence of three or more criteria defines the metabolic syndrome.

was the most predictive criterion for the metabolic syndrome (OR, 18.9; 6.8–52.7) also in this non-diabetic population. Insulin resistance (HOMA method) was significantly associated with the metabolic syndrome (OR, 2.5; 1.5–4.2; $P < 0.001$).

Liver biopsy was available in over 50% of cases, and histology was diagnostic for NASH in 74% of cases. At least one criterion for the metabolic syndrome was fulfilled in 88% of NASH patients and only in 67% of fatty liver ($P = 0.004$; Fisher's exact test). This agrees almost exactly with an earlier study in which 85% of patients with histological NASH had WHO criteria for the metabolic syndrome [10].

NASH patients were characterized by more severe liver cell necrosis, measured by 20% higher alanine and aspartate aminotransferase levels. Of the five criteria for the metabolic syndrome, only hyperglycaemia and/or diabetes was significantly associated with NASH after correction for age, gender and obesity, but the simultaneous presence of three or more criteria (a defined metabolic syndrome) was associated with a different histopathological grading, including a higher prevalence (94% versus 54%) and severity of fibrosis ($P = 0.0005$) as well as of necroinflammatory activity (97% versus 82%; $P = 0.031$), without differences in the degree of fat infiltration (Fig. 5.2). Logistical regression analysis showed that the presence of the metabolic syndrome was associated with a high risk of NASH among NAFLD subjects (OR, 3.2; 1.2–8.9;

$P = 0.026$), after correction for sex, age and body mass. In particular, the metabolic syndrome was associated with a high risk of severe fibrosis (bridging or cirrhosis: OR, 3.5; 1.1–11.2; $P = 0.032$), without differences in the degree of steatosis and necroinflammatory activity.

The study indicates that the presence of multiple metabolic disorders is associated with a potentially progressive, more severe liver disease.

Conclusions

The increasing prevalence of obesity, coupled with diabetes, dyslipidaemia, hypertension and ultimately the metabolic syndrome puts a very large population at risk of developing liver failure in the coming decades. All these diseases have insulin resistance as a common factor, and are associated with atherosclerosis and cardiovascular risk. The occurrence of diabetes may be prevented by adequate lifestyle interventions [46–48], and recent evidence indicates that the progression of the disease and its complications may also be reduced by these same lifestyle interventions [49]. Additional studies are now needed to verify the effectiveness of lifestyle changes in the progression of fatty liver to NASH and/or cirrhosis. Pilot studies support a beneficial effect [50] (and see Chapter 24).

References

1 World Health Organization. *Preventing and Managing the Global Epidemic: Report of a WHO Consultation.* World Health Organization, WHO Technical Report Series 894, 2000.

2 Mokdad AH, Ford ES, Bowman BA *et al.* Prevalence of obesity, diabetes, and obesity-related health risk factors, 2001. *J Am Med Assoc* 2003; **289**: 76–9.

3 Marceau P, Biron S, Hould FS *et al.* Liver pathology and the metabolic syndrome X in severe obesity. *J Clin Endocrinol Metab* 1999; **84**: 1513–7.

4 Ratziu V, Giral P, Charlotte F *et al.* Liver fibrosis in overweight patients. *Gastroenterology* 2000; **118**: 1117–23.

5 Dixon JB, Bhathal PS, O'Brien PE. Non-alcoholic fatty liver disease: predictors of non-alcoholic steatohepatitis and liver fibrosis in the severely obese. *Gastroenterology* 2001; **121**: 91–100.

6 Caldwell SH, Hespenheide EE. Subacute liver failure in obese women. *Am J Gastroenterol* 2002; **97**: 2058–62.

7 Creutzfeldt W, Frerichs H, Sickinger K. Liver diseases and diabetes mellitus. *Prog Liver Dis* 1970; **3**: 371–407.

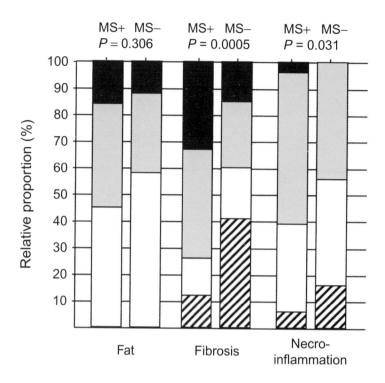

Fig. 5.2 Proportion of patients with histological lesions in relation to the presence (MS+) or absence (MS−) of the metabolic syndrome (ATPIII proposal—Expert Panel on Detection, Evaluation and Treatment of High Blood Cholesterol in Adults [43]). *Fat:* open area, mild fat infiltration (< 33% of liver cells); grey area, moderate fat infiltration (33–66%); black area, severe fat infiltration (> 66%). *Fibrosis:* dashed area, no fibrosis; open area perisinusoidal/pericellular fibrosis; grey area, periportal fibrosis; black area, bridging fibrosis or cirrhosis. *Necroinflammation:* dashed area, no necroinflammation; open area, occasional ballooned hepatocytes and no or very mild inflammation; grey area, ballooning of hepatocytes and mild to moderate portal inflammation; black area, intra-acinar and portal inflammation. The significance of differences is reported (Fisher's exact test).

8 de Marco R, Locatelli F, Zoppini G *et al.* Cause-specific mortality in type 2 diabetes: the Verona Diabetes Study. *Diabetes Care* 1999; **22**: 756–61.

9 Marchesini G, Brizi M, Morselli-Labate AM *et al.* Association of non-alcoholic fatty liver disease with insulin resistance. *Am J Med* 1999; **107**: 450–5.

10 Chitturi S, Abeygunasekera S, Farrell GC *et al.* NASH and insulin resistance: insulin secretion and specific association with the insulin resistance syndrome. *Hepatology* 2002; **35**: 373–9.

11 Pagano G, Pacini G, Musso G *et al.* Non-alcoholic steatohepatitis, insulin resistance, and metabolic syndrome: further evidence for an etiologic association. *Hepatology* 2002; **35**: 367–72.

12 Balkau B, Charles MA, for the European Group for the Study of Insulin Resistance (EGIR). Comment on the provisional report from the WHO consultation. *Diabetes Med* 1999; **16**: 442–3.

13 Comert B, Mas MR, Erdem H *et al.* Insulin resistance in non-alcoholic steatohepatitis. *Dig Liver Dis* 2001; **33**: 353–8.

14 Marchesini G, Brizi M, Bianchi G *et al.* Non-alcoholic fatty liver disease: a feature of the metabolic syndrome. *Diabetes* 2001; **50**: 1844–50.

15 Sanyal AJ, Campbell-Sargent C, Mirshahi F *et al.* Non-alcoholic steatohepatitis: association of insulin resist-ance and mitochondrial abnormalities. *Gastroenterology* 2001; **120**: 1183–92.

16 Vanni E, Bugianesi E, Gastaldelli A *et al.* Insulin resistance is an independent defect in non-alcoholic steatohepatitis (NASH). *Hepatology* 2001; **34** (suppl.): 361A.

17 Lefebvre AM, Laville M, Vega N *et al.* Depot-specific differences in adipose tissue gene expression in lean and obese subjects. *Diabetes* 1998; **47**: 98–103.

18 Walton C, Lees B, Crook D *et al.* Body fat distribution, rather than overall adiposity, influences serum lipids and lipoproteins in healthy men independently of age. *Am J Med* 1995; **99**: 459–64.

19 Caldwell SH, Hespenheide EE, Redick JA *et al.* A pilot study of a thiazolidinedione, troglitazone, in non-alcoholic steatohepatitis. *Am J Gastroenterol* 2001; **96**: 519–25.

20 Lin HZ, Yang SQ, Chuckaree C *et al.* Metformin reverses fatty liver disease in obese, leptin-deficient mice. *Nat Med* 2000; **6**: 998–1003.

21 Marchesini G, Brizi M, Bianchi G *et al.* Metformin in non-alcoholic steatohepatitis. *Lancet* 2001; **358**: 893–4.

22 Mather KJ, Verma S, Anderson TJ. Improved endothelial function with metformin in type 2 diabetes mellitus. *J Am Coll Cardiol* 2001; **37**: 1344–50.

23 Moirand R, Mortaji AM, Loreal O *et al.* A new syndrome of liver iron overload with normal transferrin saturation. *Lancet* 1997; **349**: 95–7.

24 Mendler MH, Turlin B, Moirand R *et al.* Insulin resistance-associated hepatic iron overload. *Gastroenterology* 1999; **117**: 1155–63.

25 Ferrannini E. Insulin resistance, iron, and the liver. *Lancet* 2000; **355**: 2181–2.

26 Piperno A, Trombini P, Gelosa M *et al.* Increased serum ferritin is common in men with essential hypertension. *J Hypertens* 2002; **20**: 1513–8.

27 Turlin B, Mendler MH, Moirand R *et al.* Histologic features of the liver in insulin resistance-associated iron overload: a study of 139 patients. *Am J Clin Pathol* 2001; **116**: 263–70.

28 Fernandez-Real JM, Penarroja G, Castro A, Garcia-Bragado F, Hernandez-Aguado I, Ricart W. Blood letting in high-ferritin type 2 diabetes: effects on insulin sensitivity and β-cell function. *Diabetes* 2002; **51**: 1000–4.

29 Facchini FS, Hua NW, Stoohs RA. Effect of iron depletion in carbohydrate-intolerant patients with clinical evidence of non-alcoholic fatty liver disease. *Gastroenterology* 2002; **122**: 931–9.

30 George DK, Goldwurm S, McDonald GA *et al.* Increased hepatic iron concentration in non-alcoholic steatohepatitis is associated with increased fibrosis. *Gastroenterology* 1998; **114**: 311–8.

31 Matteoni CA, Younossi ZM, Gramlich T *et al.* Non-alcoholic fatty liver disease: a spectrum of clinical and pathological severity. *Gastroenterology* 1999; **116**: 1413–9.

32 Bucala R, Makita Z, Koschinsky T, Cerami A, Vlassara H. Lipid advanced glycosylation: pathway for lipid oxidation *in vivo*. *Proc Natl Acad Sci USA* 1993; **90**: 6434–8.

33 Quinones-Galvan A, Sironi AM, Baldi S *et al.* Evidence that acute insulin administration enhances LDL cholesterol susceptibility to oxidation in healthy humans. *Arterioscler Thromb Vasc Biol* 1999; **19**: 2928–32.

34 Yuan M, Konstantopoulos N, Lee J *et al.* Reversal of obesity- and diet-induced insulin resistance with salicylates or targeted disruption of IKKβ. *Science* 2001; **293**: 1673–7.

35 Avogaro P, Crepaldi G, Enzi G, Tiengo A. Associazione di iperlipemia, diabete mellito e obesità di medio grado. *Acta Diabetol Lat* 1967; **4**: 572–90.

36 Kaplan NM. The deadly quartet: upper-body obesity, glucose intolerance, hypertriglyceridemia, and hypertension. *Arch Intern Med* 1989; **149**: 1514–20.

37 Reaven GM. (Banting Lecture 1988) Role of insulin resistance in human disease. *Diabetes* 1988; **37**: 1595–607.

38 Schmidt MI, Watson RL, Duncan BB *et al.* Clustering of dyslipidemia, hyperuricemia, diabetes, and hypertension and its association with fasting insulin and central and overall obesity in a general population. *Metabolism* 1996; **45**: 699–706.

39 Haffner SM, Valdez RA, Hazuda HP *et al.* Prospective analysis of the insulin-resistance syndrome (syndrome X). *Diabetes* 1992; **41**: 715–22.

40 DeFronzo RA, Ferrannini E. Insulin resistance: a multi-faceted syndrome responsible for NIDDM, obesity, hypertension, dyslipidemia, and atherosclerotic cardiovascular disease. *Diabetes Care* 1991; **14**: 173–94.

41 WHO Consultation. *Definition, diagnosis and classification of diabetes mellitus and its complications.* World Health Organization, WHO/NCD/NCS/99.2, 1999.

42 Bonora E, Targher G, Alberiche M *et al.* Homeostasis model assessment closely mirrors the glucose clamp technique in the assessment of insulin sensitivity: studies in subjects with various degrees of glucose tolerance and insulin sensitivity. *Diabetes Care* 2000; **23**: 57–63.

43 Expert Panel on Detection Evaluation and Treatment of High Blood Cholesterol in Adults. Executive summary of the third report of the National Cholesterol Education Program (NCEP) expert panel on detection, evaluation, and treatment of high blood cholesterol in adults (Adult Treatment Panel III). *J Am Med Assoc* 2001; **285**: 2486–97.

44 Guidelines Subcommittee. 1999 World Health Organization: International Society of Hypertension Guidelines for the Management of Hypertension. *J Hypertens* 1999; **17**: 151–83.

45 Marchesini G, Bugianesi E, Forlani G *et al.* Non-alcoholic fatty liver, steatohepatitis, and the metabolic syndrome. *Hepatology* 2003; **37**: 917–23.

46 Pan XR, Li GW, Hu YH *et al.* Effects of diet and exercise in preventing NIDDM in people with impaired glucose tolerance: the Da Qing IGT and Diabetes Study. *Diabetes Care* 1997; **20**: 537–44.

47 Tuomilehto J, Lindstrom J, Eriksson JG *et al.* Prevention of type 2 diabetes mellitus by changes in lifestyle among subjects with impaired glucose tolerance. *N Engl J Med* 2001; **344**: 1343–50.

48 Knowler WC, Barrett-Connor E, Fowler SE *et al.* Reduction in the incidence of type 2 diabetes with lifestyle intervention or metformin. *N Engl J Med* 2002; **346**: 393–403.

49 Gaede P, Vedel P, Larsen N *et al.* Multifactorial intervention and cardiovascular disease in patients with type 2 diabetes. *N Engl J Med* 2003; **348**: 457–9.

50 Ueno T, Sugawara H, Sujaku K *et al.* Therapeutic effects of restricted diet and exercise in obese patients with fatty liver. *J Hepatol* 1997; **27**: 103–7.

6

NASH is a genetically determined disease

Christopher P. Day & Ann K. Daly

Key learning points

1 Only a minority of patients with risk factors for non-alcholic fatty liver disease (NAFLD) develop non-alcoholic steatohepatitis (NASH), fibrosis and cirrhosis. Family studies suggest that genetic factors may have a role in determining susceptibility to advanced disease.

2 Candidate gene, case–control allele association-based approaches are currently the best methods available for the detection of susceptibility genes, although in future genome-wide scanning may be technically and economically feasible.

3 In future, the choice of candidate genes worthy of study seems likely to be guided by tissue expression profiling and mouse mutagenesis approaches.

4 Recent studies have reported associations between steatosis severity, NASH and fibrosis with genes encoding proteins involved in lipid metabolism, oxidative stress and endotoxin-cytokine interactions.

5 If confirmed, these associations will greatly enhance our understanding of disease pathogenesis and, accordingly, our ability to design effective therapies.

Abstract

While the vast majority of individuals with obesity and type 2 diabetes mellitus will have steatosis, only a minority will ever develop non-alcoholic steatohepatitis (NASH), fibrosis and cirrhosis. Family studies suggest that genetic factors are important in disease progression, although dissecting genetic factors having a role in NASH and fibrosis from those influencing the development of its established risk factors is clearly difficult. A variety of approaches can be used to look for genetic factors having a role in NASH. In future, genome-wide single nucleotide polymorphism (SNP) scanning of cases and controls may become feasible. However, to date studies have relied on candidate gene, case–control allele association methodology. Investigators using this approach must take care to avoid a number of pitfalls in study design likely to lead to spurious results. If these can be avoided, our increased understanding of disease pathogenesis suggests a variety of candidate genes worthy of study as susceptibility factors. Recent, and as yet preliminary studies, have reported associations between steatosis severity, NASH and fibrosis with genes whose products are involved in lipid metabolism, oxidative stress and endotoxin–cytokine interactions. If confirmed, these associations will greatly enhance our understanding of disease pathogenesis and, accordingly, our ability to design effective therapies.

Introduction

Obesity and insulin resistance are undoubtedly associated with the whole spectrum of non-alcoholic fatty liver disease (NAFLD), with the degree of obesity and the severity of insulin resistance increasing the risk of advanced disease (see Chapters 3 and 4). However, despite these strong associations, it is clear that while the majority of individuals with these risk factors will have steatosis, only a minority will ever develop NASH. An autopsy study in 351 non-drinking individuals reported that, while more than 60% of obese patients with type 2 diabetes mellitus had steatosis, only 15% had NASH [1], and a recent analysis of the Third National Health and Nutritional Examination Survey (NHANES III) database reported that only 10.6% of obese individuals with type 2 diabetes mellitus had any elevation of serum alanine aminotransferase [2]. These studies suggest that while obesity and/or insulin resistance are undoubtedly involved in the pathogenesis of steatosis and NASH, some other environmental and/or combination of genetic factors is required for progression to NASH and fibrosis. This is analogous to the situation in alcoholic liver disease (ALD) where excessive drinking leads to steatosis in the majority of individuals, but other, largely unknown, factors determine why only a minority of heavy drinkers develop hepatitis and cirrhosis [3]. With respect to environmental factors influencing the risk of NASH, diet, exercise and possibly small bowel bacterial overgrowth are obvious candidates, with the latter contributing to increased hepatic levels of tumour necrosis factor-α (TNF-α) [4]. A role for genetic factors in NASH is suggested by two recent reports of family clustering. Struben et al. [5] reported the coexistence of NASH and cryptogenic cirrhosis in seven out of eight kindreds studied, while Willner et al. [6] found that 18% of 90 patients with NASH had an affected first-degree relative. The absence of these genetic factors presumably explains the benign prognosis of simple non-alcoholic fatty liver [7,8]. It remains to be determined whether this clustering of cases is simply a reflection of the well-established heritability of the established risk factors for NAFLD—obesity and insulin resistance.

Methodology for studying genes involved in NASH susceptibility

If it is assumed that there is a genetic component to NASH, what methodology is currently available to search for genetic factors predisposing to this undoubtedly polygenic disease? Methods fall into three broad and overlapping categories: family-based linkage analysis, candidate gene studies and genome-wide SNP scanning.

Family-based studies

Allele-sharing methods involve studying affected relatives in a pedigree to determine how often a particular copy of a chromosomal region is shared identical-by-descent (IBD). The frequency of IBD sharing at a particular locus can then be compared with random expectation. Typically, this has involved linkage analysis in large cohorts of affected sibling pairs using widely spaced multiallelic markers such as microsatellites to identify chromosomal regions. Unfortunately, linkage analysis, which has been so successful in identifying genes responsible for single gene disorders, has (with few notable exceptions [9]) been generally disappointing when applied to polygenic diseases, probably because of its limited power to detect genes of moderate effect [10].

Candidate gene studies

An alternative methodological approach involves the study of candidate genes. In this method, a polymorphism (or polymorphisms) is identified by various means in a 'functional' candidate gene (a gene whose product is thought to have a role in disease pathogenesis). The polymorphism is then examined for association with disease using one of two approaches: intrafamilial allelic association studies and case–control association studies. The most commonly used test for familial association is the transmission disequilibrium test (TDT), which compares the frequency with which the allele under study is transmitted to affected offspring by each parent with the frequency expected by random transmission [11]. The major limitation of TDT testing is that the index case must have at least one surviving parent from whom to collect DNA, although variations on the TDT using siblings of affected individuals (discordant sibship) have recently been proposed [12].

The value of this test is still unclear, but, as with the TDT, when the allele frequency is low, achieving statistical significance requires very large numbers of families. Even if large enough numbers of NASH families could be collected, investigators using family-based approaches to study genetic susceptibility to NASH face two further problems:

1 Since there is currently no reliable non-invasive way of accurately determining the presence or severity of NAFLD, family members will ideally require liver biopsy for definitive diagnosis.

2 Relatives must be discordant for the established risk factors for NASH, otherwise any association with NASH observed may simply reflect an association with obesity or diabetes.

In view of these difficulties, it is perhaps not surprising that, as with ALD, studies using the candidate gene approach to look for genetic factors in NASH have thus far relied on case–control methodology [12]. In this method, the frequency of the allele(s) under study is compared in cases and controls to see whether it is associated with disease. When applying this methodology to studies in NAFLD, phenotype definition in the cases and controls is particularly important because it seems highly likely that different genetic factors will determine the development of steatosis, steatohepatitis and fibrosis. For studies specifically on NASH, controls should be individuals with steatosis only, ideally matched for body mass index (BMI), age, diabetes or insulin resistance and ethnic origin to index cases. If appropriate cases and controls can be collected, a number of criteria should be applied in selecting candidate genes worthy of study:

1 The gene product must be considered to have a key role in disease pathogenesis.

2 The polymorphism must be reasonably common, occurring in at least 1 in 20 individuals in the normal 'background' population.

3 Ideally, an effect of the polymorphism on gene expression or protein structure and/or function should be established.

4 The function of the gene product and the alteration attributable to the polymorphism should lead to a plausible *a priori* hypothesis explaining a link between the polymorphism and disease pathogenesis.

Once a candidate gene polymorphism has been selected, an adequate number of cases and controls should be recruited to give the study sufficient power to detect a predetermined magnitude of difference in allele frequencies between cases and controls. Finally, whenever possible, plans should be made to seek replication of any significant associations in a distinct set of cases and controls to reduce the risk of reporting spurious or 'chance' associations [13].

Novel approaches to candidate gene selection

Two novel approaches to identifying candidate genes worthy of study in NAFLD/NASH have recently been described. The first utilizes oligonucleotide microarray ('chip') methodology to examine global gene expression in liver biopsies from patients with NAFLD. Two groups have recently presented preliminary data that several genes involved in oxidative stress, lipid metabolism and fibrosis are either up- or downregulated in patients with NASH compared to steatosis only [14], or in NASH-related cirrhosis compared to other causes of cirrhosis [15]. Whether these changes in gene expression are a primary or secondary phenomenon is, as yet, unknown. However, these studies have already suggested a number of novel candidate genes worthy of subjecting to proximal promoter SNP screening strategies. The second approach, which has yet to be applied to NAFLD, is that of phenotype-driven mouse mutagenesis [16]. In this technique, male mice are treated with the mutagen ethyl nitrosourea and their progeny are screened for dominant mutations giving rise to the phenotypical change of interest. The mutation is then mapped to a specific gene and the human homologue is screened for SNPs that are subsequently tested for disease association using standard case–control methodology.

Whole genome scanning

An alternative to this 'hypothesis-driven' methodology based on careful selection of candidate genes, driven by the availability of a comprehensive human SNP map [17], is the possibility of looking for disease associations in polygenic diseases by performing a genome-wide survey [10]. At present, genome-wide scanning is extremely expensive, but costs may fall in the future as more efficient genotyping technologies are developed and the number of SNPs requiring genotyping falls because of the availability of haplotype maps [18]. Haplotypes are defined by multiple SNPs that cosegregate (are inherited together more often than expected by chance) and are in so-called linkage disequilibrium (LD). Recent studies of haplotype structure in the human genome have shown that the genome consists of discrete 'haplotype blocks' separated by recombination hotspots [19,20]. There appear to be limited numbers of haplotypes within each block, which can therefore be defined by the analysis of relatively small numbers of diagnostic SNPs known as haplotype tagging (ht) SNPs [20,21].

Pathogenic mechanisms of NAFLD

Given the current reliance on case–control candidate gene association methodology, it is clear that a detailed knowledge of disease mechanisms is central to the design and interpretation of studies examining genetic factors determining susceptibility to NASH. The wide variety of putative disease mechanisms is covered in Chapters 6 and 7, but the scheme depicted in Fig. 6.1 provides a rational basis for considering potential candidate genes (see also review by Day [22]).

Steatosis

An increase in adipose tissue mass, particularly in central obesity, leads to an increased release of free fatty acids (FFA). This is augmented by the increased adipose tissue expression of TNF-α in obesity, which induces insulin resistance, and leads to a further increase in lipolysis. The increased supply of FFA to a still relatively insulin-sensitive liver will initially result in increased hepatic FFA esterification and lipid storage—'the first hit'. The development of steatosis is potentially facilitated by cortisol, generated via the increased 11β hydroxysteroid dehydrogenase type 1 (11β HSD-1) activity in central adipose tissue, inhibiting FFA oxidation and by adipose tissue-derived TNF-α inhibiting the activity of microsomal triglyceride transfer protein (MTP). Hepatic resistance to the effects of the adipocyte-derived hormone leptin may also be important in the development of steatosis. The principal role of leptin appears to be to protect non-adipose tissues from steatosis and lipotoxicity during caloric excess [23]. In the liver, this effect is probably mediated through inhibition of the enzyme stearoyl CoA desaturase 1 (SCD-1) [24]. Hepatic leptin resistance is suggested by the observation that obese individuals develop severe steatosis in the face of increased serum concentrations of leptin [25].

Necroinflammation

As the severity of steatosis increases, and 'lipotoxicity' develops, the liver becomes more insulin resistant, principally because of the increasing intracellular concentrations of polyunsaturated fatty acids (PUFA) and their metabolites, and possibly also because of adipose tissue-derived TNF-α activating inhibitor of κB kinase (IKK) in hepatocytes. Gut-derived endotoxin via stimulation of TNF-α release by Kupffer cells may also contribute. The incoming FFA will then be diverted into the mitochondria and oxidized by enzymes whose genes are upregulated by FFA-induced activation of peroxisome proliferator-activated receptor α (PPARα). The increased levels of TNF-α in the liver will increase the generation of reactive oxygen species (ROS) during mitochondrial β-oxidation of FFA by impairing the flow of electrons along the mitochondrial respiratory chain. The upregulation of peroxisomal and microsomal (CYP4A family members) FFA oxidation enzymes by PPARα and insulin resistance (CYP2E1) will contribute further to oxidative stress. The resulting oxidative stress ('the second hit') in the presence of steatosis ('the first hit') will result in lipid peroxidation, further ROS production, TNF-α expression and insulin resistance, and ultimately to hepatocyte death and associated inflammation. The upregulation of uncoupling protein-2 (UCP-2) by ROS, FFA and TNF-α along with dicarboxylic acids derived from microsomal FFA oxidation may also lead to the uncoupling of oxidative phosphorylation and subsequently contribute to mitochondrial adenosine triphosphate (ATP) depletion and membrane permeability transition. These effects may increase the sensitivity of the liver to both necrotic and apoptotic cell death, with the latter a recognized feature of lipotoxicity.

Fibrosis

Until recently, fibrosis in NAFLD had been assumed to be caused by the activation of hepatic stellate cells (HSC) by cytokines released during liver injury and inflammation. However, two recent studies have suggested more NAFLD-specific mechanisms of fibrosis. The fibrogenic growth factor, connective tissue growth factor (CTGF), is overexpressed in the liver of patients with NASH, correlates with the degree of fibrosis and its synthesis by HSC is increased in response to glucose and insulin [26]. Studies in the *ob/ob* mouse

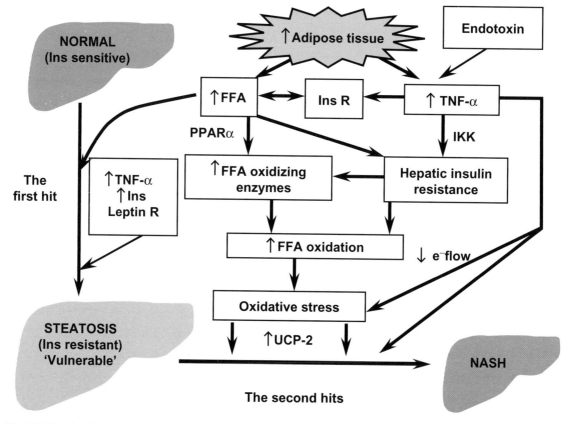

Fig. 6.1 The role of tumour necrosis factor-α (TNF-α) and free fatty acids (FFA) in the pathogenesis of non-alcoholic steatohepatitis (NASH). Expanded central adipose tissue leads to the release of FFA and TNF-α into the portal circulation. The release of FFA is largely attributable to TNF-α-induced insulin resistance in adipose tissue. FFA, free fatty acids; IKK, IκB kinase; Ins, insulin; PPARα, peroxisome proliferator activated receptor α; R, resistance; UCP-2, uncoupling protein 2.

have recently suggested that, in addition to its metabolic effects, leptin may also promote hepatic fibrogenesis [27].

Established risk factors for necroinflammation and fibrosis

This model of pathogenesis clearly explains the well-established risk factors for the development of NASH/fibrosis [28–30]. Increasing obesity, particularly central obesity, will increase the supply of FFA, TNF-α and leptin to the liver. The association between the severity of insulin resistance, the presence of type 2 diabetes mellitus and the risk of NASH and fibrosis is explained by insulin resistance increasing the supply of FFA to the liver and favouring the development of hepatic

oxidative stress and by hyperglycaemia and hyperinsulinaemia upregulating HSC synthesis of CTGF. The specific hepatic insulin resistance associated with steatosis presumably explains the universal association between NAFLD and insulin resistance. The model also provides a rational basis for the design of allele association studies aimed at elucidating why only a minority of patients with these risk factors develop NASH.

Candidate genes in NASH

Clearly, in common with most liver diseases, genes whose products are involved in the development and regulation of inflammation, apoptosis, regeneration

Table 6.1 Potential candidate genes in NASH.

Category of genes	Example(s)
Genes determining the magnitude and pattern of fat deposition	11β HSD-1 Lipodystrophic genes
Genes determining insulin sensitivity	Adiponectin, ?HFE, insulin receptor genes, PPARγ, resistin
Genes involved in hepatic lipid storage and export	Apolipoprotein E, MTP, leptin, SCD-1
Genes involved in fatty acid oxidation	PPARα, Acyl-CoA oxidase, CYP2E1, CYP4A family members
Genes influencing the generation of oxidant species	HFE, TNF-α
Genes encoding proteins involved in the response to oxidant stress	SOD-2, UCP-2
Cytokine genes	IL-10, TNF-α
Genes encoding endotoxin receptors	CD14, NOD2, TLR4
NASH-related fibrosis genes	CTGF, leptin

CTGF, connective tissue growth factor; CTLA-4, cytotoxic T lymphocyte antigen-4; 11β HSD-1, 11β hydroxysteroid dehydrogenase type 1; MTP, microsomal triglyceride transfer protein; PPAR, peroxisomal proliferator receptor; SCD-1, stearoyl CoA desaturase-1; SOD-2, superoxide dismutase-2; TLR4, toll-like receptor-4; UCP-2, uncoupling protein-2.

and fibrosis are obvious candidates for a role in susceptibility to advanced NAFLD. However, this chapter concentrates on genes considered likely to have a particular role in determining the development and progression of NASH. Potential 'functional' candidate genes are listed in Table 6.1. They can be grouped into four broad and overlapping categories:

1 Genes influencing the severity of steatosis
2 Genes influencing fatty acid oxidation
3 Genes influencing the severity of oxidative stress
4 Genes influencing the amount or effect of TNF-α.

Genes influencing the severity of steatosis

Through their influence on the supply and disposal of fatty acids to the liver, polymorphisms in genes whose products are involved in determining the pattern and magnitude of adipose tissue deposition and the development of insulin resistance will clearly have a role in determining the degree of steatosis and subsequent risk of NASH, although these will not be pure 'NASH genes' *per se*. Genes in the first category include the gene encoding the enzyme 11β HSD-1 that converts inactive cortisone to active cortisol. It is expressed at higher levels in visceral compared to peripheral adipose tissue [31] and its adipocyte-specific overexpression in

mice generates a phenotype with many features of the metabolic syndrome, including steatosis and insulin resistance [32]. At the other end of the adipose tissue spectrum are children with the various genetic lipodystrophy syndromes. These patients have a severe deficiency or absence of peripheral adipose tissue. However, they develop marked hepatic steatosis, which can be associated with NASH, and are severely insulin resistant. The 'missing' adipocyte factor responsible for the accumulation of fat in these patients is almost certainly leptin. With respect to genetic determinants of insulin resistance, children with rare mutations in the insulin receptor gene can develop NASH, and recent reports of polymorphisms in the gene encoding the transcription factor PPARγ, which has a key role in determining insulin sensitivity, suggests a further candidate gene worthy of study in NASH susceptibility [33]. Similar claims can be made for the genes encoding two recently described adipocyte-derived hormones, resistin [34] and adiponectin [35], both of which appear to influence insulin sensitivity.

Polymorphisms in genes involved in the synthesis, storage and export of hepatic triglyceride will clearly influence the magnitude of steatosis and the risk of NASH. SCD-1, which converts saturated FFA to monounsaturated FFA, is critical for the hepatic synthesis of triglyceride and the development of steatosis in *ob/ob* leptin-deficient mice [20] and is an obvious functional candidate for NAFLD. Apolipoprotein E (apoE) is an important regulator of plasma lipoprotein metabolism. The apoE gene is highly polymorphic and overexpression of one particular mutant form (apoE3-Leiden) in mice has recently been shown to lead to steatosis and altered very-low-density lipoprotein (VLDL) formation [36]. Preliminary evidence has recently been presented that patients with NAFLD homozygous for a low-activity promoter polymorphism in the MTP gene have increased steatosis and fibrosis compared to heterozygous patients or patients homozygous for the 'high' activity allele [37,38]. MTP is critical for the synthesis and secretion of VLDL in the liver and intestine and a frameshift mutation in the gene is associated with abetalipoproteinaemia. A G/T polymorphism at position -493 in the promoter significantly influences gene transcription, with the G allele associated with lower levels of transcription than the T allele. These data provide strong genetic evidence that steatosis is involved in the progression to more advanced stages of NAFLD.

Genes influencing fatty acid oxidation

Considered in light of the proposed model of NASH pathogenesis, the role of fatty acid oxidation is clearly complex. Appropriate fatty acid oxidation is required to prevent fat accumulation in the liver, while excessive fatty acid oxidation is probably responsible for the generation of oxidative stress. Accordingly, children with inherited defects in mitochondrial β-oxidation develop steatosis but not NASH, strongly suggesting that intact mitochondrial fat oxidation is required for progression to inflammation and fibrosis. With respect to peroxisomal and microsomal fat oxidation, because both are capable of generating ROS, it might be predicted that 'gain-of-function' polymorphisms in genes encoding proteins involved in these processes would predispose to NASH. However, these pathways have a role in limiting mitochondrial overload during times of excessive FFA supply and therefore it may be that 'loss-of-function' polymorphisms effecting these pathways would predispose to NASH. This latter hypothesis is supported by a study showing that mice lacking the gene encoding fatty acyl-CoA oxidase (AOX), the initial enzyme of the peroxisomal β-oxidation system, develop severe microvesicular

NASH [39]. Similar difficulties apply to interpreting a preliminary report that a mutation (*PPARA*3*) in the gene encoding PPARα is associated with NASH [40]. PPARα regulates the transcription of a variety of genes encoding enzymes involved in mitochondrial, peroxisomal β-oxidation and microsomal ω-oxidation of fatty acids and functional data on the mutation are somewhat contradictory at present [41].

Genes influencing the magnitude of oxidative stress

Other genes that may influence the magnitude and effect of oxidative stress include the *HFE* gene and genes encoding proteins involved the adaptive response to oxidative stress. With respect to *HFE*, an initial study from Australia showed that 31% of 51 patients with NASH possessed at least one copy of the C282Y *HFE* mutation, compared to only 13% of controls [42]. The mutation was also associated with an increased hepatic iron index (HII) and the severity of fibrosis. In this study there was no association with the other common *HFE* mutation, *H63D*. This was followed by a study from North America that reported no association between possession of C282Y and either the HII or the presence of NASH in 36 patients [43]. They did report a weak association between NASH and the *H63D* mutation; however, the controls were not well matched to the index cases. Most recently, an Australian study has reported an association between C282Y and NAFLD in 59 Anglo-Celts [44], but they found no association with histological severity and, similar to a previous study [45], no association between HII and histology. These data suggest that if *HFE* has any role in susceptibility to NAFLD, it may be via an association with insulin resistance rather than any effect on hepatic iron content and associated oxidative stress. With respect to the endogenous antioxidant defence systems, there has been a recent preliminary report of a polymorphism in the targeting sequence of the mitochondrial superoxide dismutase (SOD-2) being associated with the severity of fibrosis in patients with NAFLD [46] and, as a further component of the mitochondrial response to oxidative stress, the gene encoding UCP-2 is a further functional candidate worthy of study.

Genes influencing the amount or effect of TNF-α

With respect to genes influencing the amount or effects

of TNF-α, a promoter polymorphism at position -238 in the TNF-α gene has been associated with both alcoholic steatohepatitis and NASH [47,48]. However, the functional data on this polymorphism are contradictory at present [49] and further studies are required to understand the basis of this association. A number of other apparently functional TNF-α promoter polymorphisms have been described recently and all appear worthy of study in NASH susceptibility. With respect to polymorphisms in genes influencing the stimulus to TNF-α release, a study from Finland has reported an association between alcoholic steatohepatitis and a 'gain-of-function' promoter polymorphism in the endotoxin receptor CD14 [50]. A preliminary study in NASH has reported a similar association, although no association with a functional polymorphism in another endotoxin receptor, TLR4 [51]. With respect to polymorphisms in genes influencing the effect of TNF-α, studies in NASH on the low-activity promoter polymorphism in the gene encoding the anti-inflammatory cytokine IL-10, previously associated with ALD [52], are awaited with interest.

Conclusions

Investigators searching for genetic factors involved in NASH susceptibility using currently available technology face a number of potential pitfalls. However, these can undoubtedly be overcome by appropriate and careful study design, and recent advances in our understanding of basic disease mechanisms have suggested a wide range of genes worthy of subjecting to SNP screening strategies and case–control allele association studies. In future, the selection of candidate genes seems likely to be guided by mRNA and protein expression profiling of serum and liver tissue from patients with different stages of disease, and possibly by phenotype-driven mouse mutagenesis approaches. Eventually, the availability of a comprehensive SNP-based haplotype map of the human genome along with economically viable rapid throughput genotyping technology will enable genome-wide haplotype-based association studies in NASH. Together, these modern approaches are likely to lead to the identification of many as yet unknown or, at best, unsuspected susceptibility genes, which will greatly enhance our understanding of disease pathogenesis and accordingly our ability to design effective therapies.

References

1 Wanless IR, Lentz JS. Fatty liver hepatitis (steatohepatitis) and obesity: an autopsy study with analysis of risk factors. *Hepatology* 1990; **12**: 1106–10.

2 Erbey JR, Silberman C, Lydick E. Prevalence of abnormal serum alanine aminotransferase levels in obese patients and patients with type 2 diabetes. *Am J Med* 2000; **109**: 588–9.

3 Day CP. Who gets alcoholic liver disease: nature or nurture? *J R Coll Physicians London* 2000; **34**: 557–62.

4 Wigg AJ, Roberts-Thomson IC, Dymock RB et al. The role of small intestinal bacterial overgrowth, intestinal permeability, endotoxaemia, and tumour necrosis factor α in the pathogenesis of non-alcoholic steatohepatitis. *Gut* 2001; **48**: 206–11.

5 Struben VMD, Hespenheide EE, Caldwell SH. Non-alcoholic steatohepatitis and cryptogenic cirrhosis within kindreds. *Am J Med* 2000; **108**: 9–13.

6 Willner IR, Waters B, Patil SR et al. Ninety patients with non-alcoholic steatohepatitis: insulin resistance, familial tendency, and severity of disease. *Am J Gastroenterol* 2001; **96**: 2957–61.

7 Teli MR, James OFW, Burt AD et al. The natural history of non-alcoholic fatty liver: a follow-up study. *Hepatology* 1995; **22**: 1714–9.

8 Matteoni CA, Younossi ZM, Gramlich T et al. Non-alcoholic fatty liver disease: a spectrum of clinical and pathological severity. *Gastroenterology* 1999; **116**: 1413–9.

9 Hugot JP, Chamaillard M, Zouali H et al. Association of NOD2 leucine-rich repeat variants with susceptibility to Crohn's disease. *Nature* 2001; **411**: 599–603.

10 Risch N, Merikangas K. The future of genetic studies of complex human diseases. *Science* 1996; **273**: 156–7.

11 Speilman RS, Ewens WJ. The TDT and other family-based tests for linkage disequilibrium. *Am J Hum Genet* 1996; **59**: 983–9.

12 Speilman RS, Ewens WJ. A sibship test for linkage in the presence of association: the sib transmission/disequilibrium test. *Am J Hum Genet* 1998; **62**: 450–8.

13 Daly AK, Day CP. Candidate gene case–control association studies: advantages and potential pitfalls. *Br J Clin Pharmacol* 2001; **52**: 489–99.

14 Younoszai A, Ong JP, Grant G et al. Genomics of the spectrum of non-alcoholic fatty liver disease. *Hepatology* 2002; **36**: 381A.

15 Raghavakaimal S, Rosado B, Rasmussen D, Charlton M. A genomic analysis of histologically progressive NASH: evidence for a pretranscriptional basis of mitochondrial dysfunction and insulin resistance. *Hepatology* 2002; **36**: 403A.

16 Justice M, Noveroske JK, Weber JS, Zheng B, Bradley A. Mouse ENU mutagenesis. *Hum Mol Genet* 1999; **8**: 1955–63.

17 Sachidanandam R, Weissman D, Schmidt SC *et al.* A map of human genome sequence variation containing 1.42 million single nucleotide polymorphisms. *Nature* 2001; **409**: 928–33.

18 Judson R, Salisbury B, Schneider J, Windemuth A, Stephens JC. How many SNPs does a genome-wide haplotype map require? *Pharmacogenomics* 2002; **3**: 379–91.

19 Patil N, Berno AJ, Hinds DA *et al.* Blocks of limited haplotype diversity revealed by high-resolution scanning of human chromosome 21. *Science* 2001; **294**: 1719–23.

20 Daly MJ, Rioux JD, Schaffner SF, Hudson TJ, Lander ES. High-resolution haplotype structure in the human genome. *Nat Genet* 2001; **29**: 229–32.

21 Johnson GC, Esposito L, Barrat BJ *et al.* Haplotype tagging for the identification of common disease genes. *Nat Genet* 2001; **29**: 233–7.

22 Day CP. Pathogenesis of steatohepatitis. *Balliere's Best Pract Res Clin Gastroenterol* 2002; **16**: 663–78.

23 Lee Y, Wang MY, Kakuma T *et al.* Liporegulation in diet-induced obesity: the antisteatotic role of hyperleptinemia. *J Biol Chem* 2001; **276**: 5629–35.

24 Cohen P, Miyazaki M, Socci ND *et al.* Role for stearoyl-CoA desaturase-1 in leptin-mediated weight loss. *Science* 2002; **297**: 240–3.

25 Chitturi S, Farrell G, Frost L *et al.* Serum leptin in NASH correlates with hepatic steatosis but not fibrosis: a manifestation of lipotoxicity? *Hepatology* 2002; **36**: 403–9.

26 Paradis V, Perlemuter G, Bonvoust F *et al.* High glucose and hyperinsulinaemia stimulate connective tissue growth factor expression: a potential mechanism involved in progression to fibrosis in non-alcoholic steatohepatitis. *Hepatology* 2001; **34**: 738–44.

27 Marra F. Leptin and liver fibrosis: a matter of fat. *Gastroenterology* 2002; **122**: 1529–32.

28 Dixon JB, Bhathal PS, O'Brien PE. Non-alcoholic fatty liver disease: predictors of non-alcoholic steatohepatitis and liver fibrosis in the severely obese. *Gastroenterology* 2001; **121**: 91–100.

29 Angulo P, Keach JC, Batts KP *et al.* Independent predictors of liver fibrosis in patients with non-alcoholic steatohepatitis. *Hepatology* 1999; **30**: 1356–2.

30 Ratziu V, Giral P, Charlotte F *et al.* Liver fibrosis in overweight patients. *Gastroenterology* 2000; **118**: 1117–2113.

31 Bujalska IJ, Kumar S, Stewart PM. Does central obesity reflect 'Cushing's disease of the omentum'? *Lancet* 1997; **349**: 1210–3.

32 Masuzaki H, Paterson J, Shinyama H *et al.* A transgenic model of visceral obesity and the metabolic syndrome. *Science* 2001; **294**: 2166–70.

33 Kersten S, Desvergne B, Wahli W. Roles of PPARs in health and disease. *Nature* 2000; **405**: 421–4.

34 McTernan CL, McTernan PG, Harte AL *et al.* Resistin, central obesity, and type 2 diabetes. *Lancet* 2002; **359**: 46–7.

35 Berg AH, Combs TP, Du X, Brownlee M, Scherer PE. The adipocyte-secreted protein Acrp30 enhances hepatic insulin action. *Nat Med* 2001; **7**: 947–53.

36 Mensenkamp AR, van Luyn MJA, van Goor H *et al.* Hepatic lipid accumulation, altered very-low-density lipoprotein formation and apolipoprotein E deposition in apolipoprotein E3-Leiden transgenic mice. *J Hepatol* 2000; **33**: 189–98.

37 Bernard S, Touzet S, Personne I *et al.* Association between microsomal triglyceride transfer protein gene polymorphism and the biological features of liver steatosis in patients with type 2 diabetes. *Diabetologia* 2000; **43**: 995–9.

38 Day CP, Saksena S, Leathart JB *et al.* Genetic evidence supporting the two-hit model of NASH pathogenesis. *Hepatology* 2002; **36**: 383A.

39 Fan C-Y, Usuda N, Yeldandi AV *et al.* Steatohepatitis, spontaneous peroxisome proliferation and liver tumors in mice lacking peroxisomal fatty acyl-CoA oxidase: implications for peroxisome proliferator-activated receptor α natural ligand metabolism. *J Biol Chem* 1998; **273**: 15639–45.

40 Merriman, RB, Aouizerat, BE, Molloy MJ *et al.* A genetic mutation in the peroxisome proliferator-activated receptor α gene in patients with non-alcoholic steatohepatitis. *Hepatology* 2001; **34**: 441A.

41 Sapone A, Peters JM, Sakai S *et al.* The human peroxisome proliferator-activated receptor α gene: identification and functional characterization of two natural allelic variants. *Pharmacogenetics* 2000; **10**: 321–3.

42 George DK, Goldwurm S, Macdonald GA *et al.* Increased hepatic iron concentration in non-alcoholic steatohepatitis is associated with increased fibrosis. *Gastroenterology* 1998; **114**: 311–8.

43 Bonkovsky HL, Jawaid Q, Tortorelli K *et al.* Non-alcoholic steatohepatitis and iron: increased prevalence of mutations of the *HFE* gene in non-alcoholic steatohepatitis. *J Hepatol* 1999; **31**: 421–9.

44 Chitturi S, Weltman M, Farrell GC. *HFE* mutations, hepatic iron, and fibrosis: ethnic-specific associations of NASH with C282Y but not with fibrotic severity. *Hepatology* 2002; **36**: 142–9.

45 Younossi ZM, Gramlich T, Bacon BR *et al.* Hepatic iron and non-alcoholic fatty liver disease. *Hepatology* 1999; **30**: 847–50.

46 Saksena S, Daly AK, Leathart JB, Day CP. Manganese dependent superoxide dismutase (SOD-2) targeting sequence polymorphism is associated with advanced

fibrosis in patients with non-alcoholic fatty liver disease. *J Hepatol* 2003; **38** (Suppl.): 47.

47 Grove J, Daly AK, Bassendine MF, Day CP. Association of a tumour necrosis factor promoter polymorphism with susceptibility to alcoholic steatohepatitis. *Hepatology* 1997; **26**: 143–6.

48 Valenti L, Fracanzani AL, Dongiovanni P. Tumour necrosis factor α promoter polymorphisms and insulin resistance in non-alcoholic fatty liver disease. *Gastroenterology* 2002; **122**: 274–80.

49 Kaluza W, Reuss E, Grossmann S *et al.* Different transcriptional activity and *in vitro* TNF-α production is

psoriasis patients carrying the TNF-α 238A promoter polymorphism. *J Invest Dermatol* 2000; **114**: 1180–3.

50 Jarvelainen HA, Orpana A, Perolo M *et al.* Promoter polymorphism of the CD14 endotoxin receptor gene as a risk factor for alcoholic liver disease. *Hepatology* 2001; **33**: 1148–53.

51 Day CP. CD14 promoter polymorphism associated with risk of NASH. *J Hepatol* 2002; **36** (Suppl. 1): 21.

52 Grove J, Daly AK, Bassendine MF, Gilvarry E, Day CP. Interleukin 10 promoter region polymorphisms and susceptibility to advanced alcoholic liver disease. *Gut* 2000; **6**: 540–5.

7

The pathogenesis of NASH: human studies

Arun J. Sanyal

Key learning points

1 Non-alcoholic fatty liver disease (NAFLD) is associated with peripheral and hepatic insulin resistance.
2 Hepatic steatosis results when the balance between hepatic triglyceride synthesis and export is altered such that synthesis exceeds the export capacity.
3 Hepatic triglyceride synthesis may be increased by delivery of substrate (e.g. free fatty acids or 3-phosphoglycerate) from glycolysis (dietary carbohydrate excess) to the liver.
4 The development of steatohepatitis requires an additional insult such as the development of oxidative stress that can result from a multitude of pathways within the hepatocyte.
5 The precise pathways by which oxidative stress and processes that result in hepatic injury are translated into the phenotype of steatohepatitis remains to be determined.

Abstract

The pathophysiological hallmark of non-alcoholic fatty liver disease (NAFLD) is underlying insulin resistance. It is now well established that both subjects with hepatic steatosis alone as well as those with non-alcoholic steatohepatitis (NASH) have impaired metabolic clearance of glucose when compared to normal individuals. Insulin resistance is associated with impaired suppression of peripheral lipolysis by insulin. This results in an increased free fatty acid (FFA) load that is delivered to the liver. The liver adapts by increased mitochondrial fatty acid β-oxidation, re-esterification of fatty acids to triglycerides and export as very-low-density lipoproteins (VLDL). Hepatic steatosis results when the balance between delivery or synthesis of FFA exceed the capacity to oxidize these or export them as VLDL. The transition from steatosis to steatohepatitis is believed to involve several potential mechanisms, all of which result in
increased generation of free radicals and lipid peroxidation within hepatocytes. Such mechanisms include mitochondrial abnormalities, increased cytochrome P450 activity, sensitization to tumour necrosis factor (TNF)-mediated injury, and iron-mediated toxicity. The role of antioxidant defences in the pathogenesis of NASH remains to be determined.

Introduction

Non-alcoholic fatty liver disease is one of the most common causes of chronic liver disease worldwide. The two basic histological lesions in subjects with NAFLD are: (i) hepatic steatosis (NAFL); and (ii) steatohepatitis [1]. The pattern of hepatic steatosis is invariably macrovesicular, although occasionally both mixed micro- and macrovesicular steatosis may be present. When there is a mixed pattern, macrovesicular steatosis is the dominant finding. NASH is defined by the presence of macrovesicular steatosis along with a constellation of changes including cytological ballooning, Mallory bodies, pericellular fibrosis and scattered mainly lobular inflammation (see Chapter 2) [1]. In an individual case, only some of these findings are present. NASH is associated with progressive liver disease and may lead to cirrhosis.

It is now established that insulin resistance (IR) is almost always present in NASH. Because IR occurs in association with steatosis alone as well as steatohepatitis, it is generally believed that additional pathophysiological abnormalities within the liver are required to produce steatohepatitis. The intracellular sites of such abnormalities include the mitochondria, the cytochrome P450 system and peroxisomes. Abnormalities at these sites result in oxidative stress in the liver, which produces the phenotypical lesion of steatohepatitis. In this chapter, we review the human data that seeks to elucidate the mechanisms by which a fatty liver develops and also the potential roles of additional pathophysiological hits in the genesis of steatohepatitis.

Evidence to support a metabolic basis for NAFLD

Association of NAFLD with insulin resistance

There is strong evidence of an association between NAFLD and conditions known to be associated with IR (see Chapter 4). The original clinical descriptions of NAFLD noted an association between obesity and diabetes, two conditions best known to be associated with IR [2,3]. Since then, several epidemiological studies have found a direct correlation between body mass index (BMI) and the probability of having a fatty liver as defined by hepatic sonography. In an autopsy series, where liver histology was used to define the presence of a fatty liver [4], fatty liver was found in 2.7% of lean individuals and 18.5% of obese individuals. Similar data have been reported from autopsies of air-crash victims [5]. A relationship between BMI and the presence of a fatty liver has also been established in otherwise apparently healthy individuals being considered as donors for live-donor liver transplantation [6,7]. Additionally, NAFLD has been associated with a number of clinical conditions (e.g. lipodystrophy and highly active antiretroviral therapy) that are characterized by IR (see Chapter 21) [8,9].

Several recent studies have examined the relationship between NASH and the presence of the metabolic syndrome. In the first study [10], patients with NASH were found to have lower insulin sensitivity and higher insulin secretion rates compared to age and gender-matched healthy controls. In the second study [11], IR, as measured by the homeostatic model (HOMA-IR) was present in 65 of 66 (98%) subjects with NASH while the metabolic syndrome was present in 55 of 63 (87%). IR was present in lean (but centrally obese) as well as obese individuals. Importantly, the metabolic syndrome was present in 75% of patients with NASH, compared to only 8.3% of age- and gender-matched subjects with hepatitis C, indicating that the association between NASH and IR is highly specific for the condition. In another study [12], the presence of the metabolic syndrome was found to be associated with an increased risk of advanced fibrosis. Finally, the presence of IR has been confirmed using the euglycaemic–hyperinsulinaemic clamp in non-diabetic precirrhotic individuals with fatty liver as well as NASH [13].

Role of oxidative stress and the 'two-hit' hypothesis

Because both fatty liver and NASH are associated with IR and the degree of insulin resistance in these groups may overlap, it is generally believed that additional pathophysiological abnormalities are required for the development of NASH. Animal models of steatohepatitis suggest that one common denominator of liver injury in NASH is oxidative stress, which leads to lipid peroxidation of intracellular organelles (see Chapters 8, 10 and 11) [14,15]. It has recently been shown that products of lipid peroxidation (e.g. 3-nitrotyrosine [3-NT]) are increased both in fatty liver as well as NASH [13]. However, the levels of 3-NT are higher in those with NASH compared to those with fatty liver alone. These data have been corroborated in a recent study where serum thioredoxin levels, a marker of oxidative stress, was found to be significantly higher in those with NASH (mean 60.3 ng/mL) compared to those with simple fatty liver (mean 24.6 ng/mL) [16]. These features of lipid peroxidation are associated with hepatic fibrosis and steatosis in acinar zone 3, the region where the histological features of NASH predominate [17]. In addition to these observations, there is evidence of oxidative damage to DNA in persons with NASH [18].

Several metabolic pathways within hepatocytes can lead to the generation of reactive oxygen species (ROS). These include the cytochrome P450 system, nicotinamide adenine dinucleotide phosphate (NADPH) oxidase, mitochondrial and peroxisomal functional abnormalities, cycloxygenase and lipoxygenase pathways and iron overload [15,19–22]. These considerations have led to the 'two-hit' hypothesis for NASH, which proposes that, in addition to insulin resistance, a second intrahepatic abnormality, which contributes to free radical generation, is required for the genesis of NASH.

It is generally believed that steatohepatitis is the phenotypical response to a pathophysiological insult that leads to generation of a fatty liver and oxidative stress. It is therefore germane to consider the pathophysiological abnormalities in NASH in terms of factors that lead to a fatty liver and those that lead to oxidative stress. At a cellular level, the pathogenesis of NAFLD also involves abnormalities of protein synthesis, transport or disposal, leading to disruption of the actin cytoskeleton and accumulation of ubiquitin-tagged proteins in some hepatocytes producing Mallory bodies. Abnormalities of cell volume regulation lead to cytological ballooning and activation of specific pathways lead to increased apoptosis. It is probable that the production of specific cytokines resulting from hepatocyte injury induce the inflammatory response and fibrosis that occurs in NASH (see Chapters 10 and 12). While the cell biology of these abnormalities remain to be defined, such abnormalities often occur in the presence of increased ROS and lipid peroxidation. Also, these changes may be linked to IR and the development of a fatty liver. We therefore discuss the causes and consequences of IR and how these may lead to a fatty liver and oxidative stress. The development of additional 'hits' and how such hits may integrate with IR to produce oxidative stress is also be considered.

Insulin resistance and the genesis of a fatty liver

Theoretically, a fatty liver may result from excessive production (or increased uptake) of lipids by the liver or decreased metabolism and secretion of lipids by hepatocytes. In order to better appreciate the mechanisms by which IR results in hepatic steatosis, the normal metabolic pathways involving fatty acids in the hepatocyte are discussed below.

Normal hepatic fatty acid metabolism

Under normal circumstances, FFA are delivered to the liver via both the portal and arterial circulation. FFA in portal blood reflects the degree of lipolytic activity in mesenteric fat stores as well as that absorbed from the intestine. FFA undergo first-pass clearance in the liver where they are taken up by hepatocytes as well as sinusoidal endothelial cells. Not much is known of FFA metabolism in hepatic non-parenchymal cells and cross-talk between such cells and adjacent hepatocytes.

Within the liver, FFA can undergo one of four metabolic fates:

1 They can be oxidized within mitochondria to ketone bodies
2 They may undergo β-oxidation within peroxisomes
3 They may undergo oxidation within the cytochrome P450 system
4 They may be re-esterified to triglycerides or used for the synthesis of other lipids.

The relative importance of each of these pathways depends on both the nature of the fatty acid (degree of saturation and chain length) and whether the changes in FFA delivery to the liver are acute or long-standing. An important pathway regulating a hepatocyte's ability to handle an increase in FFA delivery is the peroxisome proliferator activated receptor (PPAR) transcriptional factors. Acting via the PPARα, FFA induce the expression AcylCoA oxidase, a key enzyme for peroxisomal fatty acid β-oxidation. They also induce fatty acid transport proteins and carnitine palmitoyltransferase, which results in increased mitochondrial fatty acid uptake and oxidation (see Chapter 9).

Effects of insulin on intermediary and fatty acid metabolism

Insulin is the principal anabolic hormone in the body. It increases glycogen storage, protein synthesis, glycolysis and lipogenesis, while inhibiting glycogenolysis, gluconeogenesis, lipolysis and protein breakdown. These functions are mediated by the interaction of insulin with its receptor and subsequent activation of specific signal transduction pathways related to insulin–insulin receptor binding.

The primary effect of insulin on carbohydrate metabolism is to increase glucose uptake by cells. This is accomplished by increased translocation of glucose transporters (GLUT) to the surface of individual cells [23]. Within the cells, glucose is first phosphorylated to glucose-6-phosphate. Under conditions of glucose excess, much of this glucose-6-phosphate is converted to glycogen, which can be reconverted back to glucose when required. These opposing processes are regulated by glycogen synthetase and phosphorylase [24]. Insulin regulates the phosphorylation status of these enzymes by inhibiting protein kinase A (PKA) [25]. Inhibition of PKA under conditions of high insulin : glucagon ratio also increases glycolysis by activation of phosphofructokinase-1 (PFK-1). One of the effects of hyperinsulinaemia is therefore to increase the production of glyceraldehyde-3-phosphate, a metabolic intermediate in the glycolytic pathway, which can provide the backbone for triglyceride formation. On the other hand, a high insulin : glucagon ratio inhibits gluconeogenesis. Thus, insulin stimulates glucose uptake and utilization by promoting glycogen formation as well as glycolysis. It inhibits hepatic glucose production by inhibiting glycogenolysis and gluconeogenesis.

The principal effect of insulin on lipid metabolism is to promote lipid storage and inhibit lipolysis. Insulin affects lipid storage both by its effects on the enzymes involved in lipid formation and by increasing the availability of substrates required for lipid synthesis. The effects of insulin on the transcriptional regulation of enzymes involved in lipid metabolism appear to involve the sterol regulatory element binding protein (SREBP) [26,27]. Increased PFK-1 activity promotes glycolysis and generation of pyruvate which, via conversion to acetylCoA, can provide substrates for fatty acid synthesis. AcetylCo A is also the substrate for hydroxymethylglutaryl coenzyme A (HMGCoA) reductase, the rate-limiting step in cholesterol synthesis. Also, glyceraldehyde-3-phosphate, an intermediary product of glycolysis, is a precursor for triglyceride formation.

Insulin inhibits lipolysis principally by inhibiting lipoprotein lipase in peripheral tissues [23]. Lipoprotein lipase is active in its phosphorylated state, which is increased by PKA. Insulin inhibits lipoprotein lipase activity by inhibiting PKA activity and stimulating protein phosphatase activity [28]. Conversely, factors that increase PKA activity (e.g. glucagon and growth hormone) increase lipoprotein lipase activity and peripheral lipolysis.

Free fatty acid as a metabolic integrator

The role of peripheral adipocytes in the overall regulation of metabolic homoeostasis has been the focus of intense study over the last decade, and adipocytes have emerged as a key player in the metabolic orchestra of the body. Adipocytes affect the metabolic state by serving as a site for lipid storage and lipolysis, processes that are regulated by insulin, while modulating insulin sensitivity by production of a variety of factors that affect insulin function via paracrine and endocrine mechanisms. Such substances include FFA, TNF-α, leptin, adiponectin, plasminogen activator inhibitor-1 (PAI-1), sex hormones, cortisol and resistin [29–35].

FFA, the major metabolic product of adipocytes, have both direct effects on intermediary metabolism and also indirect effects by their specific effects on insulin signalling pathways [36,37]. Approximately 40 years ago, Randle et al. [38] reported that fatty acids competed with glucose as fuel for oxidation in striated as well as cardiac muscle. The proposed mechanism was believed to be an increase in intramitochondrial acetylCoA : CoA and nicotinamide adenine dinucleotide (NAD) : reduced NAD (NADH) ratio, resulting from fatty acid oxidation. This change in redox status of cofactors inhibits pyruvate dehydrogenase activity. The production of acetylCoA from pyruvate by pyruvate dehydrogenase would therefore be decreased. The relative lack of acetylCoA for entry in to the Krebs cycle would keep this cycle from progressing beyond citrate, causing accumulation of citrate which leaked back in to the cytoplasm. Citrate is known to inhibit cytoplasmic PFK activity, thereby reducing glycolysis and producing accumulation of glucose-6-phosphate in the cell [38,39]. Glucose-6-phosphate accumulation inhibits hexokinase activity, resulting in intracellular hyperglycaemia and inhibition of glucose uptake. While these effects of fatty acids on glucose utilization have been corroborated [39,40], recent data indicate that this is mostly caused by the direct effects of fatty acids on insulin signal transduction pathways [36,41,42]. FFA also increase gluconeogenesis by the ability of acetylCoA to activate pyruvate carboxylase, which converts pyruvate to oxaloacetate, a key early step in gluconeogenesis [43].

In addition to the effects mediated by acetylCoA as described by Randle *et al.* [38], long-chain acylCoA (LC-CoA), the first product of the β-oxidation pathway of fatty acids in the cytoplasm, may modulate insulin activity and the metabolic state [39,44]. Besides undergoing oxidative degradation, LC-CoA re-esterification produces by-products such as ceramide, phosphatidic acid and diacyl glycerol, which affect the activity of numerous enzymes (e.g. pyruvate kinase) [45]. LC-CoA also increase PPARs, which, in turn, modulate fatty acid oxidation and adipocyte differentiation.

Free fatty acids: a key switch that determines insulin sensitivity and resistance

It has been shown that visceral fat is less sensitive than peripheral fat to the lipolysis-suppressing effects of insulin [46,47]. This is most likely caused by increased expression of 11β OH dehydrogenase, which converts cortisone to cortisol in visceral fat and renders it more resistant to insulin-mediated suppression of lipolysis [47,48]. The insensitivity of visceral fat stores to the lipolysis-suppressing effects of insulin is an important determinant of the metabolic consequences of IR (Fig. 7.1). In the insulin-resistant state, there is a disproportionately greater flux of FFA from visceral adipose tissue to the liver via the portal circulation. In the liver, these FFA inhibit the Krebs cycle while promoting fatty acid oxidation, which produces an oxidative stress in the liver. Simultaneously, gluconeogenesis is stimulated and glycolysis is inhibited. This results in increased hepatic glucose output. Impairment of metabolic clearance of glucose resulting from decreased uptake by striated muscle as a consequence of insulin resistance results in higher glucose levels in the blood, which in turn is sensed by the pancreatic islet cells. The pancreas responds to the increased systemic glucose load by increasing insulin output to restore glucose clearance rates to baseline values. This process continues until the pancreas is unable to keep up with the demand for insulin. At that point, diabetes develops. The central control of this metabolic cycle by FFA is also known as the 'single gateway hypothesis' and provides an unifying mechanism that links the coordinated regulation of glucose and lipid metabolism in the liver to the hormonal regulation of lipolysis in visceral adipose stores [49].

Specific metabolic abnormalities related to insulin resistance in NAFLD

Traditionally, from an operational point of view, IR has been defined by the ability of insulin to clear glucose from blood [50,51]. This is also how insulin sensitivity is defined and the two terms essentially reflect two sides of the same phenomenon. It is also important to remember that the sensitivity to insulin is measured on a continuous rather than a categorical scale. Thus, insulin sensitivity and resistance represent a 'ying–yang' that, vary along a continuous scale and there is no threshold insulin cut-off value that marks the onset of insulin resistance in a given individual.

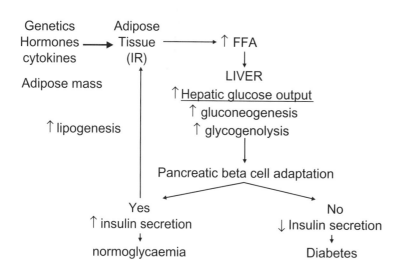

Fig. 7.1 The single gateway hypothesis demonstrating the central role of free fatty acids (FFA) in insulin resistance. The sensitivity of adipose tissue, especially visceral adipose tissue, to insulin-mediated suppression of lipolysis is impaired. As a result, fasting FFA are increased. FFA increase hepatic glucose output by increasing gluconeogenesis and decreasing glycolysis and glycogenolysis. The pancreatic islet β cells adapt to the increased glucose load by increasing insulin secretion and causing hyperinsulinaemia. Over time, the pancreas fails to keep up with the insulin requirements, producing glucose intolerance and then diabetes.

It is possible that different organs and metabolic pathways may have differential sensitivity to insulin. Thus, while IR exists almost universally in subjects with NAFLD, it is important to delineate the specific metabolic pathways that are affected. These have been evaluated using the euglycaemic–hyperinsulinaemic clamp method [13,52], which demonstrate a progressive decrease in metabolic clearance rates of glucose in patients with fatty liver and NASH compared to age- and gender-matched normal controls. As diabetes and obesity are the major risk factors for NAFLD, it may be hypothesized that the metabolic abnormalities in patients with NAFLD would mirror those seen in the classic metabolic syndrome. Thus, one would expect high baseline values of insulin and FFA. There should also be resistance to insulin-mediated suppression of lipolysis and increased hepatic glucose output.

Several studies have shown that fasting insulin as well as C-peptide levels are elevated in patients with NAFLD compared to either normal controls or age- and gender-matched subjects with other types of liver disease [10,13,53]. Further, fasting levels of FFA and glycerol, the two products of lipolysis, are elevated even in non-diabetic subjects with NAFLD compared to normal controls [13]. Of note, those with steatohepatitis have the highest levels of these substances. A priori, it is likely that similar findings are present in diabetic subjects. Using the insulin response during an

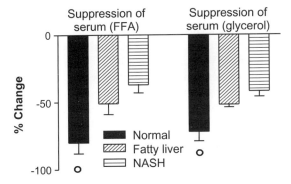

Fig. 7.2 Serum FFA and glycerol in subjects with fatty liver or NASH and in age- and gender-matched normal controls during an euglycaemic–hyperinsulinaemic clamp. There was a stepwise impairment in the ability of insulin to suppress the serum FFA and glycerol, indicating the presence of resistance to insulin actions on peripheral lipolysis. Both subjects with fatty liver and NASH were significantly different from controls. (With permission from Sanyal *et al.* [13].)

intravenous glucose tolerance test, it has recently been shown that insulin production is increased in non-obese subjects with NAFLD [10].

The ability of insulin to suppress peripheral lipolysis can be assessed by measuring the serum levels of FFA and glycerol, the products of lipolysis, during an hyperinsulinaemic–euglycaemic clamp. It has been shown that whereas serum FFA and glycerol can be markedly suppressed by insulin infusion in normal subjects, there is a stepwise progressive impairment in suppression of these products of lipolysis during a clamp in subjects with NAFLD (Fig. 7.2) [13]. These findings were further corroborated by directly measuring the rates of peripheral lipolysis from the enrichment of the glycerol pool by labelled glycerol infused during the euglycaemic clamp [13,52]. Thus, both fatty liver and NASH are associated with baseline hyperinsulinaemia and increased peripheral lipolysis as well as a marked resistance to insulin-mediated suppression of lipolysis. These abnormalities are most marked in those with NASH.

The key metabolic consequence of increased FFA delivery to the liver is an increased hepatic glucose output which, in turn, drives pancreatic hypersecretion of insulin. Hepatic glucose production was measured by enrichment of the glucose pool by exogenous labelled glucose infused during an euglycaemic–hyperinsulinaemic clamp [13]. At low-dose insulin infusion, there was little suppression of hepatic glucose output (45–60%), while high-dose infusion was able to suppress glucose output in patients with NASH (Fig. 7.3). Impaired suppression of hepatic glucose output by insulin has also been reported in another study [52].

These data clearly indicate that NAFLD is associated with increased availability of FFA for hepatic uptake because of increased baseline lipolytic activity and impaired sensitivity to insulin-mediated suppression of lipolysis. Also, NAFLD is associated with impairment of insulin-mediated suppression of hepatic glucose output. Thus, all of the key metabolic features of the insulin-resistant state are present in those with NAFLD, with the most severe findings seen in those with NASH.

Metabolic abnormalities in NAFLD and the genesis of a fatty liver

A key question is how does insulin resistance and increased delivery of FFA to the liver result in a fatty liver? A conceptual framework can be developed by

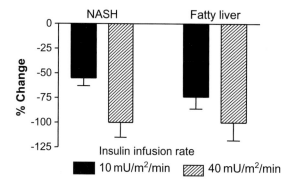

Fig. 7.3 The effects of insulin infusion on hepatic glucose output in subjects with fatty liver or NASH. At low-dose insulin infusion, there was an impairment in insulin-mediated suppression of hepatic glucose output, whereas at high-dose insulin infusion hepatic glucose output could be suppressed. (After Sanyal *et al.* [13].)

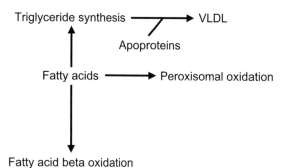

Fig. 7.4 The metabolic fate of FFA in the liver. They may either undergo oxidation or re-esterification to triglycerides or other lipids. A working hypothesis is that fatty liver can result if the amount of triglyceride formed exceeds the capacity of the liver to form very-low-density lipoprotein (VLDL). In the presence of impaired fatty acid oxidation or decreased apolipoprotein formation or microsomal formation of VLDL, fat can accumulate in the liver at relatively low levels of FFA flux through the liver.

considering the potential metabolic fate of FFA in the liver. FFA may either be oxidized in the mitochondria, peroxisomes and microsomal system or converted into other lipids (Fig. 7.4). Theoretically speaking, fat would accumulate in the liver if more triglycerides were formed than could be converted and secreted as VLDL. Thus, if large amounts of FFA were used to form triglycerides, they could potentially overwhelm the capacity of the liver to form and secrete VLDL. To examine the possibility that there might be a systemic defect in the incorporation of FFA into phospholipids and cholesterol in subjects with NAFLD, skin biopsies were performed on subjects with NASH [13]. Fibroblasts were grown in culture from these biopsies. Once the cells reached confluence, they were exposed to labelled palmitate, and its incorporation into phospholipids and cholesterol assessed by gas chromatography. There were no defects noted in either the incorporation of palmitate to triglycerides, phospholipids or cholesterol (Fig. 7.5). While these data indicate that there are no systemic defects in FFA incorporation into lipids, the possibility of a liver-specific defect remained a possibility.

Recently, using hepatic venous sampling of lipoproteins following infusion of labelled leucine, a defect in the incorporation of labelled leucine into apolipoprotein B100 was seen in patients with NASH [54]. While controversy exists about the universality of this finding and whether they represent the cause or consequence of liver disease, it does provide a potential mechanism for the genesis of a fatty liver. Increased triglyceride formation resulting from the increased availability of FFA for re-esterification, along with an impaired ability to form VLDL because of decreased apolipoprotein B formation would lead to accumulation of triglycerides in the liver. A G/T polymorphism at position 493 in the promoter region of the microsomal transfer protein, which decreases expression of this protein and inhibits VLDL formation, has been associated with features of steatohepatitis [55]. Even in the absence of such defects, if enough FFA were to be re-esterified to triglycerides, they could overwhelm the ability of the liver to form VLDL and excrete it.

Another potential mechanism by which FFA availability for triglyceride synthesis can be increased is a defect in mitochondrial fatty acid β-oxidation. In the presence of a defect in mitochondrial fatty acid β-oxidation, the substrates upstream of the site of the defect accumulate and are converted in to dicarboxylic acids. The presence of impaired mitochondrial fatty acid β-oxidation was assessed by screening early morning urine specimens of subjects with NAFLD for the presence of abnormal dicarboxylic acids [13]. There were no dicarboxylic acids noted in these urine specimens, indicating that the mitochondrial fatty acid β-oxidation pathway is functionally intact in NAFLD. While this method does not absolutely exclude the possibility of a subtle defect in mitochondrial fatty acid

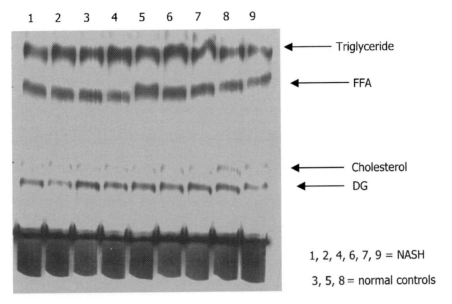

1, 2, 4, 6, 7, 9 = NASH

3, 5, 8 = normal controls

Fig. 7.5 Incorporation of labelled palmitate into triglycerides by cutaneous fibroblasts from normal individuals and subjects with NASH. There were no differences in the incorporation into triglycerides, diacylglycerol (DG) and cholesterol. (After Sanyal *et al.* [13].).

oxidation, it does exclude the possibility of a gross defect in the majority of subjects.

Increased hepatic lipid synthesis resulting from hyperinsulinaemia is another possibility that contributes to the genesis of a fatty liver. It has been observed that in subjects on peritoneal dialysis, addition of insulin to the dialysate produces a rim of steatosis in the liver. Also, it has been postulated that focal fatty change in the liver may be related to perfusion by branches of the portal vein that preferentially drain the pancreas and therefore contain high insulin concentrations. The role of hyperinsulinaemia-mediated lipid synthesis in the genesis of a fatty liver remains to be fully studied.

In summary, a fatty liver results from increased FFA flux through the liver, which exceeds the liver's ability to secrete VLDL. In most subjects with NAFLD, there are no gross abnormalities in fatty acid β-oxidation or systemic abnormalities in fatty acid incorporation into triglycerides or other lipids. However, a proportion of subjects with NASH may have decreased apolipoprotein B formation, which impairs the ability to form VLDL and allows triglycerides to accumulate in the liver. In the presence of genetic or acquired factors that impair fatty acid oxidation or formation and/or secretion of VLDL, fat accumulates in the liver at even relatively low rates of FFA flux through the liver. In the former situation, impaired fatty acid oxidation provides FFA for triglyceride formation, which may exceed the ability to form VLDL. On the other hand, if VLDL cannot be formed and secreted (e.g. in hypobetalipoproteinaemia), even normal levels of FFA flux through the liver may provide more triglycerides than can be transferred to VLDL, causing fat to accumulate in the liver. The role of increased hepatic fatty acid synthesis resulting from portal hyperinsulinaemia as a cause of hepatic steatosis remains to be fully explored.

This paradigm provides a unifying concept that can be used to understand the genesis of a fatty liver under a variety of conditions, including the various causes associated with NAFLD. For example, one might postulate that, in the presence of severe protein–calorie malnutrition, a combination of increased FFA delivery because of increased lipolysis related to the starvation state combined with a decreased availability of lipotropic factors required to form apolipoprotein B may lead to a hepatic phenotype identical to that seen in NAFLD, a disease of overnutrition.

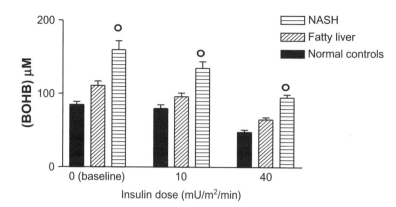

Fig. 7.6 Serum β-hydroxy butyrate (BOHB) levels at baseline and during low-dose and high-dose insulin infusion during an euglycaemic–hyperinsulinaemic clamp study in normal subjects, subjects with fatty liver and NASH. NASH was associated with the highest baseline (BOHB) and these were the most resistant to suppression by insulin infusion, indicating increased mitochondrial lipid oxidation in subjects with NASH. (After Sanyal *et al.* [13].)

From steatosis to steatohepatitis: mechanisms of increased oxidative stress

There is general consensus that oxidative stress accompanies the histological phenotype of steatohepatitis. It has been shown that both fatty liver and NASH are associated with increased hepatic 3-NT staining, which supports a role for oxidative stress and lipid peroxidation in these conditions [13]. NASH is associated with significantly higher levels of 3-NT compared to those with fatty liver. At this time, very little is known about how oxidative stress leads to cytological ballooning or to the development of Mallory bodies, which are the major morphological abnormalities associated with NASH. We will therefore limit our discussion of the potential mechanisms by which oxidative stress can occur within hepatocytes.

Role of mitochondria and peroxisomes

Mitochondria are the major site for the genesis of free radicals in hepatocytes (see Chapter 11). The mitochondria contain the electron transport chain, a series of enzymes that allow the energy released from oxidation of Krebs cycle intermediates and fatty acids to be converted to energy-rich adenosine trisphosphate (ATP). This process is not completely efficient and normally a fraction of the energy is not converted to ATP, resulting in release of oxygen free radicals in the cell. Uncoupling of oxidation and phosphorylation with increased formation of free oxygen radicals have been implicated in drug-induced steatohepatitis [56]. While fatty acids also undergo β-oxidation in peroxi-

somes, this differs from mitochondrial fatty acid oxidation in that peroxisomal fatty acid oxidation results in marked production of H_2O_2, resulting in oxidative stress. While several conditions associated with impaired peroxisomal function have been described, there are no conditions clearly associated with increased function of peroxisomes.

Mitochondrial function with respect to fatty acid oxidation can be assessed by β-OH butyrate levels because this metabolite is produced solely in mitochondria. It has been shown that baseline β-OH butyrate levels are higher in those with fatty liver and NASH compared to normal controls, with the highest values in those with NASH [13]. Further, during an euglycaemic clamp, normal individuals suppress β-OH butyrate levels, indicating that mitochondrial fatty acid oxidation is normally suppressed by insulin. On the other hand, fatty liver and NASH are associated with an impairment in insulin-mediated suppression of serum (β-OH butyrate), confirming that these conditions are associated with resistance to insulin effects on fatty acid oxidation (Fig. 7.6). These data are compatible with the known effects of increased FFA delivery on mitochondrial fatty acid oxidation.

In contrast to the relatively preserved mitochondrial fatty acid oxidation, there are severe structural abnormalities in the hepatic mitochondria of patients with NASH (Fig. 7.7) [13,57]. These findings are relatively specific for NASH and are rare in those with a fatty liver [13]. The specific abnormalities include enlargement and development of multilamellar mitochondria with loss of cristae along with the presence of intramitochondrial paracrystalline inclusions. There is no specific lobular distribution of these inclusions and

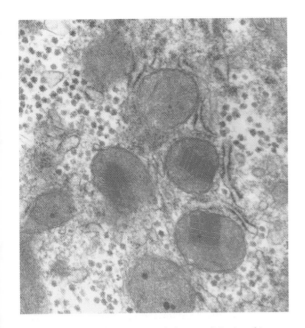

Fig. 7.7 Mitochondrial structural abnormalities in subjects with NASH. The mitochondria are ballooned, with loss of cristae and development of paracrystalline inclusions.

only a variable fraction of mitochondria within a given hepatocyte are affected. Such changes have been associated with diseases linked to mitochondrial DNA mutations (e.g. mitochondrial myopathies) [58]. We have evaluated muscle biopsies from subjects with

NASH but have not been able to document any cases of mitochondrial DNA or electron chain enzyme abnormalities in striated muscle of these subjects (unpublished work). Similarly, such abnormalities have not been detected in peripheral blood mononuclear cells in patients with NASH. Recently, we found a decrease in cytochrome oxidase functional activity in those with NASH but not in those with fatty liver [59]. This is because of decreased cytochrome oxidase subunit II (encoded by mitochondrial DNA) expression and is associated with marked mitochondrial DNA depletion in the hepatocytes of those with NASH. These are further associated with increased hepatic deoxyguanosine staining, indicating the presence of DNA damage because of oxidative stress within hepatocytes. These findings are relatively specific for NASH because they were not present in those with hepatitis C.

Based on these findings, we postulate that the development of IR causes increased FFA flux to the liver. One consequence is the development of simple steatosis. A second is increased FFA oxidation in the mitochondria (Fig. 7.8). This generates oxidative stress because of the inherent inefficiency of the coupling between oxidation and phosphorylation. The oxidative stress produces damage of mitochondrial DNA, which is inherently less able than nuclear DNA to repair oxidative damage. Over time, the cumulative damage to DNA leads to mitochondrial DNA depletion and decreased expression of electron transport chain enzymes that

Fig. 7.8 A working hypothesis linking insulin resistance to second hits that produce oxidative stress. Insulin resistance causes increased FFA to be delivered to the liver. Mitochondrial FFA oxidation causes an oxidative stress that damages mitochondrial DNA and eventually leads to mitochondrial DNA depletion. This further uncouples oxidation and phosphorylation and increases reactive oxygen species (ROS) generation. ROS also produce direct mitochondrial damage by lipid peroxidation and production of TNF, which further worsen mitochondrial function and enhance ROS production. ROS may also be produced in microsomes and in the presence of iron overload.

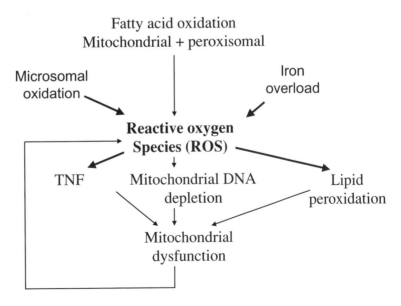

are encoded by mitochondrial DNA. This further uncouples oxidation from phosphorylation. As a result, for a given degree of fatty acid oxidation, there is marked increase in the degree of free radical generation. When the oxidative stress reaches a critical threshold or lasts long enough, it sets in motion the intracellular events that result in the phenotype of steatohepatitis.

Role of cytochrome P450 system

Another site that can produce reactive oxygen species within hepatocytes is the microsomal electron transport system which contains the cytochrome P450 (CYP) proteins. Several elements of the CYP system are capable of oxidizing lipids; of these, CYP2E1 and CYP4A are the best studied in the context of NASH. Increased CYP2E1 expression has been noted in NASH [19,60]. The increased expression is mainly seen in the pericentral regions, which correspond to the principal site of morphological changes in NASH. CYP2E1 levels have been shown to be increased in those with central

obesity and diabetes, the major risk factors for NAFLD. Increased CYP expression results in futile cycling in the absence of substrate, which results in the production of reactive oxygen species. While this has been shown to be true in experimental models, it is unclear whether this mechanism is operative in subjects with NASH. These exciting data must now be expanded to elucidate the degree to which the CYP system contributes to the oxidative stress present in NASH.

Role of tumour necrosis factor-α and other cytokines

A large body of literature has accumulated to support a key role for TNF in the genesis of alcoholic steatohepatitis. Kupffer cells are the principal site of TNF production in the liver although TNF can also be produced within hepatocytes (Fig. 7.9). TNF antagonizes insulin activity and contributes to worsening insulin sensitivity [34,61]. By activating the apoptotic pathway, TNF contributes to increased reactive oxygen species generation and oxidative stress [34,62]. TNF also has

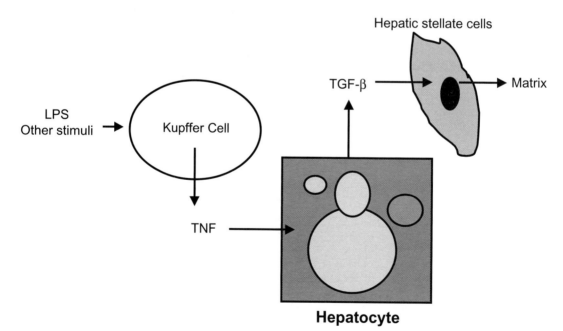

Fig. 7.9 Cross-talk between different cell types and the genesis of NASH. Kupffer cells are the principal site of TNF production. TNF can worsen the insulin-resistant state, increase oxidative stress, cause apoptosis and perpetuate

the inflammatory state by increasing the activity of the transcriptional factor NF-κB. It also increased production of cytokines (e.g. transforming growth factor-α (TGF-α) which can activate stellate cells and cause pericellular fibrosis.

a multitude of effects and induces the production of other cytokines and modulates several key hepatocyte functions (e.g. bile formation) and survival. TNF may likewise perpetuate inflammation by activation of a key transcriptional factor NF-κB, which regulates the expression of numerous genes including pro-inflammatory cytokines (e.g. interleukin-2 [IL-2] and IL-6); chemokines (e.g. IL-8); inflammatory enzymes (e.g. lipooxygenase, cyclooxygenase and inducible nitric oxide synthetase); adhesion molecules (e.g. inter-cellular adhesion molecules) and receptors (e.g. IL-2 receptor) [63]. Importantly, NF-κB increases TNF expression. Thus, TNF may set up a cycle of increased NF-κB expression, which in turn increases TNF pro-duction and perpetuates hepatic inflammation.

Much of this work has been carried out in cell lines and in experimental models. In humans, an increase in TNF messenger RNA (mRNA) has been found in the livers of those with NASH as well as in the mRNA for the p55 receptor for TNF (Fig. 7.10) [64]. These findings are most marked in those with advanced stages of NASH. Recently, an increased prevalence of polymorphisms at the 238 position of the TNF gene promoter in the liver has been found in patients with NASH (see Chapter 6) [65]. This was associated with a greater degree of insulin resistance, indicating that TNF may have a role in the genesis of NASH. How-ever, in another study [66], a correlation between IR and the polymorphism at position 238 could not be confirmed. Clearly, more work is required to elucidate the potential mechanisms by which TNF contributes

to either the genesis or perpetuation of NASH and the development of hepatic fibrosis.

Role of iron

Considerable controversy exists with respect to the potential role of iron in the pathogenesis of NASH. Bacon *et al.* [67] first identified the presence of hyperferritinaemia and increased hepatic iron in subjects with NASH. However, this was not associated with either increased Cys282Tyr mutations or an iron index greater than 1.9. Subsequently, in an Australian study [68], the Cys282Tyr mutation was found to be responsible for most cases of mild iron overload seen in association with NASH. There was an association between iron overload and increased fibrosis stages in these patients. Yet another study [69] found a greater prevalence of the HFE gene mutation in North American subjects with NASH. However, two other large studies of North American subjects with NASH failed to confirm the association with iron overload [70,71]. A recent Australian study [72] has also failed to confirm the relationship between HFE mutations and the degree of fibrosis in such patients.

Intracellular iron can impair insulin signalling and contribute to insulin resistance. It has been shown that serum ferritin levels are elevated in subjects with the metabolic syndrome [73]. Iron depletion improves parameters of insulin sensitivity even in the absence of biochemical features of iron overload [74]. It is also well known that iron overload contributes to increased

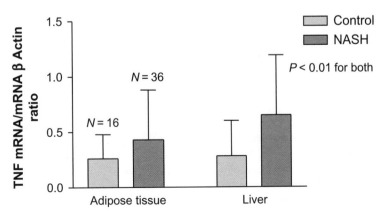

Fig. 7.10 TNF gene expression in the liver and adipose tissue of subjects with NASH and normal controls. NASH was associated with a significantly higher level of expression in both tissues. (After Crespo *et al.* [64].)

reactive oxygen species production and oxidative stress. However, the role of iron to the insulin resistance and oxidative stress associated with the metabolic syndrome and NASH remains to be defined.

Antioxidant mechanisms in NASH

The degree of oxidant stress reflects a balance between pro- and antioxidant forces within a given cell. So far, we have discussed the current state of knowledge regarding the pro-oxidant mechanisms that may be operative in the genesis of NASH. A priori, one would expect upregulation of antioxidant enzyme expression and depletion of antioxidant activity in the face of increased pro-oxidant forces. It is known that certain CYPs can induce antioxidant enzymes. However, the status of antioxidant defences in NASH is virtually unknown. Once again, more work is necessary in this area.

Conclusions

An extraordinary amount of progress has occurred in our understanding of the pathogenesis of hepatic steatosis and NASH in the last 5 years. The association of IR and NAFLD is now established. The metabolic abnormalities associated with IR have been defined in humans. This has allowed the development of a conceptual framework for understanding the genesis of a fatty liver. While all of the elements of this framework remain to be experimentally verified, it provides the foundation on which future knowledge can be built. Steatohepatitis develops as a consequence of increased oxidant stress. This may in part be caused by IR itself but in addition may involve additional pathways involving hepatic mitochondria, the cytochrome P450 system and peroxisomes. Oxidative stress and the hepatic response to this stress may be further modified by cytokines such as TNF. While much work remains to be done, progress in the last 5 years has already provided rational targets for the therapy of NASH.

Acknowledgement

This work was partially supported by a grant from the National Institutes of Health (NIH) to Dr Sanyal (K24 DK 25331 04).

References

1 Contos MJ, Sanyal AJ. The clinicopathologic spectrum and management of non-alcoholic fatty liver disease. *Adv Anat Pathol* 2002; **9**: 37–51.

2 Ludwig J, Viggiano TR, McGill DB, Oh BJ. Non-alcoholic steatohepatitis: Mayo Clinic experiences with a hitherto unnamed disease. *Mayo Clin Proc* 1980; **55**: 434–8.

3 Powell EE, Cooksley WG, Hanson R *et al.* The natural history of non-alcoholic steatohepatitis: a follow-up study of 42 patients for up to 21 years. *Hepatology* 1990; **11**: 74–80.

4 Wanless IR, Lentz JS. Fatty liver hepatitis (steatohepatitis) and obesity: an autopsy study with analysis of risk factors. *Hepatology* 1990; **12**: 1106–10.

5 Ground KEV. Prevalence of fatty liver in healthy adults accidentally killed. *Aviat Space Environ Med* 1984; **55**: 59–61.

6 Marcos A, Fisher RA, Ham JM *et al.* Selection and outcome of living donors for adult to adult right lobe transplantation. *Transplantation* 2000; **69**: 2410–5.

7 Garcia Urena MA, Colina Ruiz-Delgado F, Moreno GE *et al.* Hepatic steatosis in liver transplant donors: common feature of donor population? *World J Surg* 1998; **22**: 837–44.

8 Carr A, Samaras K, Thorisdottir A *et al.* Diagnosis, prediction, and natural course of HIV-1 protease-inhibitor-associated lipodystrophy, hyperlipidaemia, and diabetes mellitus: a cohort study. *Lancet* 1999; **353**: 2093–9.

9 Miller J, Carr A, Smith D *et al.* Lipodystrophy following antiretroviral therapy of primary HIV infection. *AIDS* 2000; **14**: 2406–7.

10 Pagano G, Pacini G, Musso G *et al.* Non-alcoholic steatohepatitis, insulin resistance, and metabolic syndrome: further evidence for an etiologic association. *Hepatology* 2002; **35**: 367–72.

11 Chitturi S, Abeygunasekera S, Farrell GC *et al.* NASH and insulin resistance: insulin hypersecretion and specific association with the insulin resistance syndrome. *Hepatology* 2002; **35**: 373–9.

12 Marchesini G, Bugianesi E, Forlani G *et al.* Non-alcoholic fatty liver, steatohepatitis, and the metabolic syndrome. *Hepatology* 2003; **37**: 917–23.

13 Sanyal AJ, Campbell-Sargent C, Mirshahi F *et al.* Non-alcoholic steatohepatitis: association of insulin resistance and mitochondrial abnormalities. *Gastroenterology* 2001; **120**: 1183–92.

14 Britton RS, Bacon BR. Role of free radicals in liver diseases and hepatic fibrosis. *Hepatogastroenterology* 1994; **41**: 343–8.

15 Berson A, De B V, Letteron P *et al.* Steatohepatitis-inducing drugs cause mitochondrial dysfunction and lipid

peroxidation in rat hepatocytes. *Gastroenterology* 1998; **114**: 764–74.

16 Sumida Y, Nakashima T, Yoh T *et al.* Serum thioredoxin levels as a predictor of steatohepatitis in patients with non-alcoholic fatty liver disease. *J Hepatol* 2003; **38**: 32–8.

17 Macdonald GA, Bridle KR, Ward PJ *et al.* Lipid peroxidation in hepatic steatosis in humans is associated with hepatic fibrosis and occurs predominantly in acinar zone 3. *J Gastroenterol Hepatol* 2001; **16**: 599–605.

18 Seki K, Kitada T, Sakaguchi H, Nakatani K, Wakasa K. *In situ* detection of lipid peroxidation and oxidative DNA damage in non-alcoholic fatty liver diseases. *J Hepatol* 2002; **37**: 56–62.

19 Weltman MD, Farrell GC, Hall P, Ingelman-Sundberg M, Liddle C. Hepatic cytochrome P450 2E1 is increased in patients with non-alcoholic steatohepatitis. *Hepatology* 1998; **27**: 128–33.

20 Leclercq IA, Farrell GC, Field J *et al.* CYP2E1 and CYP4A as microsomal catalysts of lipid peroxides in murine non-alcoholic steatohepatitis. *J Clin Invest* 2000; **105**: 1067–75.

21 Rao MS, Reddy JK. Peroxisomal β-oxidation and steatohepatitis. *Semin Liver Dis* 2001; **21**: 43–55.

22 Diehl AM. Cytokine regulation of liver injury and repair. *Immunol Rev* 2000; **174**: 160–71.

23 Anthonsen MW, Ronnstrand L, Wernstedt C, Degerman E, Holm C. Identification of novel phosphorylation sites in hormone-sensitive lipase that are phosphorylated in response to isoproterenol and govern activation properties *in vitro*. *J Biol Chem* 1998; **273**: 215–21.

24 Newgard CB, Brady MJ, O'Doherty RM, Saltiel AR. Organizing glucose disposal: emerging roles of the glycogen targeting subunits of protein phosphatase-1. *Diabetes* 2000; **49**: 1967–77.

25 Pilkis SJ, Granner DK. Molecular physiology of the regulation of hepatic gluconeogenesis and glycolysis. *Annu Rev Physiol* 1992; **54**: 885–909.

26 Shimomura I, Matsuda M, Hammer RE *et al.* Decreased IRS-2 and increased SREBP-1c lead to mixed insulin resistance and sensitivity in livers of lipodystrophic and ob/ob mice. *Mol Cell* 2000; **6**: 77–86.

27 Deng X, Cagen LM, Wilcox HG *et al.* Regulation of the Rat SREBP-1c promoter in primary rat hepatocytes. *Biochem Biophys Res Commun* 2002; **290**: 256–62.

28 Kitamura T, Kitamura Y, Kuroda S *et al.* Insulin-induced phosphorylation and activation of cyclic nucleotide phosphodiesterase 3B by the serine-threonine kinase Akt. *Mol Cell Biol* 1999; **19**: 6286–96.

29 Steppan CM, Bailey ST, Bhat S *et al.* The hormone resistin links obesity to diabetes. *Nature* 2001; **409**: 307–12.

30 Ferrannini E, Vichi S, Beck-Nielsen H *et al.* Insulin action and age: European Group for the Study of Insulin Resistance (EGIR). *Diabetes* 1996; **45**: 947–53.

31 Hube F, Hauner H. The role of TNF-α in human adipose tissue: prevention of weight gain at the expense of insulin resistance? *Horm Metab Res* 1999; **31**: 626–31.

32 Harris RB. Leptin: much more than a satiety signal. *Annu Rev Nutr* 2000; **20**: 45–75.

33 Deslypere JP, Verdonck L, Vermeulen A. Fat tissue: a steroid reservoir and site of steroid metabolism. *J Clin Endocrinol Metab* 1985; **61**: 564–70.

34 Peraldi P, Spiegelman B. TNF-α and insulin resistance: summary and future prospects. *Mol Cell Biochem* 1998; **182**: 169–75.

35 Saltiel AR, Kahn CR. Insulin signalling and the regulation of glucose and lipid metabolism. *Nature* 2001; **414**: 799–806.

36 Roden M, Price TB, Perseghin G *et al.* Mechanism of free fatty acid-induced insulin resistance in humans. *J Clin Invest* 1996; **97**: 2859–65.

37 Boden G, Chen X, Ruiz J, White JV, Rossetti L. Mechanisms of fatty acid-induced inhibition of glucose uptake. *J Clin Invest* 1994; **93**: 2438–46.

38 Randle PJ, Garland PB, Hales CN, Newholme CA. The glucose fatty-acid cycle: its role in insulin sensitivity and the metabolic disturbances of diabetes mellitus. *Lancet* 1963; **i**: 785–9.

39 Randle PJ, Priestman DA, Mistry S, Halsall A. Mechanisms modifying glucose oxidation in diabetes mellitus. *Diabetologia* 1994; **37** (Suppl. 2): S155–61.

40 Morand C, Besson C, Demigne C, Remesy C. Importance of the modulation of glycolysis in the control of lactate metabolism by fatty acids in isolated hepatocytes from fed rats. *Arch Biochem Biophys* 1994; **309**: 254–60.

41 Dresner A, Laurent D, Marcucci M *et al.* Effects of free fatty acids on glucose transport and IRS-1-associated phosphatidylinositol 3-kinase activity. *J Clin Invest* 1999; **103**: 253–9.

42 Griffin ME, Marcucci MJ, Cline GW *et al.* Free fatty acid-induced insulin resistance is associated with activation of protein kinase C theta and alterations in the insulin signaling cascade. *Diabetes* 1999; **48**: 1270–4.

43 Warren GB, Tipton KF. The role of acetyl-CoA in the reaction pathway of pig-liver pyruvate carboxylase. *Eur J Biochem* 1974; **47**: 549–54.

44 Gulick T, Cresci S, Caira T, Moore DD, Kelly DP. The peroxisome proliferator-activated receptor regulates mitochondrial fatty acid oxidative enzyme gene expression. *Proc Natl Acad Sci USA* 1994; **91**: 11012–6.

45 Prentki M, Corkey BE. Are the beta-cell signaling molecules malonyl-CoA and cystolic long-chain acyl-CoA implicated in multiple tissue defects of obesity and NIDDM? *Diabetes* 1996; **45**: 273–83.

46 Masuzaki H, Paterson J, Shinyama H *et al.* A transgenic model of visceral obesity and the metabolic syndrome. *Science* 2001; **294**: 2166–70.

47 Tomlinson JW, Stewart PM. Cortisol metabolism and the role of 11β-hydroxysteroid dehydrogenase. *Best Pract Res Clin Endocrinol Metab* 2001; **15**: 61–78.

48 Tomlinson JW, Bujalska I, Stewart PM, Cooper MS. The role of 11β-hydroxysteroid dehydrogenase in central obesity and osteoporosis. *Endocr Res* 2000; **26**: 711–22.

49 Bergman RN. New concepts in extracellular signaling for insulin action: the single gateway hypothesis. *Recent Prog Horm Res* 1997; **52**: 359–85.

50 Himsworth H. Diabetes mellitus: a differentiation into insulin-sensitive and insulin-insensitive subtypes. *Lancet* 1936; **i**: 127–30.

51 Reaven GM. Banting Lecture 1988. Role of insulin resistance in human disease, 1988. *Nutrition* 1997; **13**: 65.

52 Marchesini G, Brizi M, Bianchi G *et al*. Non-alcoholic fatty liver disease: a feature of the metabolic syndrome. *Diabetes* 2001; **50**: 1844–50.

53 Marchesini G, Brizi M, Morselli-Labate AM *et al*. Association of non-alcoholic fatty liver disease with insulin resistance. *Am J Med* 1999; **107**: 450–5.

54 Charlton M, Sreekumar R, Rasmussen D, Lindor K, Nair KS. Apolipoprotein synthesis in non-alcoholic steatohepatitis. *Hepatology* 2002; **35**: 898–904.

55 Bernard S, Touzet S, Personne I *et al*. Association between microsomal triglyceride transfer protein gene polymorphism and the biological features of liver steatosis in patients with type II diabetes. *Diabetologia* 2000; **43**: 995–9.

56 Pessayre D, Mansouri A, Fromenty B. Non-alcoholic steatosis and steatohepatitis. V. Mitochondrial dysfunction in steatohepatitis. *Am J Physiol Gastrointest Liver Physiol* 2002; **282**: G193–9.

57 Caldwell SH, Swerdlow RH, Khan EM *et al*. Mitochondrial abnormalities in non-alcoholic steatohepatitis. *J Hepatol* 1999; **31**: 430–4.

58 Sladky JT. Histopathological features of peripheral nerves and muscle in mitochondrial disease. *Semin Neurol* 2001; **21**: 293–301.

59 Haque M, Mirshahi F, Campbell-Sargent C *et al*. Non-alcoholic steatohepatitis (NASH) is associated with hepatocyte mitochondrial DNA depletion [Abstract]. *Hepatology* 2002; **36**: 403.

60 Chalasani N, Gorski JC, Asghar MS *et al*. Hepatic cytochrome P450 2E1 activity in non-diabetic patients with non-alcoholic steatohepatitis. *Hepatology* 2003; **37**: 544–50.

61 Hotamisligil GS. The role of TNF-α and TNF receptors in obesity and insulin resistance. *J Intern Med* 1999; **245**: 621–5.

62 Lancaster JR Jr, Laster SM, Gooding LR. Inhibition of target cell mitochondrial electron transfer by tumor necrosis factor. *FEBS Lett* 1989; **248**: 169–74.

63 Barnes PJ, Karin M. Nuclear factor-κB: a pivotal transcription factor in chronic inflammatory diseases. *N Engl J Med* 1997; **336**: 1066–71.

64 Crespo J, Cayon A, Fernandez-Gil P *et al*. Gene expression of tumor necrosis factor-α and TNF-receptors, p55 and p75, in non-alcoholic steatohepatitis patients. *Hepatology* 2001; **34**: 1158–63.

65 Valenti L, Fracanzani AL, Dongiovanni P *et al*. Tumor necrosis factor-α promoter polymorphisms and insulin resistance in non-alcoholic fatty liver disease. *Gastroenterology* 2002; **122**: 274–80.

66 Walston J, Seibert M, Yen C, Cheskin LJ, Andersen RE. Tumor necrosis factor-α 238 and -308 polymorphisms do not associate with traits related to obesity and insulin resistance. *Diabetes* 1999; **48**: 2096–8.

67 Bacon BR, Farahvash MJ, Janney CG, Neuschwander-Tetri BA. Non-alcoholic steatohepatitis: an expanded clinical entity. *Gastroenterology* 1994; **107**: 1103–9.

68 George DK, Goldwurm S, Macdonald GA *et al*. Increased hepatic iron concentration in non-alcoholic steatohepatitis is associated with increased fibrosis. *Gastroenterology* 1998; **114**: 311–8.

69 Bonkovsky HL, Jawaid Q, Tortorelli K *et al*. Non-alcoholic steatohepatitis and iron: increased prevalence of mutations of the HFE gene in non-alcoholic steatohepatitis. *J Hepatol* 1999; **31**: 421–9.

70 Angulo P, Keach JC, Batts KP, Lindor KD. Independent predictors of liver fibrosis in patients with non-alcoholic steatohepatitis. *Hepatology* 1999; **30**: 1356–62.

71 Younossi ZM, Gramlich T, Bacon BR *et al*. Hepatic iron and non-alcoholic fatty liver disease. *Hepatology* 1999; **30**: 847–50.

72 Chitturi S, Weltman M, Farrell GC *et al*. HFE mutations, hepatic iron, and fibrosis: ethnic-specific association of NASH with C282Y but not with fibrotic severity. *Hepatology* 2002; **36**: 142–9.

73 Mendler MH, Turlin B, Moirand R *et al*. Insulin resistance-associated hepatic iron overload. *Gastroenterology* 1999; **117**: 1155–63.

74 Valenti L, Fracanzani AL, Fargion S. Effect of iron depletion in patients with non-alcoholic fatty liver disease without carbohydrate intolerance. *Gastroenterology* 2003; **124**: 866–7.

8 Animal models of steatohepatitis

Geoffrey C. Farrell

Key learning points

1 Steatosis can be produced in animals by overnutrition, administration of diets deficient in certain lipotropic factors, physical inactivity, insulin resistance, leptin deficiency, leptin receptor dysfunction, lipoatrophy and some hepatotoxins.

2 In these models, steatosis is attributable to one or more changes in hepatic fat disposition, including enhanced fatty acid uptake and synthesis by the liver (increased fat input), impaired β-oxidation (fat burning), triglyceride formation and/or very-low-density lipoprotein secretion (decreased fat output).

3 Steatosis predisposes to oxidative forms of acute liver injury, exemplified by lipopolysaccharide stimulation of Kupffer cells, and hepatic ischaemia reperfusion.

4 Spontaneous transition to significant steatohepatitis does not occur in nutritional and metabolic models of steatosis.

5 Fatty acylCoA oxidase knockout (ko) mice, methionine adenosyltransferase-1A ko mice, and rodents fed a methionine- and choline-deficient (MCD) diet develop steatosis, severe oxidative stress and necroinflammatory change, perpetuated as steatohepatitis. Sequelae include pericellular fibrosis and disordered cell proliferation, leading to liver tumours.

6 The MCD model has allowed the mechanisms of liver cell injury, inflammatory recruitment and fibrogenesis to be studied, including the roles of redox-sensitive transcription factors (especially NF-κB) and cytokines.

7 There is an outstanding need to establish models of steatohepatitis with less nutritional depletion and similar risk factors as in humans, possibly by adapting existing models of steatosis caused by insulin resistance and dietary imbalance.

Abstract

Animal models of human disease allow disease mechanisms to be unravelled by sampling tissues during evolution of the disease, and by examining the effects of dietary, molecular or chemical interventions. Murine models have the further advantage of testing genetic factors in spontaneously mutant strains, and in transgenically manipulated animals expressing ('knock-in') or failing to express (knockout [ko]) candidate genes for disease susceptibility. However, results in animal models should be interpreted cautiously because of the confounding effects of species differences in disease-producing pathways, despite similar pathology.

There are numerous animal models of hepatic steatosis related to overnutrition and metabolic perturbations that interrupt hepatic fatty acid (FA) turnover and metabolism, favouring accumulation of triglycerides and free fatty acids (FFA) in the liver. Conditional tissue expression of liver-specific lipoprotein lipase demonstrates clearly that vectorially enhanced FA uptake by the liver can lead to steatosis; so too can transfection of molecules that enhance hepatic FA synthesis, or effect targeted deletions of pathways involved with β-oxidation (fat burning) and very-low-density lipoprotein (VLDL) formation—the latter is required for egress of triglyceride from hepatocytes. In addition, several murine models of lipoatrophy are associated with insulin resistance, glucose intolerance, hypertriglyceridaemia, hypoleptinaemia and steatosis. Irrespective of primary aetiology, the fatty liver is susceptible to oxidative forms of liver injury, including that produced by bacterial products through stimulation of Kupffer cells to release tumour necrosis factor-α (TNF-α).

Many studies on the cell biology of fatty liver disease have used leptin-deficient or lepin receptor dysfunctional animals. In the former, most or all defects can be corrected by leptin replacement. Further, while these models of steatosis are of interest to non-alcoholic fatty liver disease (NAFLD), they do not lead spontaneously to significant steatohepatitis, as found in non-alcoholic steatohepatitis (NASH). Conversely, rodents with spontaneous or diet-induced defects of FA turnover and redox balance develop liver pathology that resembles NASH. Such models of significant (or fibrosing) steatohepatitis include defects in peroxisomal β-oxidation (the acylCoA oxidase [AOX] ko mouse), and hepatic methionine deficiency produced in the methionine adenosyltransferase-1A ko (MATO) mouse, or by feeding rats or mice a lipogenic (high sucrose, 10% fat) diet deficient in both methionine and choline (MCD diet). These models allow the mechanisms of inflammatory recruitment and fibrogenesis to be studied, including the roles of redox-sensitive transcription factors (especially nuclear factor-κB [NF-κB]), TNF and other cytokines. More detailed studies in existing models will shed light on the molecular processes that initiate and perpetuate steatohepatitis; the importance of selected pathways can then be tested by studies of human liver and molecular genetics. However, there remains an outstanding need to adapt existing models of steatosis caused by insulin resistance and/or dietary lipid or carbohydrate overload to studies of steatohepatitis.

Introduction

Contemporary approaches to animal experimentation offer logistic advantages over studies in human tissues, as summarized in Table 8.1. The most cogent and powerful is the capacity to study targeted interventions that facilitate or interrupt pathogenic processes. The use of experimental animals allows multiple sampling of liver tissue, in amounts restricted only by the size of the animal, and at strategic times during the evolution, resolution or amelioration (by 'therapeutic intervention') of disease. Animal models also permit studies of the isolated perfused liver, dissection of the roles of individual cell types and subcellular fractions, profiling of tissue gene expression at the messenger RNA (mRNA) (transcriptosome) and protein (proteosome) levels, and functional elucidation of key gene products (enzyme assays, transport processes). By such composite approaches, diseases can be understood at cell biological and tissue levels, as well as in terms of molecular expression; the latter is then amenable to testing in human tissue.

Large animal models (primates, pigs, sheep, dogs) have been employed in studies of alcoholic liver disease (baboon model), liver surgery and transplantation (pig and dog models), pharmacokinetic and nutrition studies. In general, however, logistics (including cost) and investigator preference in animal experimentation favour small animal models. The ability to study human genes expressed in another (genetically manipulated) animal, or deletion of the murine homologue (ko technology) adds another powerful dimension to modelling human disease. Mice offer several advantages in this respect, and are now the preferred species for establishing models of human liver disease. The advantages include the readiness of conducting breeding experiments, the extensive knowledge base of the mouse genome and immune system, existence of a large number of genetically manipulated (knock-in and ko) lines, commercial availability of animals with spontaneous mutations (e.g. *ob/ob* mice), and lower costs of purchasing, transporting, housing and feeding.

The disadvantages of animal models are sometimes neglected. The most obvious is species differences, particularly in immune reactions but also in metabolic, pharmacological or tissue responses. A clear example of the latter is the different susceptibility of rat liver to bile duct ligation. In humans, resultant cholestatic liver injury is slowly progressive over many years, whereas

Table 8.1 Why use animal models to study questions about human liver disease?

Factor	Animal model	Humans and human tissues
Tissue availability	Multiple tissues can be sampled Time course easily constructed Liver readily obtained Amount restricted only by animal size	Blood, genomic DNA readily obtained Liver requires ethical considerations Amount restricted by safety and logistics of needle biopsy
Technical approaches	Isolated liver, cell culture, tissue subfractionation all readily available	Cell culture restricted by non-availability of healthy liver (e.g. excess donor liver) Subfractionation requires micromethodology
Genetic variation	Species differences may thwart interpretation	Most relevant species
Genetic manipulation	Possible, especially in mice Complementary approaches—'loss of function' versus 'gain of function' Cross-breeding possible	Not possible
Selective manipulation of metabolic pathways	Possible Can be coupled with tissue sampling	Difficult, especially to couple with tissue sampling
Drug interventions	Easy. Can be coupled with tissue sampling Note species differences in pharmaco-genetics and pharmacodynamics	Ethical, safety and logistic issue Hard to couple with tissue sampling
Developmental studies	Possible	Not possible/unethical
Carcinogenesis studies	Possible Rely on opportunistic observations	Toxic/unethical interventions

rats with bile duct ligation develop severe bile acid-mediated oxidative stress, acute hepatocellular injury with very high serum alanine aminotransferase (ALT) levels, high mortality (depending on strain) and development of cirrhosis within 2 months. There are also important physiological differences in eating behaviour (including coprophagy) and nutritional requirements, especially lipid intake, and in cytochrome P450 (CYP) -mediated pathways for hepatic metabolism of fatty acids, drugs, toxins and carcinogens. Finally, it should always be kept in mind that the range of hepatic lesions caused by multiple aetiologies is rather narrow; it is therefore possible that multiple causes and interactive processes can give rise to the same 'final common pathway' of liver pathology.

It seems unlikely that any animal model can provide a perfect simulation of NAFLD/NASH in humans, with identical causative factors and exhibiting the same range of pathobiological processes to arrive at identical pathology and reproducible disease outcomes (natural history). However, what animal models reveal is information on the processes that can, in some species and under some circumstances, lead to the pathological lesions of interest. This is particularly useful for testing potential therapeutic interventions. In the study of human fatty liver diseases that are not the result of alcohol, drugs or other toxic causes (NAFLD/NASH), several issues in pathogenesis and therapy are amenable to study in animal models, as summarized in Table 8.2. An overview of existing models that encapsulate some of the disease processes, together with the pathobiology involved, is presented in Table 8.3.

Animal models of steatosis

Steatosis can be produced in animals by various toxins and dietary (lipotrope) deficiencies, or by perturbations that facilitate accumulation of fat in the liver. In all these models, steatosis is the result of an imbalance of hepatic FA turnover, generated either by increased

93

Table 8.2 Issues in pathogenesis and therapy of NAFLD/ NASH amenable to study in animal models.

• Nature of insulin resistance—why it occurs, whether responsible for inflammation, cell injury and fibrogenesis, as well as hepatic triglyceride accumulation (steatosis)
• Dysregulation of hepatic FA storage and metabolism: lipotoxicity, role of leptin, adiponectin and other hormones modifying insulin sensitivity, role of individual FA, micronutrients, optimal means of reversing steatosis
• Oxidative stress: cellular and subcellular sources, mechanistic significance, therapeutic value of antioxidants
• Mechanisms for initiating and perpetuating inflammatory recruitment; role of cytokines
• Pathogenesis of fibrosis, including roles of iron, oxidative stress, cytokines, stellate cell biology
• Disordered cell proliferation, possible relationship to hepatocarcinogenesis

---

FA, fatty acid.

liver uptake of FA, increased *de novo* lipid synthesis by the liver (fat input), decreased β-oxidation (fat burning) or diminished processing into triglycerides and VLDL so that triglyceride secretion from the liver (fat output) is impaired [1,2]. The dynamic nature of hepatic FA turnover is described in more detail in Chapter 6 and summarized schematically in Fig. 8.1. Existing animal models are summarized in Table 8.4 and described in more detail here.

Hepatotoxins and virus infections

Many carcinogens and dose-dependent hepatoxins cause steatosis as part of direct hepatocellular toxicity, although in the case of carbon tetrachloride (CCl_4), mobilization of TNF has an augmenting role in causing liver injury as well as mediating recovery [3,4]. With such 'classic' hepatotoxins, liver injury is focused on cell membranes and/or mitochondria, caused either by direct solvent effects or more often as a result of CYP-generated reactive metabolites that create oxidat-

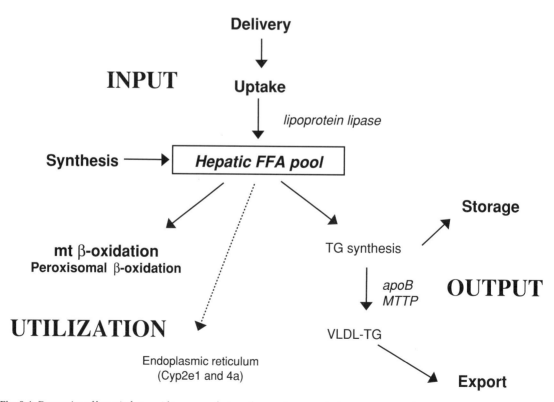

Fig. 8.1 Dynamics of hepatic fatty acid turnover: factors that can be perturbed to cause steatosis.

Table 8.3 Disease processes for which animal models can be employed to provide information about human fatty liver disease.

Disease process	Representative models	Pathobiology
Insulin resistance	*ob/ob* mouse	Leptin deficiency
	fa/fa (Zucker) rat, *db/db* mouse	Leptin receptor dysfunction
	Subcutaneous fat atrophy (specific molecular lesions; see Table 8.4)	Leptin, adiponectin deficiency; increased hepatic lipogenesis
	A^y mouse	Disordered appetite control resulting from disrupted melanocortin receptor signalling
	NZ obese mouse	Decreased activity, obesity
Steatosis	Models of insulin resistance (above)	See above
	High sucrose/fructose or high fat diets	Energy intake exceeds expenditure
	PPARα ko mouse, particularly with high fat intake	Inability to regulate hepatic lipid turnover
	Choline deficiency, particularly with high fat or sucrose intake	Abnormal phospholipid membranes
	AOX/PPARα double ko	See text
	Orotic acid, particularly with high fat or sucrose intake	?Impaired FA oxidation, VLDL trafficking
	Drug toxicity	Mitochondrial injury, impaired VLDL secretion
Initiation of inflammation/patocellular injury	Endotoxin injection into animals with steatosis	Kupffer cell release of TNF
Perpetuation of steatohepatitis	AOX ko mouse	Oxidative stress: peroxisomal H_2O_2 production and CYP4A
	MATO mouse	Oxidative stress: upregulated CYP2E1 and 4A
	MCD fed rats and mice	Oxidative stress; upregulated CYP2E1 and/or 4A; ?secondary mitochondrial injury
Fibrogenesis	MCD fed rats and mice	Roles of oxidative stress and stellate cell activation
	Iron-loaded MCD model	Facilitates fibrogenesis
Hepatocarcinogenesis	Old *ob/ob* mice	Disordered cell proliferation/tumours
	AOX ko mouse; MATO mouse; HCV core transgenic mouse	Tumors; oxidative stress and PPARα drive on cell proliferation

AOX, acylCoA oxidase; A^y, agouti mutation (melanocortin receptor); CYP, cytochrome P450; HCV, hepatitis C virus; ko, knockout; MCD, methionine and choline deficiency; MATO, methionine *S*-adenosyltransferase-1A ko; NZ, New Zealand; PPARα, peroxisome proliferator-activated receptor-α; TNF, tumour necrosis factor; VLDL, very-low-density lipoprotein.

ive stress or alkylate tissue macromolecules. Other steatogenic hepatotoxins, such as high-dose tetracycline and drugs that cause steatohepatitis in humans, perturb hepatic FA turnover by impairing VLDL formation and secretion [5–8]. Chronic ethanol favours steatosis by stimulating lipogenesis via effects on intermediary metabolism (increased NAD^+ : NADH ratio), and by impairing secretion of VLDL. However, steatosis does not occur in ethanol-fed rodents unless they are also fed a high-fat diet [9].

In general, few insights come from these early studies for understanding the pathogenesis of NAFLD/NASH. An exception is the study of amphiphilic drugs that, once protonated, concentrate in the mitochondrial matrix and cause mitochondrial injury [6–8]. These compounds include amiodarone, perhexiline maleate, tamoxifen and glucocorticoids, all potential causes of drug-induced steatohepatitis (see Chapter 21) [10]. Certain agents with carboxylic groups (aspirin, valproic acid, 2-aryl propionate anti-inflammatory drugs)

Table 8.4 Animal models of steatosis.

Type of model	Examples	Phenotype	Pathogenic factor
Drugs, toxins, hormones and virus infections	Ethanol Oestrogen antagonists; glucocorticoids; etomoxir	Steatosis with high-fat diet	Enhanced lipogenesis; inhibited VLDL release; inhibition mitochondrial β-oxidation
Lipotrope deficiency	Arginine deficient Choline deficient diet*	Steatosis with high fat or sucrose diet; may develop fibrosis	Impaired disposal of fat
	PMET ko mouse	Steatosis	Inability to synthesize choline
Dietary (overnutrition)	High sucrose/fructose; high fat (with or without high sucrose)	Steatosis (mostly macrovesicular)	Increased lipogenesis ?Purine deficiency;
	1% orotic acid (usually with high-fat or high-sucrose diet)	Microvesicular steatosis	?impaired FA oxidation and/or trafficking of VLDL
Spontaneously obese rodents (all develop insulin resistance and diabetes)	*ob/ob* mouse *db/db* mouse; *fa/fa* (Zucker) rat A^y mouse NZ obese mouse	Absent leptin Absent/dysfunctional leptin receptor (leptin resistance) Disordered appetite control Reduced spontaneous activity	Increased hepatic uptake and synthesis of FA Decreased utilization of fat
Transgenic mice with stimulated lipogenesis (all develop diabetes)	PEPCK-SREBP-1α AP2-SREBP-1c* A-bZIP/F* Fat-specific CEBPα ko* aP2-diphtheria toxin* Stat 5B ko Pancreas-specific IGF-2	*Deleted WAT (lipoatrophy); leptin deficient	Increased hepatic lipogenesis
Acquired lipoatrophy	Administration of urine from CGL patients	Lipoatrophy; leptin deficient	Increased hepatic lipogenesis
Transgenic mice with impaired oxidation of fat	PPARα ko Aromatase ko (female)	Steatosis Steatosis	Multiple defects in hepatic FA disposal

* Usually administered with high-fat diet to exacerbate steatosis
bZIP, basic leucine zipper protein; C/EBP, CCAAT enhancer binding protein; CGL, congenital generalized lipodystrophy; AP2-SREBP-1c, sterol regulatory element binding protein-1c under control of activator protein-2; FA, fatty acid; IGF, insulin-like growth factor; ko, knockout; PEPCK-SREBP-1α, sterol regulatory element binding protein-1α under control of phosphoenolpyruvate carboxykinase promoter; PMET, phosphatidylethanolamine N-methyltransferase; PPARα ko, peroxisome proliferator-activated receptor-α knockout.

can sequester coenzyme-A (CoA) or inhibit mitochondrial β-oxidation [6,7,11]. Together with the proposed effects of copper toxicity, in which the transitional metal catalyses production of reactive oxygen species (ROS) [7], they provide a paradigm whereby mitochondrial injury leads to steatosis largely because of impaired mitochondrial β-oxidation. In turn, oxidative stress results from mitochondrial production of ROS, leading to development of steatohepatitis (see Chapter 11). Feeding these drugs to mice or other small animals causes steatosis (usually microvesicular), and is universally associated with oxidative stress, but development of experimental steatohepatitis is not documented [8,10–12].

Some virus infections can cause steatosis. Of contemporary interest, the most notable is the hepatitis C virus (HCV). Thus HCV core protein transgenic mice develop steatosis [13], and older mice with this transgene go on to develop hepatocellular carcinoma without evidence of fibrotic or inflammatory liver disease [14]. The relationship between fatty liver disease and hepatic carcinogenesis is discussed in Chapter 22.

Orotic acid, usually administered to rodents with an energy-imbalanced diet (high fat, high sucrose/fructose, or both) causes purine depletion and produces striking microvesicular fatty change associated with hepatic accumulation of FFA [15–17]. Possible mechanisms include increased *de novo* hepatic synthesis of fatty acids (15), decreased mitochondrial β-oxidation (16), and impaired VLDL formation or processing [16,17]. Su *et al.* [unpublished data] have recently shown that the resultant increase in hepatic FFA induces strong (albeit submaximal) stimulation of a peroxisome proliferator-activated receptor-α (PPARα) response (see below), with resultant increased peroxisomal enzyme activities, induction of CYP4A and suppression of CYP2E1. Such studies illustrate the dynamic and highly regulated nature of hepatic FA turnover (see Chapter 9), and how the responses to lipid accumulation include upregulation of extramitochondrial pathways of FA oxidation implicated in the creation of oxidative stress (Table 8.5 and see below).

Table 8.5 Sources of oxidative stress in experimental steatohepatitis.

Source	Biochemical processes	Importance	Antioxidant protection
Hepatocytes			
Mitochondria	Leakage of electrons from respiratory chain, facilitated by uncoupling proteins, FFA, oxidative injury to respiratory chain proteins and mtDNA	Possible primary source of ROS Mitochondria also target of ROS-mediated injury, leading to secondary production of ROS (see Chapter 11)	MnSOD, glutathione peroxidase
Endoplasmic reticulum	CYP2E1 CYP4A family members	Induced in response to insulin resistance, obesity, fasting, fatty acids Under PPARα control, possible reciprocal regulation with CYP2E1	Induces glutathione synthesis, glutathione-dependent enzymes
Peroxisomes	H_2O_2	Reserve compartment when mitochondrial β-oxidation saturated/overloaded, and for products of CYP2E1/4A-mediated ω and ω-1 oxidation Increased with peroxisomal enzyme defects (e.g. AOX ko)	Catalase
Kupffer cells			
	NADPH oxidase, NO, nitroradicals, leukotrienes, TNF	Generates ROS	SOD
Recruited inflammatory cells			
Macrophages, polymorphs, lymphocytes	As above	As above	As above

AOX ko, acetylCoA oxidase knockout mouse; CYP, cytochrome P450; FFA, free fatty acids; MnSOD, manganese-superoxide dismutase; mt, mitochondrial; ROS, reduced (reactive) oxygen species; NO, nitrous oxide; SOD, superoxide dismutase; TNF, tumour necrosis factor.

Lipotrope deficiency

Certain nutrients (arginine, choline, methionine) appear essential to protect the rodent liver from accumulation of lipid. When animals are deficient in these nutrients, particularly when fed an energy-imbalanced diet (high fat, high sucrose/fructose, or both), they develop steatosis. Arginine deficiency can produce a fatty liver without obesity, possibly by causing abnormal orotic acid metabolism [18]. The potential mechanisms have been discussed elsewhere [2]. Defects in adenosine metabolism, as produced in transgenic mice by deletion of the adenosine kinase gene, gives rise to lethal neonatal steatosis [19].

Feeding rats a high-fat diet coupled with choline deficiency was developed several decades ago as a model of hepatic steatosis and 'Laennec (portal) cirrhosis' [20]. The exact mechanism of steatosis is unclear, but defective production of phosphatidylcholine, resulting in disordered membrane functions, most likely plays a crucial part. Similarly, phosphatidylethanolamine N-methyltransferase (PMET) ko mice, which are unable to synthesize choline endogenously, also develop hepatic steatosis, even during intake of a choline-supplemented diet [21]. Inflammation is not a feature of these animals, although apoptosis is present [21]. According to the author's experience, the pathology of choline deficiency does not resemble steatohepatitis found in NAFLD/NASH. Rather, macrovesicular steatosis is associated with accumulation of fat-laden macrophages in portal tracts, with progressive pericellular and portal fibrosis leading to cirrhosis [22]. Apart from the dysregulation of CYP enzymes attributable to portasystemic shunting and hormonal changes of chronic liver disease [22], there have been few metabolic studies in this model. Interest has shifted to the effects of methionine deficiency, which can result in steatohepatitis as well as steatosis (see below).

Overnutrition models

European farmers and gourmets have long known that force-feeding geese and other fowl with grain (carbohydrate) produces a fatty liver, as in the renowned delicacy of pâté de foie gras. Likewise, high carbohydrate or lipid-rich diets administered to rodents can lead to steatosis [23–50]. Mice with obesity resulting from intake of a high-fat diet exhibit leptin resistance [28]. In rats, a high-fat diet causes visceral adiposity and hepatic insulin resistance as well as steatosis [26]; these changes can be reversed by administration of ragaglitazar, a combined PPARα–γ ligand [27]. The latter studies also invoked a role for adiponectin, another adipocyte-derived insulin-sensitizing hormone as a possible mediator of hepatic lipid content and insulin action in liver and muscle [27]; the role of adiponectin is addressed in the next section.

In general, rodents are relatively resistant to developing obesity from excessive intake of a balanced diet. However, adult male Sprague–Dawley rats fed 70% sucrose for several weeks become obese and develop steatosis with a minor increase in serum ALT [2,26–28]. Studies in these models of steatosis have advanced our understanding of the pathogenesis of insulin resistance, including hyperleptinaemia and secondary leptin resistance, and the role of factors that govern hepatic FA fluxes [24–26]. However, as far as one can establish from available literature, none of the overnutritional models in rodents are associated with steatohepatitis, indicating that other factors are required for inflammatory recruitment and perpetuation in the steatotic liver.

Insulin resistance resulting from disorders of leptin production or leptin receptor function

The obese ob/ob mouse has a defect in leptin synthesis that leads to disordered appetite regulation. Resultant uncontrolled food intake results in obesity, insulin resistance, hyperglycaemia and diabetes. In younger obese mice, the phenotype is hepatic steatosis with no inflammation. The mechanism of steatosis is related to increased delivery of FA to the liver (serum triglycerides and FFA levels are increased) and enhanced hepatic lipogenesis [2]. The latter is indicated by increased nuclear binding of sterol regulatory binding protein-1c (SREBP-1c) in association with increased activity of FA synthase. Interestingly, liver-specific disruption of PPARγ in leptin-deficient ob/ob mice produces a phenotype with a smaller liver and dramatically lower hepatic triglyceride levels, associated with decreased activity of enzymes involved in FA synthesis [31]. This is despite the expected aggravation of diabetes consequent on decreased insulin sensitivity in muscle and adipose tissue. Thus, hepatic PPARγ (as well as PPARα) have a critical role in regulation of triglyceride content in steatotic diabetic mouse liver.

In some adult (particularly older) obese *ob/ob* mice, very mild inflammatory lesions and ALT elevation are observed [32–34]; these lesions appear to correspond to NAFLD type 2 rather than types 3 or 4 (NASH) (see Chapters 1 and 2). In a series of elegant experiments, Diehl *et al.* have studied pathogenesis of NAFLD in *ob/ob* mice [32,33,35–41]. Early in the course of steatosis, they detected activation of inhibitor κ kinase β (IκKβ) [38]. The downstream consequences include DNA binding (activation) of NF-κB, with synthesis of TNF. Formation of TNF was proposed as a factor that causes or accentuates and perpetuates insulin resistance [32]; in addition, it was proposed that TNF induces mitochondrial uncoupling protein-2 (UCP2) in the liver, thereby potentially rendering hepatocytes vulnerable to necrosis because of compromised adenosine triphosphate (ATP) levels [36].

Administration of metformin to *ob/ob* mice reversed these metabolic changes, corrected hepatomegaly and improved the morphological appearances of fatty liver disease [32]. Recently, Xu *et al.* [35] showed that administration of recombinant adiponectin to *ob/ob* mice decreased steatosis and ALT abnormalities; these beneficial effects were attributed to the combined effects of stimulated carnitine palmitoyltransferase-1 (CPT-1) activity with resultant enhancement of mitochondrial β-oxidation, and decreased FA synthesis via acylCoA carboxylase and FA synthase [35]. Adiponectin also suppressed hepatic TNF production in *ob/ob* mice, as well as in a model of alcohol-induced liver injury [35]. However, the role of TNF in causing insulin resistance in steatotic obese mice has been disputed by others, who found that *ob/ob* mice cross-bred with TNF receptor ko mice had identical liver disease and metabolic abnormalities as wildtype (wt) *ob/ob* mice [42]. Further, cross-breeding of *ob/ob* mice with UCP2 ko mice produced a phenotype that was identical to wt *ob/ob* mice, even after prolonged intake of a high-fat diet [34]. The finding that fatty liver disease occurs in *ob/ob* mice irrespective of the action of TNF and upregulation of UCP2, appears to negate a crucial pathogenic role for these factors in experimental NAFLD.

Leptin plays an important part in modulating the hepatic immune response. Thus, leptin-deficient obese mice exhibit disordered macrophage and hepatic lymphocyte function [40,41,43], including defective TNF secretion. Recent studies have also characterized a striking defect in the control of liver regeneration in obese *ob/ob* mice [4,39]. However, defective liver cell proliferation does not appear to be a feature of NASH in humans [44], or in models of steatosis with intact leptin responses [45]. As shown by Leclercq *et al.* [4], and discussed in Chapter 12, the defect in *ob/ob* mice is attributable to leptin deficiency, rather than fatty liver disease *per se*.

Studies in the *ob/ob* mouse have also shown that leptin is virtually essential for deposition of hepatic fibrosis [46–49]. Thus, *ob/ob* mice do not develop fibrosis spontaneously or during feeding the MCD diet to generate significant steatohepatitis [46], or after toxic or infective (schistosomiasis) challenges [46–48]. Restitution experiments are a distinct advantage of using animal models of specific adipocyte hormone deficiencies. In *ob/ob* mice, the defects in fibrogenesis and liver regeneration were readily corrected by administration of physiological levels of leptin, whereas food restriction to produce similar reversal of steatosis and metabolic abnormalities did not [4,46].

Models in which defects of lipid turnover are caused by dysfunctional leptin receptors include the *fa/fa* Zucker rat, in which the long form of the leptin receptor required for intracellular signalling is abnormal, and the *fak/fak* Zucker rat and *db/db* mouse, which are nullizygous for the leptin receptor [49–51]. The phenotype is similar to the *ob/ob* mouse, with obesity, insulin resistance and type 2 diabetes; the liver shows bland steatosis. The mechanism may be related partly to increased hepatic FA synthesis as a result of leptin resistance [52]. Thus, livers of Zucker *fa/fa* rats express increased levels of SREBP-1c mRNA compared with controls, and this is associated with increased levels of mRNA for FA synthase and other lipogenic genes. In the case of the Zucker *fa/fa* rat, near complete defects of hepatic fibrogenesis and impaired liver regeneration cannot be reversed with leptin, consistent with a role for leptin resistance [53].

Other models of insulin resistance

Mice in which atrophy of subcutaneous (white) adipose tissue (WAT) is associated with insulin resistance also develop steatosis [54]. As summarized in Table 8.4, at least six individual lines of transgenic mice have been produced with this phenotype [2,54–57]; it corresponds to the human lipodystrophic disorders (see Chapter 21). One example is the A-ZIP/F-1 transgenic mouse, which expresses a dominant-negative A-ZIP/F that prevents

DNA binding of C/EBP and Jun family transcription factors in adipose tissue. These animals have no WAT and reduced amounts of brown adipose tissue, which is metabolically inactive [56]. They develop fatty liver at an early age. A possible mechanism is that leptin deficiency and hyperinsulinaemia induce hepatic SREBP-1c [54], thereby upregulating FA synthase. Likewise, transgenic mice with SREBP-1c targeted to adipose tissue (AP2-nSREBP-1c) develop WAT atrophy and hepatomegaly attributable to steatosis; leptin treatment reverses these changes [58]. In another transgenic model, AP2-diphtheria toxin mice, an attenuated form of the diphtheria toxin is expressed in WAT [57]. Survivors develop spontaneous atrophy of WAT with concomitant hyperinsulinaemia, hyperglycaemia, hypertriglyceridaemia and steatosis.

Signal transducer and activator of transcription-5 (STAT5) is implicated in intracellular signalling from insulin and growth hormone receptors, potentially explaining the role of both hormones on lipogenesis. Some male STAT5b ko mice develop obesity and steatosis, but the metabolic explanation has not been fully evaluated [59]. In another interesting model, injection of a fraction prepared from the urine of patients with congenital generalized lipoatrophy produced lipoatrophy in mice and rabbits [60]. This was also associated with insulin resistance, glucose intolerance and hypertriglyceridaemia [60].

The metabolic consequences of having no white fat are profound. They include reduced leptin production, hence loss of appetite control. Leptin also has direct effects on FA metabolism and insulin action in the liver [61], which appear to be mediated by regulation of stearoyl-CoA desaturase-1 [62]. Together, these effects of leptin lead to insulin resistance and diabetes, increased serum triglycerides and often massive engorgement of the liver and other internal organs with lipid [56]. There do not appear to have been detailed studies of liver pathology in these models, although several authors mention the occurrence of steatosis [2,54,56].

Another transgenic mouse model of insulin resistance is produced by overexpression of insulin-like growth factor II in pancreatic β cells [63]. These mice develop hyperinsulinaemia, altered glucose and insulin tolerance, and tend to develop diabetes when fed a high-fat diet. The progeny of backcross to C57KsJ mice displayed insulin resistance and islet cell hyperplasia, and also developed obesity and hepatic steatosis [63].

Insulin signalling in the liver can be abrogated in mice lacking the insulin receptor. This results in a severe form of diabetes with ketoacidosis, hypertriglyceridaemia, increased FFA and steatosis [64]. Among several other ko mice created in attempts to understand the pathogenesis and pathobiology of insulin resistance and type 2 diabetes (reviewed by Kadowaki [64]), male mice heterozygous for the glucose transporter type 4 (GLUT4) show steatosis as well as cardiomyopathy [65].

Other transgenic models of obesity

Melanocortinergic neurons exert tonic inhibition of feeding behaviour, which is disrupted in the agouti obesity syndrome [66]. Genetically obese KKA(y) mice develop diabetes and steatosis that can be ameliorated with a disaccharidase inhibitor to prevent the postprandial rise in blood glucose after sucrose loading [67].

The New Zealand obese (NZO) mouse exhibits diminished spontaneous activity, which leads to energy intake disproportionate to bodily needs, obesity and insulin resistance [68]. The liver phenotype has not been well characterized.

Increased hepatic uptake and synthesis of fatty acids

As part of their definitive studies into mechanisms for tissue-specific insulin resistance (see Chapter 3), Kim et al. [69] produced conditional liver expression of hepatic lipoprotein lipase. The phenotype was a mouse with increased hepatic triglyceride content and liver-specific insulin resistance. This model demonstrates definitively how vectorially directed FA traffic into the liver generates both hepatic insulin resistance and steatosis.

Hepatic FA synthesis is increased in other transgenic models, including mice with conditional hepatic expression of a truncated form of SREBP-1a [70]; this form of the protein enters the nucleus without the normal requirement for proteolysis, and therefore cannot be downregulated. Transgenic mice placed on a low-carbohydrate high-protein diet to induce the phosphoenolpyruvate carboxykinase (PEPCK) promoter developed engorgement of hepatocytes with cholesterol and triglyceride, in association with upregulation of enzymes involved in synthesis of FA and cholesterol. There was a minor increase in serum ALT levels but no necroinflammatory lesions [70].

Dysregulation of hepatic FA metabolism, storage and secretion

PPARα is a nuclear receptor that has a pivotal role in control of hepatic FA turnover, particularly in governing enzymes involved in mitochondrial and peroxisomal β-oxidation. By facilitating hepatic FA uptake and oxidation, PPARα is central to management of energy stores during fasting [71]. PPARα ko mice are unable to adapt to conditions that favour accumulation of FA in the liver, including a high-fat diet or fasting [71–73], both of which exacerbate steatosis. Such accumulation of lipid accentuates steatohepatitis induced by the MCD diet (see below), indicating that while excessive storage of fat in the liver may not be sufficient to produce steatohepatitis, it is likely to be one of the factors that determines its severity.

A notable feature of studies with PPARα ko mice is sexual dimorphism [72,74]. Thus, male mice are more susceptible than females to the effects of pharmacological inhibition of mitochondrial FA oxidation (with etomoxir, an irreversible inhibitor of CPT-1), a change that could be rescued by administration of oestrogen [74]. Steatosis is also found in aromatase-deficient mice which have no intrinsic oestrogen production, and Japanese workers have demonstrated a pivotal role of oestrogen in the hepatic expression of genes involved in β-oxidation and hepatic lipid homeostasis [75]. It is not clear whether such sex differences have equivalent importance in humans, although disordered lipid homeostasis could contribute to the pathogenesis of tamoxifen-induced steatohepatitis [10].

Apolipoprotein B (ApoB) ko mice exhibit a similar phenotype to humans with a-betalipoproteinaemia (see Chapter 21) [78]. Microsomal triglyceride transfer protein (MTP) is involved with processing of triglyceride into ApoB as VLDL. MTP ko mice have a similar defect in VLDL synthesis and secretion as do ApoB ko mice, leading to lipid accumulation in the liver and spontaneous steatosis [79]. These mice are correspondingly more susceptible to liver injury from bacterial toxins [79]. It has been suggested that humans with partial deficiency in MTP expression are over-represented among those with NASH (see Chapter 6), and further studies in MTP ko mice could be of interest in defining the experimental conditions that can lead to development of steatohepatitis.

Initiation of inflammation and liver cell injury

The above nutritional or genetic models of IR and hepatic steatosis appear to simulate some of the preconditions for NAFLD/NASH in humans. However, none have been reported to undergo spontaneous transition to steatohepatitis. In an earlier hypothesis about NASH pathogenesis [78], it was proposed that steatosis provided the background (or 'first-hit') or setting for NASH, but that a 'second-hit' injury mechanism was required for induction of necroinflammatory activity and its consequences. More complex pathogenic interactions have been proposed in which steatosis is an essential precondition for steatohepatitis, but inflammatory recruitment and perpetuation and fibrosis occur by several interactive mechanisms [79]. The next section describes how experimental perturbations have confirmed that the fatty liver is susceptible to oxidative forms of liver injury as 'delivered' by an acute insult.

Susceptibility of fatty liver to endotoxin and oxidative stress

The most obvious demonstration of this phenomenon is the poor tolerance of fatty livers, irrespective of aetiology, to ischaemia–reperfusion or preservation injury prior to hepatic transplantation [80]. Both forms of liver injury are regarded as the consequence of ROS production in the liver during re-exposure to oxygen [81]. The steatotic liver provides an abundant source of unsaturated FAs, which become substrates for the autopropagative process of lipid peroxidation [11,79,82]. Lipoperoxides contribute to the state of oxidative stress in hepatocytes; they may cause mitochondrial injury and cell death by either apoptosis or necrosis [7,83]. In addition, the fatty liver is susceptible to microvascular disturbances during ischaemia–reperfusion injury [80,81].

Yang et al. [37,38] injected lipopolysaccharide (LPS, endotoxin) into leptin-deficient obese ob/ob mice or rats with steatosis attributable to leptin receptor dysfunction (Zucker rat); others have found similar results in choline-deficient rats [84]. Endotoxin administration produced foci of acute hepatocellular necrosis surrounded by focal inflammatory change, and acute mortality; it is not recorded whether these lesions resolve or transform into chronic steatohepatitis; it is

101

not known whether endotoxin can cause lesions resembling NASH (see Chapter 2). While LPS produced the expected upregulation of NF-κB and release of TNF and related cytokines, hepatocellular injury appeared more attributable to necrosis resulting from energy (ATP) depletion [39].

Analogy has been drawn between NAFLD pathogenesis in *ob/ob* mice and the proposed role of gut-derived endotoxin, Kupffer cell stimulation and release of TNF in alcohol-induced liver injury. Changing the intestinal flora with probiotics or injecting anti-TNF antibodies into *ob/ob* mice reduced insulin resistance, hepatic triglyceride accumulation and liver injury [33]. The possibility that gut-derived bacterial products contributes to the pathogenesis of steatohepatitis in NAFLD is discussed in Chapter 7 and elsewhere [85].

Spontaneous transition of steatosis to steatohepatitis, and perpetuation of steatohepatitis

To date, models of simple steatosis attributable to overnutrition (often with secondary leptin resistance), leptin deficiency (genetic or secondary to loss of WAT), leptin receptor dysfunction, or insulin resistance resulting from other causes have not been shown to develop steatohepatitis (corresponding to NAFLD types 3 or 4). This may reflect the need for multiple genetic and environmental factors to coincide for NASH pathogenesis (see Chapter 6) [79,86,87]. In contrast, animal models in which the leptin system is intact provide the dual settings of steatosis and oxidative stress; such models develop steatohepatitis. Further, the lesions can evolve into clinically relevant sequelae, such as progressive pericellular fibrosis, cirrhosis and disordered hepatocellular proliferation leading to hepatic tumour formation (hepatocarcinogenesis).

AOX knockout mouse
Long-chain fatty AOX is the first enzyme in peroxisomal β-oxidation [88]. Mice lacking AOX exhibit hepatic lipid accumulation with sustained upregulation of PPARα-dependent pathways in the liver, including CYP4A, and massively increased production of hydrogen peroxide (H_2O_2) [89]. The latter could arise from peroxisomal and/or CYP4A-catalysed microsomal lipid peroxidation. As adults, AOX ko mice exhibit florid (albeit transient) steatohepatitis, eventually leading to hepatic tumors in older mice that no longer exhibit steatosis [89]. Cross-breeding of AOX ko with PPARα

ko mice yields a phenotype with continuing steatosis but reduction in hepatic inflammation and liver injury, and correction of disordered proliferation [90].

As mentioned in relation to studies of steatosis (see also Chapter 10), activation of PPARα controls hepatic FA flux; it upregulates liver-specific FA binding protein, and enzymes involved in both mitochondrial and peroxisomal β-oxidation of FA [20,87,88]. This provides a nexus between hepatic lipid accumulation and induction of CYP-dependent lipoxygenases and/or peroxisomal oxidation of FA; such induction could have a pathogenic role in generating necroinflammatory change in steatohepatitis by increasing production of ROS in a fatty liver [79,82].

Methionine adenosyltransferase 1A ko mouse
Methionine adenosyltransferases (MAT) catalyse formation of *S*-adenosylmethionine, the principal biological methyl donor. MAT1A is the liver-specific form. In MAT1A ko (or MATO) mice, hepatic methionine, *S*-adenosylmethionine and glutathione levels are considerably depleted, despite sevenfold increase in plasma methionine levels [91,92]. While body weight of adult mice is unchanged, liver weight is increased 40% and three-quarters exhibit steatosis. This has been attributed to upregulation of genes involved with hepatic lipid and glucose metabolism, despite normal insulin levels [94]. As in the AOX ko mouse, spontaneous steatohepatitis and liver tumours are found in older MATO mice, in association with oxidative stress and upregulation of CYP2E1 and CYP4A genes [92]. In keeping with these metabolic findings, the MATO mouse is highly susceptible to CCl_4-induced liver injury [92], while administration of a choline-deficient diet produced striking steatohepatitis [91]. As in the MCD dietary model (see below), hepatic methionine deficiency in the MATO mouse is associated with lowered hepatic glutathione levels and upregulation of antioxidant genes, reflecting the operation of oxidative stress in this form of steatohepatitis [92].

Methionine- and choline-deficient dietary model
Several groups have confirmed that rats or mice fed a lipogenic and lipid-rich (10% of energy as fat, versus 4% in normal chow) MCD diet develop steatohepatitis characterized by progressive pericellular and pericentral fibrosis ('fibrosing steatohepatitis') [20,46,73,93–99]. The diet can be obtained commercially as the base diet, to which methionine and choline

can be supplemented for control studies [73,94]. Rats and mice fed the MCD diet acclimatize to it within a few days and generally remain physically active with good coat colour and apparently normal physiological functioning. However, a striking feature of the dietary regimen is loss of weight and failure to store fat in subcutaneous adipose tissues. In mice, weight loss may be as great as 40% of starting body weight. Animals therefore need to be monitored daily to detect loss of well-being and to avoid cannibalism of weakened animals. There also appear to be gender differences, with injury, fibrosis and mortality seemingly higher in male mice, and steatosis and steatohepatitis more severe in females (unpublished observations). Metabolic studies in male mice have shown enhanced insulin sensitivity by 5 weeks of MCD dietary intake, possibly because of loss of subcutaneous fat [99]. Thus, a criticism of this model is that it is associated with weight loss, insulin sensitivity and low serum triglyceride levels, rather than with obesity, insulin resistance and hypertriglyceridaemia as is found in subjects with clinically significant NASH [86,87]. More recently, however, studies of insulin receptor signaling intermediates indicate the operation of hepatic insulin resistance in the MCD model, most likely caused by CYP2E1-induced oxidative stress (M. Czaja et al., unpublished data, 2003).

The MCD model has allowed the evolution of steatohepatitis to be studied in relation to oxidative stress. In mice fed the MCD diet, lipid peroxides accumulate from day 2, reaching massive (up to 100-fold) levels by day 10 (A. de la Peña et al., unpublished data, 2003). Lipid peroxidation persists throughout the course of dietary feeding, albeit with slight amelioration later (A. de la Peña et al., unpublished data, 2003). Steatosis becomes evident by day 2 or 3, with increasing numbers of perivenous hepatocytes exhibiting microvesicular or macrovesicular fatty change by day 10. By 3 weeks, virtually all hepatocytes show steatosis. The first inflammatory cells, sparse polymorphs, are evident between days 2 and 3, at which time serum ALT levels become elevated (A. de la Peña et al., unpublished data, 2003). These generally reach almost fivefold the upper limit of normal by day 10 and persist throughout 10 weeks of dietary feeding. Inflammation becomes more diffuse by day 10, and by 3 weeks of dietary feeding the lobular necroinflammatory changes are similar to, but recognizably different from NASH (NAFLD types 3 and 4) (P. Hall, personal communication).

At 5 weeks, the livers of MCD diet-fed mice show upregulation of multiple antioxidant genes compared with control mice (I.A. Leclercq et al., unpublished data). At this time, increased expression of collagen-1 mRNA is also readily detected [97]. By 8 weeks, extensive fine strands of collagen can be seen in a pericellular and pericentral distribution on liver sections stained with Sirius red.

In rats, MCD-induced steatohepatitis is less 'florid', but fibrosis is evident from 12 weeks of dietary feeding (Plate 11, facing p. 22), and can lead to cirrhosis in some animals by 18 weeks. George et al. [95] have characterized the role of activated hepatic stellate cells (HSC) and other cell types in hepatic fibrogenesis in this model. Oxidative stress appears to originate from hepatocytes, which are also the source of preformed transforming growth factor-β1 (TGF-β1), a pivotal profibrogenic cytokine. Together with studies in MCD-fed mice, a clear role for oxidative stress in mediating fibrosis has come from interventional studies with vitamin E [97]. However, despite a reduction in hepatic cytosolic and mitochondrial reduced glutathione (GSH) levels, cysteine precursors had no antifibrotic efficacy in this model [97].

The basis of oxidative stress has been studied in the MCD model. As in humans with NASH [100,101], both rats and mice fed the MCD diet exhibit induction of hepatic microsomal CYP2E1 [93,94], with particularly high levels in females (unpublished observations); in microsomal fractions, CYP2E1 catalyses abundant NADPH-dependent lipid peroxidation [94]. After 10 weeks of dietary feeding, mitochondrial injury is clearly evident, resembling that found in human liver of NASH patients (see Chapter 7). Early lesions are apparent after 3 weeks of dietary feeding, but to date there is no evidence that mitochondria generate ROS at this time (N. Phung, unpublished observations). Taken together, these findings are consistent with one or more extramitochondrial sites being an important source of pro-oxidants in the MCD model of steatohepatitis.

In CYP2E1 knockout mice, CYP4A proteins are recruited as alternative microsomal lipid oxidases in MCD-fed mice [94]. Because CYP4A proteins are partly governed by PPARα, stimulation of PPARα-responsive pathways carries potential for overproduction of ROS. However, PPARα also governs hepatic FA flux by upregulation of liver-specific FA binding protein and enzymes involved in mitochondrial and peroxisomal β-oxidation. In contrast to the findings

103

attributed to PPARα stimulation in AOX ko mice [89], Ip *et al.* [73] have shown that pharmacological stimulation of PPARα with the potent non-toxic inducer Wy-14,643 actually prevents (and later reverses [98]) development of steatohepatitis in the MCD murine model, despite induction of CYP4A proteins. The most likely explanation is that prevention of hepatic accumulation of FFA removes substrates for lipid peroxidation, thereby preventing oxidative stress and its downstream consequences for inflammatory recruitment, liver injury and fibrogenesis [20,73,79].

It has recently been shown that oxidative stress in the MCD dietary model is associated with early (day 3) activation of NF-κB (A. de la Peña *et al.*, unpublished data; I.A. Leclercq, unpublished data). The downstream consequences are transient expression of proinflammatory molecules like vascular cell adhesion molecule-1 (VCAM-1), and apparently sustained upregulation of intercellular adhesion molecule-1 (ICAM-1) and cyclooxygenase-2 (COX-2). Conversely, there was minimal increase in hepatic TNF expression during the first 10 days of MCD dietary feeding, and identical pathology was observed in TNF ko mice fed the MCD diet (A. de la Peña *et al.*, unpublished data, 2003).

Because differences in activation of NF-κB between MCD deficient and control diet-fed animals appear to wane by week 5 of dietary feeding (unpublished data), the factors that operate to perpetuate inflammation in established steatohepatitis may differ from those that activate inflammatory recruitment during the initiation phase. This added complexity to NASH pathogenesis, the existence of more than one pro-inflammatory pathway, would be difficult to establish from studies of human liver that, by their nature, are single 'snapshots in time'. Further, it indicates that it may be an oversimplification to conceptualize NASH pathogenesis in a 'two-hit' model [78,79,87]. Rather, as articulated more than 25 years ago by Hans Popper, pathogenesis of chronic liver disease is more likely to be the outcome of complex networks of processes, some facilitating, others curbing or countering pathobiological mechanisms.

The MCD model has also been used to study potential treatments for NASH. Thus, vitamin E but not *N*-acetylcysteine prevented fibrogenesis in MCD-fed mice [97], while Wy14,643 (PPARα agonist) both prevented development of steatosis and steatohepatitis [73], and caused resolution of established fibrosing steatohepatitis [98]. In human liver, PPARα may be a less important transcription factor for lipid turnover

than in rodents, indicating how caution needs to be exercised in extrapolating results from animal models to the human clinical context. None the less, the results of these studies indicate the powerful effect that can be obtained by 'correcting at source' defects leading to steatosis and steatohepatitis: thus, reducing hepatic FA accumulation corrects all facets of liver pathology in this experimental form of fibrosing steatohepatitis, including near total reversal of hepatic fibrosis within 12 days [98].

Role of iron

Use of the MCD diet model has also allowed the potential role of hepatic iron to be studied in relation to NASH pathogenesis [78,86,87]. In iron-loaded rats, MCD dietary feeding caused greater hepatocellular injury and liver inflammation at week 4, and facilitated fibrosis so that dense fibrosis was present at 14 weeks [96]. The proposed mechanism is the known pro-oxidant effect of iron in the liver.

Role of antioxidant depletion

The conditions associated with most 'florid' steatohepatitis in humans, alcoholic steatohepatitis and jejuno-ileal bypass (see Chapter 20), are associated with nutritional depletion and lowered GSH levels. Depletion of mitochondrial GSH (mtGSH) is particularly important in the pathogenesis of hepatocyte injury because it predisposes to mitochondrial injury with secondary enhancement of ROS production [6,7]. In mice fed the MCD diet, steatohepatitis with fibrosis follows a decrease in hepatocellular and mtGSH. Likewise, methionine deficiency in the MATO mouse lowers GSH and predisposes to oxidative stress. Perturbation of hepatic antioxidant mechanisms in models of steatosis would be of interest for the proposed oxidative stress mechanism of transition to steatohepatitis.

Conclusions

Nutritional and transgenetic models of insulin resistance and hepatic steatosis appear to simulate preconditions for NAFLD/NASH in humans. However, a noteworthy feature is that, to date, none has been reported to undergo spontaneous transition to steatohepatitis, or to develop hepatic fibrosis. This is consistent with the emerging concept of NASH pathogenesis as being multifactorial [79,86,87], perhaps requiring more than a background of steatosis (the 'first-hit') and a single 'second-hit' injury mechanism [78]. It seems likely that there are multiple factors, some genetic (see Chapter 6), and others environmental; the latter may include dietary composition and changes in lifestyle leading to central obesity and insulin resistance [86,87,102]. Much has been learnt about the potential of lipid peroxidation to advance steatohepatitis in the MCD model, with parallels from AOX and MATO mice. The importance of selected pro-inflammatory and profibrotic pathways can now be tested by molecular genetics or studies of human liver. However, development of new experimental models of significant steatohepatitis based on existing models of steatosis caused by insulin resistance would be a useful objective towards understanding the pathogenesis of NASH [87].

References

1 Fong DG, Nehra V, Lindor K, Buchman AL. Metabolic and nutritional considerations in non-alcoholic fatty liver. *Hepatology* 2000; **32**: 3–10.

2 Koteish A, Diehl AM. Animal models of steatosis. *Semin Liver Dis* 2002; **21**: 89–104.

3 Czaja MJ, Xu J, Alt E. Prevention of carbon tetrachloride-induced rat liver injury by soluble tumor necrosis factor receptor. *Gastroenterology* 1995; **108**: 1849–54.

4 Leclercq IA, Field J, Farrell GC. Leptin-specific mechanisms for impaired liver regeneration in *ob/ob* mice after toxic injury. *Gastroenterology* 2003; **124**: 1451–64.

5 Hansen CH, Pearson LH, Schenker S, Combes B. Impaired secretion of triglycerides by the liver: a cause of tetracycline-induced fatty liver. *Proc Exp Biol Med* 1968; **128**: 143–6.

6 Fromenty B, Pessayre D. Impaired mitochondrial function in microvesicular steatosis: effects of drugs, ethanol, hormones and cytokines. *J Hepatol* 1997; **26** (Suppl. 2): 43–53.

7 Pessayre D, Mansouri A, Fromenty B. Non-alcoholic steatosis and steatohepatitis. V. Mitochondrial dysfunction in steatohepatitis. *Am J Physiol Gastrointest Liver Physiol* 2002; **282**: G193–9.

8 Lettéron P, Sutton A, Mansouri A, Fromenty B, Pessayre D. Inhibition of microsomal triglyceride transfer protein: another mechanism for drug-induced steatosis in mice. *Hepatology* 2003; **38**: 133–40.

9 Lieber CS, DeCarli LM. Quantitative relationship between amount of dietary fat and severity of alcoholic fatty liver. *Am J Clin Nutr* 1970; **23**: 474–8.

10 Farrell GC. Drugs and steatohepatitis. *Semin Liver Dis* 2002; **22**: 185–94.

11 Letteron P, Fromenty B, Terris B, Degott C, Pessayre D. Acute and chronic hepatic steatosis lead to *in vivo* lipid peroxidation in mice. *J Hepatol* 1996; **24**: 200–8.

12 Pirovino M, Müller O, Zysset T, Honeggar U. Amiodarone-induced hepatic phospholipidosis: correlation of morphological and biochemical findings in an animal model. *Hepatology* 1988; **8**: 591–8.

13 Moriya K, Yotsuyanagi H, Shintani Y *et al.* Hepatitis C virus core protein induces hepatic steatosis in transgenic mice. *J Gen Virol* 1997; **78**: 1527–31.

14 Moriya K, Fujie H, Shintani Y *et al.* The core protein of hepatitis C virus induces hepatocellular carcinoma in transgenic mice. *Nat Med* 1998; **4**: 1065–7.

15 Miyazawa S, Furuta S, Hashimoto T. Reduction of β-oxidation capacity of rat liver mitochondria by feeding orotic acid. *Biochim Biophys Acta* 1982; **711**: 494–502.

16 Cartwright IJ, Hebbachi AM, Higgins JA. Transit and sorting of apolipoprotein B within the endoplasmic reticulum and Golgi compartments of isolated hepatocytes from normal and orotic acid-fed rats. *J Biol Chem* 1993; **268**: 20937–52.

17 Hebbachi AM, Seelaender MCL, Baker PW, Gibbons GF. Decreased secretion of very-low-density lipoprotein triacylglycerol and apolipoprotein B is associated with decreased intracellular triacylglycerol lipolysis in hepatocytes derived from rats fed orotic acid or n-3 fatty acids. *Biochem J* 1997; **325**: 711–9.

18 Milner JA, Hassan AS. Species specificity of arginine deficiency-induced hepatic steatosis. *J Nutr* 1981; **111**: 1067–73.

19 Boison D, Scheurer L, Zumsteg V *et al.* Neonatal hepatic steatosis by disruption of the adenosine kinase gene. *Proc Natl Acad Sci USA* 2002; **99**: 6985–90.

20 Green RM. NASH: hepatic metabolism and not simply the metabolic syndrome. *Hepatology* 2003; **38**: 14–7.

21 Zhu X, Song J, Mar M-H, Edwards LJ, Zeisel SH. Phosphatidylethanolamine *N*-methyltransferase (PMET) knockout mice have hepatic steatosis and abnormal hepatic choline metabolite concentrations despite ingesting a recommended dietary intake of choline. *Biochem J* 2003; **370**: 987–93.

22 Murray M, Cantrill E, Mehta I, Farrell GC. Impaired expression of microsomal cytochrome P450 2C11 in choline-deficient rat liver during the development of cirrhosis. *J Pharmacol Exp Ther* 1992; **261**: 373–80.

23 Novikoff PM. Fatty liver produced in Zucker 'fatty' (ff) rats by a semisynthetic diet rich in sucrose. *Proc Natl Acad Sci USA* 1977; **74**: 3550–4.

24 Bogin E, Avidar Y, Merom M. Biochemical changes in liver and blood during liver fattening in rats. *J Clin Chem Clin Biochem* 1986; **24**: 621–6.

25 Poulsom R. Morphological changes of organs after sucrose or fructose feeding. *Prog Biochem Pharmacol* 1986; **21**: 104–34.

26 Storlein LH, James DE, Burleigh KM, Chisholm DJ, Kraegen EW. Fat feeding causes widespread *in vivo* insulin resistance, decreased energy expenditure, and obesity in rats. *Am J Physiol Endocrinol Metab* 1986; **251**: E576–83.

27 Ye J-M, Iglesias MA, Watson DG *et al.* PPARα/γ ragaglitazar eliminates fatty liver and enhances insulin action in fat-fed rats in the absence of hepatomegaly. *Am J Physiol Endocrinol Metab* 2003; **284**: E531–40.

28 El-Haschimi K, Pierroz DD, Hileman SM, Bjorbaek C, Flier JS. Two defects contribute to hypothalamic leptin resistance in mice with diet-induced obesity. *J Clin Invest* 2000; **105**: 1827–32.

29 Leclercq I, Horsmans Y, Desager JP, Delzenne N, Geubel AP. Reduction in hepatic cytochrome P450 is correlated to the degree of liver fat content in animal models of steatosis in the absence of inflammation. *J Hepatol* 1998; **28**: 410–6.

30 Harrold JA, Widdowson PS, Clapham JC *et al.* Individual severity of dietary obesity in unselected Wistar rats: relationship with hyperphagia. *Am J Physiol* 2000; **279**: E340–7.

31 Matsusue K, Haluzik M, Lambert G *et al.* Liver-specific disruption of PPARγ in leptin-deficient mice improves fatty liver but aggregates diabetic phenotypes. *J Clin Invest* 2003; **111**: 737–47.

32 Lin HZ, Yang SQ, Kujhada F *et al.* Metformin reverses fatty liver disease in obese, leptin-deficient mice. *Nat Med* 2000; **6**: 998–1003.

33 Li Z, Yang S, Lin H *et al.* Probiotics and antibodies to TNF inhibit inflammatory activity and improve non-alcoholic fatty liver disease. *Hepatology* 2003; **37**: 343–50.

34 Baffy G, Zhang C-Y, Glickman JN, Lowell BB. Obesity-related fatty liver is unchanged in mice deficient for mitochondrial uncoupling protein 2. *Hepatology* 2002; **35**: 753–61.

35 Xu A, Wang Y, Keshaw H *et al.* The fat-derived hormone adiponectin alleviates alcoholic and non-alcoholic fatty liver diseases in mice. *J Clin Invest* 2003; **112**: 91–100.

36 Yang SQ, Zhu H, Li Y *et al.* Mitochondrial adaptations to obesity-related oxidant stress. *Arch Biochem Biophys* 2000; **378**: 259–68.

37 Yang SQ, Lin H, Lane MD, Clemens M, Diehl AM. Obesity increases sensitivity to endotoxin liver injury: implications for pathogenesis of steatohepatitis. *Proc Natl Acad Sci USA* 1997; **94**: 2557–62.

38 Yang SQ, Lin H, Diehl AM. Fatty liver vulnerability to endotoxin-induced damage despite NF-κB induction and

inhibited caspase 3 activation. *Am J Physiol Gastrointest Liver Physiol* 2001; **281**: G382–92.

39 Yang SQ, Lin HZ, Mandal AK, Huang J, Diehl AM. Disrupted signaling and inhibited regeneration in obese mice with fatty livers: implications for non-alcoholic fatty liver disease pathophysiology. *Hepatology* 2001; **34**: 694–706.

40 Diehl AM. Non-alcoholic steatosis and steatohepatitis. IV. Non-alcoholic fatty liver disease abnormalities in macrophage function and cytokines. *Am J Physiol Gastrointest Liver Physiol* 2002; **282**: G1–5.

41 Guebre-Xabier M, Yang SQ, Lin HZ *et al.* Altered hepatic lymphocyte subpopulations in obesity-related murine fatty livers: potential mechanism for sensitization to liver damage. *Hepatology* 2000; **31**: 633–40.

42 Memon RA, Grunfeld C, Feingold KR. TNF-α is not the cause of fatty liver disease in obese mice. *Nat Med* 2001; **7**: 2–3.

43 Faggioni R, Fantuzzi G, Gabay C *et al.* Leptin deficiency enhances sensitivity to endotoxin-induced lethality. *Am J Physiol* 1999; **276**: R136–42.

44 Hussein O, Svalb S, Van den Akker-Berman LM, Assy N. Liver regeneration is not altered in patients with non-alcoholic steatohepatitis (NASH) when compared with chronic hepatitis C infection with similar grade of inflammation. *Dig Dis Sci* 2002; **47**: 1926–31.

45 Farrell GC, Robertson G, Leclercq I, Horsmans Y. Liver regeneration in obese mice with fatty livers: does the impairment have relevance for other types of fatty liver disease? [Letter]. *Hepatology* 2002; **35**: 731–2.

46 Leclercq IA, Farrell GC, Shriemer R, Robertson GR. Leptin is essential for the hepatic fibrogenic response to chronic liver injury. *J Hepatol* 2002; **37**: 206–13.

47 Honda H, Ikejima K, Hirose M *et al.* Leptin is required for fibrogenic responses induced by thioacetamide in the murine liver. *Hepatology* 2002; **36**: 12–21.

48 Potter JJ, Mezey E. Leptin deficiency reduces but does not eliminate the development of hepatic fibrosis in mice infected with *Schistosoma mansoni*. *Liver* 2002; **22**: 173–7.

49 Chen H, Charlat O, Tartaglia LA *et al.* Evidence that the diabetes gene encodes the leptin receptor: identification of a mutation in the leptin receptor gene in *db/db* mice. *Cell* 1996; **84**: 491–5.

50 Phillips MS, Liu Q, Hammond HA *et al.* Leptin receptor missense mutation in the fatty Zucker rat. *Nat Genet* 1996; **13**: 18–9.

51 Lee GH, Proenca M, Montez JM *et al.* Abnormal splicing of the leptin receptor in diabetic mice. *Nature* 1996; **379**: 632–5.

52 Kakuma T, Lee Y, Higa M *et al.* Leptin, troglitazone, and the expression of sterol regulatory element binding

proteins in liver and pancreatic islets. *Proc Natl Acad Sci USA* 2000; **97**: 8536–41.

53 Ikejima K, Takei Y, Honda H *et al.* Leptin receptor-mediated signaling regulates hepatic fibrogenesis and remodeling of extracellular matrix in the rat. *Gastroenterology* 2002; **122**: 1399–410.

54 Reitman ML, Mason MM, Moitra J *et al.* Transgenic mice lacking white fat: models for understanding human lipoatrophic diabetes. *Ann NY Acad Sci* 1999; **892**: 289–96.

55 Shimomura I, Hammer RE, Richardson JA *et al.* Insulin resistance and diabetes mellitus in transgenic mice expressing nuclear SREBP-1c in adipose tissue: model for generalized lipodystrophy. *Genes Dev* 1998; **12**: 3182–94.

56 Moitra J, Mason MM, Olive M *et al.* Life without white fat: a transgenic mouse. *Genes Dev* 1998; **12**: 3168–81.

57 Ross SR, Graves RA, Spiegelman BM. Targeted expression of a toxin gene to adipose tissue: transgenic mice resistant to obesity. *Genes Dev* 1993; **7**: 1318–24.

58 Shimomura I, Hammer RE, Ikemoto S, Brown MS, Goldstein JL. Leptin reverses insulin resistance and diabetes mellitus in mice with congenital lipodystrophy. *Nature* 1999; **401**: 73–6.

59 Udy GB, Towers RP, Snell RG *et al.* Requirement of STAT5b for sexual dimorphism of body growth rates and liver gene expression. *Proc Natl Acad Sci USA* 1997; **94**: 7239–44.

60 Foss I, Trygstad O. Lipoatrophy produced in mice and rabbits by a fraction prepared from the urine from patients with congenital generalized lipodystrophy. *Acta Endocrinol* 1975; **80**: 398–416.

61 Barzilai N, Wang J, Massilon D *et al.* Leptin selectively decreases visceral adiposity and enhances insulin action. *J Clin Invest* 1997; **100**: 3105–10.

62 Cohen P, Miyazaki M, Socci ND *et al.* Role for stearoyl-CoA desaturase-1 in leptin-mediated weight loss. *Science* 2002; **297**: 240–3.

63 Devedjian JC, George M, Castellas A *et al.* Transgenic mice overexpressing insulin-like growth factor-II in β cells develop type 2 diabetes. *J Clin Invest* 2000; **105**: 731–40.

64 Kadowaki T. Insights into insulin resistance and type 2 diabetes from knockout mouse models. *J Clin Invest* 2000; **106**: 459–65.

65 Rossetti L, Stenbit AE, Chen W *et al.* Peripheral but not hepatic insulin resistance in mice with one disrupted allele of the glucose transporter type 4 (GLUT4). *J Clin Invest* 1997; **100**: 1831–9.

66 Fan W, Boston BA, Kesterson RA, Hruby VJ, Cone RD. Role of melanocortinergic neurons in feeding and the agouti obesity syndrome. *Nature* 1997; **385**: 165–8.

67 Odaka H, Shino A, Ikeda H, Matsuo T. Antiobesity and antidiabetic actions of a new potent disaccharidase inhibitor in genetically obese-diabetic mice, KKA(y). *J Nutr Sci Vitaminol* 1992; **38**: 27–37.

68 Andrikopoulos S, Prietto J. The biochemical basis of increased hepatic glucose production in a mouse model of type 2 (non-insulin dependent) diabetes mellitus. *Diabetologia* 1995; **38**: 1389–96.

69 Kim JK, Fillmore JJ, Chen Y *et al.* Tissue-specific over-expression of lipoprotein lipase causes tissue-specific insulin resistance. *PNAS* 2001; **98**: 7522–7.

70 Shimano H, Horton JD, Hammer RE *et al.* Overproduction of cholesterol and fatty acids causes massive liver enlargement in transgenic mice expressing truncated SREBP-1a. *J Clin Invest* 1996; **98**: 1575–84.

71 Kersten S, Seydoux J, Peters JM *et al.* Peroxisome proliferator-activated receptor α mediates the adaptive response to fasting. *J Clin Invest* 1999; **103**: 1489–98.

72 Coste P, Legendre C, More J *et al.* Peroxisome proliferator-activated receptor α isoform deficiency leads to progressive dyslipidemia with sexually dimorphic obesity and steatosis. *J Biol Chem* 1998; **273**: 29577–85.

73 Ip E, Farrell GC, Robertson GR *et al.* Central role of PPARα-dependent hepatic lipid turnover in dietary steatohepatitis in mice. *Hepatology* 2003; **38**: 123–32.

74 Djouadi F, Weinheimer CJ, Saffitz JE *et al.* A gender-related defect in lipid metabolism and glucose homeostasis in peroxisome proliferator-activated receptor α-deficient mice. *J Clin Invest* 1998; **102**: 1083–91.

75 Nemoto Y, Toda Y, Ono M *et al.* Altered expression of fatty acid-metabolizing enzymes in aromatase-deficient mice. *J Clin Invest* 2000; **105**: 1819–25.

76 Chen Z, Fitzgerald RL, Averna MR, Schonfeld G. A targeted apolipoprotein B-38.9-producing mutation causes fatty liver in mice due to the reduced ability of apolipoprotein B-38.9 to transport triglycerides. *J Biol Chem* 2000; **275**: 32807–15.

77 Björkegren J, Beigneux A, Bergo MO, Maher JJ, Young SG. Blocking the secretion of hepatic very low density lipoproteins renders the liver more susceptible to toxin-induced injury. *J Biol Chem* 2002; **277**: 5476–83.

78 Day CP, James OFW. Steatohepatitis: a tale of two 'hits'? *Gastroenterology* 1998; **114**: 842–5.

79 Chitturi S, Farrell GC. Etiopathogenesis of non-alcoholic steatohepatitis. *Semin Liver Dis* 2001; **21**: 27–41.

80 Selzner M, Clavien PA. Fatty liver in liver transplantation and surgery. *Semin Liver Dis* 2001; **21**: 105–13.

81 Teoh NC, Farrell GC. Hepatic ischemia reperfusion injury: pathogenic mechanisms and basis for hepatoprotection. *J Gastroenterol Hepatol* 2003; **18**: 891–902.

82 Robertson G, Leclercq I, Farrell GC. Non-alcoholic steatosis and steatohepatitis. II. Cytochrome P450 and

oxidative stress. *Am J Physiol Gastrointest Liver Physiol* 2001; **281**: G1135–9.

83 Kaplowitz N. Biochemical and cellular mechanisms of toxic liver injury. *Semin Liver Dis* 2002; **22**: 137–44.

84 Eastin CE, McClain CJ, Lee EY, Bagby GJ, Chawla RK. Choline deficiency augments and antibody to tumor necrosis factor-α attenuates endotoxin-induced hepatic injury. *Alcoholism Clin Exp Res* 1997; **21**: 1037–41.

85 Farrell GC. Is bacterial ash the flash that ignites NASH? *Gut* 2001; **48**: 148–9.

86 Angulo P. Non-alcoholic fatty liver disease. *N Engl J Med* 2002; **16**: 1221–31.

87 Neuschwander-Tetri BA, Caldwell SH. Non-alcoholic steatohepatitis: summary of an AASLD single topic conference. *Hepatology* 2003; **37**: 1202–19.

88 Reddy JK. Non-alcoholic steatosis and steatohepatitis III. Peroxisomal β-oxidation, PPARα, and steatohepatitis. *Am J Physiol Gastrointest Liver Physiol* 2001; **281**: G1333–9.

89 Fan C-Y, Pan J, Usuda N *et al.* Steatohepatitis, spontaneous peroxisomal proliferation and liver tumors in mice lacking peroxisomal fatty acyl-CoA oxidase: implications for peroxisomal proliferator-activated receptor a natural ligand metabolism. *J Biol Chem* 1998; **273**: 15639–45.

90 Hashimoto T, Fujita T, Usuda N *et al.* Peroxisomal and mitochondrial fatty acid β-oxidation in mice nullizygous for both peroxisome proliferator-activated receptor α and peroxisomal fatty acyl-CoA oxidase: genotype correlation with fatty liver phenotype. *J Biol Chem* 1999; **274**: 19228–36.

91 Lu SC, Alvarez L, Huang Z-Z *et al.* Methionine adenosyltransferase 1A knockout mice are predisposed to liver injury and exhibit increased expression of genes involved in proliferation. *Proc Natl Acad Sci USA* 2001; **98**: 5560–5.

92 Martinez-Chantar ML, Corrales FJ, Martinez-Cruz LA *et al.* Spontaneous oxidative stress and liver tumors in mice lacking methionine adenosyltransferase 1A. *FEBS J* 2002; **16**: 1292–4.

93 Weltman MD, Farrell GC, Murray M, Liddle C. Increased hepatocyte CYP2E1 expression in a rat nutritional model of hepatic steatosis with inflammation. *Gastroenterology* 1996; **111**: 1645–53.

94 Leclerq IA, Farrell GC, Field J *et al.* CYP2E1 and CYP4A as microsomal catalysts of lipid peroxides in murine non-alcoholic steatohepatitis. *J Clin Invest* 2000; **105**: 1067–75.

95 George J, Pera N, Phung N *et al.* Lipid peroxidation, stellate cell activation and hepatic fibrogenesis in a rat model of chronic steatohepatitis. *J Hepatol* 2003; **39**: 756–64.

96 Kirsch R, Verdonk RV, Twalla M *et al.* Iron potentiates liver injury in the rat nutritional model of non-alcoholic steatohepatitis (NASH). *J Hepatol* 2002; **36** (Suppl. 1): 148 (A534).

97 Phung N, Farrell G, Robertson G, George J. Antioxidant therapy with vitamin E ameliorates hepatic fibrosis in MCDD-associated NASH. *J Gasterenterol Hepatol* 2001; **16**: A52.

98 Ip E, Farrell G, Robertson G *et al.* Central role of PPAR α-dependent hepatic lipid turnover in dietary steatohepatitis in mice. *Hepatology* 2003; **38**: 123–32.

99 Rinella ME, Green RM. The methionine-choline deficient (MCD) diet model of NASH is associated with relative hypoglycemia and diminished serum insulin levels. *Hepatology* 2002; **36**: 402A.

100 Weltman MD, Farrell GC, Ingelman-Sundberg M, Liddle C. Hepatic cytochrome P4502E1 is increased in patients with non-alcoholic steatohepatitis. *Hepatology* 1998; **27**: 128–33.

101 Chalasani N, Gorski JC, Asghar MS *et al.* Hepatic cytochrome P4502E1 activity in non-diabetic patients with non-alcoholic steatohepatitis. *Hepatology* 2003; **37**: 544–50.

102 Musso G, Gambino R, De Michieli F *et al.* Dietary habits and their relations to insulin resistance and postprandial lipemia in non-alcoholic steatohepatitis. *Hepatology* 2003; **37**: 909–16.

9 Fatty acid metabolism and lipotoxicity in the pathogenesis of NAFLD/NASH

Nathan M. Bass & Raphael B. Merriman

Key learning points

1 The fundamental principles of hepatic fatty acid metabolism and the mechanisms of steatosis and lipotoxicity.
2 The concept of fatty acid overload and the molecular and biochemical adaptive responses in the liver to fatty acid overload.
3 The value and limitations of *in vitro* and *in vivo* research models in investigating and understanding the mechanisms of hepatic lipotoxicity.
4 The likely contribution of polygenic variations in structure and function of the genes of fatty acid metabolism and transport to the pathogenesis and the evolution of fatty liver diseases.

Abstract

Lipid accumulation in the hepatocyte (steatosis) is a defining histological feature of non-alcoholic fatty liver disease (NAFLD). This chapter provides an overview of the fundamental principles of hepatic lipid metabolism relevant to understanding the mechanisms of hepatic steatosis and discusses the evidence for a role for intracellular fat and fatty acid traffic in the progression of simple steatosis to more severe histological disease typified by non-alcoholic steatohepatitis (NASH). Steatosis results from increased fatty acid flux or impaired fatty acid utilization in the liver cell. Triglyceride droplets provide a substrate for lipid peroxidation which may initiate and perpetuate cell injury. Increased fatty acid flux may produce direct cytotoxic effects to the cell as well. Several protective mechanisms exist to deal with fatty acid overload in the hepatocyte and evidence of their deployment is a clue to the presence of fatty acid overload in NASH. Current concepts of the cellular toxicity produced by fatty acids suggest an extremely varied and complex mechanistic spectrum. Cytotoxicity attributed to fatty acids (lipotoxicity) may be produced by a complex array of derivatives and via a large number of mechanisms implicated by both *in vitro* and *in vivo* evidence. The range of effects produced by fatty acids includes subtle modulation of physiological cellular signalling pathways to the promotion of apoptotic and necrotic cell death and, over the long term, the development of hepatocellular cancer.

Indeed, over the past decade there has been increasing interest in the contribution of disordered fatty acid homeostasis to several major diseases, including in addition to liver disease, diabetes, obesity, cardiovascular disease and cancer [1,2,3] all of which bear epidemiological and pathophysiological relationship to NASH.

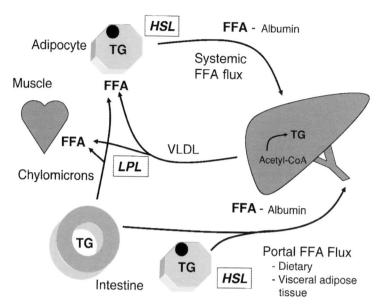

Fig. 9.1 Schematic of free fatty acid (FFA) flux. The liver receives fatty acids from endogenous synthesis (lipogenesis) and import from the circulation. Fatty acids in the circulation derive from the hydrolysis (lipolysis) of triglycerides (TG) in adipocytes in the post-absorptive state and to a lesser extent from the postprandial lipolysis of triglyceride-rich particles (chylomicrons and very-low-density lipoproteins [VLDL]). Fatty acids are released from triglyceride stores in adipose tissue through the action of adipocyte hormone-sensitive lipase (HSL). Following their release into the circulation, fatty acids are bound to albumin. The peripheral tissues, in turn, receive fatty acids as substrate for oxidation and storage through the action of endothelial lipoprotein lipase (LPL) on circulating triglyceride-rich particles—either VLDL secreted by the liver, or chylomicrons delivered into the circulation via the lymphatics following intestinal fat absorption. During fat digestion, medium- and short-chain fatty acids are absorbed directly into the portal circulation. Long-chain fatty acids (C > 14) are mainly re-esterified into chylomicrons, but a proportion of unsaturated long-chain FFA enter the portal circulation.

Hepatic fatty acid metabolism

Long-chain fatty acids in simple non-esterified form are known as free fatty acids (FFA) or non-esterified fatty acids (NEFA). Fatty acids serve several important and biologically diverse functions, which include serving as cell structural components in membrane phospholipids, providing a key source of caloric energy, and also having a role in intracellular signalling and the regulation of gene transcription. Fatty acids are chemically active amphipathic molecules with a complex physical chemistry and are packaged in cells and lipoproteins as relatively inert triacylglycerol esters (triglycerides). Triglyceride is the most abundant lipid that accumulates in hepatocytes in NAFLD. Triglyceride is synthesized through several enzymatic steps from glycerol and fatty acids following the activation of the latter to their acylCoA esters (for reviews see

[4,5]). The liver has two modes of access to fatty acids (Fig. 9.1): endogenous synthesis (lipogenesis) from acetylCoA (derived mainly from carbohydrate substrate) and import from the circulation.

The liver receives fatty acids from the circulation from the hydrolysis (lipolysis) of triglycerides in adipocytes in the post-absorptive state and to a lesser extent from the postprandial lipolysis of triglyceride-rich particles (chylomicrons and very-low-density lipoproteins [VLDL]). Fatty acids are released from triglyceride stores in adipose tissue through the action of adipocyte hormone-sensitive lipase. Following their release into the circulation, fatty acids are bound to albumin (Fig. 9.1). The peripheral tissues, in turn, receive fatty acids as substrate for oxidation (mainly muscle) and storage (adipose tissue), through the action of endothelial lipoprotein lipase on circulating triglyceride-rich particles—either VLDL secreted by the liver, or chylomicrons delivered into the circulation via the lymphatics following intestinal fat absorption [6]. During fat digestion, medium- and short-chain fatty acids are absorbed directly into the portal circulation. Long-chain fatty acids (C > 14) are mainly re-esterified into chylomicrons, but a proportion of long-chain FFA, particularly unsaturated FFA, may enter the portal circulation as well [7]. Direct hepatic exposure to high concentrations of FFA via the portal circulation occurs predominantly as a result of lipolysis of triglyceride in visceral adipose tissue [6]. FFA dissociate from albumin in the space of Disse and cross the liver cell plasma membrane via a mechanism that is still poorly understood, although several candidate membrane transporters have been identified [8,9]. Once in the cell, FFA is bound, at least in part, to a liver cytoplasmic fatty acid binding protein (L-FABP) [10]. Under normal physiological circumstances, FFA undergo oxidation in the mitochondria or are esterified to triglyceride, phospholipids and cholesteryl esters (Fig. 9.2a).

Under conditions of increased FFA influx into the hepatocyte, or impairment of the mitochondrial β-oxidation pathway, a number of consequences occur (Fig. 9.2b). Fatty acids are increasingly directed towards triglyceride synthesis. When this exceeds the capacity of the liver cell to assemble and/or export triglyceride-rich VLDL particles, hepatocellular steatosis results. This increases the substrate for hepatocellular lipid peroxidation [3,11,12]. It is also postulated that the increased intracellular flux or accumulation of FFA may produce more direct cytotoxic effects. This cytotoxic potential is kept at bay by several protective mechanisms that appear both constitutive and orchestrated by the nuclear receptor peroxisome proliferator activated receptor α (PPARα) [13–15].

PPARα serves as a sensor of increased intracellular FFA in the hepatocyte. It is activated principally by unsaturated and polyunsaturated fatty acids. Activated PPARα forms a heterodimeric transactivating complex with the RXR nuclear receptor. This heterodimer binds to specific response elements in the promoter region of a number of genes that regulate fatty acid metabolism, modulating increased transcription of these genes. These 'fatty acid response' genes include carnitine palmitoyltransferase I (CPT-1), which is rate limiting for mitochondrial long-chain fatty acid transport; CYP4A1, which initiates the omega oxidation of fatty acids in the microsomes; and several genes specifying enzymes of the peroxisomal β-oxidation

pathway [14]. L-FABP is constitutively abundantly expressed in the liver, but is also transcriptionally upregulated via PPARα. The net result of PPARα-mediated increase gene transcription is an adaptation strategy that enhances intracellular protein binding and metabolic disposal of fatty acids via mitochondrial and extramitochondrial pathways of oxidation. A potentially negative consequence of this adaptation process is the increased production of dicarboxylic fatty acids via the microsomal ω-oxidation pathway. Long-chain dicarboxylic fatty appear to be a particularly toxic derivative of FFA and are preferentially catabolized in the peroxisomes, where their disposal may be relatively inefficient [16,17]. Their presence in the urine and circulation is recognized as a marker of fatty acid overload states, particularly in conditions characterized by microvesicular fatty liver disorders secondary to mitochondrial β-oxidation impaired by either acquired toxic states or inborn errors of the enzymes of mitochondrial β-oxidation [16,18,19].

The mechanisms recognized for the accumulation of triglyceride in the liver are summarized in Fig. 9.3. These include increased fatty acid influx from peripheral sites (adipose tissue and portal flux from intestinal uptake), decreased fatty acid oxidation (e.g. secondary to impaired mitochondrial β-oxidation), increased fatty acid synthesis and decreased VLDL assembly and secretion. Factors recognized or postulated to promote several of these mechanisms include obesity, insulin resistance and hyperinsulinaemia, leptin deficiency and resistance, excess dietary fat and carbohydrate consumption, certain drugs, and genetic deficiencies in key enzymes of fatty acid metabolism.

Mechanisms of fatty acid toxicity

Current concepts emphasize two major potential mechanisms of fatty acid toxicity in the pathogenesis of steatohepatitis. The direct mechanism invokes cytotoxic effects of fatty acids on the liver cell, through an excess of intracellular fatty acid (fatty acid overload). The most important indirect mechanism is lipid peroxidation of polyunsaturated fatty acids either in the free or esterified state [3,11].

The view of a simple, dual mechanism of fatty acid cytotoxicity that is either direct or peroxidative is simplistic. Table 9.1 lists the potential fatty acyl mediators of cellular toxicity. Fatty acids are extremely versatile

(a)

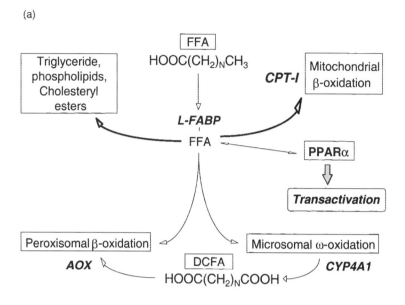

(b)

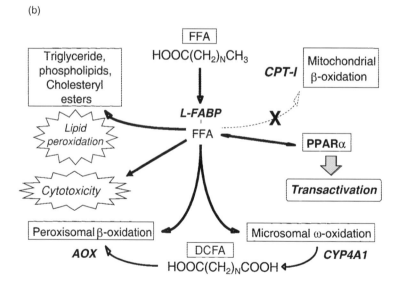

Fig. 9.2 Schematic of hepatic fatty acid metabolism under conditions of normal and increased fatty acid flux. (a) Normal hepatic fatty acid metabolism. Long-chain free fatty acids (FFA) dissociate from albumin in the space of Disse and cross the liver cell plasma membrane. In the cell, FFA are bound to liver fatty acid binding protein (L-FABP). Under conditions of normal flux, FFA largely undergo oxidation in the mitochondria or are esterified to triglyceride, phospholipids and cholesteryl esters. (b) Under conditions of increased FFA influx into the hepatocyte, or impairment (X) of mitochondrial β-oxidation, FFA are increasingly directed towards triglyceride synthesis. When the capacity of the liver cell to assemble and/or export triglyceride-rich VLDL particles is exceeded, hepatocellular steatosis results. This increases the substrate for hepatocellular lipid peroxidation, while the increased flux of FFA may also produce direct cytotoxic effects. Increased FFA flux activates peroxisome proliferator activated receptor α (PPARα), a nuclear receptor that increases the transcription of 'fatty acid response' genes including L-FABP, mitochondrial carnitine palmitoyltransferase I (CPT-1), CYP4A1, which initiates the ω-oxidation of fatty acids in the microsomes, and several enzymes of the peroxisomal β-oxidation pathway including acylCoA oxidase (AOX). Increased activity of CYP4A1 results in production of dicarboxylic fatty acids (DCFA) via the microsomal ω-oxidation pathway. DCFA are preferentially catabolized in the peroxisomes and appear in the urine and circulation in fatty acid overload states.

in the mechanisms whereby they can ultimately produce disruptive and toxic effects upon cellular physiology, while direct and peroxidative mechanisms of toxicity may not always be easily separable experimentally.

Cytotoxic effects may be mediated directly by fatty acids or by a variety of derivatives produced either enzy-matically through physiological pathways, or arising spontaneously through non-enzymatic mechanisms. The primary FFA include saturated, unsaturated and polyunsaturated FFA, trans-isomers of polyunsaturated fatty acids [20] and dicarboxylic fatty acids [16]. Dicarboxylic fatty acids produced via microsomal

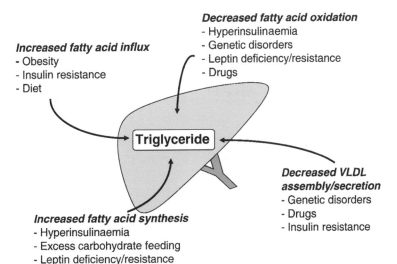

Fig. 9.3 Factors influencing hepatic triglyceride accumulation NASH.

Table 9.1 Mediators of fatty acid toxicity.

Primary non-esterified fatty acids
Saturated, unsaturated and polyunsaturated non-esterified
  fatty acids
Trans-isomers of PUFA
Dicarboxylic fatty acids
Very-long-chain fatty acids
Eicosanoids

Peroxidation products
Lipid hydroperoxides and derivatives (aldehydes
  [malondialdehyde, 4-hydroxynonenal, acrolein], epoxy
  fatty acids)

Esters
Long-chain acylCoA
Long-chain acylcarnitines
Diacylglycerols (DAG)
Fatty acid esters (ethyl esters, xenobiotic conjugates)

Complex lipids
Sphingolipids
Ceramides
Ether lipids

PUFA, polyunsaturated fatty acids.

ω-oxidation of long-chain fatty acids are disruptive of mitochondrial function *in vitro*, and are potential mediators of fatty acid toxicity in overload states [17]. Very-long-chain fatty acids are neurotoxic and accumulate in certain inborn errors such as adreno-leukodystrophy [21]. Oxidized derivatives of fatty acid including eicosanoids, produced via intracellular enzyme pathways or non-enzymatic lipid peroxidation, are particularly important mediators of fatty acid cytotoxicity [3,11,12]. Lipid hydroperoxides and reactive aldehydes formed from the spontaneous oxidation of polyunsaturated fatty acids (PUFA) may cause cell death either by signalling apoptosis or through promotion of necrotic cell death [3,12,22,23]. Arachidonic acid (AA) is a special case of a PUFA cytomodulator and potential cytotoxin [3,24,25]. Lipid peroxidation of cellular AA and other PUFA has been implicated in the pathogenesis of many disease states as well as the aging process [3]. Natural fatty acid esters that are biologically active and potentially disruptive of cellular homoeostasis include long-chain acylCoA, long-chain acylcarnitines and diacylglycerol [26]. Fatty acids are esterified with ethanol *in vivo* to produce fatty acid ethyl esters, neutral molecules that can accumulate in mitochondria and impair cell function. Fatty acid ethyl esters have been implicated in the onset or pathogenesis of myocardial, hepatic and pancreatic diseases occurring in association with alcohol [27]. Conjugates of fatty acids may also form with a broad array of xenobiotics and these may also mediate tissue damage

Table 9.2 Mechanisms of fatty acid toxicity.

Direct toxicity
Detergent effect
Inhibition of Na^+/K^+ ATPase
Modulation of $Na^+ K^+ Cl^-$ ion channels
Ca^{2+} ionophore activity
Inhibition of glycolysis
Uncoupling of oxidative phophorylation
Mitochondrial ROS toxicity and ATP depletion
Genotoxicity (aldehydes)

Signalling
PPAR signalling (ROS, carcinogenesis)
Non-PPAR signalling (PKC, HNF4, LXRa, T3R, SREBP-1c, ChREBP)
Modulation of MAPK, Fos/Jun, RAS

Complex actions
Cellular insulin resistance
Lipoapoptosis

ATP, adenosine triphosphate; PPAR, peroxisome proliferator activated receptor; ROS, reactive oxygen species.

under certain circumstances [28]. Complex lipids derived from fatty acids including sphingomyelins and ceramides may have an important role in cell signalling and programmed cell death.

There also exists a variety of mechanisms of fatty acid toxicity within the cell, mediated either by FFA or their more complex lipid derivatives, or the two acting in concert (Table 9.2). Direct mechanisms include detergent effects at very high concentrations (which may be typically achieved in some *in vitro* cell culture experiments), inhibition of ion pumps and channels, and calcium ionophor activity [29–31]. Fatty acids and fatty acylCoA have been strongly implicated in producing mitochondrial toxicity and in initiating mitochondrial events that lead to both necrotic and apoptotic cell death pathways [23,25,26]. Toxicity may be produced through overstimulation of signalling pathways. Prolonged activation of PPARα, for example, may result in generation of reactive oxygen species accumulation as well as carcinogenesis [14,15]. In addition to PPARα, there are several transcriptional factors and regulatory proteins for which there is evidence for activation or inhibition by fatty acids. These include PPARs γ, β/δ protein kinase C, HNF-4, LXRα, the T3R and SREBP-1c, a key regulatory pro-

tein that modulates the pathways of lipogenesis and fatty acid oxidation [32–34]. Recent evidence supports an important role for fatty acids in apoptosis, cellular insulin resistance and pancreatic β-cell failure in diabetes mellitus [1,3,12,23,35,36]. The mechanisms underlying these effects are complex and may be the result of both direct effects of fatty acids as well as their derivatives, particularly ceramide, acylCoA esters and diacylglycerides [36,37].

The role of lipid peroxidation in NASH and alcoholic liver disease has been a focus of considerable research [11,38,39] and is further discussed in Chapter 8. Recent work using liver tissue from patients with NASH has suggested that lipid peroxidation occurs predominantly in the centrilobular area of the hepatic lobule adjacent to the most fat-laden hepatocytes and is associated with inflammation and fibrosis in this region [40].

Fatty acid overload and cellular defence mechanisms

In terms of biological evidence, the cytotoxic potential of FFA is supported by the existence of several defence mechanisms.
1 Binding proteins—both extracellular (serum albumin) and intracellular fatty acid binding proteins (FABP) serve to transport and sequester fatty acid. *In vitro* evidence supports a role for these proteins in preventing fatty acid cytotoxicity and PPARα activation [41].
2 Efficient microsomal triglyceride synthesis from fatty acids for storage and transport as triglyceride-rich lipoproteins.
3 Efficient mitochondrial β-oxidation and 'back-up' extramitochodrial pathways for fatty acid oxidation.
4 Soluble receptors (PPAR) to sense overload and mediate transcriptional expression of compensatory metabolic pathways for fatty acid catabolism.
5 Enzymatic (catalase, superoxide dismutase, glutathione S-transferases) and non-enzymatic (vitamins A and E) antioxidant mechanisms to prevent lipid peroxidation [3].

The concept of fatty acid overload has emerged from the evidence for intrinsic fatty acid toxicity and the evidence for cellular adaptive responses to increased fatty acid flux [1,14,41,42]. The best example of the latter is PPARα-mediated transcriptional induction of genes that metabolize and transport fatty acids [13,14,41]. Fatty acid overload typically results under conditions of increased fatty acid delivery to non-adipose tissues (as may occur in obesity and diabetes) and/or reduced metabolism. Impaired mitochondrial function appears to have a key role in fatty acid overload-induced hepatotoxicity, both in terms of potentiating fatty acid accumulation and mediating pathways of cell death [18,23,25]. The most dramatic examples of hepatic steatosis and dysfunction occurring as a consequence of impaired mitochondrial β-oxidation of fatty acids are the microvesicular fatty liver disorders characterized by Reye's syndrome, acute fatty liver of pregnancy and toxic microvesicular hepatitis [19,43,44]. It has been suggested from this evidence that more subtle disorders of mitochondrial function may underlie a component of the macrovesicular fat accumulation of NAFLD and NASH. Mitochondrial dysfunction, which may be initiated by a variety of toxins, drugs or metabolic derangements, results in impairment of β-oxidation that leads to a combination of fatty acid accumulation and loss of energy production. Despite PPARα-mediated metabolic adaptation, or perhaps because of the magnitude of FFA overload overwhelming this response, accumulated NEFA may potentiate mitochondrial and general cellular toxicity either directly or via secondary oxidized metabolites (lipid hydroperoxides, aldehydes and dicarboxylic acids). Fatty acid alteration of mitochondrial function or production of mitochondrial damage may result in initiation of the mitochondrial permeability transition or decreased mitochondrial membrane potential that results in hepatocyte apoptosis or necrosis [23,25].

Experimental systems and models

The main experimental systems and models that have contributed to our understanding of fatty acid cellular toxicity are summarized in Table 9.3. There are numerous examples of *in vitro* fatty acid exposure and toxicity ranging from prokaryotes [45–47] through cultured mammalian cells and tissue culture [42,48–53] as well as experiments exposing subcellular components to fatty acids [29,54]. There are several key caveats in interpreting the data from these experiments. It is apparent that the type and severity of observed toxic phenomena depend upon at least six determinants:

1 Characteristics of the exposed cell type
2 Concentration of fatty acids to which cells or cellular components are exposed
3 Fatty acid chain length

4 Degree of unsaturation
5 Class of polyunsaturation (e.g. ω3 versus ω6)
6 Relative (to fatty acid) and absolute concentration of albumin in the medium.

Long-chain fatty acids are poorly soluble in water, and depend on specialized proteins for their binding and transport circulation and intercellular environment. These include serum albumin, and approximately eight or nine distinct tissue-specific 15-kd soluble cytoplasmic FABP [10]. Several plasma membrane transporters have also been described [8,9].

The role of these binding proteins, an important role for albumin in limiting access of FFA to the cell and in protecting various aspects of cell structure and function from high ambient concentrations of long-chain FFA has been demonstrated repeatedly *in vitro* [55,56] as well as *in vivo* [57,58]. Thus, when hypoalbuminaemia occurs in end-stage liver disease, nephrotic syndrome and malnutrition, the capacity of the serum to efficiently buffer long-chain fatty acids may be compromised. The beneficial effects of intravenous albumin in patients with complications of advanced end-stage liver disease is commonly attributed to benefits derived from circulatory oncotic support [59], but the ligand-binding role of albumin may also serve a purpose in this setting.

A similar protective part may be played by cytoplasmic FABP inside the cell. The relative importance

Table 9.3 Experimental and clinical models of fatty acid toxicity.

Model	Example
In vitro **FFA exposure**	Prokaryotes, cell culture, etc.
Animal models	
Toxicological	Oleic acid lung injury
Nutritional	Intragastric ethanol/PUFA
Genetic	
Transgenic	Lipotoxic myopathy
Knockout	Acyl-CoA oxidase (–/–)
Human disease	
	Hyperlipidaemic pancreatitis
	Impaired β-oxidation and microvesicular fatty liver disease
	Disorders of peroxisomal β-oxidation

FFA, free fatty acids; PUFA, polyunsaturated fatty acids.

of a binding/buffering versus transport function of these proteins remains an interesting and unresolved question [41,60–63]. Several knockout mice for the cytoplasmic FABP now exist with interesting phenotypes, suggesting a still poorly understood role in fatty acid compartmentalization and transport to sites of utilization [62,64,65].

Animal models of fatty acid toxicity

Animal models that have been used to study NASH are described in detail in Chapter 8. However, a few that are highly illustrative of the potential role of fatty acids in producing cellular injury are briefly considered here. Animal models that have studied FFA-mediated cellular injury include *toxicological models* in which large amounts of fatty acids are injected to produce specific organ injury (e.g. the model of oleic-acid-induced lung injury [66]). Examples of *nutritional models*, in the case of liver, include models of dietary deficiency of lipotropic agents [39] and the intragastric ethanol/ polyunsaturated fatty acid fed rat (Tsukamoto–French– Nanji) model of steatohepatitis [38]. The importance of lipid peroxidation of PUFA in the production of liver injury in alcoholic fatty liver disease is suggested by the intragastric ethanol/fat-fed rat models. Animals fed PUFA with alcohol develop severe liver injury, while those fed saturated fat are protected [38]. Also, clofibrate can prevent the liver injury caused by hepatic lipid peroxidation produced by a variety of insults [67] including PUFA/alcohol feeding [68], supporting the importance of the protective role of PPARα-mediated gene activation in fatty acid-mediated liver toxicity. Finally, there are *genetic models* that have explored the two main experimental types of gene dosage variation: overexpression (transgenic models) or underexpression (knockout models).

In humans, direct FFA-mediated cytotoxicity has long been implicated in hyperlipidaemic pancreatitis. Interestingly, experimental data are not uniformly supportive of the role of FFA in this classic scenario [69]. There are excellent examples of the consequences of impaired mitochondrial β-oxidation in humans in producing liver disease and severe hepatic fatty acid toxicity [8,19,44].

Among the most convincing experimental animal models supporting the concept of fatty acid overload and the capability of fatty acids to produce serious tissue injury *in vivo* are two transgenic mouse models of fatty acid-induced myotoxicity. This has been reported in mice overexpressing lipoprotein lipase on skeletal muscle, which develop a severe myopathy and increased peroxisomes in skeletal muscle (MCK LPL mouse) [70] and in transgenic mice overexpressing membrane-bound acylCoA synthetase in heart muscle, which develop a lipotoxic cardiomyopathy (the MHCACS mouse) [71]. These models appear to produce fatty acid toxicity through massively increased delivery or import; essentially 'anterograde' fatty acid overload.

The MCK LPL transgenic mouse expresses the human lipoprotein lipase on the skeletal myocyte plasma membrane [70]. This leads to a massive increase in a triglyceride hydrolysis at the myocyte surface with enhanced fatty acid delivery into the myocytes. In part, this traffic is directed into triglyceride synthesis and lipid droplets accumulate in the muscle. The increase in fatty acid flux is also associated with insulin resistance that is restricted to muscle tissue expressing the transgene. In time, MCK LPL transgenic mice develop a profound myopathy associated with a marked increase in myofibrillar mitochondria and peroxisomes. This sequence of events strongly suggests that the sustained increase in FFA delivery produces a functional metabolic disorder (insulin resistance), steatosis, a toxic structure–function disruption of muscle (myopathy) and an adaptive compensation mediated by PPARα activation (mitochondrial and peroxisomal proliferation) [37,70]. A hepatocyte-specific equivalent of the MCK LPL model has been described in which the albumin promoter was used to target hepatocytes. This mouse model develops liver-specific insulin resistance, but morphological or functional disruptive effects have not been described to date [72].

In the MHCACS mouse, long-chain acylCoA synthetase is transgenically overexpressed 9–11-fold on cardiac myocytes [71]. This results in increased vectorial uptake and oversupply of FFA in excess of utilization in heart muscle. As these animals grow, they develop progressive cardiac hypertrophy accompanied by increased cardiac myocyte apoptosis and eventually disrupted cardiac function. This sequence of events occurs in the absence of derangements in plasma FFA, serum glucose, insulin or global triglyceride transport. This model is thus relatively simple in terms of demonstrating the tissue effects of a marked increase in tissue delivery of FFA and the structural and functional consequences of this on the target organ tissue. Additional experimental data support a primary role for palmitate and the FFA-mediated generation of reactive oxygen species in producing the pathological changes in this model. Ceramide synthesis is also increased in this model but appears to have a permissive or amplifying role as opposed to a primary role in the observed apoptosis, but detailed mechanisms remain to be determined [73].

In the case of the liver, lipotoxic models developed to date have been more complex, and no convincing anterograde fatty acid overload models have been described. For a detailed discussion of these models see Chapter 8. It is important to note that available models are interesting and valuable for the study of the pathogenesis and treatment of NASH, but are usually too complex to dissect out the specific part played by fatty acids in producing tissue injury. Fatty liver models include those produced by nutritional deficiency of lipotropic factors [9], nutritional oversupply of fat and alcohol [38], and models based on obesity [74], increased hepatic lipogenesis or lipoatrophy [75,76]. There are also models of decreased or impaired fatty acid oxidation in mitochondria and peroxisomes, which differ with respect to the myotoxic models described above in expressing a disruption in fatty acid metabolism at a relatively downstream site ('retrograde' fatty acid overload model). One interesting such model is the acylCoA oxidase (AOX) –/– mouse, which has a disruption of the gene specifying AOX, the rate-limiting enzyme in peroxisomal β-oxidation of fatty acids [77]. The AOX null mouse sequentially develops steatosis, peroxisome proliferation and eventually liver tumours [77,78]. This sequence of events has been interpreted to show evidence for both early toxicity from accumulated long-chain fatty acids and very-long-chain fatty acids, and the carcinogenic potential for chronic activation of PPARα. These mice suffer from growth failure and develop steatohepatitis at an early age. Later, the steatotic hepatocytes become replaced by hepatocytes in which there is significant proliferation of peroxisomes. By 15 months of age, these mice develop adenomas as well as non-metastatic liver cancers.

Interpretation of the phenotype of this model offers a fascinating and challenging exercise because of its downstream or 'retrograde' overloaded nature of the model. For example, according to current understanding, the loss of the peroxisomal β-oxidation pathway would mainly impair the catabolism of more peroxisome-dependent very-long-chain fatty acids and polyunsaturated fatty acids, as well as dicarboxylic

fatty acids produced by the microsomal ω-oxidation pathway. Microsomal ω-oxidation, in turn, would be expected to increase substantially as a result of the accumulation of fatty acyl activators of PPARα. Increased cytotoxicity from the accumulation of conventional long-chain fatty acids and, to a greater extent, very-long-chain fatty acids, polyunsaturated fatty acids and dicarboxylic fatty acids may be responsible for the early onset of steatohepatitis in this model [78]. The hepatic neoplasms in this mouse model appear to arise not as a result of a genotoxic effect of accumulated fatty acids and fatty acid derivatives, but as direct result of chronic PPARα activation stimulation by the accumulated fatty acyl ligands.

When AOX –/– mice are cross-bred with PPARα –/– mice to produce a double knockout, liver histology tends to be more benign, simple steatosis and the tendency to form tumours is abolished [78,79]. This supports the interesting hypothesis that intact PPARα signalling is necessary for the production of steatohepatitis under conditions of fatty acid overload, and is essential for the production of liver neoplasms in the overload state extant under conditions of disrupted peroxisomal β-oxidation of fatty acids.

Evidence for fatty acid overload in human NASH

Serum and tissue fatty acids in fatty liver diseases

Several studies have documented the presence of increased serum FFA in patients with NAFLD [80,81] and, in this respect, the data are similar to that in patients with obesity and diabetes [6]. In one recent study, patients with NASH and severe fibrosis on liver biopsy had significantly greater serum concentrations of FFA than patients without severe fibrosis [80]. Other authors have reported increased hepatic peroxisomes—indirect evidence for fatty acid overload—in the livers of patients with alcoholic and NAFLD, but also in a variety of other hepatic diseases [82,83]. There are very few data concerning fatty acid levels in the liver under normal conditions or in NAFLD/NASH.

Table 9.4 shows the data from human studies. Lipid analyses in patients with acute fatty liver of pregnancy have reported increased levels of NEFA measured in liver [84,85]. The very high level of 250 μmol/g of liver reported in the earlier of the two studies [84] probably represents an artefact of phospholipolysis in

Table 9.4 Measurements of hepatic FFA levels.

	mol/g liver (wet weight)
Rat liver	
Bass & Manning (unpublished)	0.040–0.158
Human liver	
Mavrelis *et al.* [87]	
Normal	1.6 ± 0.7
Obesity	13.7 ± 1.6
Alcoholic liver disease	19.9 ± 2.4
Eisele *et al.* [84]	
Acute fatty liver of pregnancy	250
Ockner *et al.* [85]	
Acute fatty liver of pregnancy	21.6

tissue obtained at autopsy. Using snap-freeze methods and enzyme inhibitors to minimize phospholipolysis [86], normal rat liver contains only between 40 and 158 nmol/g of non-esterified long-chain fatty acid (wet weight) of liver (Bass and Manning, unpublished data). Mavrellis *et al.* [87] found that normal fatty acid content was at about 1.6 μmol/g of liver, about an order of magnitude higher than our laboratory found in rat liver, and that levels were increased in obesity and alcoholic liver disease. These studies used careful preservation and extraction techniques on liver biopsies from patients and normal controls. A real increase in hepatic FFA in obese individuals and patients with NAFLD is thus supported by these data.

Genetic studies

The pathogenesis of NASH is likely to depend on a complex interaction of environmental and genetic factors. The role of genes involved in fatty acid metabolism are of major importance (see Chapter 6); a role for variants in hepatic gene expression and gene product function in determining hepatic flux of FFA and triglycerides and contributing to the spectrum of clinical and histopathological injury seen in NASH ('central model'; Fig. 9.4). However, the recurrence of NASH in up to 25% of patients who undergo liver transplantation for either NASH or cryptogenic cirrhosis [88], many of whom appear to have evolved from NASH, suggests that extrahepatic mechanisms must also be important in at least some individuals who develop this disease, especially the most severe forms. In terms

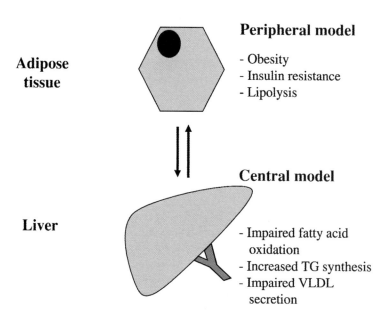

Adipose tissue

Liver

Peripheral model

- Obesity
- Insulin resistance
- Lipolysis

Central model

- Impaired fatty acid oxidation
- Increased TG synthesis
- Impaired VLDL secretion

Fig. 9.4 Illustration of the theory of central and peripheral genetic models of disordered fatty acid metabolism in the pathogenesis of NASH. The central model of pathogenesis of NASH emphasizes the contribution of critical functional mutations (rare familial or monogenic NASH) or sets of polymorphisms (common varieties of NASH) in genes of hepatic fatty acid metabolism and transport to the pathogenesis and the evolution of liver disease. The peripheral model emphasizes the role of genes expressed outside of the liver, particularly those that orchestrate insulin action and fatty acid traffic in adipose tissue. Although isolated central or peripheral factors may be important in rare genetic diseases, the common type of NASH associated with the metabolic syndrome is likely polygenic, involving both centrally and peripherally expressed genes.

of the role of fatty acids in the pathogenesis of NASH, this phenomenon compels us to focus attention on the extrahepatic peripheral tissues, and in particular the adipocyte, in our search for functionally significant variations in the structure of genes that control fatty acid metabolism and flux (peripheral model; Fig. 9.4). Indeed, preliminary data from our group support the idea that variants in genes that influence adipocyte mobilization of fatty acids, including adiponectin and hormone-sensitive lipase, may in part affect the contribution of fatty acids to the pathogenesis of NAFLD (Merriman *et al.*, unpublished data).

Fatty acids in hepatocellular carcinoma and other liver diseases

In the case of NASH, a major question yet to be answered satisfactorily by experimental models is whether the process of liver injury depends on inflammatory pathways with secondary fat accumulation, direct fatty acid-induced toxicity, toxic damage resulting from the oxidized products of accumulated fatty acid/triglycerides, or some combination of these pathogenetic pathways acting in concert or sequentially. A relatively unexplored but potentially extremely important long-term consequence of fatty acid toxicity is carcinogenesis [89]. A high incidence of hepatocellular carcinoma is reported in obesity-associated cirrhosis [90,91], and there is strong evidence from rodent models that chronic activation of PPARα by fatty acid can result in liver tumours [78]. Other mechanisms whereby fatty acids may produce carcinogenic effects in the long term include the genotoxicity of certain products such as aldehydes produced thorough lipid peroxidation [92].

Finally, there is increasing evidence that the presence of fundamental risk factors for NASH, mainly obesity and diabetes, are associated with more severe disease in the case of liver disease associated with alcohol [93] and chronic hepatitis C [94]. The implication of these observations is that disordered fatty acid traffic and metabolism may be important, not only in the production of microvesicular fatty liver diseases NAFLD/NASH, but in the pathogenesis of a wider spectrum of liver diseases.

References

1 Unger RH, Zhou YT. Lipotoxicity of β-cells in obesity and in other causes of fatty acid spillover. *Diabetes* 2001; 50 (Suppl 1): S118–21.

2 Poitout V, Robertson RP. Minireview: secondary β-cell failure in type 2 diabetes: a convergence of glucotoxicity and lipotoxicity. *Endocrinology* 2002; 143: 339–42.

3 Mylonas, C, Kouretas, D. Lipid peroxidation and tissue damage. *In Vivo* 1999; 13: 295–309.

4 Vance DE, Vance JE, eds. *Biochemistry of Lipids, Lipoproteins, and Membranes*, Vol 20. *New Comprehensive Biochemistry*. Elsevier, 1991.

5 Bass NM. Organization and zonation of hepatic lipid metabolism. In: Gumucio JJ, ed. *Hepatocyte Heterogeneity and Liver Function, Cell Biology Reviews*. 1989; 19: 61–86.

6 Castro Cabezas M, Halkes CJ, Erkelens DW. Obesity and free fatty acids: double trouble. *Nutr Metab Cardiovasc Dis* 2001; 11: 134–4.

7 McDonald GB, Weidman M. Partitioning of polar fatty acids into lymph and portal vein after intestinal absorption in the rat. *Q J Exp Physiol* 1987; 72: 153–9.

8 Brinkmann JF, Abumrad NA, Ibrahimi A, Van Der Vusse GJ, Glatz JF. New insights into long-chain fatty acid uptake by heart muscle: a crucial role for fatty acid translocase/CD36. *Biochem J* 2002; 367: 561–70.

9 Berk PD, Stump DD. Mechanisms of cellular uptake of long-chain free fatty acids. *Mol Cell Biochem* 1999; 192: 17–31.

10 Zimmerman AW, Veerkamp JH. New insights into the structure and function of fatty acid-binding proteins. *Cell Mol Life Sci* 2002; 59: 1096–116.

11 Jaeschke H, Gores GJ, Cederbaum AI *et al*. Mechanisms of hepatotoxicity. *Toxicol Sci* 2002; 65: 166–76.

12 Tang DG, La E, Kern J, Kehrer JP. FA oxidation and signaling in apoptosis. *Biol Chem* 2002; 383: 425–42.

13 Kersten S. Peroxisome proliferator activated receptors and obesity. *Eur J Pharmacol* 2002; 440: 223–34.

14 Kliewer SA, Xu HE, Lambert MH, Willson TM. Peroxisome proliferator-activated receptors: from genes to physiology. *Recent Prog Horm Res* 2001; 56: 239–63.

15 Bocher V, Pineda-Torra I, Fruchart JC, Staels B. PPARs: transcription factors controlling lipid and lipoprotein metabolism. *Ann N Y Acad Sci* 2002; 967: 7–18.

16 Mortensen PB. Formation and degradation of dicarboxylic acids in relation to alterations in fatty acid oxidation in rats. *Biochim Biophys Acta* 1992; 1124: 71–9.

17 Kaikaus RM, Chan W, Lysenko N *et al*. Induction of peroxisomal fatty acid oxidation and liver fatty acid binding protein by peroxisome proliferators: mediation via the cytochrome P450 IVA1-hydroxylase pathway. *J Biol Chem* 1993; 268: 9593–603.

18 Fromenty B, Pessayre D. Impaired mitochondrial function in microvesicular steatosis: effects of drugs, ethanol,
hormones and cytokines. *J Hepatol* 1997; **26** (Suppl 2):
43–53.

19 Pessayre D, Berson A, Fromenty B, Mansouri A. Mitochondria in steatohepatitis. *Semin Liver Dis* 2001; **21**:
57–69.

20 Balazy M. Trans-arachidonic acids: new mediators of
inflammation. *J Physiol Pharmacol* 2000; **51**: 597–607.

21 Khan M, Pahan K, Singh AK, Singh I. Cytokine-induced
accumulation of very long-chain fatty acids in rat C6
glial cells: implication for X-adrenoleukodystrophy. *J
Neurochem* 1998; **71**: 78–87.

22 Parola M, Bellomo G, Robino G, Barrera G, Dianzani
MU. 4-Hydroxynonenal as a biological signal: molecular
basis and pathophysiological implications. *Antioxid
Redox Signal* 1999; **1**: 255–84.

23 Ockner RK. Apoptosis and liver diseases: recent concepts
of mechanism and significance. *J Gastroenterol Hepatol*
2001; **16**: 248–60.

24 Heller A, Koch T, Schmeck J, van Ackern K. Lipid mediators in inflammatory disorders. *Drugs* 1998; **55**: 487–96.

25 Wu D, Cederbaum AI. Cyclosporine A protects against
arachidonic acid toxicity in rat hepatocytes: role of CYP2E1
and mitochondria. *Hepatology* 2002; **35**: 1420–30.

26 Ventura FV, Ruiter JP, Ijlst L, Almeida IT, Wanders RJ.
Inhibition of oxidative phosphorylation by palmitoyl-
CoA in digitonin permeabilized fibroblasts: implications
for long-chain fatty acid β-oxidation disorders. *Biochim
Biophys Acta* 1995; **1272**: 14–20.

27 Laposata M. Fatty acid ethyl esters: current facts and
speculations. *Prostaglandins Leukot Essent Fatty Acids*
1999; **60**: 313–5.

28 Ansari GA, Kaphalia BS, Khan MF. Fatty acid conjugates
of xenobiotics. *Toxicol Lett* 1995; **75**: 1–17.

29 Bass NM, Raghupathy E, Manning JA, Rhoads DE,
Ockner RK. Partial purification of Mr 12 000 fatty
acid binding proteins from rat brain and their effect on
synaptosomal Na⁺-dependent amino acid transport. *Biochemistry* 1984; **23**: 6539–44.

30 Schonfeld P, Wieckowski MR, Wojtczak L. Long-chain
fatty acid-promoted swelling of mitochondria: further
evidence for the protonophoric effect of fatty acids in the
inner mitochondrial membrane. *FEBS Lett* 2000; **471**:
108–12.

31 Nguyen N, Glanz D, Glaesser D. Fatty acid cytotoxicity
to bovine lens epithelial cells: investigations on cell viability,
ecto-ATPase, Na⁺, K⁺-ATPase and intracellular sodium
concentrations. *Exp Eye Res* 2000; **71**: 405–13.

32 Clarke SD, Gasperikova D, Nelson C, Lapillonne A,
Heird WC. Fatty acid regulation of gene expression: a
genomic explanation for the benefits of the Mediterranean
diet. *Ann N Y Acad Sci* 2002; **967**: 283–98.

33 Jump DB. Dietary polyunsaturated fatty acids and regulation
of gene transcription. *Curr Opin Lipidol* 2002; **13**: 155–64.

34 Duplus E, Forest C. Is there a single mechanism for fatty
acid regulation of gene transcription? *Biochem Pharmacol*
2002; **64**: 893–90.

35 Bosello O, Zamboni M. Visceral obesity and metabolic
syndrome. *Obes Rev* 2000; **1**: 47–56.

36 Chen HC, Farese RV Jr. Fatty acids, triglycerides, and
glucose metabolism: recent insights from knockout mice.
Curr Opin Clin Nutr Metab Care 2002; **5**: 359–63.

37 Pulawa LK, Eckel RH. Overexpression of muscle lipoprotein lipase and insulin sensitivity. *Curr Opin Clin Nutr
Metab Care* 2002; **5**: 569–74.

38 Nanji AA, Jokelainen K, Tipoe GL, Rahemtulla A,
Dannenberg AJ. Dietary saturated fatty acids reverse
inflammatory and fibrotic changes in rat liver despite
continued ethanol administration. *J Pharmacol Exp Ther*
2001; **299**: 638–44.

39 Chitturi S, Farrell GC. Etiopathogenesis of non-alcoholic
steatohepatitis. *Semin Liver Dis* 2001; **21**: 27–41.

40 MacDonald GA, Bridle KR, Ward PJ *et al.* Lipid peroxidation in hepatic steatosis in humans is associated with
hepatic fibrosis and occurs predominantly in acinar zone
3. *J Gastroenterol Hepatol* 2001; **16**: 599–606.

41 Bass NM. Interaction of fatty acid-binding proteins
(FABP) with the peroxisome proliferator-activated receptor α (PPARα): evidence for FABP modulation of the
gene response to fatty acid overload. In: Vanderhoek JY,
ed. *Frontiers in Bioactive Lipids. Proceedings of the
XXVI Washington International Spring Symposium on
Bioactive Lipids*. Plenum Press, 1996: 67–72.

42 Janero DR, Burghardt C, Feldman D. Amphiphile-induced
heart muscle-cell (myocyte) injury: effects of intracellular
fatty acid overload. *J Cell Physiol* 1988; **137**: 1–13.

43 Hautekeete ML, Degott C, Benhamou JP. Microvesicular
steatosis of the liver. *Acta Clin Belg* 1990; **45**: 311–26.

44 Ibdah JA, Yang Z, Bennett MJ. Liver disease in pregnancy
and fetal fatty acid oxidation defects. *Mol Genet Metab*
2000; **71**: 182–9.

45 Knapp HR, Melly MA. Bactericidal effects of polyunsaturated fatty acids. *J Infect Dis* 1986; **154**: 84–94.

46 Garg AP, Muller J. Fungitoxicity of fatty acids against
dermatophytes. *Mycoses* 1993; **36**: 51–63.

47 Palmer CN, Axen E, Hughes V, Wolf CR. The repressor
protein, Bm3R1, mediates an adaptive response to toxic
fatty acids in *Bacillus megaterium*. *J Biol Chem* 1998;
273: 18109–16.

48 Siegel I, Liu TL, Yaghoubzadeh E, Keskey TS, Gleicher N.
Cytotoxic effects of free fatty acids on ascites tumor cells.
J Natl Cancer Inst 1987; **78**: 271–7.

49 Grammatikos SI, Subbaiah PV, Victor TA, Miller WM.
Diverse effects of essential (n-6 and n-3) fatty acids on
cultured cells. *Cytotechnology* 1994; **15**: 31–50.

50 Noding R, Schonberg SA, Krokan HE, Bjerve KS. Effects of polyunsaturated fatty acids and their n-6 hydroperoxides on growth of five malignant cell lines and the significance of culture media. *Lipids* 1998; 33: 285–93.

51 Lieberthal W, Sheridan AM, Schwartz JH. Fatty acid-induced cytotoxicity: differences in susceptibility between MDCK cells and primary cultures of proximal tubular cells. *J Lab Clin Med* 1997; 129: 260–5.

52 Tronstad KJ, Berge K, Flindt EN, Kristiansen K, Berge RK. Optimization of methods and treatment conditions for studying effects of fatty acids on cell growth. *Lipids* 2001; 36: 305–13.

53 Cnop M, Hannaert JC, Pipeleers DG. Troglitazone does not protect rat pancreatic β cells against free fatty acid-induced cytotoxicity. *Biochem Pharmacol* 2002; 63: 1281–5.

54 Singh AK, Yoshida Y, Garvin AJ, Singh I. Effect of fatty acids and their derivatives on mitochondrial structures. *J Exp Pathol* 1989; 4: 9–15.

55 Mitchell LA, Moran JH, Grant DF. Linoleic acid, *cis*-epoxyoctadecenoic acids, and dihydroxyoctadecadienoic acids are toxic to Sf-21 cells in the absence of albumin. *Toxicol Lett* 2002; 126: 187–96.

56 Trimborn M, Iwig M, Glanz D, Gruner M, Glaesser D. Linoleic acid cytotoxicity to bovine lens epithelial cells: influence of albumin on linoleic acid uptake and cytotoxicity. *Ophthalmic Res* 2000; 32: 87–93.

57 Hoak JC. Fatty acids in animals: thrombosis and hemostasis. *Am J Clin Nutr* 1997; 65 (Suppl. 5): 1683–6S.

58 John M, Glaesser D. Concentrations of serum albumin and non-sterified fatty acids in bovine aqueous humor with regard to the fatty acid sensitivity of bovine lens epithelial cells. *Ophthalmic Res* 2000; 32: 151–6.

59 Bass NM. Intravenous albumin in the treatment of spontaneous bacterial peritonitis in cirrhosis. *N Engl J Med* 1999; 341: 443–5.

60 Zimmerman AW, Veerkamp JH. Fatty-acid-binding proteins do not protect against induced cytotoxicity in a kidney cell model. *Biochem J* 2001; 360: 159–65.

61 Burczynski FJ, Fandrey S, Wang G, Pavletic PA, Gong Y. Cytosolic fatty acid binding protein enhances rat hepatocyte [3H]palmitate uptake. *Can J Physiol Pharmacol* 1999; 77: 896–901.

62 Newberry EP, Kennedy SM, Xie Y, Luo J, Davidson NO. Liver fatty acid binding protein (L-FABP) modulates hepatic steatosis in fasted mice. *Gastroenterology* 2003; 124 (Suppl. 1): A–8.

63 Akiyama TE, Ward JM, Gonzalez FJ. Regulation of the liver fatty acid-binding protein gene by hepatocyte nuclear factor 1α (HNF1α): alterations in fatty acid homeostasis in HNF1α-deficient mice. *J Biol Chem* 2000; 275: 27117–22.

64 Binas B, Danneberg H, McWhir J, Mullins L, Clark AJ. Requirement for the heart-type fatty acid binding protein in cardiac fatty acid utilization. *FASEB J* 1999; 13: 805–12.

65 Maeda K, Uysal KT, Makowski L et al. Role of the fatty acid binding protein mal1 in obesity and insulin resistance. *Diabetes* 2003; 52: 300–7.

66 Beilman G. Pathogenesis of oleic acid-induced lung injury in the rat: distribution of oleic acid during injury and early endothelial cell changes. *Lipids* 1995; 30: 817–23.

67 Nicholls-Grzemski FA, Belling GB, Priestly BG, Calder IC, Burcham PC. Clofibrate pretreatment in mice confers resistance against hepatic lipid peroxidation. *J Biochem Mol Toxicol* 2000; 14: 335–45.

68 Nanji AA, Dannenberg AJ, Jokelainen K, Bass NM. Experimental alcoholic liver disease is associated with reduced expression of peroxisome proliferator-activated receptor-α (PPARα) regulated genes and is ameliorated by PPARα activation. *Hepatology* 2001; 34: 241A.

69 Paye F, Presset O, Chariot J, Molas G, Rozé C. Role of non-esterified fatty acids in necrotizing pancreatitis: an *in vivo* experimental study in rats. *Pancreas* 2001; 23: 341–48.

70 Levak-Frank S, Radner H, Walsh A et al. Muscle-specific overexpression of lipoprotein lipase causes a severe myopathy characterized by proliferation of mitochondria and peroxisomes in transgenic mice. *J Clin Invest* 1995; 96: 976–86.

71 Chiu HC, Kovacs A, Ford DA et al. A novel mouse model of lipotoxic cardiomyopathy. *J Clin Invest* 2001; 107: 813–22.

72 Kim JK, Fillmore JJ, Chen Y et al. Tissue-specific overexpression of lipoprotein lipase causes tissue-specific insulin resistance. *Proc Natl Acad Sci USA* 2001; 98: 7522–27.

73 Listenberger LL, Schaffer JE. Mechanisms of lipoapoptosis: implications for human heart disease. *Trends Cardiovasc Med* 2002; 12: 134–8.

74 Leibel RL, Chung WK, Chua SC Jr. The molecular genetics of rodent single gene obesities. *J Biol Chem* 1997; 272: 31937–40.

75 Shimomura I, Bashmakov Y, Horton JD. Increased levels of nuclear SREBP-1c associated with fatty livers in two mouse models of diabetes mellitus. *J Biol Chem* 1999; 274: 30028–32.

76 Moitra J, Mason MM, Olive M et al. Life without white fat: a transgenic mouse. *Genes Dev* 1998; 12: 3168–81.

77 Fan CY, Pan J, Chu R et al. Hepatocellular and hepatic peroxisomal alterations in mice with a disrupted peroxisomal fatty acyl-coenzyme A oxidase gene. *J Biol Chem* 1996, 271: 24698–710.

78 Rao MS, Reddy JK. Peroxisomal β-oxidation and steatohepatitis. *Semin Liver Dis* 2001; 21: 43–55.

79 Hashimoto T, Fujita T, Usuda N *et al*. Peroxisomal and mitochondrial fatty acid β-oxidation in mice nullizygous for both peroxisome proliferator-activated receptor α and peroxisomal fatty acyl-CoA oxidase: genotype correlation with fatty liver phenotype. *J Biol Chem* 1999; **274**: 19228–36.

80 Nehra V, Angulo P, Buchman AL, Lindor KD. Nutritional and metabolic considerations in the etiology of non-alcoholic steatohepatitis. *Dig Dis Sci* 2001; **46**: 2347–52.

81 Tavares De Almeida IH, Cortez-Pinto H, Fidalgo G, Rodrigues D, Camilo ME. Plasma total and free fatty acids composition in human non-alcoholic steatohepatitis. *Clin Nutr* 2002; **21**: 219–23.

82 De Craemer D, Pauwels M, Van den Branden C. Alterations of peroxisomes in steatosis of the human liver: a quantitative study. *Hepatology* 1995; **22**: 744–52.

83 De Craemer D, Pauwels M, Van den Branden C. Morphometric characteristics of human hepatocellular peroxisomes in alcoholic liver disease. *Alcohol Clin Exp Res* 1996; **20**: 908–13.

84 Eisele JW, Barker EA, Smuckler EA. Lipid content in the liver of fatty metamorphosis of pregnancy. *Am J Pathol* 1975; **81**: 545–60.

85 Ockner SA, Brunt EM, Cohn SM *et al*. Fulminant hepatic failure caused by acute fatty liver of pregnancy treated by orthotopic liver transplantation. *Hepatology* 1990; **11**: 59–64.

86 van der Vusse GJ, Roemen TH, Reneman RS. The content of non-esterified fatty acids in rat myocardial tissue: a comparison between the Dole and Folch extraction procedures. *J Mol Cell Cardiol* 1985; **17**: 527–31.

87 Mavrelis PG, Ammon HV, Gleysteen JJ, Komorowski RA, Charaf UK. Hepatic free fatty acids in alcoholic liver disease and morbid obesity. *Hepatology* 1983; **3**: 226–23.

88 Contos MJ, Cales W, Sterling RK *et al*. Development of non-alcoholic fatty liver disease after orthotopic liver transplantation for cryptogenic cirrhosis. *Liver Transpl* 2001; **7**: 363–73.

89 Ockner RK, Kaikaus RM and Bass NM. Fatty acid metabolism and the pathogenesis of hepatocellular carcinoma: an hypothesis. *Hepatology* 1993; **18**: 669–76.

90 Bugianesi E, Leone N, Vanni E *et al*. Expanding the natural history of non-alcoholic steatohepatitis: from cryptogenic cirrhosis to hepatocellular carcinoma. *Gastroenterology* 2002; **123**: 134–40.

91 Ratziu V, Bonyhay L, Di Martino V *et al*. Survival, liver failure, and hepatocellular carcinoma in obesity-related cryptogenic cirrhosis. *Hepatology* 2002; **35**: 1485–93.

92 Pandey M, Shukla VK. Fatty acids, biliary bile acids, lipid peroxidation products and gallbladder carcinogenesis. *Eur J Cancer Prev* 2000; **9**: 165–71.

93 Raynard B, Balian A, Fallik D *et al*. Risk factors of fibrosis in alcohol-induced liver disease. *Hepatology* 2002; **35**: 635–8.

94 Monto A. Hepatitis C and steatosis. *Semin Gastrointest Dis* 2002; **13**: 40–6.

10 Cytokines and inflammatory recruitment in NASH: experimental and human studies

Zhiping Li & Anna-Mae Diehl

Key learning points

1 Data in humans and animal models indicate that abnormalities in the immune system are involved in the development of NAFLD/NASH; both directly and indirectly through a cytosine mechanism.

2 The major immunologic abnormality (currently identified) is a decreased number of natural killer T (NKT) cells mediated through a deficiency in norepinephrine (NE) and increased apoptosis of these NKT cells.

3 Consequent to the diminished NKT cells in the liver, the cytokine milieu in the liver is pro-inflammatory (Th-1 polarized) which causes hepatocyte injury; particularly when cytokine production is induced by a secondary stimulus such as lipopolysaccharide.

4 Therapies directed against both the immunologic (NE administration) and cytokine (neutralizing anti-TNF antibodies and probiotics) mechanisms of injury have been shown to improve hepatic histology and hepatocyte damage in animal models of NAFLD/NASH.

Abstract

Immunological mechanisms mediate many chronic liver diseases, including non-alcoholic steatohepatitis (NASH). Patients with NASH often have elevated serum tumour necrosis factor-α (TNF-α) values. Moreover, in obese humans, the severity of liver disease and insulin resistance correlates well with the level of TNF-α in adipose tissue and liver. Obese *ob/ob* mice also overexpress TNF-α in adipose tissue and liver and, like many obese humans, develop insulin resistance and NASH. Treating *ob/ob* mice with agents that inhibit TNF-α activity improves both conditions, extending previous evidence that this inflammatory cytokine promotes the pathogenesis of these disorders.

Additional studies of *ob/ob* mice suggest that chronic hepatic inflammation is an indirect consequence of leptin deficiency, and that it occurs, at least in part, secondary to decreased levels of norepinephrine. The latter reduces hepatic natural killer T (NKT) cells, unbalancing local production of pro-inflammatory (Th-1) and anti-inflammatory (Th-2) cytokines, such that Th-1 polarization of hepatic cytokine producing cells ensues. Preliminary evidence suggests that the livers of mice that have been fed methionine- and choline-deficient (MCD) diets to induce NASH are also depleted of NKT cells. If Th-1 cytokine polarization proves to be a common pathogenic mechanism for hepatic insulin resistance and NASH, then therapies that inhibit inflammatory activity may be beneficial for these disorders.

Cytokines and NASH

Because the histopathology of NASH resembles that of alcohol-induced steatohepatitis (ASH) [1], common pathogenic mechanisms may mediate both of these diseases. Immunological mechanisms have a pivotal role in the pathogenesis of ASH [2]. This has been remarkably well demonstrated by studies of patients and experimental animals. In hospitalized patients with severe ASH, serum levels of several pro-inflammatory cytokines, including TNF-α, are increased significantly [3,4]. Cytokine levels correlate well with liver disease severity, generally falling in those who recover but remaining elevated in those who do not [5]. These seminal observations stimulated subsequent studies in small animal models for ASH to determine if inflammatory cytokines directly mediate alcohol-related hepatotoxicity. The results strongly support this concept. For example, various therapies that inhibit gut-derived lipopolysaccharide (LPS) endotoxaemia or that block the activity of TNF-α, an LPS-induced cytokine, provide mice and rats nearly complete protection from ASH [6–8]. This chapter reviews human and animal data concerning potential involvement of inflammatory cytokines and intestinal endotoxins in the pathogenesis of NASH.

NASH is strongly associated with obesity in humans, mice and rats [9,10]. Once considered to be a relatively inert storage depot for fat, adipose tissue is now known to produce many different hormones and cytokines, including TNF-α [11]. Thus, the increased adipose tissue mass of obese individuals provides a major source of serum TNF-α. Recent evidence suggests that resident immune cells in organs such as the liver may also contribute to obesity-related increases in pro-inflammatory cytokine production [12]. Table 10.1 summarizes the human data supporting the role of TNF in the pathogenesis of non-alcoholic fatty liver disease (NAFLD).

Increased TNF-α in obese patients with NASH

While it is widely acknowledged that TNF-α expression increases in obesity [11], the mechanisms driving chronic overproduction of TNF-α in obese humans remain obscure. However, the resultant chronic inflam-

Table 10.1 Evidence supporting the pathophysiological role of tumour necrosis factor (TNF) in non-alcoholic fatty liver disease (NAFLD) in humans.

Serum TNF levels increased in obese [11] and NASH patients [16]

TNF gene expression is increased in adipose and liver tissue of obese patients [14]

TNF mRNA expression higher in NASH patients with hepatic fibrosis [14]

Increased prevalence of TNF polymorphisms in NAFLD patients [15]

Liver histology similar between NASH and alcoholic steatohepatitis (ASH); a disease in which TNF is known to be an important pathophysiological factor [1]

Numbers in parentheses refer to the specific articles cited in the references.

matory state has been implicated in the pathogenesis of the dysmetabolic syndrome (cardiovascular disease, dyslipidaemia and insulin resistance) that often accompanies obesity. The robustness of the relationship between chronic inflammation and end-organ damage in individuals with the dysmetabolic syndrome is illustrated by recent recommendations that serum C-reactive protein levels should be tested to assess risk for adverse cardiovascular events [13]. Increased TNF-α production has also been described in obese patients with NASH. A recent Spanish study correlated liver disease severity with TNF-α gene expression in adipose and liver tissues of 52 obese patients [14]. TNF-α mRNA was overexpressed in adipose tissues and livers of patients with NASH, and was higher in patients with than in those without significant hepatic fibrosis. Another study of 99 Italian patients with NAFLD noted an increased prevalence of TNF-α polymorphism in subjects with NAFLD than in controls [15]. In that study, subjects who had the TNF-α polymorphism had greater insulin resistance, and were more likely to exhibit glucose intolerance. In addition, they were less likely to have other risk factors for hepatic steatosis. Thus, the authors concluded that TNF-α polymorphism represents a susceptibility genotype for insulin resistance, NAFLD and NASH.

In mice and rats with ASH, products of intestinal bacteria, particularly LPS endotoxin, are key inducers of hepatic TNF-α expression. Similar mechanisms appear to contribute to hepatic insulin resistance and

NASH in at least one murine model for NAFLD (see below). However, whether or not the intestinal flora promote pro-inflammatory cytokine production, insulin resistance and/or NASH in obese patients is uncertain. Wigg *et al.* [16] investigated the prevalence of small intestinal bacterial overgrowth, increased intestinal permeability, elevated endotoxin and TNF-α levels in 22 patients with NASH and 23 control subjects. Patients with NASH were more than twice as likely as controls to have small intestinal bacterial overgrowth. Serum TNF-α levels were also approximately twofold greater in the NASH group than controls. However, intestinal permeability (as measured by a dual lactulose–rhamnose sugar test) and serum endotoxin levels (as measured by the limulus lysate assay) were similar in the two groups. Hence, the authors concluded that intestinally derived endotoxin is not likely to be the factor that increases TNF-α production in patients with NASH. However, because endotoxin levels were not assessed in portal blood and gut-derived endotoxin is efficiently cleared during its first-pass through the liver, differences in hepatic endotoxin exposure may have been underestimated. Therefore, the possibility that intestinal bacterial products contribute to hepatic TNF-α induction in human NASH has not been excluded. Indeed, a role for the gut bacteria in human NASH pathogenesis is supported by the results of a recent small study that demonstrated improved liver enzymes in NASH patients who were treated with oral probiotics (mixtures of 'non-pathogenic' bacterial strains) to modify their intestinal flora [17]. Potentially pertinent to this debate is recent evidence that in Scandanavian alcoholics, promoter polymorphisms of the CD14 endotoxin receptor gene significantly increase the risk of developing steatohepatitis and cirrhosis [18].

Increased TNF-α in animal models of obesity-related NAFLD

Inbred strains of mice and rats provide convenient tools to study the pathogenesis of NAFLD because they provide opportunities to control genetic and environmental factors that might influence the natural history of NAFLD. A number of small animal models of NAFLD have emerged [10]. The fact that various genetic alterations or environmental stresses produce a similar phenotype proves that many different immuno-logical, neuronal and hormonal factors are involved in the pathogenesis of NAFLD. Therefore, any one of these animal models could be used to clarify how altered cross-talk among immune cells, neurons and endocrine cells promotes NAFLD. Unfortunately, an in-depth analysis of the inter-relationships among these systems has been lacking in all but a few of these models. The immunopathogenesis of obesity-related NASH has been studied most extensively in *ob/ob* mice. Like obese humans with NASH, *ob/ob* mice over-express TNF-α in adipose tissue and liver. The ensuing discussion focuses on the mechanisms that promote abnormal cytokine production in this model. Additional work is needed to determine if results in genetically obese *ob/ob* mice have general relevance to NASH pathogenesis in other animal models and humans.

Immunological mechanisms for NASH in leptin-deficient mice (Fig. 10.1)

Ob/ob mice have a naturally occurring mutation in the *ob* gene that prevents the synthesis of leptin, the *ob* gene product [19]. Leptin regulates feeding behaviour and energy homoeostasis. Congenital leptin deficiency results in obesity, insulin resistance, hyperinsulinaemia, glucose intolerance, dyslipidaemia and hepatic steatosis. Similar to obese or alcoholic patients with fatty livers, leptin-deficient *ob/ob* mice are unusually sensitive to liver injury induced by a secondary inflammatory stress, such as bacterial LPS endotoxin [20]. LPS-induced liver injury is generally mediated by Th-1, pro-inflammatory cytokines, while Th-2, anti-inflammatory cytokines, protect the liver from LPS-toxicity. Therefore, *ob/ob* mice have been evaluated before and after LPS exposure to determine how leptin deficiency enhances sensitivity to cytokine-mediated hepatotoxicity. Surprisingly, as discussed in subsequent sections, work with the *ob/ob* mouse model has uncovered conserved mechanisms that may regulate hepatic cytokine production in both leptin-deficient and leptin-sufficient states.

Immune cells express leptin and leptin receptors

It has gradually become apparent that leptin is a potent immunomodulator [21]. Lymphocytes and macrophages express leptin receptors [22,23] and some immune cells can produce leptin [24]. Interactions between leptin and its receptors on immune cells regu-

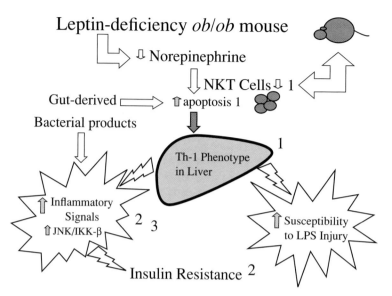

Fig. 10.1 A hypothesis for the pathophysiology of non-alcoholic fatty liver disease (NAFLD) derived from the *ob/ob* mouse model. It emphasizes the interactions among cytokines, the immune system and intestinal bacteria. The numbers 1, 2 and 3 denote abnormalities in the *ob/ob* mouse that are corrected by norepinephrine infusions, anti-tumour necrosis factor antibodies and probiotics, respectively. The inflammatory signals are Jun N-terminal kinase (JNK) and inhibitor of κ kinase-β (IKK-β). LPS, lipopolysaccharide; NKT, natural killer T cells.

late immune cell functions, including phagocytosis [25] and cytokine production [12]. Leptin deficiency also sensitizes T cells to corticosteroid-induced apoptosis and this promotes thymic atrophy in *ob/ob* mice [26]. Defects in the innate immune system, including selective reductions in hepatic NKT cell populations, also develop during leptin deficiency [27]. We have suggested that the latter may be particularly relevant to LPS hepatotoxicity, because NKT cells regulate local pro-inflammatory and anti-inflammatory cytokine production by other liver mononuclear cells. Interestingly, infection with *Propionibacterium acnes* is thought to sensitize normal livers to subsequent LPS-induced injury by reducing hepatic NKT cells and causing Th-1 polarization of other cytokine-producing cells in the liver [28].

Leptin deficiency alters the hypothalamic–pituitary–adrenal axis

Leptin deficiency also profoundly alters the hypothalamic–pituitary–adrenal (HPA) axis, increasing certain stress-related factors (e.g. corticosteroids) [29], while decreasing others (e.g. norepinephrine) [30]. Recent seminal studies in *ob/ob* mice demonstrate that many of the effects of leptin deficiency are mediated by changes in the activity of neurohumoral factors that are regulated by leptin. Indeed, Dr Friedman's group recently proved that leptin-regulated neuronal factors

have a role in the pathogenesis of NAFLD. They generated mice with a neuronal-specific deletion of *Ob-Rb* [31]. These mice produce leptin and are capable of receiving the signals that result when leptin interacts with its receptors on all other types of cells. Amazingly, mice with neuronal-specific deletion of *Ob-Rb* resemble *ob/ob* mice. Particularly relevant to the present discussion, these mice (which cannot receive leptin signals in neurons) develop insulin-resistance and NAFLD. Therefore, although leptin is clearly a key inhibitory factor for NAFLD pathogenesis, this does *not* mean that other factors are unimportant. In fact, it is likely that these other factors are the proximal mediators of obesity-related diseases in both leptin-deficient and leptin-sufficient states.

Reduced neurotransmitters and immune dysfunction

This, in turn, suggests novel, generally applicable, mechanisms for obesity-related steatohepatitis because neurotransmitters can regulate the immune system. The regulation may be mediated indirectly, as when neurotransmitters influence the release of corticosteroids and other immunomodulatory hormones from the hypothalamus, pituitary and adrenal glands. In addition, direct regulation of immune cells by neuronal factors is possible because some immune cells express neurotransmitter receptors. For example, Kupffer cells and certain types of liver lymphocytes, including NKT cells, express adrenergic receptors and respond to norepinephrine (NE) by producing various cytokines [32–35]. Neurotransmitters may also regulate the hepatic accumulation of certain lymphocyte subpopulations. Minagawa *et al.* [36] reported that pretreatment with adrenergic receptor antagonists virtually abolished the accumulation of NKT cell populations in the livers of mice that were subjected to partial hepatectomy.

The latter finding intrigued us because *ob/ob* mice are known to have both reduced NE levels and decreased hepatic NKT cells. Therefore, we decided to evaluate the hypothesis that *ob/ob* mice are sensitized to LPS hepatotoxicity because reduced NE inhibits the hepatic accumulation of NKT cells and results in Th-1 polarization of hepatic cytokine production in leptin-deficient mice. If NE proves to be a major proximal regulator of hepatic NKT cell populations, then changes in NE activity may alter hepatic NKT cell numbers and influence hepatic cytokine production independently of leptin. This, in turn, suggests a mechanism for sensitization to LPS hepatotoxicity that may have general relevance to the pathogenesis of steatohepatitis.

Norepinephrine increases hepatic NKT cells in leptin-deficient mice

Because leptin deficiency induces multiple neuronal, hormonal, metabolic and immunological abnormalities, including relative deficiency of NE, it is difficult to predict which factors are predominately responsible for decreasing NKT cells in the livers of leptin-deficient mice. To assess the significance of NE deficiency to the hepatic depletion of NKT cells that occurs in leptin-deficient mice, we implanted minipumps containing NE or saline vehicle subcutaneously into *ob/ob* mice. Three weeks later, hepatic mononuclear cells were isolated and fluorescent antibody cell sorting (FACS) analysis was performed to determine if NE altered hepatic mononuclear cell populations. NE significantly increased hepatic NKT cells in the leptin-deficient mice, demonstrating that reduced NE has an important role in decreasing hepatic NKT cells during leptin deficiency. Moreover, evidence that supplemental NE restores hepatic NKT cell populations despite persistent leptin deficiency demonstrates that this sympathetic neurotransmitter does not require leptin to increase hepatic NKT cells.

Norepinephrine reduces hepatic NKT cell apoptosis in leptin-deficient mice

To gain insight into the mechanisms by which NE increases hepatic NKT cells, we assessed the effects of NE on NKT cell apoptosis. Similar to obese humans with NASH, *ob/ob* mice overexpress TNF-α, a factor that causes NKT cell apoptosis. Therefore, we suspected that NKT cell apoptosis might be increased in *ob/ob* livers. To assess this possibility, we isolated hepatic mononuclear cells from NE-treated *ob/ob* mice and vehicle-treated *ob/ob* and lean mice and measured the levels of apoptotic cells using Annexin V. We found that hepatic NKT cell apoptosis is increased significantly in *ob/ob* mice. Moreover, 3 weeks of NE treatment decreased hepatic NKT cell apoptotic activity to normal levels. To determine if interleukin 15 (IL-15), another factor that increases NKT cells, also reduces hepatic NKT cell apoptosis, these studies were repeated in *ob/ob* mice that were treated with IL-15. Compared to NE, IL-15 is a much less effective inhibitor of hepatic NKT cell apoptosis. This finding suggests that IL-15 and NE may act by different mechanisms to promote hepatic accumulation of NKT cells.

Norepinephrine reverses Th-1 polarization of hepatic cytokine production during leptin deficiency

The livers of leptin-deficient mice are unusually sensitive to LPS-induced injury, a process that is mediated by Th-1 cytokines, such as TNF-α and interferon-γ (IFN-γ). Studies with TNF-α neutralizing antibodies demonstrate that TNF-α is required for LPS liver injury. However, IFN-γ sensitization to TNF-α is also critically important, because mice that are genetically deficient in IFN-γ are completely protected from LPS hepatotoxicity despite persistent TNF-α expression [37]. NKT cell populations produce both IFN-γ and IL-4. While the former exacerbates TNF-α toxicity, the latter is a key inducer of anti-inflammatory (Th-2) cytokines, which generally attenuate the toxic effects of TNF-α. Therefore, it is difficult to predict the ultimate effects of hepatic NKT cell depletion on hepatic cytokine production and LPS sensitivity.

ELLISPOT assays of mononuclear cells harvested from *ob/ob* livers demonstrate significantly reduced production of IL-4 [27]. This suggested that in liver, as in other epithelial tissues, reducing NKT cell populations promotes unbalanced overproduction of Th-1 cytokines. To evaluate this possibility, we treated *ob/ob* mice with NE or vehicle, isolated hepatic mononuclear cells and measured intracellular cytokines. Results from both *ob/ob* groups were also compared to those of lean control mice. Production of IFN-γ and TNF-α are increased significantly in total liver mononuclear cells from *ob/ob* mice compared to controls. These differences reflect increases in Th-1 cytokine production by several different cell populations, as demonstrated by increased IFN-γ and/or TNF-α expression in hepatic T cells and NK cells. Treatment with doses of NE that restore hepatic NKT cell numbers reduced Th-1 cytokine production by all of the hepatic mononuclear cell populations evaluated.

TNF-α, hepatic insulin resistance and NASH in *ob/ob* mice

The aforementioned studies clearly demonstrate that cytokine-producing cells in *ob/ob* livers are Th-1 polarized. This microenvironment favours the perpetuation of inflammatory signals. Sustained activation of inflammatory kinases, including Jun N-terminal kinase (JNK) [38] and inhibitor of κ kinase-β (IKK-β) [39,40], was recently found to cause cellular insulin resistance. The latter information identifies a potential mechanism for hepatic insulin resistance in leptin-deficient mice, because both kinases are targets for TNF-α-initiated activation [41]. Others have already reported that breeding *ob/ob* mice with mice that are genetically deficient in TNF function generates offspring with improved systemic sensitivity to insulin [42]. However, the role of TNF-α in NAFLD pathogenesis has remained controversial. To evaluate the role of TNF-α in hepatic insulin resistance, we treated obese adult *ob/ob* mice with vehicle or neutralizing anti-TNF antibodies for 1 month and compared hepatic activities of JNK and IKK-β in the two groups [43]. Inhibiting TNF-α significantly reduced the hepatic activities of both kinases, thereby supporting the concept that excessive TNF-α activity contributes to hepatic insulin resistance in leptin-deficient mice.

A strong positive correlation has been noted between hepatic insulin resistance and NAFLD in many experimental animals and humans. Also, increased TNF-α activity has a major role in the pathogenesis of ASH. To determine if antibodies that inhibit TNF-α activity and improve hepatic insulin resistance in *ob/ob* mice also reduce NASH, we compared histological and bio-chemical parameters of liver injury in *ob/ob* mice that had been treated with vehicle or neutralizing TNF-α antibodies for 4 weeks. Inhibition of TNF-α activity with anti-TNF antibodies significantly improved liver histology and serum aminotransferases in *ob/ob* mice [43]. Hence, as in humans with NASH, TNF-α activity and the severity of NASH are well-correlated in leptin-deficient mice.

Intestinal bacterial products and hepatic Th-1 cytokine activity

In experimental animal models of ASH, products of intestinal bacteria induce TNF-α and enhance alcohol-related liver damage. To determine if products of the intestinal flora might also be one of the endogenous signals that trigger hepatic cytokine production, insulin resistance and NASH, we fed probiotics (a mixture of live lactobacillus and bifidobacteria) to another group of *ob/ob* mice. Although probiotics did not inhibit hepatic expression of TNF-α mRNA, they did significantly downregulate JNK and IKK-β activities. Similar to anti-TNF antibodies, probiotics also improved histological and biochemical evidence of steatohepatitis [43]. These findings suggest that intestinal bacterial products might regulate TNF-α activity by post-transcriptional mechanisms in *ob/ob* mice. One such mechanism might involve altered production of other cytokines that are known to enhance (e.g. IFN-γ) or inhibit (e.g. IL-10, IL-15, transforming growth factor-β) TNF-α activity. Further study is needed to evaluate this possibility directly.

Hepatic innate immune system abnormalities in leptin-sufficient models for NAFLD

There has been considerable controversy about the relevance of findings in leptin-deficient mice to NAFLD pathogenesis in mice and humans with normal leptin genes. To address this issue, we evaluated another widely studied mouse model of NAFLD to determine if hepatic NKT cell depletion also occurs in mice that develop NAFLD despite having normal genes for leptin and leptin receptors. Normal adult mice of the same genetic background (C57BL-6) as *ob/ob* mice were fed MCD diets to increase TNF-α production and induce steatohepatitis [44]. Age- and gender-matched control C57BL-6 mice were fed a nutritionally replete diet from the same manufacturer. Liver mononuclear cells were isolated from both groups and analysed by FACS. Compared to normal controls, mice fed MCD diets have reduced numbers of NKT cells, including CD4[+] NKT cells. Indeed, the degree of NKT-cell depletion in the MCD diet model of NAFLD is similar to that noted in *ob/ob* mice with NAFLD. These findings suggest that defects in the hepatic innate immune system are likely to be conserved among different NAFLD models. This supports the concept that the early stages of NALFD (steatosis and steatohepatitis) may be a common end-point of diverse insults that promote excessive hepatic sensitivity to Th-1 cytokines.

Conclusions

Immunological mechanisms mediate most kinds of chronic liver disease, including NAFLD/NASH. Studies in genetically obese leptin-deficient *ob/ob* mice, a murine model for NAFLD, demonstrate some of these immunological alterations and also suggest mechanisms that might be driving them. In this model, the cytokine milieu of the liver is pro-inflammatory (Th-1 polarized). Thus, when cytokine production is induced by secondary stimuli (e.g. LPS), pro-inflammatory cytokines (e.g. TNF-α, IFN-γ) accumulate and their activities become sustained because anti-inflammatory (Th-2) cytokines (which normally inhibit Th-1 cytokines) are relatively deficient. Th-1/Th-2 cytokine imbalance develops because hepatic NKT cell populations are reduced significantly during leptin deficiency.

Liver NKT cell depletion results from excessive apoptosis in this cell population. Apoptosis increases because leptin deficiency inhibits the production of factors, such as norepinephrine, that are required for hepatic NKT cell viability. When *ob/ob* mice are treated with supplemental norepinephrine, NKT cell populations are restored in the liver and production of Th-1 cytokines is downregulated to normal levels.

Treatments (e.g. anti-TNF-α antibodies) that inhibit Th-1 cytokine activity directly also improve hepatic insulin resistance and NASH in *ob/ob* mice.

It remains to be seen if similar immunological abnormalities occur in other animal models of fatty liver disease, and in humans with NASH. The following evidence supports the concept that common immune mechanisms mediate the pathogenesis of NASH:

- The livers of mice that have been fed MCD diets to induce NASH are also depleted in NKT cells and overexpress TNF-α.
- Excessive hepatic activity of Th-1 cytokines, such as TNF-α, mediates steatohepatitis that is induced by alcohol in mice and rats.
- Gene polymorphisms that enhance TNF-α activity have been associated with NASH (and ASH) in patients.
- In humans with ASH, certain anti-inflammatory agents (e.g. corticosteroids, pentoxifyline) are beneficial.
- Inhibition of TNF-α activity is also a common property of diverse drugs (e.g. metformin, thiazolidendiones, betaine, vitamin E) that have been reported to improve NASH in obese insulin-resistant patients.

Thus, a growing body of evidence supports a role for hepatic Th-1 cytokine polarization in the pathogenesis of hepatic insulin resistance and NASH. These results suggest various therapeutic strategies that might be utilized to improve these conditions in obese individuals.

References

1 Ludwig J, Viggiano RT, McGill DB. Non-alcoholic steatohepatitis: Mayo Clinic experiences with a hitherto unnamed disease. *Mayo Clin Proc* 1980; **55**: 342–8.

2 Kamimura S, Tsukamoto H. Cytokine gene expression by Kupffer cells isolated from ethanol-fed rats. *Hepatology* 1995; **22**: 1304–9.

3 Bird GLA, Sheron N, Goka AKJ, Alexander GL, Williams RS. Increased plasma tumor necrosis factor in severe alcoholic hepatitis. *Ann Intern Med* 1990; **112**: 917–20.

4 McClain CJ, Cohen DA. Increased tumor necrosis factor production by monocytes in alcoholic hepatitis. *Hepatology* 1989; **9**: 349–51.

5 Hill D, Marsano L, Cohen D *et al*. Increased plasma interleukin-6 activity in alcoholic hepatitis. *J Lab Clin Med* 1992; **119**: 507–12.

6 Iimuro Y, Gallucci RM, Luster MI, Kono H, Thurman RG. Antibodies to tumor necrosis factor-α attenuates hepatic necrosis and inflammation caused by chronic exposure to ethanol in the rat. *Hepatology* 1997; **26**: 1530–7.

7 Adachi Y, Moore LE, Bradford BU, Gao W, Thurman RG. Antibiotics prevent liver injury in rats following long-term exposure to ethanol. *Gastroenterology* 1995; **108**: 218–24.

8 Nanji AA, Khettry U, Sadrzadeh SM. Lactobacillus feeding reduces endotoxemia and severity of experimental

alcoholic liver disease. *Proc Soc Exp Biol Med* 1994; **205**: 243–7.

9 Wanless IR, Lentz JS. Fatty liver hepatitis (steatohepatitis) and obesity: an autopsy study with analysis of risk factors. *Hepatology* 1990; **12**: 1106–10.

10 Koteish A, Diehl AM. Animal models of steatosis. *Semin Liver Dis* 2001; **21**: 89–104.

11 Kern PA, Saghizaheh M, Ong JM *et al.* The expression of tumor necrosis factor in human adipose tissue: regulation by obesity, weight loss, and relationship to lipoprotein lipase. *J Clin Invest* 1995; **95**: 2111–9.

12 Li Z, Lin HZ, Yang SQ, Diehl AM. Murine leptin deficiency alters Kupffer cell production of cytokines that regulate the innate immune system. *Gastroenterology* 2002; **123**: 1304–10.

13 Ridker PM, Rifai N, Rose L, Buring JE, Cook NR. Comparison of C-reactive protein and low-density lipoprotein cholesterol levels in the prediction of first cardiovascular events. *N Engl J Med* 2002; **347**: 1557–65.

14 Crespo J, Cayon A, Fernandez-Gil P *et al.* Gene expression of tumor necrosis factor α and TNF-receptors, p55 and p75, in non-alcoholic steatohepatitis patients. *Hepatology* 2001; **34**: 1158–63.

15 Valenti L, Fracanzani AL, Dongiovanni P *et al.* Tumor necrosis factor α promoter polymorphisms and insulin resistance in non-alcoholic fatty liver disease. *Gastroenterology* 2002; **122**: 274–80.

16 Wigg AJ, Roberts-Thomson IC, Dymock RB *et al.* The role of small intestinal bacterial overgrowth, intestinal permeability, endotoxaemia, and tumour necrosis factor α in the pathogenesis of non-alcoholic steatohepatitis. *Gut* 2001; **48**: 206–11.

17 Loguercio C, DeSimone T, Federico A *et al.* Gut-liver axis: a new point of attack to treat chronic liver damage? *Am J Gastroenterol* 2002; **97**: 2144–6.

18 Jarvelainen HA, Orpana A, Perola M *et al.* Promoter polymorphism of the CD14 endotoxin receptor gene as a risk factor for alcoholic liver disease. *Hepatology* 2001; **33**: 1148–53.

19 Zhang Y, Proenca R, Maffei M *et al.* Positional cloning of the mouse obese gene and its human homologue. *Nature* 1994; **372**: 425–32.

20 Yang SQ, Lin HZ, Lane MD, Clemens M, Diehl AM. Obesity increases sensitivity to endotoxin liver injury: implications for pathogenesis of steatohepatitis. *Proc Natl Acad Sci USA* 1997; **94**: 2557–62.

21 Faggioni R, Feingold KR, Grunfeld C. Leptin regulation of the immune response and the immunodeficiency of malnutrition. *FASEB J* 2001; **15**: 2565–71.

22 Zarkesh-Esfahani H, Pockley G, Metcalfe RA *et al.* High-dose leptin activates human leukocytes via receptor expression on monocytes. *J Immunol* 2001; **167**: 4593–9.

23 Lord GM, Matarese G, Howard JK *et al.* Leptin modulates the T-cell immune response and reverses starvation-induced immunosuppression. *Nature* 1998; **394**: 897–901.

24 Sanna V, Di Giacomo A, La Cava A *et al.* Leptin surge precedes onset of autoimmune encephalomyelitis and correlates with development of pathogenic T cell responses. *J Clin Invest* 2003; **111**: 241–50.

25 Loffreda S, Yang SQ, Lin HZ *et al.* Leptin regulates proinflammatory immune responses. *FASEB J* 1998; **12**: 57–65.

26 Howard JK, Lord GM, Matarese G *et al.* Leptin protects mice from starvation-induced lymphoid atrophy and increases thymic cellularity in *ob/ob* mice. *J Clin Invest* 1999; **104**: 1051–9.

27 Guebre-Xabier M, Yang SQ, Lin HZ *et al.* Altered hepatic lymphocyte subpopulations in obesity-related fatty livers. *Hepatology* 1999; **31**: 633–40.

28 Matsui K, Yoshimoto T, Tsutsui H *et al.* *Propionibacterium acnes* treatment diminishes CD4+ NK1.1+ T cells but induces type 1 T cells in the liver by induction of IL-12 and IL-18 production from Kupffer cells. *J Immunol* 1997; **159**: 97–106.

29 Makimura H, Mizuno TM, Roberts J *et al.* Adrenalectomy reverses obese phenotype and restores hypothalamic melanocortin tone in leptin-deficient *ob/ob* mice. *Diabetes* 2000; **49**: 1917–23.

30 Knehans AW, Romsos DR. Reduced norepinephrine turnover in brown adipose tissue of *ob/ob* mice. *Am J Physiol* 1982; **242**: E253–61.

31 Cohen P, Zhao C, Cai X *et al.* Selective deletion of leptin receptor in neurons leads to obesity. *J Clin Invest* 2001; **108**: 1113–21.

32 Spengler RN, Chensue SW, Giacherio DA, Blenk N, Kunkel SL. Endogenous norepinephrine regulates tumor necrosis factor-α production from macrophages *in vitro*. *J Immunol* 1994; **152**: 3024–31.

33 Kalinichenko VV, Mokyr MB, Graf LH Jr, Cohen RL, Chambers DA. Norepinephrine-mediated inhibition of antitumor cytotoxic T lymphocyte generation involves a β-adrenergic receptor mechanism and decreased TNF-α gene expression. *J Immunol* 1999; **163**: 2492–9.

34 Elenkov IJ, Chrousos GP, Wilder RL. Neuroendocrine regulation of IL-12 and TNF-α/IL-10 balance: clinical implications. *Ann NY Acad Sci* 2000; **917**: 94–105.

35 Zhou M, Yang S, Koo DJ *et al.* The role of Kupffer cell 2-adrenoceptors in norepinephrine-induced TNF-α production. *Biochim Biophys Acta* 2001; **1537**: 49–57.

36 Minagawa M, Oya H, Yamamoto S *et al.* Intensive expansion of natural killer T cells in the early phase of hepatocyte regeneration after partial hepatectomy in mice and its association with sympathetic nerve activation. *Hepatology* 2000; **31**: 907–15.

37 Shimizu Y, Margenthaler JA, Landeros K *et al*. The resistance of *P. acnes*-primed interferon-γ-deficient mice to low-dose lipopolysaccharide-induced acute liver injury. *Hepatology* 2002; **35**: 805–14.

38 Hirosumi J, Tuncman G, Chang L *et al*. A central role for JNK in obesity and insulin resistance. *Nature* 2002; **420**: 333–6.

39 Kim JK, Kim YJ, Fillmore JJ *et al*. Prevention of fat-induced insulin resistance by salicylate. *J Clin Invest* 2001; **108**: 437–46.

40 Yuan M, Konstantopoulos N, Lee J *et al*. Reversal of obesity- and diet-induced insulin resistance with salicylates or targeted disruption of IKK-β. *Science* 2001; **293**: 1673–7.

41 Aggarwal BB. Tumour necrosis factors receptor associated signalling molecules and their role in activation of apoptosis, JNK and NK-κB. *Ann Rheum Dis* 2000; **59** (Suppl. 1): I6–I16.

42 Uysal KT, Wiesbrock SM, Marino MW, Hotamisligil GS. Protection from obesity-induced insulin-resistance in mice lacking TNF-α function. *Nature* 1997; **389**: 610–4.

43 Li Z, Yang S, Lin H *et al*. Probiotics and antibodies to TNF inhibit inflammatory activity and improve non-alcoholic fatty liver disease. *Hepatology* 2003; **37**: 343–50.

44 Chitturi S, Farrell GC. Etiopathogenesis of non-alcoholic steatohepatitis. *Semin Liver Dis* 2001; **21**: 27–41.

11 Mitochondrial injury and NASH

Bernard Fromenty & Dominique Pessayre

Key learning points

1 High mitochondrial fatty acid β-oxidation increases the delivery of electrons to the mitochondrial respiratory chain.
2 Reactive oxygen species (ROS) oxidize fat deposits to release lipid peroxidation products that react with mitochondrial DNA (mtDNA) and proteins to partially block the flow of electrons in the respiratory chain.
3 The imbalance between high electron input and restricted electron flow may cause over-reduction of respiratory chain components, which react with oxygen to generate ROS.
4 Increased mitochondrial ROS formation further damages mtDNA, proteins and lipids, increases tumour necrosis factor formation and can deplete antioxidants.
5 In steatohepatitis, mitochondria exhibit ultrastructural lesions, mtDNA depletion and decreased activity of respiratory chain complexes.

Abstract

Rich diet and lack of exercise can result in obesity, insulin resistance and steatosis, which may evolve into non-alcoholic steatohepatitis (NASH). Patients with this 'primary' (metabolic) form of NASH have high levels of hepatic free fatty acids (FFA), and sometimes high blood glucose levels. Enhanced mitochondrial fatty acid β-oxidation increases the delivery of electrons to the mitochondrial respiratory chain. The resultant reduction of oxygen forms reactive oxygen species (ROS), which oxidize fatty acids to release lipid peroxidation products. In turn, these react with mitochondrial DNA (mtDNA) and proteins to partially block the flow of electrons in the respiratory chain. The imbalance between high electron input and restricted electron flow may cause over-reduction of respiratory chain components, which react with oxygen to generate ROS. Increased mitochondrial ROS formation further damages mtDNA, proteins and lipids, depletes antioxidants, and stimulates the formation of tumour necrosis factor-α (TNF-α). In patients with NASH, mitochondria exhibit ultrastructural lesions, mtDNA depletion and decreased activity of respiratory chain complexes. The *in vivo* ability to resynthesize adenosine triphosphate (ATP) after a fructose challenge is decreased. Hepatic lipid peroxidation products are increased. Blood vitamin E can be decreased, and liver tests can improve after vitamin E supplementation. In steatohepatitis resulting from other causes such as drugs and alcohol, mitochondrial ROS formation increases to a greater extent because of the direct toxic effects of the aetiological agent. This exaggerated ROS formation promotes more lipid peroxidation and cytokine induction, triggering more pronounced apoptosis, inflammation and fibrogenesis than in steatohepatitis resulting from metabolic causes (NASH).

Introduction

As a result of a lipid-rich diet and lack of exercise, the populations of affluent countries are becoming increasingly obese. This thrifty trend in energy storage as fat is associated with a parallel surge in prevalence of hepatic steatosis characterized by an accumulation of fat droplets within the cytoplasm of hepatocytes [1–3]. In some patients, this hepatic steatosis remains isolated (without other liver injury; see Chapter 2), while in others it triggers mild hepatocyte injury (ballooning degeneration, apoptosis and necrosis) and a mild inflammatory cell infiltrate, termed steatohepatitis; there may be a slow development of hepatic fibrosis which can progressively evolve over a period of years or decades into cirrhosis [2].

In addition to steatohepatitis associated with obesity, type 2 diabetes and insulin resistance (NASH), there are also several 'secondary' forms of steatosis and steatohepatitis, including jejuno-ileal bypass, total parenteral nutrition, alcohol abuse, Wilson's disease and administration of some drugs [2]. Steatohepatitis tends to be more severe in these cases with a known cause (see Chapters 20 and 21).

Accumulating evidence suggests a major role for lipid peroxidation, mitochondrial dysfunction, ROS formation, cytokine induction and apoptosis in steatohepatitis (see Chapters 8 and 10). To understand these mechanisms, it may be useful to first recall the normal role of mitochondria in fat metabolism, energy production and formation of ROS.

Normal role of mitochondria in hepatic fat metabolism, energy production and reactive oxygen species formation

Hepatic fat metabolism

Hepatic FFA are taken up by the liver from the plasma FFA that are released by adipose tissue, or generated in the liver from the hydrolysis of chylomicrons coming from the intestine, or are directly synthesized *de novo* within hepatocytes [2]. These hepatic FFA either enter the mitochondria to undergo mitochondrial β-oxidation, or are esterified into triglycerides (a storage form of lipid in which FFA molecules are esterified to glycerol).

Hepatic triglycerides, surrounded by a single monolayer of phospholipids, either accumulate as fat droplets within the cytoplasm of hepatocytes, or are secreted as very-low-density lipoproteins (VLDL). Plasma VLDL particles comprise lipid (triglycerides and cholesterol esters) surrounded by phospholipids and a large protein termed apolipoprotein B (apo B; see Chapter 9). Apo B is co-translationally lipidated in the endoplasmic reticulum lumen by microsomal triglyceride transfer protein (MTP) and is further lipidated in the Golgi apparatus [4]. The extent of lipidation directs the fate of apo B molecules. Fully lipidated apo B quickly follows vesicular flow, to be secreted into the plasma. In contrast, incompletely lipidated apo B molecules fail to completely translocate into the endoplasmic reticulum lumen and/or undergo retrotranslocation to the cytosol where they are ubiquitinated, and finally digested by the proteasome [5]. For a detailed discussion of fat metabolism (see Chapter 9).

Mitochondrial fatty acid oxidation

The entry of long-chain FFA into the mitochondria is critically dependent on carnitine palmitoyltransferase 1 (CPT-1), an outer membrane enzyme whose activity is inhibited by malonyl-CoA [6]. Malonyl-CoA is formed by acetyl-CoA carboxylase and is the first step in the synthesis of fatty acids from acetyl-CoA [6].

After a carbohydrate meal, high blood glucose and insulin levels stimulate brisk hepatic synthesis of fatty acids [6]. This produces abundant malonyl-CoA, which inhibits CPT-1, thereby blocking FFA entry into mitochondria and β-oxidation [6]. The undegraded FFA are directed towards the formation of triglycerides, which are secreted as VLDL [6].

In contrast, in the fasting state, FFA are released by adipose tissue and taken up by the liver. During fasting, hepatic FFA synthesis and thus malonyl-CoA levels are low, permitting extensive mitochondrial import of FFA and extensive β-oxidation. Successive β-oxidation cycles split FFA into acetyl-CoA subunits. Acetyl-CoA can then be completely degraded to CO_2 by the tricarboxylic acid cycle. However, during fasting conditions, acetyl-CoA is mostly condensed into ketone bodies, which are secreted by the liver to be oxidized in muscles and other peripheral tissues [6].

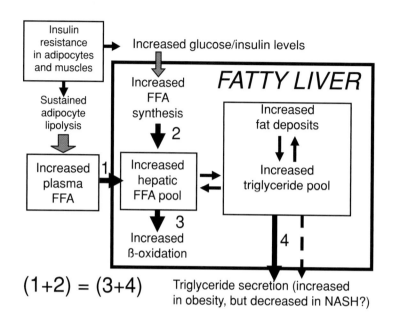

Fig. 11.1 Insulin resistance and hepatic steatosis in obese subjects. Insulin resistance in adipocytes increases adipocyte lipolysis, which increases plasma free fatty acids (FFA) and hepatic FFA uptake. Insulin resistance in myocytes increases glucose and/or insulin levels, which may increase hepatic FFA synthesis. Hepatic FFAs are increased because of increased uptake and increased synthesis, in equilibrium with an expanded pool of triglycerides, with triglyceride deposits in the cytoplasm. A new steady state is achieved whereby these increased input pathways are compensated by an increased oxidation of fatty acids. The hepatic secretion of triglycerides is also increased in obese patients without NASH, but might be decreased in patients with NASH. (Modified from Pessayre [3].)

Mitochondrial energy production

The oxidation of FFA in mitochondria, and the oxidation of other fuels both elsewhere and in mitochondria, are associated with the conversion of oxidized cofactors (NAD^+ and FAD) into reduced cofactors (NADH and $FADH_2$) (Fig. 11.1) [7]. These reduced cofactors are then re-oxidized by the mitochondrial respiratory chain, which is attached to the mitochondrial inner membrane. This re-oxidation regenerates the NAD^+ and FAD necessary for other cycles of fuel oxidation [7].

During their re-oxidation, NADH and $FADH_2$ transfer their electrons to the first complexes of the respiratory chain. Electrons then migrate along the repiratory chain and this flow of electrons is coupled with the extrusion of protons from the mitochondrial matrix into the mitochondrial intermembranous space. Proton extrusion creates a large electrochemical potential across the inner membrane, thus creating a reservoir of latent potential energy.

When energy is needed, protons re-enter the matrix through the F_0 portion of ATP synthase, causing the rotation of a molecular rotor in the F_1 portion of ATP synthase and the conversion of adenosine diphosphate (ADP) into ATP. The adenine nucleotide trans-locator then extrudes the formed mitochondrial ATP, in exchange for cytosolic ADP [2]. Cytoplasmic ATP is then used to power all the cell processes that require energy.

Mitochondrial reactive oxygen species formation

Most of the electrons, which are donated to the respiratory chain, migrate all the way along the respiratory chain, to finally reach cytochrome *c* oxidase (the terminal oxidase), where they safely combine with oxygen and protons to form water [2]. However, at several upstream sites of the respiratory chain, a fraction of these electrons can react directly with oxygen, to form the superoxide anion radical. This radical is then dismutated by mitochondrial manganese superoxide dismutase (MnSOD) into hydrogen peroxide, which is detoxified into water by mitochondrial glutathione peroxidase [2].

Due to the intermediate formation of the superoxide anion radical and hydrogen peroxide, which can form the hydroxyl radical, mitochondria are the main site of ROS formation in the cell [7]. This high basal rate of mitochondrial ROS formation is further increased whenever the electron flow in the respiratory chain is partially hampered [2]. This may occur when hepatic steatosis develops as a result of diverse causes, including obesity.

Obesity, insulin resistance and steatosis

Obesity

In the past, prolonged overeating was self-regulating, as excess weight soon impaired the physical fitness required to gather food and handle predators or foes [1]. For the first time in history, a large fraction of the population in affluent countries can concomitantly indulge in rich food and physical idleness, causing a surge in obesity. About 22.5% of US citizens are obese, and this prevalence could reach 40% by the year 2025 [8] unless drastic lifestyle changes can curb present trends.

Obesity involves the accumulation of fat not only in adipocytes, but also in muscle cells, and this accumulation can cause insulin resistance in adipocytes and muscles.

Insulin resistance in adipocytes and muscles

After a meal in lean persons, a mild increase in blood glucose causes a minor increase in insulin. Insulin acts on its receptor on the surface of adipocytes and myocytes to trigger the phosphorylation of insulin receptor substrates (IRS), which activate phosphatidyl inositol 3-kinase and Akt/protein kinase B, to eventually cause the translocation of GLUT-4 glucose transporters from intracellular storage vesicles to the plasma membrane [9]. Abundant expression of GLUT-4 transporter on the membrane causes efficient glucose uptake, which limits the increase in blood glucose and insulin levels.

In obese people, however, adipocytes may produce less GLUT-4 transporter [9]. More importantly, both fat-engorged adipocytes and fat-laden myocytes are resistant to the signalling effects of the insulin receptor [9]. It is suggested that acyl-CoA or other derivatives of FFA may limit the activation of IRS and phosphatidyl inositol 3-kinase [9]. The mechanism could involve the activation of Jun N-terminal kinase and, hence, the serine phosphorylation and thus inactivation of IRS [10]. Whatever the mechanism, insufficient translocation of GLUT-4 to the plasma membrane limits glucose uptake by adipocytes and myocytes [9]. This insufficient uptake results in an increase of blood glucose and a compensatory increase in the release of

insulin by pancreatic β cells (the insulin-secreting cells of the pancreas) [11]. In some subjects, however, this compensatory insulin increase is not enough, or secondarily fails, and frank diabetes develops. Therefore, insulin resistance in adipocytes and muscles tends to result in increased C-peptide, insulin and blood glucose levels (after eating).

Another normal effect of the activation of Akt/protein kinase B by the insulin receptor in adipocytes, is to activate a phosphodiesterase, which degrades cyclic adenosine monophosphate (AMP) [12]. This degradation prevents the cyclic AMP-mediated activation of protein kinase A and then hormone-sensitive lipase, which otherwise would hydrolyse triglycerides into fatty acids. As a final consequence, a normal effect of insulin is to block adipose tissue lipolysis. However, this normal effect of insulin is hampered during insulin resistance. Indeed, whereas the adipocytes of lean insulin-sensitive persons release FFA during fasting but then store fat after meals, in contrast, the fat-engorged insulin-resistant adipocytes of obese people keep releasing FFA after meals, causing a sustained increase in plasma FFA [13].

Thus, in obese persons, insulin resistance causes not only high blood insulin and glucose levels, but also high plasma FFA. Both effects may be involved in the development of hepatic steatosis in obese persons [3].

Hepatic steatosis

High plasma FFA levels increase hepatic FFA uptake, while high glucose and insulin levels may increase hepatic FFA synthesis in some obese patients (Fig. 11.1) [3]. Indeed, insulin increases the transcription of sterol regulatory element-binding protein-1 (SREBP-1), and genetically obese ob/ob mice have increased levels of SREBP-1 mRNA and protein [14]. SREBP-1 upregulates the expression of acetyl-CoA carboxylase and fatty acid synthase, to increase hepatic fatty acid synthesis [14]. Interestingly, stearoyl-CoA desaturase is also increased in ob/ob mice, resulting in a considerable increase in oleic acid [14], an unsaturated fatty acid that is a substrate for lipid peroxidation.

In obese persons, the increased uptake and synthesis of FFA expand the hepatic FFA pool [3]. These increased input pathways are compensated by an increased rate of hepatic mitochondrial FFA β-oxidation (Fig. 11.1) [15]. By contrast, the hepatic secretion of triglyceride might be differently affected in obese persons without NASH and obese patients with NASH (Fig. 11.1). Thus, in obese persons without NASH, the secretion of apo B tended to be slightly increased [16], which may explain why these patients tend to have hyper-triglyceridaemia. Likewise, in obese *ob/ob* mice, MTP expression and hepatic lipoprotein secretion were both increased [17]. However, in obese persons with NASH, hepatic apo B secretion was decreased [16], which infers decreased secretion of VLDL.

The reasons for the differences in apo B secretion in patients with and without NASH are unknown. There are two possible mechanisms. First, NASH may be associated with even higher insulin and TNF levels, which both downregulate MTP production [18,19]. Although insulin resistance in the liver could perhaps hamper insulin effects, increased TNF may decrease MTP-mediated apo B lipidation and thus the secretion of triglyceride-rich VLDL particles in patients with NASH. Secondly, subjects with an inborn partial deficiency in MTP expression could excrete less hepatic VLDL and could therefore store more fat in the liver, to be at increased risk of developing NASH [20].

Although a new equilibrium is achieved between input and output pathways in insulin-resistant persons (with or without NASH), this new equilibrium is achieved at the expense of expanded pools of hepatic FFA and triglycerides, thus causing steatosis (Fig. 11.1) [3].

Harmful effects of fat in the liver

Although the reasons for the deleterious effects of steatosis are still incompletely understood, there is growing evidence that the presence of oxidizable fat in the liver can trigger lipid peroxidation, mitochondrial dysfunction and increased mitochondrial ROS formation.

Lipid peroxidation

Even in the basal (fat-free) state, hepatocytes produce large amounts of ROS. These ROS are formed mainly in mitochondria, but also at other sites, including microsomal cytochrome P450 (CYP). Yet another potential source of ROS is the NADPH oxidase of Kupffer cells (Fig. 11.2) [21].

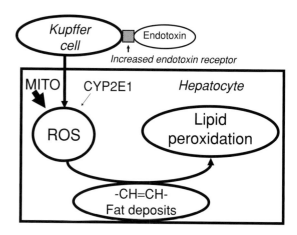

Fig. 11.2 The presence of fat in the liver triggers lipid peroxidation. Mitochondria (MITO) and cytochrome P450 2E1 (CYP2E1) generate reactive oxygen species (ROS). In several models of steatosis, the endotoxin receptors of Kupffer cells are increased, which might trigger ROS formation by these cells. When fat accumulates in the liver, ROS oxidize the unsaturated lipids of fat deposits to cause lipid peroxidation. (Modified from Pessayre [3].)

This large basal ROS formation is further enhanced in steatotic livers. First, mitochondrial ROS formation is increased (see below). Secondly, CYP2E1 is also increased [22], which further increases ROS formation in hepatocytes. Finally, endotoxin receptors on Kupffer cells are upregulated in animals with either obesity- or alcohol-mediated hepatic steatosis [23,24]. Increased sensitivity of Kupffer cells to bacterial endotoxin may increase ROS formation by these cells (Fig. 11.2). This abundant formation of ROS may start to oxidize the unsaturated lipids of fat deposits to cause lipid peroxidation (Fig. 11.2) [1,2].

Indeed, 11 different treatments causing acute or chronic steatosis always increased hepatic thiobarbituric acid reactants and ethane exhalation, an *in vivo* index of lipid peroxidation, in mice [25]. After a single dose of tetracycline or ethanol, there was a parallel time course in the rise and fall of hepatic triglycerides, and the rise and fall of lipid peroxidation products. This is consistent with a cause-and-effect relationship between the presence of oxidizable fat in the liver and lipid peroxidation [25]. Extensive lipid peroxidation also occurs in animals with hepatic steatosis resulting from a methionine- and choline-deficient diet [26], genetically obese leptin-deficient *ob/ob* mice (personal unpublished results) and patients

Fig. 11.3 Electron overflow and reactive oxygen species (ROS). In the normal liver, the electrons that are given to the respiratory chain mostly flow along this chain, up to cytochrome *c* oxidase (the terminal oxidase), where they safely combine with oxygen and protons to form water. In the fatty liver of insulin-resistant patients, high β-oxidation rates increase the delivery of electrons to the respiratory chain, while ROS and lipid peroxidation products, such as 4-hydroxynoneal (HNE), may partially block the flow of electrons within this chain. The imbalance between a high input and a restricted flow of electrons may cause over-reduction of respiratory chain components, which directly transfer their electrons to oxygen to form the superoxide anion radical and other ROS. (Adapted from Pessayre [3].)

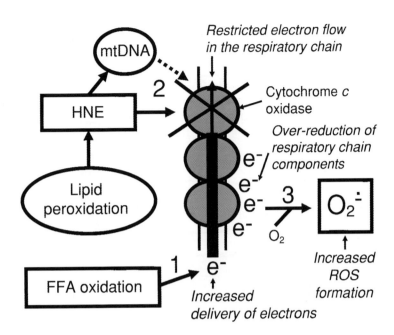

with NASH [15]. This extensive lipid peroxidation releases several reactive substances that can damage mitochondria.

Mitochondrial dysfunction

Restricted electron flow

The peroxidation of hepatic triglycerides releases reactive aldehydes, such as 4-hydroxynonenal and malondialdehyde, that damage mtDNA (Fig. 11.3) [27]. This may secondarily impair the flow of electrons in the respiratory chain, because mtDNA encodes some of the respiratory chain polypeptides [1]. Lipid peroxidation products also directly attack and inactivate respiratory chain polypeptides, including cytochrome *c* oxidase, the terminal oxidase of the respiratory chain [28]. These two effects of lipid peroxidation products could thus partially hamper the flow of electrons in the respiratory chain (Fig. 11.3) [1].

The livers of patients with NASH have been shown to exhibit ultrastructural mitochondrial lesions, with the presence of crystalline inclusions in megamitochondria [15] (see Chapte 2, Fig. 2.1). These patients have mtDNA depletion and decreased expression of a mtDNA-encoded cytochrome oxidase subunit II [29]. The *ex vivo* activity of mitochondrial respiratory chain complexes is decreased [30], as is the *in vivo* resynthesis of ATP after a fructose challenge [31].

Increased input of electrons

Contrasting with this partial block in the flow of electrons in the respiratory chain, the input of electrons into this chain may be enhanced by the increased mitochondrial β-oxidation of FFA [15], which forms NADH and $FADH_2$, that transfer their electrons to the respiratory chain (Fig. 11.3). In diabetic patients, increased blood glucose levels and enhanced glucose oxidation could further increase this influx of electrons.

Increased mitochondrial reactive oxygen species formation

The imbalance between an increased electron input into the respiratory chain and a partially hampered flow of electrons within this chain may cause over-reduction of respiratory chain components. These can then react with oxygen to form the superoxide anion radical, thus increasing mitochondrial ROS formation (Fig. 11.3) [3]. An increased mitochondrial ROS formation has indeed been demonstrated in genetically obese *ob/ob* mice [32] and in mice fed a choline-deficient diet [33]. This increased mitochondrial ROS formation will in turn cause several vicious cycles (see below).

137

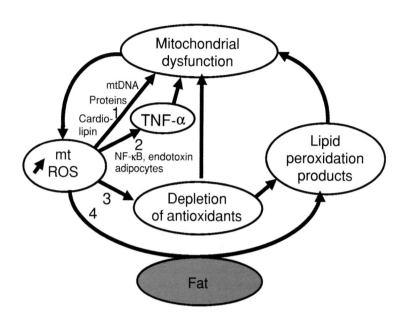

Fig. 11.4 Vicious cycles involving reactive oxygen species (ROS) and mitochondria. The increased formation of mitochondrial ROS (mtROS) can further damage mitochondria and further increase mtROS formation through several vicious cycles. 1. ROS directly damage mitochondrial DNA, proteins and cardiolipin to impair the flow of electrons in the respiratory chain and increase mitochondrial ROS formation. 2. ROS activate NF-κB, which increases TNF-α and further damages mitochondria. 3. ROS deplete antioxidants such as vitamin E. 4. ROS trigger further lipid peroxidation, whose products impair the flow of electrons in the respiratory chain to further increase mitochondrial ROS formation. (Adapted from Pessayre [3].)

Reactive oxygen species-dependent vicious cycles

Because ROS themselves damage mitochondria to further increase mitochondrial ROS formation (Fig. 11.4), an increase in mitochondrial ROS production can trigger the following processes that amplify injury:

1 ROS directly damage mtDNA, respiratory chain polypeptides and mitochondrial cardiolipin [1].
2 ROS cause NF-κB activation, which induces the synthesis of TNF [34]. TNF is also synthesized by fat-engorged adipocytes and is released by Kupffer cells stimulated by endotoxin. TNF damages mitochondria and increases mitochondrial ROS formation (see below).
3 ROS may deplete some tissue antioxidants, thereby further aggravating ROS-induced damages. Thus, low serum vitamin E levels are found in some obese children with steatohepatitis [35] and supplementation with vitamin E can decrease serum aminotransaminase (AT) levels in obese children [36].
4 Increased mitochondrial ROS formation further increases lipid peroxidation, thereby releasing more reactive aldehydes that further damage mtDNA and respiratory chain polypeptides [1].

These vicious cycles can damage mitochondria and enhance ROS formation in patients with NASH secondary to obesity, type 2 diabetes and insulin resist-ance. In other causes of steatohepatitis, the situation is exacerbated because the causative disease process itself directly increases ROS formation [1]. This subject has been reviewed elsewhere [7,37].

From reactive oxygen species formation to the development of NASH

ROS cause lipid peroxidation, which releases reactive aldehydes, such as malondialdehyde, and 4-hydroxynonenal [1]. ROS also increase the expression of several cytokines, including transforming growth factor-β (TGF-β), interleukin-8 (IL-8), TNF and Fas ligand [1]. Both lipid peroxidation products and cytokines seem to be involved in steatohepatitis liver injury [1].

Inflammation and Mallory bodies

TGF-β, IL-8 and 4-hydroxynonenal are chemoattractants for human neutrophils, which may account for the neutrophilic infiltrate in steatohepatitis [1]. TGF-β also induces tissue transglutaminase [1]. This enzyme is associated with the cytoskeleton, including intermediary filaments. Transglutaminase catalyses the formation of ε-lysine–gamma-glutamyl cross-links between a lysine on one polypeptide chain and a

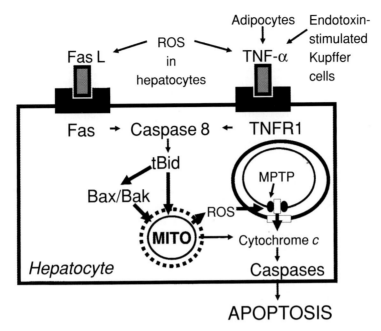

Fig. 11.5 Death receptors, mitochondria and apoptosis. In hepatocytes, ROS trigger the expression of Fas ligand (Fas L) and TNF-α. The latter is also formed by the adipocytes of obese subjects and by endotoxin-stimulated Kupffer cells. The interaction of Fas L with Fas, or TNF-α with TNF-α receptor 1 (TNFR1), activates procaspase 8 into caspase 8, which cuts BH3 interacting domain death agonist (Bid). Truncated Bid (tBid) enters the outer mitochondrial membrane to permeabilize this membrane. Bid also induces a conformational change in Bcl-2-associated x protein (Bax) and its analogue Bak, which translocate to the outer mitochondrial membrane to permeabilize this membrane. This increased permeability causes the release of cytochrome *c* from the intermembranous space, thus blocking the flow of electrons into the respiratory chain and increasing mitochondrial ROS formation. ROS could then act on the same or other mitochondria to open an inner membrane pore called the mitochondrial permeability transition pore (MPTP). Pore opening causes matrix expansion and outer membrane rupture. As a result of both increased permeability and rupture of the outer membrane, cytochrome *c*, procaspases and other pro-apoptotic factors leave the mitochondrial intermembrane space to activate caspase 9 and effector caspases in the cytosol and trigger apoptosis. (Adapted from Pessayre [3].)

glutamine on another polypeptide chain. The induction of tissue transglutaminase by TGF-β could polymerize cytokeratins to form Mallory bodies, which are formed of cross-linked cytoskeletal proteins, in particular cytokeratins [1].

Death receptors, mitochondria and apoptosis

Normally, hepatocytes express Fas (a membrane receptor), but not Fas ligand, preventing them from killing their neighbours [38]. However, several conditions leading to increased ROS formation, such as drugs, alcohol abuse or Wilson's disease, cause Fas ligand expression by hepatocytes, so that Fas ligand on one hepatocyte can now interact with Fas on another hepatocyte to cause fratricidal apoptosis (Fig. 11.5) [38]. ROS also increase the synthesis of TNF, and patients with steatohepatitis have high hepatic TNF mRNA levels [39]. TNF is also synthesized by fat-engorged adipocytes in obese people, and may be released in excess by Kupffer cells stimulated by bacterial endotoxin, because of the overexpression of endotoxin receptors on these cells (Fig. 11.5).

The interaction of Fas ligand with Fas, or the interaction of TNF with TNF receptor 1 (TNFR1), activates procaspase 8 into caspase 8, which cuts BH3 interacting domain death agonist (Bid) [38]. Truncated Bid enters the outer mitochondrial membrane to permeabilize this membrane. Bid also induces a conformational change in Bcl-2-associated x protein (Bax)

139

and its analogue Bak, which translocate to mitochondria to form channels in the outer mitochondrial membrane (Fig. 11.5).

Increased permeability of the outer mitochondrial membrane may release cytochrome c from the intermembranous space of some mitochondria, thus blocking the flow of electrons into the respiratory chain and increasing mitochondrial ROS formation. ROS could then act on the same or other mitochondria to open an inner membrane pore, whose opening causes matrix expansion and outer membrane rupture (Fig. 11.5) [40].

Because of increased permeability and rupture of the outer membrane, cytochrome c and other pro-apoptotic factors leave the mitochondrial intermembranous space to activate caspase 9 in the cytosol. Caspase 9 activates effector caspases, which trigger apoptosis (Fig. 11.5) [40]. It is therefore noteworthy that apoptosis seems to have an important role in both NASH and alcoholic steatohepatitis [41,42].

Implications for genetic susceptibility

In hepatic steatosis, the tendency of different subjects to develop steatohepatitis varies considerably [2]. For the same amount of excess weight, or the same alcohol consumption, some subjects only have steatosis while others develop cirrhosis.

Genetic polymorphisms could also be in involved (see Chapter 6). For example, in obesity-related NASH, a genetic polymorphism, which decreases MTP activity, may cause less hepatic VLDL secretion and thus more fat accumulation, more lipid peroxidation, more ROS formation and more liver lesions [20]. Also, a genetic dimorphism affects the mitochondrial targeting sequence of MnSOD. The alanine-containing sequence confers an α-helical structure to the import peptide, causing better mitochondrial import than the valine sequence, which confers a β-sheet structure to the peptide [43]. The genetic polymorphism therefore modulates the mitochondrial import of MnSOD, which may affect the mitochondrial detoxication of ROS [43]. Although this MnSOD dimorphism has been implicated in susceptibility to severe alcoholic liver disease in a French population, this finding was not confirmed in a larger English study [44]. Other studies are required to evaluate further the role of this dimorphism in both NASH and alcoholic liver disease.

Implications in clinical management

Although overweight patients should lose weight, severe dieting or total fasting increases peripheral lipolysis and the release of FFA, which uncouple and inhibit mitochondrial respiration [1]. Fasting may also cause glutathione depletion [45], which enhances lipid peroxidation and cytokine-mediated cell death [46]. It is therefore not surprising that rapid weight loss resulting from starvation, severe dieting, jejuno-ileal bypass or gastroplasty paradoxically increases liver inflammation and fibrosis in obese patients (for a detailed discussion see Chapter 20) [1].

Instead, the combination of physical exercise and a moderately hypocaloric diet (high in vegetables but low in sugar, starch and fat) can progressively decrease adipocyte fat stores, improve liver tests and stop fibrogenesis [1]. The role of hypolipidaemic peroxisome proliferator receptor-α agonists, metformin, vitamin E and betaine (to improve VLDL secretion) are discussed in Chapter 16.

Conclusions

In affluent countries, new lifestyle habits combining rich diet and lack of physical activity have resulted in an ever-increasing prevalence of obesity. Excess weight can trigger insulin resistance in adipocytes and muscle. Insulin resistance increases blood glucose and insulin levels and causes persistent adipocyte lipolysis, which can cause a fatty liver. As insulin resistance causes hepatic steatosis, and steatosis can develop into NASH, there is an almost universal association of primary NASH with insulin resistance. Insulin resistance can also be present in patients with hepatic steatosis but without NASH [15] and, conversely, steatohepatitis can occur when hepatic steatosis is triggered by mechanisms other than insulin resistance. During chronic hepatic steatosis, several vicious cycles involving lipid peroxidation, mitochondrial damage, ROS formation, depletion of antioxidants and cytokine release may cause necroinflammation and fibrogenesis in genetically susceptible patients. Further studies are required to understand better how these diverse effects interact with each other, which genetic or environmental factors are involved in individual susceptibility, and which treatments or combinations of treatments are best used in patients who fail to lose weight, despite medical advice.

References

1 Pessayre D, Berson A, Fromenty B, Mansouri A. Mitochondria in steatohepatitis. *Semin Liver Dis* 2001; **21**: 57–69.

2 Pessayre D, Mansouri A, Fromenty B. Mitochondrial dysfunction in steatohepatitis. *Am J Physiol Gastrointest Liver Physiol* 2002; **282**: G193–9.

3 Pessayre D. Mitochondrial injury in steatohepatitis. In: Suchy FJ, Gregory FJ, Maher JJ. American Association for the Study of Liver Diseases Postgraduate Course 2002. *Mechanisms of Acute and Chronic Liver Diseases: Implications for Diagnosis, Pathogenesis and Treatment*. AASLD Postgraduate Course, 2002: 97–103.

4 Tran K, Thorne-Tjomsland G, DeLong CJ *et al.* Intracellular assembly of very-low-density lipoproteins containing apolipoprotein B100 in rat hepatoma McA-RH777 cells. *J Biol Chem* 2002; **277**: 31187–200.

5 Liao W, Yeung SCJ, Chan L. Proteasome-mediated degradation of apolipoprotein B targets both nascent peptides cotranslationally before translocation and full-length apolipoprotein B after translocation into the endoplamic reticulum. *J Biol Chem* 1998; **273**: 27225–30.

6 McGarry JD, Foster DW. Regulation of hepatic fatty acid oxidation and ketone body production. *Ann Rev Biochem* 1980; **49**: 395–420.

7 Fromenty B, Pessayre D. Inhibition of mitochondrial β-oxidation as a mechanism of hepatotoxicity. *Pharmacol Ther* 1995; **67**: 101–54.

8 Kopelman PG. Obesity as a medical problem. *Nature* 2000; **404**: 635–43.

9 Shepherd PR, Kahn BB. Glucose transporters and insulin action: implications for insulin resistance and diabetes mellitus. *N Engl J Med* 1999; **341**: 248–57.

10 Hirosumi J, Tuncman G, Chang L *et al.* A central role for JNK in obesity and insulin resistance. *Nature* 2002; **420**: 353–6.

11 Chitturi S, Abeygunasekera S, Farrell GC *et al.* NASH and insulin resistance: insulin hypersecretion and specific association with the insulin resistance. *Hepatology* 2002; **35**: 373–9.

12 Valet P, Tavernier G, Castan-Laurell I *et al.* Understanding adipose tissue development from transgenic animal models. *J Lipid Res* 2002; **43**: 835–60.

13 Gorden ES. Non-esterified fatty acids in blood of obese and lean subjects. *Am J Clin Nutr* 1960; **8**: 740–7.

14 Shimomura I, Bashmakov Y, Horton JD. Increased levels of nuclear SREBP-1c associated with fatty livers in two mouse models of diabetes mellitus. *J Biol Chem* 1999; **274**: 30028–32.

15 Sanyal AJ, Campbell-Sargent C, Mirshahi F *et al.* Non-alcoholic steatohepatitis: association of insulin resistance and mitochondrial abnormalities. *Gastroenterology* 2001; **120**: 1183–92.

16 Charlton M, Sreekumar R, Rasmussen D, Lindor K, Nair S. Apolipoprotein synthesis in non-alcoholic steatohepatitis. *Hepatology* 2002; **35**: 898–904.

17 Bartels ED, Lauritsen M, Nielsen LB. Hepatic expression of microsomal triglyceride transfer protein and *in vivo* secretion of triglyceride-rich lipoproteins are increased in obese diabetic mice. *Diabetes* 2002; **51**: 1233–9.

18 Lin MCM, Gordon DC, Wettereau JR. Microsomal triglyceride transfer protein (MTP) regulation in HepG2 cells: insulin negatively regulates MTP gene expression. *J Lipid Res* 1995; **36**: 1073–81.

19 Navasa M, Gordon DA, Hariharan N *et al.* Regulation of microsomal triglyceride transfer protein mRNA expression by endotoxin and cytokines. *J Lipid Res* 1998; **39**: 1220–30.

20 Day CP, Saksena S, Leathart J *et al.* Genetic evidence supporting the two-hit model of NASH pathogenesis. *Hepatology* 2002; **36**: 82A.

21 Kono H, Rusyn I, Yin M *et al.* NADPH oxidase-derived free radicals are key oxidants in alcohol-induced liver disease. *J Clin Invest* 2000; **106**: 867–72.

22 Weltman MD, Farrell GC, Hall P, Ingelman-Sundberg M, Liddle C. Hepatic cytochrome P450 2E1 is increased in patients with non-alcoholic steatohepatitis. *Hepatology* 1998; **27**: 128–33.

23 Fiorini RN, Shafizadeh SF, Chavin KD. Primary non-function in steatotic livers is due to differential Toll-like expression and endotoxin sensitivity. *Hepatology* 2002; **36**: 198A.

24 Enomoto N, Takei Y, Hirose M *et al.* Thalidomide prevents alcoholic liver injury in rats through suppression of Kupffer cell sensitization and TNF-α production. *Gastroenterology* 2002; **123**: 291–300.

25 Lettéron P, Fromenty B, Terris B, Degott C, Pessayre D. Acute and chronic steatosis lead to *in vivo* lipid peroxidation in mice. *J Hepatol* 1996; **24**: 200–8.

26 Leclercq IA, Farrell GC, Field J *et al.* CYP2E1 and CYP4A as microsomal catalysts of lipid peroxides in murine non-alcoholic steatohepatitis. *J Clin Invest* 2001; **105**: 1067–75.

27 Hruszkewycz AM. Evidence for mitochondrial DNA damage by lipid peroxidation. *Biochem Biophys Res Commun* 1988; **153**: 191–7.

28 Chen J, Schenker S, Frosto TA, Hensderson GI. Inhibition of cytochrome *c* oxidase activity by 4-hydroxynonenal (HNE): role of HNE adduct formation with the enzyme catalytic site. *Biochem Biophys Acta* 1998; **1380**: 336–44.

29 Haque M, Mirshahi F, Campbell-Sargent C *et al.* Non-alcoholic steatohepatitis (NASH) is associated with hepatocyte mitochondrial DNA depletion. *Hepatology* 2002; **36**: 403A.

30 Perez-Carrera M, Del Hoyo P, Martin M et al. Activity of the mitochondrial respiratory chain enzymes is decreased in the liver of patients with non-alcoholic steatohepatitis. *Hepatology* 1999; **30**: 379A.

31 Cortez-Pinto H, Chatham J, Chacko VP et al. Alterations in liver ATP homeostasis in human non-alcoholic steatohepatitis: a pilot study. *J Am Med Assoc* 1999; **282**: 1659–64.

32 Yang SQ, Zhu H, Li Y et al. Mitochondrial adaptations to obesity-related oxidant stress. *Arch Biochem Biophys* 2000; **378**: 259–68.

33 Hensley K, Kotake Y, Sang H et al. Dietary choline restriction causes complex I dysfunction and increased H_2O_2 generation in liver mitochondria. *Carcinogenesis* 2000; **21**: 983–9.

34 Yin M, Gäbele E, Wheeler MD et al. Alcohol-induced free radicals in mice: direct toxicants or signaling molecules? *Hepatology* 2001; **34**: 935–42.

35 Strauss RS. Comparison of serum concentrations of α-tocopherol and β-carotene in a cross-sectional sample of obese and non-obese children (NHANES III). *J Pediatr* 1999; **134**: 160–5.

36 Lavine JE. Vitamin E treatment of non-alcoholic steatohepatitis in children: a pilot study. *J Pediatr* 2000; **136**: 739–43.

37 Berson A, De Beco V, Leteron P et al. Steatohepatitis-inducing drugs cause mitochondrial dysfunction and lipid peroxidation in rat hepatocytes. *Gastroenterology* 1998; **114**: 764–74.

38 Pessayre D, Feldmann G, Haouzi D et al. Hepatocyte apoptosis triggered by natural substances (cytokines, other endogenous substances and foreign toxins). In: Cameron RG, Feuer G, eds. *Apoptosis and its Modulation by Drugs: Handbook of Experimental Pharmacology.* Heidelberg: Springer Verlag, 2000, **142**: 59–108.

39 Crespo J, Cayon A, Fernadez-Gil P et al. Gene expression of tumor necrosis factor-α and TNF-receptors p55 and p75 in non-alcoholic steatohepatitis patients. *Hepatology* 2001; **34**: 1158–63.

40 Feldmann G, Haouzi D, Moreau A et al. Opening of the mitochondrial permeability transition pore causes matrix expansion and outer membrane rupture in Fas-mediated hepatic apoptosis in mice. *Hepatology* 2000; **31**: 674–83.

41 Natori S, Rust C, Stadheim LM et al. Hepatocyte apoptosis is a pathologic feature of human alcoholic hepatitis. *J Hepatol* 2001; **34**: 248–53.

42 Rodriguez CM, Cortez-Pinto H, Sola S et al. Apoptosis is a prominent feature of human alcoholic and non-alcoholic steatohepatitis. *Hepatology* 2001; **34**: 672A.

43 Sutton A, Khoury H, Prip-Buus C et al. The Ala-9Val dimorphism modulates the import of human manganese superoxide dismutase into rat liver mitochondria. *Pharmacogenetics* 2003; **13**: 145–57.

44 Stewart SF, Leathart JB, Chen Y et al. Valine-alanine manganese superoxide dismutase polymorphism is not associated with alcohol-induced oxidative stress or liver fibrosis. *Hepatology* 2002; **36**: 1355–60.

45 Pessayre D, Dolder A, Artigou JY et al. Effect of fasting on metabolite-mediated hepatotoxicity in the rat. *Gastroenterology* 1979; **77**: 264–71.

46 Haouzi D, Lekehal M, Tinel M et al. Prolonged, but not acute, glutathione depletion promotes Fas-mediated mitochondrial permeability transition and apoptosis in mice. *Hepatology* 2001; **33**: 1181–8.

12 Cell biology of NASH: fibrosis and cell proliferation

Isabelle A. Leclercq & Yves Horsmans

Key learning points

1 In the liver, injury triggers a physiological wound healing response that contains the injurious agent, isolates damaged cells and effects wound closure, leading to restoration of normal hepatic structure and function. The process requires coordination of the inflammatory reaction, cell proliferation, differentiation and death (apoptosis), fibrogenesis and matrix remodelling.

2 Activation of the fibrotic cascade is part of the response to liver injury. The organized sequence of responses include activation of hepatic stellate cells (HSC) and other cell types (Kupffer cells and endothelial cells), migration and proliferation of HSC, synthesis and deposition of extracellular matrix, remodelling and degradation of scar tissue, and deactivation or apoptosis (cell deletion) of the effector cells.

3 Pathological examination of liver tissue from non-alcoholic steatohepatitis (NASH) patients reveals increased numbers of α-smooth muscle actin-reactive HSC, mainly located in the perivenular area, confirming the presence of activated HSC in this setting.

4 Fibrosis associated with NASH can be understood as the physiological consequence of chronic hepatic injury, necrosis and inflammation (steatohepatitis). However, profibrotic mechanisms specifically related to the context of NASH are emerging: steatosis and insulin resistance, oxidative stress generated by CYP2E1 and 4A or from other sources, dysregulation of leptin expression and signalling, peroxisome proliferator-activated receptor-α and -γ expression and signalling, inflammation and release of cytokine and fibrogenic mediators.

5 Clinical observations suggest an impairment of hepatocyte proliferation in non-alcoholic fatty liver disease (NAFLD)/NASH. However, it remains to be confirmed that such altered adaptive response to liver injury participate in the pathogenesis of the disease.

6 From animal studies, it has been shown that liver regeneration and hepatocyte proliferation are normal in several models of fatty liver as well as in fibrosing steatohepatitis. In contrast, liver regeneration is markedly impaired in fatty liver because of disrupted leptin signalling. To date, the parts played by altered lipid metabolism, insulin resistance and/or leptin deficiency in the control of liver regeneration remain to be established.

Abstract

Fibrosis is the most significant pathological consequence associated with non-alcoholic steatohepatitis (NASH). Activation of hepatic stellate cells (HSC) into extracellular matrix (ECM) producing myofibroblasts, the central event in hepatic fibrosis, is recognized in NASH. Hepatic fibrogenesis could represent the healing and tissue repair response to chronic necroinflammatory injury associated with NASH. However, there is no strict link between the intensity of the necroin-flammation and the intensity of fibrosis.

Recently, profibrotic mechanisms specifically related to the context of NASH have been identified and might explain the propensity for fibrosis progression in this metabolic disorder. These include oxidative stress and lipid peroxidation, imbalanced intrahepatic lipid metabolism, and insulin resistance. Hormones and transcription factors involved in the control of glucose and/or lipid metabolism have been implicated in fibrogenesis. They operate directly by stimulating HSC activation and collagen synthesis, or indirectly by modulating the inflammatory response and the release of profibrotic cytokines and mediators. Fundamental insights into leptin biology and its dysregulation associated with the insulin resistance (metabolic) syndrome (IRS), peroxisome proliferator-activated receptor (PPAR) transcription factors and their dual effects on the control of insulin sensitivity and biology of HSCs, and cytokine signalling are all likely to benefit our understanding of NASH-associated fibrosis.

NASH is characterized by chronic hepatocellular injury. Clinical observations suggest an impairment of hepatocyte proliferation in non-alcoholic fatty liver disease (NAFLD)/NASH. Animal studies provide evidence that intrahepatic lipid overload *per se* does not appear to compromise the proliferative response of the liver. However, liver regeneration is impaired in animals with disrupted leptin signalling, resistance to insulin and immune perturbations, a phenotype that closely resembles that of patients with NASH. Conceptually, these factors, alone or together, could potentially dampen the adaptive response of the liver to injury and could contribute to NASH pathogenesis, but this remains to be confirmed.

Introduction

The wound healing process is integral to any organ's response to injury. In the liver, injury triggers a physiological wound healing response that operates containment of the injurious agent, isolation of damaged cells and wound closure, leading to restoration of normal hepatic structure and function. The entire process requires precise coordination of several important cellular actions: the inflammatory reaction, cell proliferation and differentiation, fibrogenesis and matrix remodelling, as well as apoptosis. In response to an acute injury, the effectiveness of the wound healing process is mostly dependent on the ability of the liver to isolate the damage and reconstitute functional liver mass by hepatocyte proliferation, the process known as liver regeneration. When the injury is chronic or repeated, as in NASH, there are multiple cycles of tissue repair and deposition of ECM or scarring (fibrosis). Chronic activation of the scarring response leads to hepatic fibrosis, which can be considered as the highly integrated response to any type of chronic liver injury, irrespective of aetiology. Hepatic complications develop when fibrosis has progressed to cirrhosis. They result from portal hypertension and loss of hepatic cell mass, which leads to hepatocellular failure, or from imbalance between hepatocellular proliferation and apoptosis, which can result in tumour formation. This review discusses these tissue and cell biological responses to chronic liver injury, and considers mechanisms and outcomes relevant to NAFLD/NASH.

Hepatic fibrosis

Fibrosis is the most significant pathological consequence of liver disease associated with hepatic steatosis. It is therefore important to identify profibrotic stimuli associated with fatty liver disease.

The mechanism of the fibrotic process in chronic metabolic steatohepatitis is likely to be similar in nature to that in response to other forms of chronic liver injury. Considerable insight into these mechanisms has been gained in the past decade, as reviewed elsewhere [1,2]. Fibrosis associated with NASH can be understood as the physiological consequence of chronic hepatic injury, necrosis and inflammation (steatohepatitis). However, profibrotic mechanisms specifically related to the context of NASH have emerged recently. The activation of these pathways might determine or at least partly explain the propensity for fibrosis progression between individuals with NASH. This section briefly recalls the general features of the fibrogenic process, and discusses special aspects pertaining to fibrogenesis in NASH.

Role of hepatic stellate cells

The hepatic scar consists of a broad accumulation of ECM. In turn, this comprises macromolecules from three main families: collagens, glycoproteins and proteoglycans. As the liver becomes fibrotic, production and accumulation of collagen and non-collagen compounds increases and there are qualitative changes in the composition of the ECM [1–3]. More interstitial type matrix molecules are produced: fibril-forming collagens (types I and III) become prominent, proteoglycans and structural glycoproteins such as laminin and fibronectin are deposited and accumulate in the subendothelial space (space of Disse).

An additional factor is that excessive matrix deposition is no longer compensated by enhanced degradation because of an imbalance between expression of matrix metalloproteinases (MMP) and their inhibitors (tissue inhibitors of metalloproteinases, TIMP) [1,3,4]. The accumulation of matrix and the formation of fibrous septa disrupts the normal architecture of the vascular and cellular compartments in the liver, impairing the ready exchange of oxygen and nutrients and progressively leading to cirrhosis.

As part of the acute response to liver injury, the fibrotic cascade is activated. The short duration of the stimulus allows recognition of an organized sequence of responses. These include the activation of HSC and other cell types (Kupffer cells and endothelial cells), migration and proliferation of HSC, synthesis and deposition of ECM, remodelling and degradation of the scar tissue and deactivation or apoptosis (cell deletion) of the effector cells. It is yet to be determined whether these events represent a continuum or are independent but interconnected phenomena triggered by specific or multiple factors. During chronic liver injury, injurious and healing processes evolve simultaneously; thus, organization of the fibrotic cascade is disrupted, leading to scar formation and distortion of liver architecture [1,2].

ECM deposition in perivascular and pericellular areas is the hallmark of hepatic fibrosis. Hepatic matrix producing cells are diverse populations that exist in both the normal and injured liver [5–7]. They differ by their content in vitamin A, the expression of intermediate filaments and other characteristics of myogenic or neural crest cells, and their location (perisinusoidal HSC or perivascular and periportal fibroblasts). The embryological origin of these cells and the way they participate in the fibrogenic process is still debated [4–7].

HSC and myofibroblasts have been identified as the principal cell types in the liver responsible for ECM production during fibrogenesis [4,5,8]. In normal liver, HSC are found in the space of Disse and beneath the endothelial cells. They emit multiple star-like projections and establish direct contacts via gap junctions with other stellate cells, hepatocytes and probably endothelial cells [5,8]. Regardless of the nature of the insult, liver injury provides stimuli that transform HSC from a quiescent retinoid-storing phenotype into a proliferative migrating ECM-producing and contractile myofibroblast-like phenotype [1,2,5,8]. This process, characterized by morphological and functional changes of the HSC, is known as 'activation'; it is a programmed response occurring in a reproducible sequence at the onset of injury. Stellate cell activation is initiated by paracrine stimuli from injured and neighbouring parenchymal and non-parenchymal cells, recruited inflammatory cells as well as subtle changes in ECM composition. Activation is then perpetuated through enhanced cytokine expression and responsiveness to cytokines mediated by autocrine and paracrine stimuli and by accelerated ECM remodelling [1,4,5,9,10]. It follows that, if the injurious factor is not removed, the fibrotic process is perpetuated. Alternatively, if the injurious process is interrupted or if the injury is self-limited, loss of activated stellate cells through phenotypical reversion or apoptosis may occur with resultant resolution of fibrosis [10,11].

Amongst the best-studied paracrine stimuli for HSC activation are fibronectin, lipid peroxides and cytokines. The latter include platelet-derived growth factor (PDGF), transforming growth factor-β1 (TGF-β1), endothelin-1 (ET-1) and epidermal growth factor (EGF) [1,4,5,10,12,13]. Transcription factors involved in HSC activation include c-myb, nuclear factor-κB (NF-κB), activator protein-1 (AP-1), signal transducer and activator of transcription-1 (STAT-1) and members of the Krüppel-like transcription factors family, such as KLF6 or SP-1 [9,13]. Once activated, stellate cells undergo phenotypical changes that concur with the accumulation of ECM, as summarized in Fig. 12.1.

1 HSC proliferate under the action of paracrine and autocrine mediators, such as PDGF, ET-1, and TGF-β1.

2 They gain contractile capability; this can increase resistance to portal blood flow resulting in portal hypertension. The key contractile mediator is ET-1, but vasopressin and/or eicosanoids also participate in this action.

3 HSC are stimulated to produce large amounts of fibril-forming collagen. The most potent stimulus for

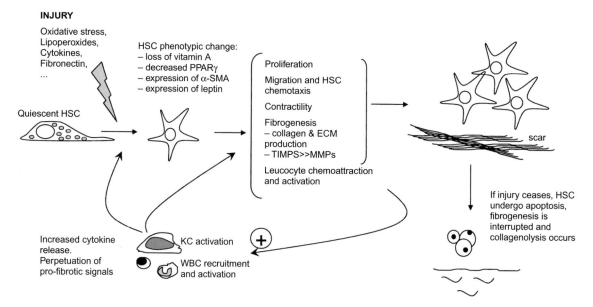

INJURY

Fig. 12.1 Schematic representation of hepatic fibrogenesis and hepatic stellate cells (HSC) activation during liver injury and resolution. In response to injury to the liver, HSC undergo activation, characterized by phenotypical changes from quiescent, vitamin A storing cells to proliferative, migrating, contractile and extracellular matrix (ECM) producing cells. α-SMA, α-smooth muscle actin; KC, Kupffer cells; MMP, metalloproteinase; PPARγ, peroxisome proliferator-activated receptor γ; TIMP, tissue inhibitors of metalloproteinases; WBC, white blood cells (mainly lymphocytes, polymorphonuclear neutrophils and recruited macrophages).

fibrogenesis is TGF-β1, but other factors such as interleukin 1β (IL-1β), tumour necrosis factor (TNF) and lipid peroxides can induce synthesis of ECM.

4 PDGF and monocyte chemoattractant peptide-1 (MCP-1) direct migration of HSC. This process, together with HSC proliferation, participates in recruitment of active matrix-depositing cells at the site of injury.

5 The production of MMP and their inhibitors (TIMP) modifies the fibrolytic activity and the remodelling of the matrix.

6 Cytokines acting at the site of injury are critical for the perpetuation of HSC activation.

Fibrosis in NASH

Ten to 20% of patients with NAFLD will progress to NASH (see Chapters 1 and 3). Patients with steatosis and minimal or no inflammation appear to exhibit a benign course. In contrast, in patients with NASH, fibrotic evolution of the disease seems to be the rule and can lead to cirrhosis (see Chapter 2). Once this process is initiated, spontaneous histological improvement is uncommon (but see Chapter 24), although reversion of fibrosis has been described in other types of liver disease following treatment that removes the cause of injury [11]. Interestingly, the recurrence of NASH following liver transplantation for cryptogenetic cirrhosis implicates the operation of an underlying extrahepatic or metabolic abnormality that may account for the disease in both native and transplanted livers (see Chapter 17).

Fibrosis in a characteristic chicken-wire pericellular distribution has long been recognized as a hallmark of NASH and a criterion for severity of the disease (see Chapter 2). Pathological examination of liver tissue from NASH patients, compared to normal controls, reveals increased numbers of α-smooth muscle actin (α-SMA)-reactive HSC, mainly located in the perivenular area, confirming the presence of activated HSC in this setting [14,15]. To date, there are no true indicators for fibrosis progression in NAFLD. However, increasing obesity and type 2 diabetes correlate with severity of fibrosis and risk of cirrhosis (see Chapter 3). Other risk factors for fibrosis in NASH include necroinflammatory activity, increased alanine aminotransferase (ALT) above twice the normal value or inversion of the aspartate aminotransferase : alanine aminotransferase (AST : ALT) ratio, age [16] and systemic hypertension [17], possibly reflecting the IRS (see Chapter 5).

The grading and staging systems used for evaluation of NASH on liver biopsy allow the assessment of fibrosis, but have no value for predicting the risk for fibrosis development or fibrosis progression (see Chapter 2). One study performed on 15 NASH biopsies and five controls showed a significant association between the labelling index for activated HSC and portal and lobular inflammation, but not with severity of fibrosis [14]. This suggests that a worse prognosis in NASH is determined by the presence of inflammation. By contrast, another study of a larger number of patients found that the degree of HSC activation correlated with severity of fibrosis but not with inflammatory activity, severity of steatosis or stainable iron [15]. Further, in one-third of these patients (25 out of 76) the degree of HSC activation was greater than expected on the basis on fibrosis intensity, raising the question as to whether these patients are at higher risk of disease progression.

In a study of 551 morbidly obese patients undergoing antiobesity surgery, steatosis was found in 86%, fibrosis in 74%, with cirrhosis in 2%; mild inflammation was present in only 24% of cases. There was a strong correlation between fibrosis and extent of steatosis. Further, the risk of fibrosis increased sevenfold among patients with insulin resistance or type 2 diabetes [18]. It is therefore possible that the IRS, via impaired glucose tolerance or insulin resistance, could be linked directly to fibrosis, and necroinflammation might not always be essential for HSC activation and fibrosis progression.

This hypothesis is supported by immunohistochemical studies. Washington et al. [15] demonstrated that HSC activation and fibrosis occur not only in NASH but also in fatty liver in the absence of significant necroinflammation. Likewise, in alcoholic liver disease, Reeves et al. [19] have shown a correlation between severity of steatosis and degree of fibrosis in the absence of hepatic inflammation.

Pathogenesis of fibrosis associated with NAFLD/NASH

No clear picture has yet emerged from studies investigating the source and nature of fibrotic stimuli in NAFLD/NASH. It is unclear whether fibrogenesis is sustained by steatosis, metabolic factors (especially insulin resistance and altered lipid metabolism), hepatocyte injury, the inflammatory response or a combination of several of these factors. It is essential to address these issues in order to identify potential therapeutic targets for the prevention and the treatment of NAFLD-related fibrosis. Several pathways could contribute to fibrogenesis in NAFLD/NASH:

1 Steatosis and insulin resistance
2 Oxidative stress generated by CYP2E1 and 4A, or other sources (see Chapters 7, 8 and 10)
3 Dysregulation of leptin expression and signalling
4 PPARα and γ expression and signalling
5 Inflammation and release of cytokine and other fibrogenic mediators (summarized in Table 12.1).

These factors are inter-related but, for clarity, are described separately.

Steatosis and insulin resistance

Obesity, and in particular truncal (central) obesity, is associated with hepatic steatosis and insulin resistance. It is increasingly recognized as an important risk factor for fibrosis progression in many chronic liver diseases [20–22]. A growing body of evidence suggests that steatosis and insulin resistance have a causal role in the progression from steatosis to NASH. In NASH, as well as in alcohol-induced liver disease, activation of HSC and early fibrosis can been evidenced in the absence of demonstrable inflammation or hepatocyte necrosis [15,18,19]. Together with the recognition of obesity as a risk factor for fibrosis, this observation suggests that the presence of fat might be directly fibrogenic. In hepatitis C, the amelioration of fibrosis and resolution of hepatic steatosis achieved by weight reduction [23] is further support for a causal link between steatosis and fibrosis.

Using animal models, the importance of dietary fat on liver disease induced by alcohol intake has been well documented [24, and references therein]. Together with intragastric administration of alcohol, a high dietary fat content (25% of energy intake) is necessary for hepatic fibrosis to develop. There is also a correlation between the dietary content of unsaturated fatty acids and the severity of fibrosis. Thus, rats fed unsaturated fat (corn oil) develop severe liver disease and hepatic fibrosis, while those fed pork or bovine fat develop substantially less or no injury, respectively. This has been shown to be directly related to the

Table 12.1 Possible pathways for NASH-related fibrogenesis.

Steatosis	↑ Polyunsaturated FA ↑ FA beyond metabolic oxidative capabilities Mitochondrial dysfunction	Prone to lipid peroxidation ↑ Non-oxidative metabolism ↑ Production of lipoperoxides, ceramides and lipid mediators of inflammation Generate ROS
Insulin resistance	↑ Hepatic availability of free FA High insulin and high glucose	↑ Substrate for lipid peroxidation and ROS Stimulate HSC proliferation and collagen production Stimulate CTGF expression
Oxidant stress	Generated by altered lipid metabolism, microsomal enzymes (CYP2E1, CYP4A), mitochondrial dysfunction, inflammatory reaction	Direct fibrogenic stimulation of HSC Stimulate inflammatory reaction
Leptin	Altered leptin signalling ↑ Circulating and intrahepatic leptin and altered leptin signalling	Associated with insulin resistance, altered intrahepatic lipid metabolism and steatosis Increase TGF-β1 activity Modulate paracrine/autocrine regulation of the cytokine microenvironment conducive to fibrotic response
PPARγ	PPARγ signalling Dysregulation of PPARγ pathway	Modulate the response to insulin Could lead to loss of the maintenance of the quiescent phenotype of HSC
Inflammatory reaction	Paracrine and autocrine release of inflammatory and fibrogenic mediators such as TGF-β1, leptin, CTGF, chemokines and TNF	Stimulate profibrotic response Perpetuation of pro-inflammatory and profibrotic signals

FA, fatty acids; CTGF, connective tissue growth factor; HSC, hepatic stellate cells; PPARγ, peroxisome proliferator-activated receptor-γ; ROS, reactive oxygen species; TGF-β, transforming growth factor β; TNF, tumour necrosis factor.

amount of linoleic acid in the diet (18 : 2, n-6). Rats fed ethanol with fish oil develop even more severe fibrosis than those fed ethanol with corn oil. Fish oil contains the highest percentage of polyunsaturated fatty acids (more than two double bounds) and hence is highly susceptible to lipid peroxidation. It therefore appears that an increased amount of peroxidable fatty acids is associated with greater severity of liver injury and fibrosis in alcohol-induced liver injury.

Steatosis has been conceptualized as the background upon which steatohepatitis develops [25]. *In vivo* animal experiments have demonstrated that stimulation of fatty acid β-oxidation by PPARα agonists increases fat combustion and thereby reduces intrahepatic storage of fat. In an experimental model of steatohepatitis, induced by a lipogenic diet deficient in methionine and choline (MCD), administration of a

PPARα agonist prevented steatosis and also oxidative stress, necroinflammation and fibrosis [26]. Further, this treatment reversed steatohepatitis and fibrosis in well-established steatohepatitis [27]. It is therefore likely that accumulation of triglyceride and free fatty acids (FFA) in the liver beyond the oxidative and transport capabilities of the liver (see Chapter 9) provides substrate for reserve pathways of lipid metabolism. In turn, these can result in the formation of profibrotic lipoperoxides, ceramides and other lipid mediators of inflammation. These observations reveal a relationship between the quantity and the quality of fatty acids accumulating in the liver and fibrogenesis. The balance between the amount and nature of intrahepatic lipids, and the capacity for their oxidative and non-oxidative intrahepatic metabolism, appears to be a determinant for NASH progression and fibrogenesis.

Insulin resistance is a risk factor for fibrosis and fibrosis progression in NASH (see Chapters 3, 5, 14 and 24). The consequences of insulin resistance on intrahepatic lipid metabolism are numerous (see Chapter 9). In particular, availability of FFA for intrahepatic metabolism is increased in the insulin resistance state. This potentially leads to increased production of reactive oxygen species (ROS) and non-oxidative metabolites that have consequences for fibrogenesis (see below). Insulin may also have direct effects on HSC biology. Both insulin and insulin-like growth factors stimulate HSC mitogenesis and collagen synthesis [28]. Increased glucose levels slightly induced collagen expression in cultured HSC [29]. Moreover, in cultured HSC, high glucose concentrations and insulin stimulate the expression of connective tissue growth factor (CTGF), a profibrogenic molecule [29].

CTGF expression has also been detected in liver biopsies from patients with NASH, but not in normal liver. The induction of profibrogenic CTGF provides one possible direct link between metabolic features associated with NASH and fibrosis. However, the observation that CTGF is also upregulated in hyperinsulinaemic and hyperglycaemic Zucker rats [29], in which fatty liver has no propensity for fibrosis, indicates that an increase of CTGF is not sufficient to induce fibrosis. Rather, it might act as a surrogate factor to enhance the fibrotic process in the context of type 2 diabetes.

Oxidative stress

Oxidative stress is associated with important pathobiological processes in a variety of liver diseases, and in particular with hepatic fibrosis. It has been proposed that free radicals and lipid peroxidation products may modulate injury and fibrosis by their ability to damage cellular components, such as membranes, proteins and DNA, to recruit inflammatory cells, and/or to directly modulate collagen gene expression in HSC [30, and references therein].

It is now established that oxidative stress is present in several animal models of NAFLD and steatohepatitis (see Chapter 8), including rodents fed a MCD diet [31], and acyl-CoA deficient mice [32]. Oxidative stress is also prominent in the liver of humans with NASH [33–35]. Adducts between proteins and 4-hydroxynonenal (HNE), an end-product of lipid peroxidation, could be are detected by immunohistochemistry in 80% of cases of uncomplicated NAFLD and 100% of NASH biopsises. Also, 8-hydroxydeoxyguanosine, a DNA base modified by oxygen-derived free radicals, was detected in 20–30% of NASH biopsies, but not in NAFLD [33]. These indices appear to correlate with the grade of necroinflammation and the stage of fibrosis. Hence, oxidative stress has been proposed as an important pathogenic factor for disease progression and fibrosis in NASH [25,31,36]. The possible sources for oxidative stress in NAFLD and NASH are discussed in Chapters 8–11.

In the rodent MCD diet model of steatohepatitis, intrahepatic oxidative stress and lipid peroxidation occur as early events, preceding necroinflammatory changes, HSC activation and collagen deposition [31,37]. The causal link between oxidative stress and fibrosis is further supported by the observation that vitamin E, a potent antioxidant, decreases oxidative stress and also ameliorates the severity of fibrosis in experimental steatohepatitis [38]. A reduction of fibrosis scores has also been obtained in humans with NASH with such antioxidant therapies as α-tocopherol, combination of vitamins E and C, or betaine (see Chapter 16) [39].

Although it has been questioned whether HSC are directly subjected to oxidative stress in experimental fibrosis, exposure of cultured human or rat HSC to pro-oxidant systems or to medium containing products released from hepatocytes undergoing oxidative stress is followed by increased gene expression and synthesis of collagen type I [30]. Antioxidants and nitric oxide (NO) donors prevented this effect. Collagen gene expression in HSC is also strongly elicited by very low levels of end-products of lipid peroxidation (HNE, malondialdehydes and related hydroxyalkenals) in the culture medium, as well as by H_2O_2 [30].

Microsomal metabolism has been proposed as a possible source for oxidative stress and lipoperoxidation in NASH [31]. In particular, CYP2E1 and 4A exhibit high NADPH oxidase activities and extensively release O_2, H_2O_2 and hydroxyethyl radicals. These enzymes also possess an endogenous lipoperoxidase activity. A role for either intracellular and extracellular reactive intermediates (such as ROS) as profibrogenic mediators has been confirmed in HSC transfected with human CYP2E1 cDNA, as well as in co-culture experiments of HSC and CYP2E1-transfected hepatocytes [40,41]. In these *in vitro* systems, collagen type I expression was found to be proportional to CYP2E1 levels. Morevover, CYP2E1-transfected HSC overexpressed collagen type I after exposure to ethanol or arachidonic acid, an effect prevented by antioxidants or by specific inhibition of CYP2E1 activity [42].

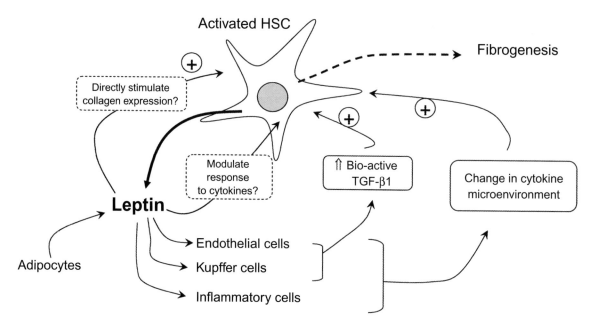

Fig. 12.2 Profibrogenic effect of leptin: possible mechanisms of action. Leptin, derived from adipocytes or produced locally during fibrogenesis by activated HSC, participates in the paracrine–autocrine regulation of the cytokine microenvironment of the liver. Leptin increases the release and the bioactivation of the most potent fibrogenic cytokine, TGF-β1. Leptin is involved in the maturation and activation of immune cells, and thereby modulates cytokine balance. Also, leptin regulates the expression of several cytokine receptors and responsiveness to cytokines. In addition, a direct effect of leptin on collagen I expression has been proposed.

There are few data available on the molecular mechanisms involved in oxidative stress-mediated activation of HSC and upregulation of collagen. Nieto *et al.* [42] have shown that CYP2E1-generated oxidative stress acts at the post-transcriptional level to increase the efficiency of translation of type I collagen mRNA. HNE and ROS can also activate transcription factors involved in the control of HSC activation, such as NF-κB and AP-1 [8,13,30]. In addition, H_2O_2 may act as an intracellular mediator of the profibrotic action of TGF-β1 [30]. Some experimental results also suggest that oxidative stress may modulate collagen synthesis through activation of the Na^+/H^+ exchanger and the resultant increase in intracellular pH [30].

Dysregulation of leptin expression and signalling
Leptin, an adipocyte-derived cytokine, has a wide range of biological actions. Recently, the essential role of leptin in fibrogenesis has been elucidated [43–45]. Leptin-deficient *ob/ob* obese mice are protected from experimental hepatic fibrosis caused by repeated administration of carbon tetrachloride (CCl_4) or thio-acetamide [43,44]. More pertinent to this discussion, leptin-deficient mice also fail to develop fibrosis during the evolution of MCD diet-induced steatohepatitis, despite equivalent levels of oxidative stress and inflammatory infiltration as in leptin-competent controls [43]. Importantly, these experiments clearly demonstrate that fibrogenic capability could be restored by administration of recombinant leptin in physiological amounts [43]. This confirms that leptin is directly involved in the control and modulation of the profibrogenic process in steatohepatitis. Conversely, a pharmacological increase in leptin levels enhanced fibrosis severity during the wound healing response to toxic liver injury [46].

Several mechanisms could underlie the role of leptin in steatosis-related hepatic fibrosis (Fig. 12.2). First, in leptin-deficient animals, the absence of fibrotic response to CCl_4 administration is associated with a defect in the production of TGF-β1 [43], the most potent profibrotic cytokine [12]. Ikejima *et al.* [44] have further shown that leptin upregulates TGF-β1 production by endothelial cells and Kupffer cells.

Secondly, HSC express and produce leptin during their *in vitro* transformation to the activated phenotype [47]. Leptin expression has also been demonstrated in HSC isolated from liver of rats with MCD diet-induced steatohepatitis (Leclercq *et al.*, unpublished data), and in rat fibrotic liver [44]. Thus, leptin produced locally at the site of injury is likely to participate in the paracrine–autocrine regulation of the fibrotic response. In addition, it has been proposed that leptin might act directly on HSC to increase collagen gene expression via activation of STAT-3 by ligand-binding activation to the long form of the leptin receptor [45]. However, others have not reproduced these results [44; Leclercq *et al.*, unpublished data]. Finally, in experimental animals, expression of CYP2E1 appears to be dependent on leptin [48], so the profibrogenic activity of leptin could also be partly mediated through its ability to induce oxidant stress via CYP2E1 activity.

Hyperleptinaemia is usually encountered in the IRS and is observed in NASH patients (see Chapter 5). The increased risk of fibrosis and fibrosis progression observed in these patients could therefore be attributable to leptin. However, hyperleptinaemia is thought to be the consequence of a resistance to leptin action. Central resistance to leptin has been demonstrated but little is known about leptin signalling in peripheral tissues in this setting [49]. To reconcile this apparent paradox, there is still much to be learnt from studies of leptin receptor expression, function and leptin signalling in peripheral tissues. In particular, the threshold of stimulation for central leptin receptors might be different from that of peripheral receptors; the level of leptin-receptor expression in specific cell types could then allow signalling events despite central leptin resistance. Alternatively, local production of leptin could be sufficient to increase local concentrations, thereby effecting receptor signalling at the specific site of fibrogenesis by autocrine and paracrine pathways of humoral regulation.

On the contrary, because leptin acts to prevent excessive fat accumulation and its consequences in non-adipose tissues [50,51], it is possible that intrahepatic resistance to leptin protects the liver against the deleterious effects of steatosis and steatohepatitis.

With normal leptin signalling, the prevalence of fibrosis and the rate of fibrosis progression in NAFLD and NASH could be significantly increased. Detailed studies of hepatic leptin-receptor expression and function in humans with obesity and hyperleptinaemia are therefore mandatory to address the leptin paradox, and to exploit it therapeutically.

PPARα and γ expression and signalling

PPARs are a family of ligand-activated transcription factors that regulate cell differentiation and proliferation, control the metabolism of glucose and lipids and modulate the response to insulin. They are of particular interest here because NASH is clearly part of the IRS (see Chapter 5). PPARα in rodents is known to stimulate fatty acid β-oxidation (see Chapter 11), thereby preventing accumulation of lipid substrates for non-oxidative metabolism as well as steatosis, inflammation and fibrosis [26].

PPARγ is expressed at high levels in adipose tissue where it controls adipocyte differentiation and metabolism. By stimulating PPARγ, thiazolidinedione drugs induce triglyceride storage in adipocytes. As a consequence, there is a decrease in FFA available for hepatic uptake, and the response to insulin is improved (see Chapter 4). Quiescent HSC express PPARγ, and this transcription factor is thought to participate in the maintenance of the quiescent phenotype [52]. Thus, PPARγ stimulation by specific agonists prevents activation of HSC *in vitro* and prevents fibrosis in several experimental models [52].

Thiazolidinedione drugs (PPARγ ligands—rosiglitazone and pioglitazone), which are currently used as insulin-sensitizers in the treatment of type 2 diabetes, could have additional effects in preventing fibrosis in NASH [39,53]. However, transformation of the HSC phenotype is associated with decreased or loss of PPARγ expression [54]. Therefore, HSC already activated and involved in fibrogenesis become insensitive to PPARγ agonists. Current animal studies and clinical trials will determine whether these drugs, by inhibiting *de novo* recruitment of HSC for fibrogenesis, are effective in the treatment of fibrosing NASH or whether they are only effective in preventing fibrosis (see Chapters 16 and 24).

Inflammation and release of cytokines and other fibrogenic mediators

Infiltration of inflammatory cells into the hepatic parenchyma is a key feature of fibrosing steatohepatitis, although to date it has not been resolved whether inflammation is the cause or a consequence of hepatocellular injury. Any chronic inflammatory process in the liver is associated with fibrosis, largely attributable to profibrogenic cytokines released by infiltrating lymphocytes and neutrophils, as well as by activated Kupffer cells. Injured hepatocytes also release profibrogenic cytokines [1,2,8,9]. Enhanced hepatocyte synthesis of TGF-β1 has been documented in the MCD model of fibrosing steatohepatitis in rats [37].

A vast array of cytokines and chemokines has been implicated in the various steps of fibrogenesis, and no inflammatory mediators are thought to be unique to NAFLD/NASH. Thus, any cytokine that contributes to the perpetuation of inflammation in NASH could also ensure an ongoing profibrotic stimulus via paracrine activation of HSC. Particular attention has been paid to TNF-α because of its links with the IRS and steatosis, and also because of its role in mediating hepatocyte injury initiated by endotoxin and other bacterial products (see Chapters 4, 5 and 10). However, there is no evidence that TNF itself initiates chronic inflammation in the fatty liver (steatohepatitis) (see Chapter 8), or that TNF has a direct profibrogenic effect.

Matrix remodelling and reversion of NASH-associated fibrosis

The chapter has so far concentrated on profibrogenic mechanisms in NASH. However, it is well known that fibrosis progression in the liver results from an imbalance between matrix production and matrix degradation [1–3,10].

The ECM has an important regulatory role in fibrogenesis [3]. First, it constitutes a large reservoir for cytokines and other mediators of fibrosis and inflammation that are variably released and activated upon degradation and remodelling of the matrix. Secondly, ECM is in close contact and has specific interactions with all cell types involved in the fibrotic process. ECM remodelling and matrix turnover have not yet been studied in human NASH, and animal studies to date provide scarce and fragmented data. In MCD diet-induced steatohepatitis, TIMP 1 and 2 are upregulated [37]. This increased expression occurs several weeks after the initiation of the fibrotic process and at a stage where significant fibrosis is already present [37]. Studies are needed to determine the level of activation of fibrogenic and fibrolytic processes in NASH-associated fibrosis and whether stimulation of fibrolytic processes would have a beneficial effect in this setting.

Similarly, nothing is known of the fate of activated HSC in NASH. Clinical studies suggest that progression of steatosis-associated fibrosis can be interrupted and even reversed (see Chapter 24). However, it is unknown whether all forms of fibrosis are reversible, or whether the clinical setting and severity of the process can determine a 'point of no return' for fibrosis. This is a key issue as antifibrotic therapies are most effective when administered to patients with reversible fibrosis. Alternatively, patients identified as having irreversible hepatic fibrosis might be more suitably directed towards aggressive therapy, such as liver transplantation. Another point that has not been developed here is the existence and identification of systemic or genetic factors responsible for NASH (see Chapter 6), as inferred by the possibility of rapidly fibrosing NASH recurring after liver transplantation (see Chapter 17).

Consequences of steatosis (NAFLD/NASH) on liver regeneration

Hepatocyte proliferation is an adaptive response to liver injury in an attempt to preserve functional mass, and is an important factor in pathogenesis and prognosis in all chronic liver diseases. NASH is associated with hepatocellular injury, commonly in the form of ballooning degeneration and lytic necrosis, but also as acidophilic apoptotic bodies signing apoptosis. Impaired liver regeneration with failure to replace damaged hepatocytes could exacerbate the noxious consequences of liver injury. Understanding the mechanisms controlling hepatocyte proliferation and liver regeneration has been the subject of intense research over several decades, as reviewed elsewhere [55,56]. The aim here is to review the impact of NAFLD and NASH on the regenerative response of the liver.

Human data

Steatosis has been associated with increased morbidity and mortality after liver resection. Thus, the mortality after hepatic resection in patients with moderate to severe steatosis exceeded 10% in one series, whereas this figure was below 2% for those whose livers did not contain fat [57]. The increased mortality was attributable to postoperative liver failure occurring between days 3 and 7, a delay that is consistent with the proposal that dysfunction of the regenerative response may be an important mechanism for liver failure. However, the true impact of NAFLD and NASH on the ability of hepatocytes to regenerate after surgical removal or pathological destruction of hepatocellular mass has not yet been carefully evaluated in humans.

In hepatitis C, chronic hepatocellular injury is accompanied by compensatory cell proliferation in order to maintain liver mass [58]. Studies on a limited number of patients with NASH have identified some hepatocellular proliferative activity, as determined by immunohistochemical determination of the Ki67 labelling index, a marker of cell proliferation [58]. Susca et al. [59] mentioned that, in spite of similar hepatocellular injury (based on similar ALT levels), hepatocyte proliferation was lower in steatohepatitis than in viral hepatitis C. This observation might suggest impaired hepatocyte proliferation in NASH. However, the relationship between the extent of hepatocellular injury and the regenerative response has not yet been carefully addressed.

Insights from animal models

Most of the data pertaining to the capacity of the fatty liver to regenerate have been derived from animal studies, as summarized in Table 12.2. Two models are commonly used to study liver regeneration [55]. The first involves surgical removal of 70% of the liver (partial hepatectomy). This induces a synchronous proliferative response, with 95% of the remaining hepatocytes entering the cell cycle within 24 h. In rats, this process leads to restoration of the original liver mass in 7 days. The second model is based on the destruction of hepatic parenchyma by a toxic agent. In the CCl_4 model, the proliferative response is less synchronous than in the partial hepatectomy model [55]. Compared to the partial hepatectomy model, the toxic damage induced by CCl_4 is associated with an inflammatory reaction and release of cytokines that are able to influence the proliferative process.

The hepatic proliferative response consists schematically of three successive phases [55]. The first is the priming phase. It is characterized by the activation of proto-oncogenes (c-fos, c-jun, c-myc) and intracellular signalling pathways such as NF-κB, STAT-3, AP-1 and C/EBPβ. Priming is necessary to confer replicative competence to hepatocytes, but is generally insufficient to drive the proliferative response to completion. The second phase is the proliferative phase, in which the mechanisms required for DNA synthesis and cell division are activated. Control mechanisms involve

cytokines and co-mitogens. The third, post-replicative phase ensures termination of the proliferative process and final adjustment of liver mass, with cell deletion by apoptosis.

Effect of steatosis and steatohepatitis on liver regeneration

The hepatic regenerative response after partial hepatectomy has been shown to be normal in several models of fatty liver. Thus, hepatocyte proliferation is normal in models of steatosis resulting from impaired very-low-density lipoprotein (VLDL) export [60,61]. Likewise, PPARα null mice develop a mild steatosis because of the inability to adapt PPARα-dependent fatty acid β-oxidation metabolism pathways to hepatic lipid load; in such mice, the proliferative response after partial hepatectomy was similar to their PPARα +/+ littermates [62]. This indicates that neither the physiological inability to induce β-oxidation of fatty acids for metabolic needs, nor the PPARα are essential for enhanced cell proliferation after partial hepatectomy. However, in another study, Anderson et al. [63] reported that the onset of DNA synthesis was slightly delayed in these mice. Acyl-CoA oxidase is the rate-limiting enzyme for peroxisomal β-oxidation of fatty acids. As a consequence of its absence, long-chain fatty acids accumulate in the liver. In mice lacking acyl-CoA oxidase, DNA synthesis and mitotic index after partial hepatectomy were similar to those of control littermates [64]. It is interesting to note that, in the long term, acyl-CoA oxidase-deficient mice develop steatohepatitis (see Chapter 8) [32]. In the MCD model of fibrosing steatohepatitis, Zhang et al. [65] as well as Picard et al. [60] did not find any impairment of cyclin expression, DNA synthesis or restoration of liver mass after partial hepatectomy. It therefore appears that neither fatty infiltration of the liver, nor experimental steatohepatitis that pathologically resembles human NAFLD type 4 (steatohepatitis with pericellular fibrosis) are associated with diminished regenerative potential after reduction of hepatic mass.

Effects of leptin deficiency and leptin receptor dysfunction on liver regeneration

Contrasting with the normal hepatocyte proliferation found in models of steatosis or steatohepatitis, the regenerative potential of the fatty liver is severely

Table 12.2 Effect of steatosis and steatohepatitis on liver regeneration in animal models.

Model	Liver pathology	Metabolic alteration	Model for liver regeneration	Liver regeneration	Comments	Reference
Orotic acid	Confluent microvesicular steatosis	Impaired VLDL export	70% PH	Normal		60
Choline-deficient diet	Steatosis, mild inflammation and, ultimately, carcinogenesis	Impaired VLDL export	70% PH	Normal		61
PPARα −/− mice	Steatosis	Inability to upregulate β-oxidation in response to lipid load	70% PH	Normal		62
				Delayed	Increased IL-6 and IL-1β, delayed onset for DNA synthesis	63
Acyl-CoA oxidase −/− mice	Steatosis, mild steatohepatitis in the long term	Inability to upregulate β-oxidation in response to lipid load and induction of CYP4A	70% PH	Normal		64
MCD diet-induced steato-hepatitis	Severe macrovesicular steatosis, necroinflammation, pericellular and perivascular fibrosis	Depleted hepatic antioxidants Intrahepatic oxidative stress Altered intrahepatic flux of lipids	70% PH	Normal		60,65
fa/fa Zucker rats	Severe steatosis hyperinsulinaemia and insulin resistance Dyslipidaemia Altered immune function	Obesity, leptin resitance,	70% PH	Impaired block at G1/S transition	No effect of recombinant IL-6 on DNA synthesis or proliferation	66
ob/ob mice	Severe steatosis	Obesity, leptin deficiency, hyperinsulinaemia and insulin resistance Dyslipidemia Altered mitochondrial function Altered immune function	70% PH	Impaired block at G1/S transition	Altered priming phase, STAT3 hyperstimulation Defect in cyclin D1 expression	67,68
			Acute CCl$_4$-induced liver injury	Impaired block at G1/S transition	Altered priming phase, STAT3 hyperstimulation Defect in cyclin D1 expression Defect of TNF and IL-6 expression Rescued by recombinant leptin and by TNF injection	69

CCl$_4$, carbon tetrachloride; IL, interleukin; MCD, methionine- and choline-deficient; PH, partial hepatectomy; PPARα, peroxisome proliferator-activated receptor-α; STAT, signal transducer and activator of transcription; TNF, tumour necrosis factor; VLDL, very-low-density lipoprotein.

impaired in animals with disrupted leptin signalling. Fatty (*fa/fa*) Zucker rats and obese (*ob/ob*) mice spontaneously develop severe hepatic steatosis as a consequence of uncontrolled food intake resulting from leptin receptor dysfunction and deficiency in leptin production, respectively. Zelzner and Clavien [66] found liver regeneration was significantly delayed and impaired in fatty Zucker rats compared with lean littermates. Similarly, Diehl *et al.* [67,68] showed increased mortality in *ob/ob* mice after 70% partial hepatectomy, and severe impairment of the regenerative response among survivors. The regenerative response is also profoundly impaired in *ob/ob* mice after acute toxic injury to the liver [69]. In all cases, a block in hepatocyte cell cycle at the transition between G_1 and S phases (the G_1 restriction points has been observed).

Impaired proliferation observed in conditions where steatosis is associated with altered leptin signalling, but not in other forms of steatosis that respect the integrity of this pathway, suggests that factors directly related to leptin signalling rather than to intrahepatic lipid overload are implicated. This proposition is supported by the observation that exogenous recombinant leptin restores normal proliferative response to acute CCl_4-induced liver injury in *ob/ob* mice [69].

The priming phase, which confers replicative competence to hepatocytes [55], is altered after partial hepatectomy in *ob/ob* mice [67]. Activation of the mitogen-activated kinases ERK1 and 2 is enhanced, while induction of the stress-activated kinase, JNK, is abolished, activation of nuclear factor NF-κB is impaired, whereas STAT-3 is hyperactivated [67,68]. All these changes, by different processes, might act in concert to block activation of the cyclin D_1–cyclin dependent kinase complex and trap hepatocytes in the late G_1 phase. Consistent with the proposal that overexpression of STAT-3 could be mechanistically related to defective hepatocyte replication, leptin replacement to *ob/ob* mice has been reported to restrain the exuberance of STAT-3 activation following CCl_4 injection to the levels found in lean mice, as well as normalizing cyclin D_1 expression and the proliferative response [69]. The observation that direct injection of IL-6, a potent STAT-3 activator, was ineffective at restoring DNA synthesis and cell proliferation after partial hepatectomy in the leptin-resistant Zucker rat [66] is also consistent with this proposition.

Metabolic factors and insulin resistance have been proposed to explain the proliferative defect in animals

with disrupted leptin signalling [67,68]. Replicating cells consume energy generated by mitochondrial β-oxidation [56]. It has been shown that stimulation of mitochondrial energy production by supplementing rats with FFA and carnitine, the carrier required for fatty acid transport into mitochondria (see Chapter 11), increases hepatocellular proliferation after partial hepatectomy [56]. Thus, in leptin-deficient or leptin-resistant livers, altered lipid metabolism and mitochondrial function leading to ATP depletion could render the cells unable to meet the increased energy demands required for the proliferative process [67,70]. Increased mortality after surgery to leptin-deficient mice correlates with profound hypoglycaemia [67]. Therefore, metabolic dysfunction or failure of hepatocytes to adapt in the face of increased metabolic demands imposed by cell replication could, at least partly, account for impaired proliferation in this setting.

Leptin deficiency induces severe resistance to insulin action [49]. Insulin is considered to be a secondary mitogen that enhances liver sensitivity to other complete mitogens but does not have full mitogenic activity. The role of insulin in liver regeneration is supported by the blunting of intermediate–early gene response and DNA synthesis after partial hepatectomy in animals with type 1 diabetes [56]. In *ob/ob* mice, injection of exogenous leptin at the time of CCl_4 injection restores hepatic regenerative capacity [69]. This intervention ameliorates insulin sensitivity and intrahepatic lipid metabolism but does not resolve all the metabolic consequences of long-term leptin deficiency. To our knowledge, the impact of hyperinsulinaemia, insulin resistance and/or glucose intolerance on liver regeneration have not been studied, but decreased insulin sensitivity is likely to interfere with the replicative capacity of hepatocytes. As NAFLD and NASH are usually associated with insulin resistance (see Chapter 5), it would be interesting to understand whether this interferes with cell proliferation, and the consequences for this on progression of fatty liver diseases.

Another important function of leptin relevant to liver regeneration is its immunomodulatory properties. *Ob/ob* mice exhibit immune dysregulation, and monocyte–macrophage function is altered (see Chapter 10). In these mice, hepatic TNF and IL-6 mRNA expression was altered after partial hepatectomy [67], and production of TNF and IL-6 was defective after acute CCl_4 toxicity [69]. Leptin repletion in this context normalized the pattern of cytokine expression. The importance of cytokine release in conferring replicative competence to leptin-deficient animals was further demonstrated by low-dose TNF injection prior to toxin administration, a treatment that restored liver regeneration in the same manner as observed with leptin repletion [69]. Taken together, these observations are consistent with the concept that altered cytokine production in *ob/ob* mice is part of the mechanism responsible for impaired hepatocyte proliferation in response to liver injury.

In summary, in the context of leptin deficiency, several factors, either directly or indirectly leptin-dependent, can influence the proliferative response in the liver. These include alteration in the priming phase of liver regeneration and in the expression of proteins involved in the control of cell cycle and apoptosis, alteration of energy metabolism and resistance to insulin, and dysregulation of the cytokine network. To date, the parts played by altered lipid metabolism, insulin resistance and/or leptin deficiency in the control of hepatocyte poliferation and, most importantly, the causal links between their alteration and impaired liver regeneration remains to be established.

Conclusions

In light of the growing prevalence of NAFLD and NASH, progress in elucidating pathogenic mechanisms and in defining appropriate treatment is sorely needed. As the increased morbidity and mortality of NASH is associated with fibrosis progression, clarifying the basis for fibrogenesis in NAFLD and NASH is essential. New evidence on the profibrogenic effects of oxidative stress and lipid peroxidation, imbalanced intrahepatic lipid metabolism and insulin resistance are emerging as important factors. Fundamental insights into leptin biology and its dysregulation associated with the metabolic syndrome, PPAR transcription factors and their dual effects on the control of insulin sensitivity and biology of HSC, and cytokine signalling are likely to benefit our understanding of the pathogenesis of NASH.

NASH is associated with chronic hepatocellular injury. As a result, decreased proliferative capacity could alter the adaptive response of fatty liver to chronic injury, thereby participating in NASH pathogenesis. Animal studies provide evidence that intrahepatic lipid overload *per se* does not appear to compromise the proliferative response of the liver. However, liver regeneration is impaired in animals with disrupted leptin signalling, resistance to insulin and immune perturbations, a phenotype that closely resembles that of patients with NASH. These factors, separately or together, could potentially decrease the adaptive response of the liver to injury and participate in progression of NAFLD to NASH to cirrhosis and hepatocarcinogenesis (see Chapter 22). Additional studies are needed to explore whether inappropriately dampened or unrestrained proliferative responses are a pathogenic factor in fatty liver diseases.

References

1 Friedman, SL. Molecular regulation of hepatic fibrosis, an integrated cellular response to tissue injury. *J Biol Cell* 2000; **275**: 2247–50.

2 Rojkind M, Greenwel P. Pathophysiology of liver fibrosis. In: Arias IM, ed. *The Liver: Biology and Pathobiology*, 4th edn. Philadelphia: Lippincott Williams & Wilkins, 2001: 721–38.

3 Shuppan D, Ruehl M, Somasundaram R *et al.* Matrix as modulator of hepatic fibrogenesis. *Semin Liver Dis* 2001; **21**: 351–72.

4 Li D, Friedman SL. Hepatic stellate cells: morphology, function, and regulation. In: Arias IM, ed. *The Liver: Biology and Pathobiology*, 4th edn. Philadelphia: Lippincott Williams & Wilkins, 2001: 455–68.

5 Knittel T, Kobold D, Saile B *et al.* Rat liver myofibroblasts and hepatic stellate cells: different cell populations of the fibroblast lineage with fibrogenic potential. *Gastroenterology* 1999; **117**: 1205–21.

6 Cassiman D, Roskams T. Beauty is in the eye of the beholder: emerging concepts and pitfalls in hepatic stellate cell research. *J Hepatol* 2002; **37**: 527.

7 Geerts A. History, heterogeneity, developmental biology and function of quiescent hepatic stellate cells. *Semin Liver Dis* 2001; **21**: 311–35.

8 Eng FJ, Friedman SL. Fibrogenesis: new insights into hepatic stellate cell activation—the simple becomes complex. *Am J Physiol Gastrointest Liver Physiol* 2000; **279**: G7–11.

9 Maher JJ. Interactions between hepatic stellate cells and the immune system. *Semin Liver Dis* 2001; **21**: 417–26.

10 Benyon RC, Arthur MJ. Extracellular matrix degradation and the role of hepatic stellate cells. *Semin Liver Dis* 2001; **21**: 373–84.

11 Wanless IR, Nakashima E, Sherman M. Regression of human cirrhosis: morphologic features and the genesis of

incomplete septal cirrhosis. *Arch Pathol Lab Med* 2000; **124**: 1599–607.

12 Bissell DM, Roulot D, George J. Transforming growth factor β and the liver. *Hepatology* 2001; **34**: 859–67.

13 Mann DA, Smart DE. Transcriptional regulation of hepatic stellate cell activation. *Gut* 2002; **50**: 891–6.

14 Cortez-Pinto H, Baptista A, Camilo ME *et al*. Hepatic stellate cell activation occurs in non-alcoholic steatohepatitis. *Hepatogastroenterology* 2001; **48**: 87–90.

15 Washington K, Wright K, Shyr Y *et al*. Hepatic stellate cell activation in non-alcoholic steatohepatitis and fatty liver. *Hum Pathol* 2000; **31**: 822–88.

16 Angulo P, Keach JC, Batts KP *et al*. Independent predictors of liver fibrosis in patients with non-alcoholic steatohepatitis. *Hepatology* 1999; **30**: 1356–62.

17 Dixon JB, Bhathal PS, O'Brien PE. Non-alcoholic fatty liver disease: predictors of non-alcoholic steatohepatitis and liver fibrosis in the severely obese. *Gastroenterology* 2001; **121**: 91–100.

18 Marceau P, Biron S, Hould FS *et al*. Liver pathology and metabolic syndrome X in severe obesity. *J Clin Endocrinol Metab* 1999; **84**: 1513–7.

19 Reeves HL, Burt AD, Wood S, Day CP. Hepatic stellate cell activation occurs in the absence of hepatitis in alcoholic liver disease and correlates with the severity of steatosis. *J Hepatol* 1996; **25**: 677–83.

20 Naveau S, Giraud V, Borotto E *et al*. Excess weight is a risk factor for alcoholic liver disease. *Hepatology* 1997; **25**: 108–11.

21 Hourigan LF, McDonald GA, Purdic D *et al*. Fibrosis in chronic hepatitis C correlates significantly with body mass index and steatosis. *Hepatology* 1999; **29**: 1215–29.

22 Adolfini LE, Gambardela M, Andreana A *et al*. Steatosis accelerates the progression of liver damage of chronic hepatitis C patients and correlates with specific HCD genotype and visceral obesity. *Hepatology* 2001; **33**: 1358–64.

23 Hickman IJ, Clouston AD, Macdonald GA *et al*. Effect of weight reduction on liver histology and biochemistry in patients with chronic hepatitis C. *Gut* 2002; **51**: 89–94.

24 Mezey E. Dietary fat and alcoholic liver disease. *Hepatology* 1998; **28**: 901–5.

25 Day CP, James OF. Steatohepatitis: a tale of two 'hits'? *Gastroenterology* 1998; **114**: 842–5.

26 Ip E, Farrell GC, Hall P *et al*. Administration of the potent PPARα against, Wy-14,643, reverses nutritional fibrosis and steatohepatitis in mice *Hepatology* 2004; **39**: 1286–96.

27 Ip E, Farrell GC, Robertson G *et al*. Activation of PPARα-dependent pathways causes rapid regression of fibrosing steatohepatitis in MCD-fed mice. *J Hepatol* 2003; **38**: A83.

28 Svegliati-Baroni G, Ridolfi F, Di Sario A *et al*. Insulin and insulin-like growth factor-1 stimulate proliferation and type I collagen accumulation by human hepatic stellate cells: differential effects in signal transduction pathways. *Hepatology* 1999; **29**: 1743–51.

29 Paradis V, Perlemuter G, Bonvoust F *et al*. High glucose and hyperinsulinemia stimulate connective tissue growth factor expression: a potential mechanism involved in progression to fibrosis in non-alcoholic steatohepatitis. *Hepatology* 2001; **34**: 738–44.

30 Parola M, Robino G. Oxidative stress-related molecules and liver fibrosis. *J Hepatol* 2001; **35**: 297–306.

31 Leclercq IA, Farrell GC, Field J *et al*. CYP2E1 and CYP4A as microsomal catalysts of lipid peroxides in murine non-alcoholic steatohepatitis. *J Clin Invest* 2000; **105**: 1067–75.

32 Fan C, Pan J, Chu R *et al*. Hepatocellular and hepatic peroxisomal alterations in mice with a disrupted peroxisomal fatty acyl-coenzyme A oxidase gene. *J Biol Chem* 1996; **271**: 24698–710.

33 Seki S, Kitada T, Yamada T *et al*. *In situ* detection of lipid peroxidation and oxidative DNA damage in non-alcoholic fatty liver diseases. *J Hepatol* 2002; **37**: 56–62.

34 MacDonald GA, Bridle KR, Ward PJ *et al*. Lipid peroxidation in hepatic steatosis in humans is associated with hepatic fibrosis and occurs predominately in acinar zone 3. *J Gastroenterol Hepatol* 2001; **16**: 599–606.

35 Sanyal A, Campbell-Sargent C, Mirshahi F *et al*. Non alcoholic steatohepatitis: association of insulin resistance and mitochondrial abnormalities. *Gastroenterology* 2001; **120**: 1183–92.

36 Robertson G, Leclercq IA, Farrell GC. Non-alcoholic steatosis and steatohepatitis: cytochrome P450 enzymes and oxidative stress. *Am J Physiol Gastrointest Liver Physiol* 2001; **281**: G1135–9.

37 George J, Pera N, Phung N *et al*. Lipid peroxidation, stellate cell activation and hepatic fibrogenesis in a rat model of chronic steatohepatitis. *J Hepatol* 2003; **39**: 756–64.

38 Phung N, Farrell GC, Robertson G, George J. Vitamin E but not glutathione precursors inhibits hepatic fibrosis in experimental NASH exhibiting oxidative stress and mitochondrial abnormalities. *Hepatology* 2001; **34**: 361A.

39 Angulo P. Current best treatment for non-alcoholic fatty liver disease. *Exp Opin Pharmacother* 2003; **4**: 611–23.

40 Nieto N, Friedman SL, Cerderbaum AI. Cytochrome P450 2E1-derived oxygen species mediate paracrine stimulation of collagen I protein synthesis by hepatic stellate cells. *J Biol Chem* 2002; **277**: 9853–64.

41 Nieto N, Friedman SL, Cerderbaum AI. Stimulation and proliferation of primary rat hepatic stellate cells by cytochrome P450 2E1-derived reactive oxygen species. *Hepatology* 2002; **35**: 62–73.

42 Nieto N, Greenwel P, Friedman SL *et al*. Ethanol and arachidonic acid increase α2(I) collagen expression in rat

hepatic stellate cells overexpressing cytochrome P450 2E1. *J Biol Chem* 2000; **275**: 20136–45.

43 Leclercq IA, Farrell GC, Schriemer R *et al*. Leptin is essential for hepatic fibrogenic response to chronic liver injury. *J Hepatol* 2002; **37**: 206–13.

44 Ikejima K, Takei Y, Honda H *et al*. Leptin receptor-mediated signaling regulates hepatic fibrogenesis and remodeling of extracellular matrix in the rat. *Gastroenterology* 2002; **122**: 1399–410.

45 Saxena NK, Ikeda K, Rockey DC *et al*. Leptin in hepatic fibrosis: evidence for increased collagen production in stellate cells and lean littermates of *ob/ob* mice. *Hepatology* 2002; **35**: 762–71.

46 Ikejima K, Honda H, Yoshikawa M *et al*. Leptin augments inflammatory and profibrogenic responses in the murine liver induced by hepatotoxic chemicals. *Hepatology* 2001; **34**: 288–97.

47 Potter JJ, Womack L, Mezey E, Anania FA. Transdifferentiation of rat hepatic stellate cells results in leptin expression. *Biochem Biophys Res Commun* 1998; **244**: 178–82.

48 Enriquez A, Leclercq I, Farrell GC *et al*. Altered expression of hepatic CYP2E1 and CYP4A in obese, diabetic *ob/ob* mice, and *fa/fa* Zucker rats. *Biochem Biophys Res Commun* 1999; **255**: 300–6.

49 Friedman JM. The function of leptin in nutrition, weight, and physiology. *Nutr Rev* 2002; **60**: S1–14; discussion S68–87.

50 Chitturi S, Farrell G, Frost L *et al*. Serum leptin in NASH correlates with hepatic steatosis but not fibrosis: a manifestation of lipotoxicity? *Hepatology* 2002; **36**: 403–9.

51 Lee Y, Wang MY, Kakuma T *et al*. Liporegulation in diet-induced obesity: the antisteatotic role of hyperleptinemia. *J Biol Chem* 2001; **276**: 5629–35.

52 Galli A, Crabb DW, Ceni E *et al*. Antibiabetic thiazolidinediones inhibit collagen synthesis and hepatic stellate cell activation *in vivo* and *in vitro*. *Gastroenterology* 2002; **122**: 1924–40.

53 Neuschwander-Tetri BA, Sponseller C, Brunt E *et al*. Rosiglitazone improves insulin sensitivity, ALT and hepatic steatosis in patients with non-alcoholic steatohepatitis. *Gastroenterology* 2002; **122**: 5A.

54 Miyahara T, Schrum L, Rippe R *et al*. Peroxisome proliferator-activated receptors and hepatic stellate cell activation. *J Biol Chem* 2000; **46**: 35715–22.

55 Fausto N. Liver regeneration. In: Arias IM, ed. *The Liver: Biology and Pathobiology*, 4th edn. Philadelphia: Lippincott Williams & Wilkins, 2001: 591–610.

56 Michalopoulos GK, DeFrances MC. Liver regeneration. *Science* 1997; **276**: 60–6.

57 Behrns KE, Tsiotos GG, De Souza NF *et al*. Hepatic steatosis as a potential risk factor for major hepatic resection. *J Gastrointest Surg* 1998; **2**: 292–8.

58 Hussein O, Szvalb S, Van Den Akker-Berman LM *et al*. Liver regeneration is not altered in patients with non-alcoholic steatohepatitis (NASH) when compared to chronic hepatitis C infection with similar grade of inflammation. *Dig Dis Sci* 2002; **47**: 1926–31.

59 Susca M, Grassi A, Zauli D *et al*. Liver inflammatory cells, apoptosis, regeneration and stellate cell activation in non-alcoholic steatohepatitis. *Dig Dis Sci* 2001; **33**: 768–77.

60 Picard C, Lambotte L, Starkel P *et al*. Steatosis is not sufficient to cause an impaired regenerative response after partial hepatectomy in rats. *J Hepatol* 2002; **32**: 645–52.

61 Rao MS, Papreddy K, Abecassis M *et al*. Regeneration of liver with marked fatty change following partial hepatectomy in rats. *Dig Dis Sci* 2001; **46**: 1821–6.

62 Rao MS, Peters JM, Gonzalez FJ *et al*. Hepatic regeneration in peroxisome proliferator-activated receptor α-null mice after partial hepatectomy. *Hepatol Res* 2002; **22**: 52–7.

63 Anderson SP, Yoon L, Richard EB. Delayed liver regeneration in peroxisome proliferator-activated receptor-α-null mice. *Hepatology* 2002; **36**: 544–54.

64 Rao MS, Reddy JK. The effect of microvesicular fatty change on liver regeneration after partial hepatectomy. *Hepatogastroenterol* 2000; **47**: 912–5.

65 Zhang BH, Weltman M, Farrell GC. Does steatohepatitis impair liver regeneration? A study in a dietary model of steatohepatitis in rats. *J Gastroenterol Hepatol* 1999; **14**: 133–7.

66 Zelzner M, Clavien PA. Failure of regeneration of the steatotic rat liver: disruption at two different levels in the regeneration pathway. *Hepatology* 2000; **31**: 35–42.

67 Yang SQ, Lin HZ, Mandal AK *et al*. Disrupted signaling and inhibited regeneration in obese mice with fatty livers: implications for non-alcoholic fatty liver disease pathophysiology. *Hepatology* 2001; **34**: 694–706.

68 Torbenson M, Yang SQ, Liu HZ *et al*. STAT-3 overexpression and p21 up-regulation accompany impaired regeneration of fatty livers. *Am J Pathol* 2002; **161**: 155–61.

69 Leclercq IA, Field J, Farrell GC. Leptin-specific mechanisms for impaired liver regeneration in *ob/ob* mice after toxic liver injury: roles of TNF and STAT3. *Gastroenterology* 2003; **124**: 1451–64.

70 Chavin KD, Yang S, Lin HZ *et al*. Obesity induces expression of uncoupling protein-2 in hepatocytes and promotes liver ATP depletion. *J Biol Chem* 1999; **274**: 5692–700.

13 Clinical manifestations and diagnosis of NAFLD

Stephen A. Harrison & Brent Neuschwander-Tetri

Key learning points

1 Patients with NAFLD usually present without symptoms in the 4th or 5th decade of life.
2 Although NAFLD may occur in any type of individual, the typical patient profile is a white or Hispanic middle-aged female with obesity, hypertension, dyslipidaemia and diabetes.
3 There is no single serum liver chemistry or radiologic test that will distinguish the less serious forms of NAFLD from NASH, which is a type of NAFLD that may progress to cirrhosis.
4 Certain clinical characteristics used in combination such as age, obesity and/or diabetes, the AST-ALT ratio and the metabolic syndrome increases the reliability of predicting advanced fibrosis in NASH.
5 Only a liver biopsy accurately predicts the histologic form of NAFLD. However, the decision to perform a liver biopsy should be individualized for each patient.
6 An algorithm is provided as a suggested diagnostic approach to patients with NAFLD.

Abstract

Non-alcoholic fatty liver disease (NAFLD) typically manifests itself clinically in the 4–5th decade of life. Patients usually present with asymptomatic elevations in their serum aminotransferases that are detected on routine clinical and laboratory evaluations. All ethnic groups are at risk, but white people and Hispanics appear to represent the majority of patients with this condition. This disease appears to be related to long-standing insulin resistance and likely represents the hepatic manifestation of the metabolic syndrome. The prevalence is increasing as the prevalence of obesity and diabetes mellitus increases in our society. Most patients with NAFLD are obese and are likely to have hypertension, diabetes mellitus or hyperlipidaemia. However, with the exception of hepatomegaly, which is seen in up to 50% of patients, specific findings are lacking on physical examination. On laboratory evaluation, patients usually have mild elevations in their aminotransferase levels, with an alanine aminotransferase (ALT) predominance. Occasionally, the alkaline phosphatase may be slightly elevated. Imaging studies are helpful in detecting NAFLD, but are not effective in distinguishing simple fatty liver from non-alcoholic steatohepatitis (NASH), a potentially more aggressive form of NAFLD. Subsequently, a liver biopsy is often necessary to determine the severity of the fatty liver disease. The decision to perform liver biopsies in patients with NAFLD is still controversial, and therefore recent study has focused on evaluating clinical data for predictors of advanced liver disease. These clinical data are presented here and may assist the clinician in deciding whether or not to proceed with a liver biopsy.

Introduction

The purpose of this chapter is to highlight the clinical manifestations of NAFLD. This is accomplished by separating the clinical data into several categories to include historical data, physical examination, laboratory data, and potential imaging modalities, and concluding with a discussion on the role of liver biopsy in assisting in disease management. Potential future directions are also discussed.

Clinical history

When examining a patient with suspected NAFLD, the time invested in obtaining a good history can be very helpful. While occurring in all age groups, NAFLD in adults typically becomes recognized clinically in the 4–5th decade of life [1]. This is usually the result of incidentally discovered elevated aminotransferase levels, which prompts further evaluation leading to the diagnosis. Earlier studies suggested a female predominance [2–4], but more recent data suggest an equal to slight male predominance [5–8]. However, females may have an increased tendency to progress to more advanced disease [6,7]. NAFLD has been reported in all ethnic groups, but data tend to support a white and Hispanic over-representation [9]. Interestingly, while several cross-sectional studies demonstrate a low prevalence among African Americans [10], evaluation of the recent Third National Health and Nutrition Examination Survey (NHANES III) data showed that African Americans may be more likely to have NAFLD than white people [8].

The clinical association of obesity, diabetes mellitus, hyperlipidaemia and hypertension with NAFLD is well characterized (Table 13.1) [3,6,11–14] and seems to be related to underlying insulin resistance [15,16]. Obesity, as defined by a body mass index (BMI) of > 30 kg/m^2 in the US population, is the most frequent clinical association seen in cross-sectional population studies, occurring in 40–100% of patients [17]. Diabetes mellitus is found in 21–75%, hyperlipidaemia in 21–83% and hypertension in 15–68% [3,6,18]. It is now known that the combination of these variables in patients with NAFLD is associated with more advanced liver disease at the time of presentation [13,19]. It is important to note, however, that NAFLD may occur in the absence of any these clinical variables [12]. These patients have been termed 'normal weight, metabolically obese' and the majority of such people may have insulin resistance as well.

Typically, patients will be asymptomatic, having been referred for further evaluation of incidentally discovered abnormal aminotransferases. Some patients may present with progressive fatigue or right upper quadrant discomfort [12]. The abdominal discomfort is usually vague, non-descript and thought to be related to distention of the hepatic capsule (Fig. 13.1). Recently, it has been suggested anecdotally that obstructive sleep apnoea is more prevalent in this patient population given the increased weight of most patients; the authors' experience supports this finding.

In addition, other historical data obtained should include questions about previous bariatric surgery, such as jejuno-ileal bypass; previous or current drugs that are well known to be associated with NAFLD (Table 13.2); and menstrual irregularities, infertility, and/or hirsutism,

Table 13.1 Patient demographics and characteristics.

Author	N	Mean age	Male (%)	HLP (%)	DM (%)	Obesity (%)	HTN (%)	ALT (U/L)	AST (U/L)
Ludwig *et al.* [3]	20	54	35	67	25	90	15	38	72
Powell *et al.* [11]	42	49	17	62	36	95	ND	96	70
Bacon *et al.* [12]	33	47	58	21	21	39	18	ND	ND
Angulo *et al.* [13]	144	51	33	27	28	60	ND	82	63
Harrison & Hayashi [6]	102	51	57	74	42	73	58	89	63
Chitturi *et al.* [49]	93	49	60	ND	29	57	ND	90	53

ALT, alanine aminotransferase; AST, aspartate aminotransferase; DM, diabetes mellitus; HLP, hyperlipidaemia; HTN, hypertension; ND, no data.

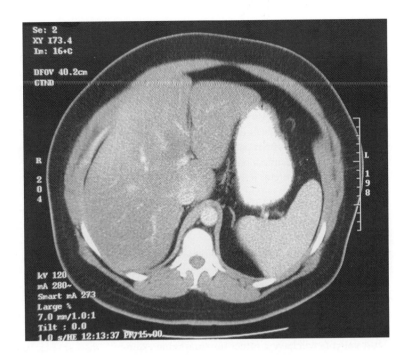

Fig. 13.1 An abdominal computerized tomography (CT) image of a patient with right upper quadrant abdominal fullness and pain. The image shown reveals that the liver has a lower density than the spleen, indicating hepatic steatosis. The liver also appears enlarged anteriorly, a finding that probably explains her pain. A liver biopsy showed moderate mixed macro- and microsteatosis involving 33–66% of hepatocytes. There was mild inflammatory activity (grade 1) and no significant fibrosis (stage 1).

Table 13.2 Medications associated with hepatic steatosis.

Macrovesicular steatosis
Isoniazid
Methotrexate
Allopurinol
Halothane
α-Methyldopa
Corticosteroids

Microvesicular steatosis
Tamoxifen
Valproic acid
Tetracycline
Salicyclic acid
Ibuprofen
Fialuridine
Didanosine

Mixed macrovesicular/microvesicular
Amiodarone
Perhexiline

suggesting polycystic ovarian syndrome (PCOS). PCOS is associated with insulin resistance [20] and may be associated with NAFLD, although this has yet to be formally reported.

Furthermore, questions about family history of diabetes or NAFLD are important. One small study showed that out of eight families, 18 family members with NAFLD were discovered [21]. Another study found that 16 out of 90 patients with NASH had a first-degree relative with the disease [22]. While no familial inheritance pattern emerged, this suggests that environmental as well as genetic factors are likely to have a role in this disease. These findings have prompted the search for genetic abnormalities that may predispose susceptible individuals to NAFLD. Some of the genes currently being evaluated include those that influence development of hepatic steatosis such as leptin [23], apolipoprotein E [24] and microsomal triglyceride transfer protein (MTP) [25], genes encoding proteins involved in the adaptive response to oxidative stress such as manganese superoxide dismutase (MnSOD) [26] and genes influencing tumour necrosis factor α (TNF-α) expression, such as CD14 [27].

The relationship of dietary habits to insulin resistance and hepatic triglyceride metabolism is currently being investigated. A recent study evaluated the dietary habits of 25 NASH patients compared with 25 age-, gender- and BMI-matched controls. Each patient was required to keep a 7-day alimentary record followed by oral glucose and oral fat load testing. The results

161

demonstrated that the patients with NASH ate diets higher in saturated fats with less polyunsaturated fatty acids, fibre and the antioxidant vitamins C and E. Interestingly, this study also showed that the NASH cohort had higher postprandial total triglyceride and very-low-density lipoprotein (VLDL) triglyceride levels when compared with controls. Also, the postprandial apolipoprotein B48 and B100 levels did not rise with elevated triglyceride levels in NASH patients, as they did in the control group, suggesting a possible defect in the generation of apolipoproteins in NASH patients [28].

Physical examination

Clinical stigmata of chronic liver disease such as the characteristic peripheral muscle wasting, gynaecomastia, spider telangiectasias or caput medusa are rarely seen on initial presentation. Interestingly, while spider telangiectasias are well described in alcoholic liver disease, they do not seem to be as prevalent in NAFLD. Most patients will have a rather unremarkable examination. Cross-sectional studies suggest that up to 50% of patients may have hepatomegaly on initial presentation [3,12]. The majority of patients will be overweight (BMI > 25 kg/m²), and are likely to have an elevated waist : hip ratio, indicating abdominal adiposity. The ratio is calculated by dividing the waist circumference by the hip circumference. A recent study demonstrated that NAFLD patients, even in the presence of normal body weight, have increased visceral adiposity [29]. Hypertension is found in 15–68% of cases reported to date [3,6,12]. Occasionally, female patients may exhibit increased acne and hirsutism, suggesting the underlying endocrine abnormality of PCOS. Finally, one should pay attention to the physical findings suggestive of underlying lipodystrophies. Lipodystrophies are typically characterized by an abnormal fat distribution.

Acanthosis nigricans (hyperpigmented, velvety plaques found in body folds) is recognized as a clinical marker of insulin resistance and diabetes mellitus, and is frequently identified in patients with excessive weight gain [30]. Given that patients with NAFLD have insulin resistance as a general rule and tend to be overweight, it would stand to reason that acanthosis nigricans would be found with increasing prevalence in patients with NAFLD. While this has been noted in children with NAFLD, there are no data explicitly stating the prevalence of this skin finding in adults with NAFLD.

Right upper quadrant tenderness is sometimes found. This is likely related to capsular extension by the hepatic parenchyma (Fig. 13.1). Some evidence suggests that this occurs in up to 30% of patients [12], although the pain is vague and often not specifically sought or noted in the patient's history.

Laboratory data

Typically, the ALT and aspartate aminotransferase (AST) will be raised, but usually less than four times the upper limit of normal. Some patients may have normal liver enzymes [31,32]. Patients with NAFLD have an ALT predominance over AST, in contrast to alcoholic liver disease. However, if advanced fibrosis or cirrhosis is present, the AST : ALT ratio may approach or even exceed 1. It is important to note that several studies indicate that aminotransferase values do not correlate with underlying histological activity, and in fact enzymes may be within the normal range despite advanced liver disease [31]. While the aminotransferases are typically the only liver enzyme abnormality, occasionally the alkaline phosphatase may be mildly elevated. Unless the patient is presenting with advanced disease, the serum bilirubin, albumin and coagulation studies are normal.

Hyperlipidaemia is found in 21–83% of patients and is usually a result of elevated triglycerides. Given that up to 75% of patients will have diabetes, the fasting glucose levels and haemoglobin A_{1C} may also be elevated. The relevance of hyperglycaemia to the pathogenesis of NAFLD is uncertain.

Serum iron studies, to include ferritin, are often abnormal in patients with NAFLD. In fact, ferritin levels have been reported to be elevated in 40–62% of patients [7,12,13,33]. Some studies evaluating iron overload and abnormal iron indices in NAFLD patients demonstrate collectively that while serum iron indices and ferritin may be abnormal, hepatic iron concentration is usually normal [13,34]. By comparison, the majority of iron-overloaded patients have some degree of insulin resistance, similar to the mechanism of fat accumulation within the liver [35,36]. Mendler recently evaluated 161 patients with iron overload and found that 28% had NASH, with a mean ferritin of 698 [37]. More recently, with the advent of genetic testing for hereditary haemochromatosis, studies have demonstrated that mutations in the *HFE* gene can be seen in up to 60% of patients with NAFLD [33,34,38].

Subsequently, several investigators have attempted to correlate the prevalence of *HFE* mutations with iron overload and advanced stages of NAFLD. Two studies, both performed at iron-overload referral centres, suggested an association between *HFE* mutations, iron overload and severity of underlying histopathology [33,34]. However, neither study controlled for age, obesity or diabetes; all factors which have been shown to be independent predictors of advanced stages of NAFLD. Furthermore, there have been two subsequent studies that did not demonstrate an association between iron overload and advanced fibrosis in NAFLD [7,39].

As interest in this field grows, it is becoming clear that NAFLD can be found in the presence of other liver disease such as hepatitis B and C, autoimmune hepatitis, primary biliary cirrhosis, α_1-antitrypsin deficiency and haemochromatosis [40]. Consequently, it is important that other concomitant causes of chronic liver disease are considered when patients are evaluated for suspected NAFLD. Serological testing obtained at the time of initial presentation should include a chronic viral hepatitis panel for B and C, fasting iron levels, antinuclear and antismooth muscle antibodies, antimitochondrial antibody, serum protein electrophoresis and, if under the age of 40 years, ceruloplasmin assessment should also be made.

Imaging studies

Various imaging modalities have been utilized to detect fatty liver, with differing levels of success. Ultrasound is likely to be the most available option, but computerized tomography (CT) and magnetic resonance imaging (MRI) also are useful. On ultrasound, the fatty liver is diffusely echogenic, the so-called 'bright' liver. CT scans can detect low-density liver parenchyma that is contrasted to that of the spleen, indicating steatosis. While typically a diffuse process, occasionally hepatic steatosis can be localized. Alternatively, the opposite may hold true, when the entire liver is fatty with focal areas of spared normal hepatic parenchyma. This may give the appearance of a high-density lesion that could be mistaken for a potential neoplastic process [41]. MRI scanning is sometimes utilized, but the cost and availability of this imaging technique limits its usefulness.

A recent trial by Saadeh *et al.* [42] prospectively evaluated ultrasound, CT and MRI for the diagnosis of NAFLD. This study demonstrated that all three of these modalities had good sensitivity for detecting NAFLD, as long as there was more than 30% fat deposition in the liver. However, none of these imaging studies were able to different simple steatosis from NASH. This study demonstrated that using a cut-off of 33% fat deposition in the liver, ultrasound had a sensitivity of 100% and CT scan had a sensitivity of 93%. However, the positive predictive values were only 62% and 76%, respectively [42]. An additional study evaluating ultrasound detection of fatty liver demonstrated a sensitivity of 67%, a specificity of 77% and a positive predictive value of 67% [43]. The imaging modality with the most promise in differentiating simple fatty liver from more advanced stages of disease is nuclear magnetic resonance (NMR). Interestingly, there is close to 100% correlation between hepatic triglyceride content obtained via NMR and liver biopsy [44]. Moreover, newer techniques using ^{31}P have been able to differentiate varying degrees of fibrosis in patients with hepatitis C virus, suggesting a possible similar benefit in patients with more advanced NAFLD [45].

Liver biopsy

The decision of when to perform a liver biopsy in patients with NAFLD can sometimes be quite difficult and is certainly not without debate. Recent studies have looked at the utility of performing a liver biopsy in asymptomatic patients with chronically elevated aminotransferases. One study, in more than 350 patients without serological evidence of other forms of liver disease, found NAFLD or NASH in 66% of cases [46]. Additionally, management decisions were altered 18% of the time. This work was corroborated by a similar study in 81 'marker negative' patients that showed NAFLD or NASH in 83% of the biopsy specimens [47]. Recent data suggest that at the time of initial biopsy, up to 30–40% of NASH patients will have advanced fibrosis [2,12] and cirrhosis may be found in up to 20% of cases. In fact, there is some suggestion that many obese patients with NASH will have normal aminotransferases at the time of presentation, but will have advanced fibrosis or cirrhosis found on the biopsy [31]. Currently, non-invasive imaging modalities are unable to distinguish between NAFLD and NASH, making a liver biopsy the only way to differentiate between these two entities. Some authors suggest that because there is little specific or definitive treatment for NAFLD at

Table 13.3 Non-invasive predictors of significant fibrosis in NASH patients.

Author	N	Histological staging system	Mean BMI	Mean age	Female (%)	Stage 0–2 (%)	Stage 3–5 (%)	Non-invasive predictors of fibrosis
Angulo et al. [13]	144	Brunt [51]	31.2	50.5	67	73	27	Age, obesity, DM
Marceau et al. [48]	93	METAVIR [52]	47	36	80	88	12	Age, steatosis, FBS, with histological evaluation WHR, BMI, DM
García-Monzón [31]	32	Brunt	50.5	41	65	84	16	Age, steatosis, Inflammation grade
Ratziu et al. [5]	93	METAVIR	29.1	49	34	84	16	Age, BMI, ALT, triglycerides, inflammation grade
Dixon et al. [19]	26	Brunt	47.2	44	58	59	41	HTN, ALT, C-peptide, Homa%B
Chitturi et al. [7]	93	Brunt	32	49	40	67	33	Female, DM, inflammation grade
Harrison & Hayashi [6]	102	Brunt	33.9	51.3	43	81	19	BMI, AST : ALT ratio, HgbA$_1$C

ALT, alanine aminotransferase; BMI, body mass index; DM, diabetes mellitus; FBS, fasting blood sugar; Homa%B, homoeostasis model assessment, a validated method of estimating insulin resistance and B islet cell function; WHR, waist : hip ratio.

the present time, liver biopsies should be reserved for those patients willing to enter clinical trials. Interestingly, performing a biopsy and establishing a diagnosis may favourably impact a person's outcome independent of specific treatment [48].

While long-term natural history studies in NAFLD are lacking, data at present suggest that patients with simple fatty liver alone have a much lower likelihood of progression to cirrhosis than if there is histological evidence of ballooning degeneration or necrosis, or perisinusoidal fibrosis. When these abnormalities are present, up to 20% of patients may progress to cirrhosis.

Given this debate over whether or not to perform liver biopsies in patients presenting with a high clinical suspicion of NAFLD, several authors have evaluated clinical data obtained on routine clinic visits to determine independent predictors of advanced fibrosis to guide the clinician to proceed more aggressively and perform a liver biopsy, or take a more conservative approach and defer the liver biopsy and treat with current standard therapy for the associated comorbid associated metabolic disorders [5,6,13,19,31,49,50].

The studies outlined in Table 13.3 demonstrate the independent predictors of fibrosis found in NAFLD patients. Age at the time of diagnosis, obesity and diabetes are found in the majority of the studies to be predictors of advanced fibrosis or cirrhosis. Work is currently in progress in large cohorts of NAFLD patients to develop a simple scoring system for detecting advanced fibrosis, non-invasively, based on clinical variables readily obtainable.

In summary, the decision to perform a liver biopsy should be individualized, taking into account how the information gained might influence patient and physician decisions. If excluding less likely diagnoses and establishing a diagnosis of NASH is important, then obtaining these important diagnostic data can outweigh the risks involved.

Conclusions

The prevalence of NAFLD is increasing in our society. While most patients with NAFLD are thought to have a benign natural history, some patients—particularly those

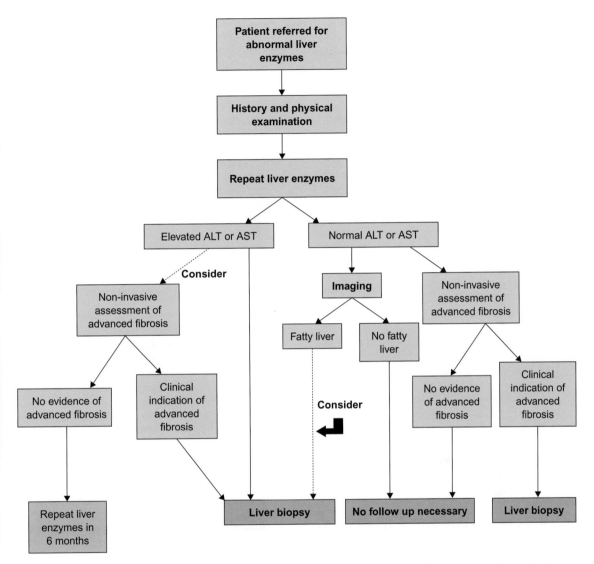

Fig. 13.2 An algorithm summarizing common diagnostic decisions encountered during the management of suspected non-alcoholic fatty liver disease (NAFLD). Patients are often identified initially by elevations of the alanine aminotransferase (ALT) or aspartate aminotransferase (AST), although the enzymes may be normal despite advanced liver disease resulting from non-alcoholic steatohepatitis (NASH). If the enzymes are elevated without known reversible causes such as medication-induced elevations, then a liver biopsy is often considered. If the enzymes are normal and imaging studies show the presence of fat (NAFLD), then the approach is less certain and continued observation during lifestyle modification may be warranted.

with NASH—may progress to cirrhosis and end-stage liver disease. This chapter provides the clinician with clues as to the underlying histopathological diagnosis based on historical facts, physical examination, laboratory data and imaging studies. Additionally, a review of independent clinical predictors of advanced NAFLD is provided to assist the clinician in making a decision to pursue further evaluation with a liver biopsy. An algorithmic approach to diagnosis is provided (Fig. 13.2), in the hope of assisting the clinician in making these decisions.

165

References

1 Harrison SA, Diehl AM. Fat and the liver: a molecular overview. *Semin Gastrointest Dis* 2002; **13**: 3–16.

2 Lee RG. Non-alcoholic steatohepatitis: a study of 49 patients. *Hum Pathol* 1989; **20**: 594–8.

3 Ludwig J, Viggiano TR, McGill DB, Ott BJ. Non-alcoholic steatohepatitis. *Mayo Clinic Proc* 1980; **55**: 434–8.

4 Sheth SG, Gordon FD, Chopra S. Non-alcoholic steatohepatitis. *Ann Intern Med* 1997; **126**: 137–45.

5 Ratziu V, Giral P, Charlotte F *et al.* Liver fibrosis in overweight patients. *Gastroenterology* 2000; **118**: 1117–23.

6 Harrison SA, Hayashi P. Clinical factors associated with fibrosis in 102 patients with non-alcoholic steatohepatitis [Abstract]. *Hepatology* 2002; **36**: 412A.

7 Chitturi S, Weltman M, Farrell GC *et al.* HFE mutations, hepatic iron, and fibrosis: ethnic-specific association of NASH with C282Y but not with fibrotic severity. *Hepatology* 2002; **36**: 142–9.

8 Clarke JM, Brancati FL, Diehl AM. Non-alcoholic fatty liver disease. *Gastroenterology* 2002; **122**: 1649–57.

9 Santos L, Molina EG, Jeffers LJ, Reddy KR, Schiff ER. Prevalence of non-alcoholic steatohepatitis among ethnic groups [Abstract]. *Gastroenterology* 2001; **120**: A630.

10 Caldwell SH, Harris DM, Patrie JT, Hespenheide EE. Is NASH underdiagnosed among African Americans? *Am J Gastrorenterol* 2002; **97**: 1496–500.

11 Powell EE, Cooksley WG, Hanson R *et al.* The natural history of non-alcoholic steatohepatitis: a follow-up study of 42 patients for up to 21 years. *Hepatology* 1990; **11**: 74–80.

12 Bacon BR, Farahvash MJ, Janney CG, Neuschwander-Tetri BA. Non-alcoholic steatohepatitis: an expanded clinical entity. *Gastroenterology* 1994; **107**: 1103–9.

13 Angulo P, Keach JC, Batts KP, Lindor KD. Independent predictors of liver fibrosis in patients with non-alcoholic steatohepatitis. *Hepatology* 1999; **30**: 1356–62.

14 Chitturi S, Farrell GC. Etiopathogenesis of non-alcoholic steatohepatitis. *Semin Liver Dis* 2001; **21**: 27–41.

15 Marchesini G, Bugianesi E, Forlani G *et al.* Non-alcoholic fatty liver, steatohepatitis, and the metabolic syndrome. *Hepatology* 2003; **37**: 917–23.

16 DeFronzo RA, Ferrannini E. Insulin resistance: a multifaceted syndrome responsible for NIDDM, obesity, hypertension, dyslipidemia, and atherosclerotic cardiovascular disease. *Diabetes Care* 1991; **14**: 173–94.

17 Harrison SA, Kadakia S, Lang KA, Schenker S. Non-alcoholic steatohepatitis: what we know in the new millennium. *Am J Gastroenterol* 2002; **97**: 2714–24.

18 Kumar KS, Malet PF. Non-alcoholic steatohepatitis. *Mayo Clinic Proc* 2000; **75**: 733–9.

19 Dixon JB, Bhathal PS, O'Brien PE. Non-alcoholic fatty liver disease: predictors of non-alcoholic steatohepatitis and liver fibrosis in the severely obese. *Gastroenterology* 2001; **121**: 91–100.

20 Sir-Petermann T, Angel B, Maliqueo M *et al.* Prevalence of type 2 diabetes mellitus and insulin resistance in parents of women with polycystic ovary syndrome. *Diabetologia* 2002; **45**: 959–64.

21 Struben VMD, Hespenheide EE, Caldwell S. Non-alcoholic steatohepatitis and cryptogenic cirrhosis within kindreds. *Am J Med* 2000; **108**: 9–13.

22 Willner IR, Waters B, Patil SR *et al.* Ninety patients with non-alcoholic steatohepatitis: insulin resistance, familial tendency, and severity of disease. *Am J Gastroenterol* 2001; **96**: 2957–61.

23 Lee Y, Wang MY, Kakuma T *et al.* Liporegulation in diet-induced obesity: the antisteatotic role of hyperleptinemia. *J Biol Chem* 2001; **276**: 5629–35.

24 Mensenkamp AR, van Luyn MJ, van Goor H *et al.* Hepatic lipid accumulation, altered very low density lipoprotein formation and apolipoprotein E deposition in apolipoprotein E3-Leiden transgenic mice. *J Hepatol* 2000; **33**: 189–98.

25 Bernard S, Touzet S, Personne I *et al.* Association between microsomal triglyceride transfer protein gene polymorphism and the biological features of liver steatosis in patients with type 2 diabetes. *Diabetologia* 2000; **43**: 995–9.

26 Degoul F, Sutton A, Mansouri A *et al.* Homozygosity for alanine in the mitochondrial targeting sequence of superoxide dismutase and risk for severe alcoholic liver disease. *Gastroenterology* 2001; **120**: 1468–74.

27 Day C. CD14 promoter polymorphism associated with risk of NASH. *J Hepatol* 2002; **36** (Suppl. 1): 21.

28 Musso G, Gambino R, De Michieli F *et al.* Dietary habits and their relations to insulin resistance and postprandial lipemia in non-alcoholic steatohepatitis. *Hepatology* 2003; **37**: 909–16.

29 Marchesini G, Brizi M, Bianchi G *et al.* Non-alcoholic fatty liver disease: a feature of the metabolic syndrome. *Diabetes* 2001; **50**: 1844–50.

30 Braverman IM. Skin signs in gastrointestinal disease. *Gastroenterology* 2003; **124**: 1595–614.

31 García-Monzón C, Martín-Pérez E, Iacono OL *et al.* Characterization of pathogenic and prognostic factors of non-alcoholic steatohepatitis associated with obesity. *J Hepatol* 2000; **33**: 716–24.

32 Schaffner F, Thaler H. Non-alcoholic fatty liver disease. In: Popper H, Shaffner F, eds. *Progress in Liver Diseases*, Vol. 8. New York: Grune & Stratton, 1986: 283–98.

33 George DK, Goldwurm S, MacDonald GA *et al.* Increased hepatic iron in non-alcoholic steatohepatitis is associated with increased fibrosis. *Gastroenterology* 1998; **114**: 311–8.

34 Bonkovsky HL, Jawaid Q, Tortorelli K *et al.* Non-alcoholic steatohepatitis and iron: increased prevalence of mutations of the *HFE* gene in non-alcoholic steatohepatitis. *J Hepatol* 1999; **31**: 421–9.

35 MacDonald GA, Powell LW. More clues to the relationship between hepatic iron and steatosis: an association with insulin resistance? [Editorial; comment]. *Gastroenterology* 1999; **117**: 1241–4.

36 Facchini FS, Hua NW, Stoohs RA. Effect of iron depletion in carbohydrate-intolerant patients with clinical evidence of non-alcoholic fatty liver disease. *Gastroenterology* 2002; **122**: 931–9.

37 Mendler MH, Turlin B, Moirand R *et al.* Insulin resistance-associated hepatic iron overload. *Gastroenterology* 1999; **117**: 1155–63.

38 Fargion S, Mattioli M, Fracanzani AL *et al.* Hyperferritinemia, iron overload, and multiple metabolic alterations identify patients at risk for non-alcoholic steatohepatitis. *Am J Gastroenterol* 2001; **96**: 2448–55.

39 Younossi ZM, Gramlich T, Bacon BR *et al.* Hepatic iron and non-alcoholic fatty liver disease. *Hepatology* 1999; **30**: 847–50.

40 Brunt EM, Ramrahkiani S, Cordes BG *et al.* Concurrence of histologic features of steatohepatitis with other forms of chronic liver disease. *Mod Pathol* 2003; **16**: 49–56.

41 Neuschwander-Tetri BA. Non-alcoholic steatohepatitis. *Clin Liver Dis* 1998; **2**: 149–73.

42 Saadeh S, Younossi ZM, Remer EM *et al.* The utility of radiological imaging in non-alcoholic fatty liver disease. *Gastroenterology* 2002; **123**: 745–50.

43 Graif M, Yanuka M, Baraz M *et al.* Quantitative estimation of attenuation in ultrasound video images: correlation with histology in diffuse liver disease. *Invest Radiol* 2000; **35**: 319–24.

44 Szczepaniak LS, Babcock EE, Schick F *et al.* Measurement of intracellular triglyceride stores by H spectroscopy: validation *in vivo*. *Am J Physiol* 1999; **276**: E977–89.

45 Lim AK, Patel N, Hamilton G *et al.* The relationship of *in vivo* ^{31}P MR spectroscopy to histology in chronic hepatitis C. *Hepatology* 2003; **37**: 788–94.

46 Skelly MM, James PD, Ryder SD. Findings on liver biopsy to investigate abnormal liver function tests in the absence of diagnostic serology. *J Hepatol* 2001; **35**: 195–9.

47 Daniel S, Ben-Menachem T, Vasudevan G, Ma CK, Blumenkehl M. Prospective evaluation of unexplained chronic liver transaminase abnormalities in asymptomatic and symptomatic patients. *Am J Gastroenterol* 1999; **94**: 3010–4.

48 Lindor KD, on behalf of the UDCA/NASH Study Group. Ursodeoxycholic acid for treatment of non-alcoholic steatohepatitis: results of a randomized, placebo-controlled trial. *Gastroenterology* 2003; **124** (Suppl.): A708.

49 Marceau P, Biron S, Hould F-S *et al.* Liver pathology and the metabolic syndrome X in severe obesity. *J Clin Endocrinol Metab* 1999; **84**: 1513–7.

50 Chitturi S, Abeygunasekera S, Farrell GC *et al.* NASH and insulin resistance: insulin hypersecretion and specific association with the insulin resistance syndrome. *Hepatology* 2002; **35**: 373–9.

51 Brunt EM, Janney CJ, Di Bisceglie AM, Neuschwander-Tetri BA, Bacon BR. Non-alcoholic steatohepatitis: a proposal for grading and staging the histologic lesions. *Am J Gastroenterol* 1999; **94**: 2467–74.

52 French METAVIR Cooperative Study Group. Intraobserver and interobserver variations in liver biopsies in patients with chronic hepatitis C. *Hepatology* 1994; **20**: 15–20.

14 The clinical outcome of NAFLD including cryptogenic cirrhosis

Stephen H. Caldwell & Anita Impagliazzo Hylton

Key learning points

1 The long-term prognosis for patients with NASH appears to depend on the initial histology. NAFLD types 1 and 2 (simple steatosis and steatosis with mild inflammation) are relatively stable conditions. However, NAFLD types 3–4 (NASH, characterized by the presence of fibrosis, balloon cells and Mallory bodies) is potentially progressive, with approximately 20% having increased fibrosis and up to 20% progressing to cirrhosis over 5–7 years.

2 Data regarding the natural course of NAFLD are limited. Furthermore, the potential progression to cirrhosis is often obscured by the insidious nature of NASH and the effects of medications for associated conditions (obesity, diabetes and hyperlipidaemia). Some medications such as tamoxifen, methotrexate and amiodarone may accelerate the condition.

3 Although vascular disease remains a predominant clinical concern, the development of cirrhosis produces substantial and often unrecognized morbidity. Common problems, which may be confused with depression, heart disease or intrinsic lung disease, include subtle encephalopathy, fluid retention and hepatopulmonary physiology.

4 Cirrhosis may also present as 'cryptogenic cirrhosis' with loss of characteristic fatty infiltration on biopsy. It commonly remains silent and goes unrecognized until the onset of a major complication of portal hypertension such as ascites or variceal bleeding. Hepatocellular cancer is increasingly observed in these patients.

Abstract

The natural history of non-alcoholic fatty liver disease (NAFLD) ranges from a stable long-term condition to a progressive disease leading to cirrhosis, portal hypertension and hepatocellular cancer. Cirrhosis often becomes evident at approximately 60 years, although it may develop at a much younger age and even in adolescence. It may be associated with histological steatohepatitis (non-alcoholic steatohepatitis [NASH] with cirrhosis) but it may also present as 'cryptogenic' cirrhosis with loss of characteristic steatosis. Preliminary data indicate that the risk for progression of NASH to cirrhosis varies with the histological characteristics of the initial biopsy. Simple steatosis (NAFLD type 1) and steatosis with only inflammation (NAFLD type 2) appear to be stable. In contrast, steatosis with inflammation *plus* fibrosis, balloon cells and/or Mallory bodies (NAFLD types 3–4 or NASH) carries a substantial risk for progression to cirrhosis (up to 20% over 5–7 years). If future studies confirm these estimates, the high prevalence of NAFLD and NASH in industrialized countries points to a tremendous increase in the incidence of cirrhosis over the foreseeable future. Although patients may rarely present with subacute liver failure, NASH is more typically an insidious process; liver disease is often unsuspected until a major complication develops such as ascites, variceal bleeding or hepatocellular cancer. While death in NAFLD is commonly the result of diabetes-associated vascular disease, the development of cirrhosis carries substantial but often unrecognized morbidity, and cirrhosis-related problems may eventually dominate the clinical course. In addition, the hepatic effects of concomitant therapy for obesity, diabetes and hyperlipidaemia present the clinician with additional uncertainty and as yet unresolved issues of long-term risk versus benefit.

Introduction

Although it is one of the most common of all liver disorders [1,2], the natural history of NAFLD remains in large part unclear. It is apparent that for many people with fatty liver, the condition is stable for years without overt symptoms. It may be a minor concern to their physician and lead to additional testing for viral hepatitis and admonitions regarding alcohol use. If associated with abnormal liver enzymes, it may be a hindrance to purchasing life insurance and may produce confusion over medication side-effects but it often remains static indefinitely. However, it is now apparent that a substantial proportion of these patients will ultimately develop more severe liver injury presenting with new-onset ascites or variceal bleeding many years after the diagnosis of 'fatty liver'. In addition, biopsy performed for abnormal liver enzymes frequently reveals NASH with bridging fibrosis or even silent cirrhosis. It has also become common to see older patients with cryptogenic cirrhosis in the setting of prior known fatty liver, long-standing obesity and type 2 diabetes. Advanced liver disease may become the dominant clinical problem in these patients, overtaking diabetes-related vascular disease. Not uncommonly, these patients eventually develop hepatocellular cancer. We review the current understanding of this remarkably broad spectrum of clinical severity associated with NAFLD (Fig. 14.1).

Historical perspective

An association between obesity and liver injury has been known since at least the mid-nineteenth century [3,4]. A number of papers in the mid-twentieth century further reported a relationship between steatosis, potentially progressive liver injury and obesity [5]. Later, the association between intestinal bypass and progressive steatohepatitis further raised awareness of this disease [6]. However, even after the publication of several landmark papers in the 1980s (including that of Ludwig which provided the disease with its most common appellation 'NASH') [7], it became commonly accepted that 'fatty liver' was a benign condition warranting little concern for the patient, the primary care physician, the endocrinologist or even the gastroenterologist. While these misconceptions have largely faded, there remains a good deal of lingering doubt about the overall prognosis of fatty liver.

Outcome of NAFLD based on initial histological classification

A conceptual division of NAFLD into 'big' and 'little' NASH was proposed at a consensus conference in 1998. McCullough noted at that time that there existed a spectrum of disorders which appropriately fall under the broad term 'fatty liver disease'. Since then, this same group has published a refined classification of NAFLD [8]. The authors ascertained 132 patients with long-term follow-up and whose baseline biopsy, performed between 1979 and 1987, had NAFLD. The biopsies were grouped into classes (Table 14.1): NAFLD type 1 or simple steatosis; type 2 or steatosis with inflammation; and types 3 and 4 characterized by steatosis, inflammation and fibrosis, balloon cells or Mallory bodies. A recent paper [9] has shown a high degree of correlation between types 3 and 4, such that these are now typically put together as one group representing 'NASH'. The primary outcomes of cirrhosis, mortality and liver-related mortality were determined with an average follow-up of 8 years.

The groups consisted of 49 type 1, 10 type 2, 19 type 3 and 54 type 4 subjects. Testing for hepatitis C virus (HCV) polymerase chain reaction (PCR) in a subset of the biopsies excluded HCV as a significant factor in most patients. No age or gender differences were noted between these groups. Combining types 1 and 2 and comparing these to the combined type 3 and 4 groups, the authors noted no difference in overall mortality, but a substantial difference in the frequency of cirrhosis was observed. Clinically defined cirrhosis developed

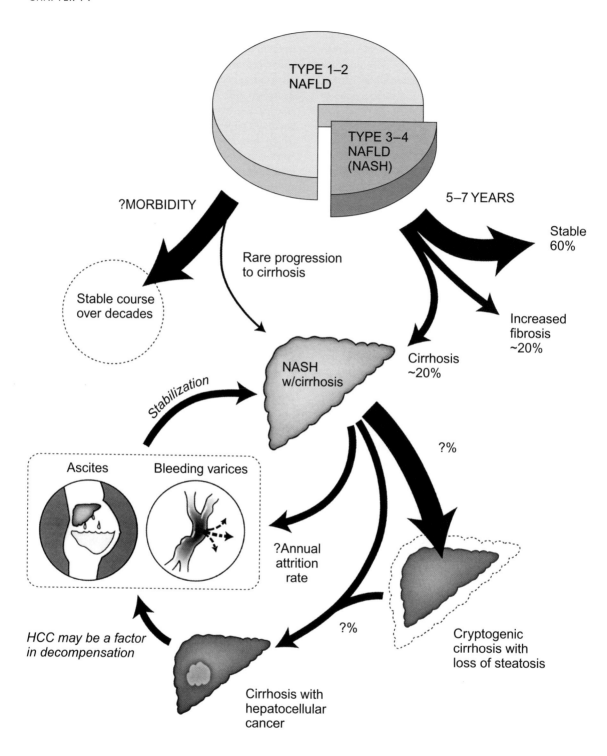

Table 14.1 NAFLD classification.

Modified NAFLD classification (After Matteoni *et al.* [8] and
Saadeh *et al.* [9].) All classes include the presence of steatosis
> 5%. Mallory bodies are not included as these generally
correlate with the presence of balloon cells and are variably
identified
Type 1 Simple steatosis. No inflammation and no evidence
of fibrosis on collagen stain
Type 2 Steatosis plus inflammation. No fibrosis by collagen
stain or balloon cells
Type 3–4 Steatosis, inflammation and fibrosis of any degree
or balloon cells (NASH). Note that the presence of balloon
cells and fibrosis generally correlate with each other. This
group constitutes NASH and imparts a more significant
prognosis with potential for progression over subsequent
years to decades

much more commonly in the combined type 3–4 group
(25%) than in the combined type 1–2 group (3%). In
the combined type 3–4 group, the crude liver-related
mortality rate was also higher than in the combined
type 1–2 group and it was also substantially higher than
the published crude death rate from US census data.
While limited by its retrospective nature and the lack
of histological follow-up, this work offers a convincing
explanation for the long-held perception of 'fatty liver'
as a reassuringly benign condition in some patients
and a potentially progressive disease in others.

The age of the patients with different types of NAFLD
as defined in this work warrants some additional comment. The similar age between the two major groups
(type 1–2 versus type 3–4) suggests that these groups
do not represent different stages in the evolution of

Fig. 14.1 (*opposite*) The natural history of NAFLD
based on the initial histological classification (see text and
Table 14.1). Estimations of progression are based on
currently available literature. NAFLD type 1–2 appears to
be stable with rare progression. NAFLD type 3–4 (NASH)
may remain stable in many but also carries a substantial
risk of progression to cirrhosis estimated at the figures
shown based on limited available studies. Cirrhosis is
often silent and may progress to a 'bland' stage with loss
of markers of steatohepatitis (cryptogenic cirrhosis).
Once cirrhosis develops, the patient may remain stable,
develop decompensation or further progress to
hepatocellular cancer.

NAFLD but rather that they represent two distinct
groups. In other words, it is unlikely that there is progression from type 1–2 over time to type 3–4. If there
was such a progression, it can be reasoned that there
would be either an age difference between the two
groups (the more severely afflicted would be older)
or there would be no detectable difference in the prognosis between the two groups. However, there does
appear to be a substantial difference in the long-term
prognosis between these two broad divisions of NAFLD
and there appears to be no age difference between them.
Thus, it is more likely that the individual who develops
fatty infiltration of the liver, soon thereafter either controls the problem (through as yet inadequately understood mechanisms) and remains stable indefinitely,
or the individual develops cellular injury manifested
histologically as steatohepatitis. To resolve this issue,
the histological course of the liver would need to be
assessed before and after the development of conditions,
such as obesity, associated with steatosis—a study that
is unlikely to be performed.

Other studies have supported the validity of this classification scheme and its associated prognosis. Hilden
et al. [10] reported on 58 patients with mild fatty liver
followed for up 33 years. The study antedated the proposed classification scheme but appears to largely
comprise types 1 and 2 patients because the presence
of Mallory bodies was used as an exclusion criterion.
Only one of these patients was known to have progressed to cirrhosis. In another retrospective study,
Teli *et al.* [11] demonstrated similar results. They
studied 40 patients with non-alcoholic steatosis and
absent inflammation or fibrosis on the index biopsy
(NAFLD type 1). Although inclusion of six patients
with cancer-related cachexia and secondary steatosis
limits the interpretation, the overall results were very
similar to those noted above. None of the patients
developed clinical cirrhosis after an average follow-up
of 11 years. Approximately half had persistent liver
enzyme abnormalities but among those undergoing
repeat biopsy, only one showed the development of
mild perivenular fibrosis after almost 10 years.

Because these data point towards the prognostic
importance of the baseline liver biopsy, it follows that
some knowledge of the prevalence of these various
types of NAFLD in high-risk groups would be of substantial practical value. Unfortunately there is a dearth
of histological prevalence data among type 2 diabetic
patients and hyperlipidaemic patients. More is known

171

about the patient with high body mass index (BMI). Although much has to be conjectured because of the lack of common terminology, it can be concluded from a number of series of obese patients that approximately 60% of obese individuals have relatively stable 'simple steatosis' or at most NAFLD type 2, while approximately 30% have type 3–4 NAFLD or frank NASH with fibrosis or balloon degeneration (marking them as more likely to develop cirrhosis) [12–16]. Only approximately 5% of such individuals have normal histology and, strikingly, approximately 5% have silent and previously unrecognized cirrhosis. Whether or not these prevalence figures can be extrapolated to diabetic and hyperlipidaemic patients is unknown but warrants additional study. What is known is that a substantial proportion of type 2 diabetic patients and hyperlipidaemic patients have fatty infiltration by non-invasive testing (a mode of testing that is likely to underdiagnose the problem) [17,18].

Histological progression: studies with serial biopsies

Knowledge of the risk of histological progression is essential to making recommendations and developing a prognosis for an individual patient. While NAFLD type 3–4 (NASH) appears to have a more severe long-term course compared to type 1 or 2, there are only a few studies utilizing serial biopsies to assess the rate of progression to increased fibrosis or cirrhosis (Table 14.2). Each of these studies is small and limited by lack of information on potential confounding variables such as changes in weight or lifestyle and concomitant medication use (see below). None the less, the available information indicates a substantial risk

of histological disease progression when the baseline biopsy shows features of NAFLD type 3–4 (NASH).

Lee [19] reported follow-up biopsies on 13 patients over an average of 3.5 years (1.2–6.9 years) after the baseline biopsy. Among these, 12 patients with features of NASH did not have cirrhosis at baseline. Follow-up histology revealed increased fibrosis in five and the development of cirrhosis in two patients. Similarly, Powell *et al.* [20] reported follow-up biopsy in 13 NASH patients with a median follow-up of 4.5 years. Repeat biopsy revealed worsening fibrosis in three, progression to cirrhosis in three, absent change in six and decreased fibrosis in one patient. Of note, this study also demonstrated the progression of NASH with fibrosis or cirrhosis to cryptogenic cirrhosis with loss of the histological hallmarks of steatohepatitis. Bacon *et al.* [21] reported serial biopsy in two patients studied over approximately 5 years; one of these patients developed cirrhosis. Finally, Ratziu reported serial biopsy in 14 patients with NAFLD [14]. Four of these had NASH at baseline while 10 had only steatosis with minimal or no necroinflammatory activity or fibrosis. Among the four with baseline NASH (necroinflammatory activity and some degree of fibrosis), one progressed to cirrhosis over approximately 5 years whereas none of the 10 patients without fibrosis progressed to cirrhosis.

Compiling these results provides a crude estimate of the histological progression from baseline NASH (NAFLD type 3–4) to advanced fibrosis or cirrhosis (Figs 14.1 & 14.2). From these series, it is estimated that approximately 40% had worsening histology: as many as 20% developed worsening fibrosis and up to 20% progressed to cirrhosis over approximately 5–7 years. Risk factors for progression remain unclear although a number of studies have examined predictors of more advanced fibrosis on the *baseline* biopsy.

Table 14.2 Serial biopsy studies.

Study [Reference]	n^*	F/U† (years)	Cirrhosis	Fibrosis	No change	Improved
Lee [19]	12	3.5	2	3	7	–
Powell *et al.* [20]	13	4.5	3	3	6	1
Bacon *et al.* [21]	2	5	1	–	1	–
Ratzui *et al.* [52]	4	5	1	1	2	–

* *n* represents the number of patients with baseline NASH without cirrhosis. Several of these publications also reported on patients with NAFLD types 1–2 or with cirrhosis (see text).
† The approximate duration of follow-up is expressed as a median.

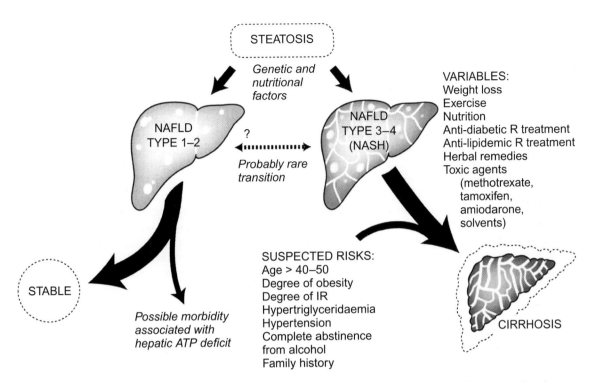

Fig. 14.2 Factors affecting the development and progression of NAFLD. Based on similar age at presentation and the long-term stability of NAFLD type 1–2 compared to the risk of progression in NAFLD type 3–4, it is likely that these two entities originate separately and probably diverge early without substantial transformation from one to the other. Whether or not there is morbidity associated with type 1–2 remains unclear. For those with fibrosis (NAFLD type 3–4), there are a number of risks for more severe disease and a number of variables that likely alter these risks.

Age over 40–50 years is prominent in this regard [22]. Of note, this relationship is consistent with the 10-year age difference between NASH patients and those with cryptogenic cirrhosis (see below). Other factors include the degree of obesity, the degree of diabetes or insulin resistance, hypertriglyceridaemia, hypertension, family history of NASH or cryptogenic cirrhosis, complete abstinence from ethanol, transaminase elevation and an aspartate aminotransferase : alanine aminotransferase (AST : ALT) ratio > 1 [23–26]. Female gender has not been a consistent predictor of more advanced histology on baseline biopsy; however, the preponderance of older females in most series of cryptogenic cirrhosis (see below) suggests a possible gender-based difference in prognosis.

It should be emphasized that all of these predictive factors have been shown to have relevance in predicting more severe histology on the *baseline* diagnostic biopsy. Similar predictors may eventually be identified that are associated with the risk of progression of disease after the baseline diagnosis of NASH has been established.

Mortality

Among people with major risks for NAFLD such as obesity and type 2 diabetes, liver-related mortality has largely been overshadowed by the high rate of cardio- and cerebrovascular death [27]. Nevertheless, cirrhosis has been shown to be an unexpectedly common cause of death among type 2 diabetics [28]. In this study, the authors reported on mortality in 1939 type 2 diabetic patients followed for over 9 years. Not unexpectedly, vascular disease was the most common cause of death, with heart disease accounting for 19%, cerebrovascular disease for 16% and renal disease for 13% of deaths. Cirrhosis was determined to be the cause of death in 6% of these patients, but the observed : expected ratio was actually higher (O : E = 2.67) for cirrhosis than for cerebro- and cardiovascular disease overall (O : E = 2.12). This indicates a substantial risk for liver-related mortality in these patients. Because of the growing epidemic of obesity, it is likely that the liver has become an even more significant factor among these patients in the interval since publication of this paper (see also Chapter 3). Liver-related morbidity is also likely an under-recognized factor in the management of diabetes and obesity.

The existence of cirrhosis in the obese diabetic patient without major outward signs of liver disease is not in doubt. Prior studies of liver disease among obese patients have demonstrated consistently that approximately 5% will have occult cirrhosis (see above). A small percentage of these patients come to medical attention with rapid development of overt and progressive signs of liver failure over a period of weeks to months [29]. More commonly, the disease is evident only by the presence of subtle abnormalities such as spider angiomas or thrombocytopenia. Eventually, approximately half of the patients with occult cirrhosis will present with a major complication of portal hypertension such as ascites or variceal bleeding (see Cryptogenic cirrhosis below).

Morbidity of advanced NASH in the metabolic syndrome

Silent cirrhosis is commonly diagnosed during the evaluation of some other problem in patients with long-standing obesity, type 2 diabetes or hyperlipidaemia [30]. The surprise discovery may occur during gallbladder surgery, the evaluation of thrombocytopenia or the evaluation of new-onset gastrointestinal bleeding or ascites. Its presence has significant implications for

the overall management of these patients. In particular, there are a number of potential drug interactions and adverse clinical scenarios in a patient with unrecognized cirrhosis.

Because cirrhosis fundamentally changes the physiology of the individual to that of the low systemic resistance (hyperdynamic) state, medication response is potentially altered. These patients frequently (perhaps invariably) have features of the 'metabolic syndrome' such as hypertension and diabetes and associated renal changes as well as increased risk for the development of cardiovascular disease. It is now common practice to employ a number of preventive treatments in this setting. However, in the presence of cirrhosis these interventions may have unexpected side-effects. For instance, angiotensin-converting enzyme (ACE) inhibitors can promote salt retention and ascites formation. In addition, aspirin and other antithrombotic medications can promote fluid retention and/or gastrointestinal bleeding (often from gastric antral vascular ectasia, GAVE).

The silent development of cirrhosis may also provide an alternative and potentially treatable explanation for certain symptoms (Table 14.3). For instance, fatigue in the obese diabetic patient with occult cirrhosis may actually reflect subclinical encephalopathy treatable with typical ammonia-lowering regimens. Gut dysmotility, either as a result of associated diabetes or as part of NAFLD [31], may contribute to constipation, making these patients especially prone to bouts of encephalopathy. Dyspnea may reflect the development of hepatopulmonary syndrome rather than intrinsic lung disease (without a high index of suspicion hepatopulmonary syndrome may be missed and the symptom attributed to some other process). These conditions indicate a need for increasing awareness of NASH among primary care providers, endocrinologists and cardiologists.

Symptom/sign	Common diagnosis	Possible explanation
Fatigue	Depression	Encephalopathy
SOB	Lung disease	Hepatopulmonary syndrome
Oedema	Heart failure	Cirrhosis-related oedema
Thrombocytopenia	ITP	Hypersplenism
Gastrointestinal bleeding	Ulcer, gastritis	Varices, GAVE
Ascites	Malignancy	Cirrhosis-related ascites

Table 14.3 Common misdiagnoses in occult cirrhosis. When cirrhosis develops silently in the obese diabetic patient, common complaints need to be re-interpreted as possibly related to underlying portal hypertension and portosystemic shunting.

GAVE, gastric antral vascular ectasia; ITP, idiopathic thrombocytopenia purpura; SOB, shortness of breath.

Furthermore, an expanded point of view of NAFLD is warranted based on the systemic nature of the metabolic syndrome. In this regard, it is interesting to speculate on the potential role of the mitochondria in NASH [32,33] and its associated conditions. The existence of variation in mitochondrial integrity in different tissues offers a possible explanation (mitochondrial heteroplasmy) [34] for both the primary liver injury and the systemic manifestations of the metabolic syndrome. Gut motility disorders, common in patients with NAFLD, may be an example of this hypothetical process. In addition, a unique and little described ocular gaze disorder (intermittent disconjugate gaze, IDG) seen in approximately 15% of NASH patients lends support to the hypothesis [35]. Vision impairment is typically absent in IDG but simple examination demonstrates disconjugate left or right lateral gaze which fluctuates in severity and may at times be undetectable suggesting easy muscle fatigue as the likely mechanism. Its increased presence in NAFLD patients and the association of similar ocular motor disorders in patients with primary mitochondrial myopathies point to a common pathogenesis in some patients.

Disease modifiers and confounding variables

There are a number of variables that may alter the natural course of NAFLD and which are likely to play some part in patients encountered day to day with this condition. Patients with NASH are often candidates for treatment with various agents aimed specifically at the components of the metabolic syndrome including obesity, diabetes and hyperlipidaemia. These agents may also have effects on the expression of NAFLD—their overall impact has not yet been fully elucidated.

Several studies have reported that thiazolidinediones alter the histological expression of NASH by decreasing inflammation. We previously demonstrated reduction in the inflammatory score with only a short course of troglitazone of 3–6 months in patients with NASH [36]. More recently, treatment with rosiglitazone resulted in a reduction of the pericentral vein inflammation resulting in predominantly periportal residual inflammation [37]. Similarly, pioglitazone has been shown to reduce inflammation in NASH [38,39]. The statin drugs, commonly used for coexisting hyperlipidaemia in NASH patients, have also had some positive effects histologic-

ally but have not been as well studied [40] (see also Chapter 24). Dietary plans, exercise, over-the-counter herbal remedies and modest ethanol use (which may actually be protective) also introduce variables that have not been very well studied. In contrast, other agents that these patients may require for comorbid conditions (e.g. tamoxifen for breast cancer, amiodarone for cardiac dysrhythmias or methotrexate for psoriasis) may accelerate cellular injury and require careful consideration of the risk : benefit ratio. The effects of these common and potentially confounding variables complicate the assessment of prognosis in NAFLD.

Cryptogenic cirrhosis

Cryptogenic cirrhosis—defined as cirrhosis of unknown cause after exhaustive diagnostic evaluation—remains a common problem accounting for 5–15% of cirrhosis patients in different series. While there are clearly a number of disease processes involved with the development of cryptogenic cirrhosis (including NASH, occult ethanol, subclinical autoimmune hepatitis and non-B non-C hepatitis), several studies have demonstrated a close association between NASH and cryptogenic cirrhosis. Based on the studies discussed below and a recent detailed histological analysis of explanted livers by Ayata et al. [41], it is estimated that NASH constitutes the underlying disease process in 30–70% of cryptogenic cirrhosis patients.

The seminal observation linking cryptogenic cirrhosis and NASH was that of Powell et al. [20] in a 1990 report in which serial biopsy of NASH patients demonstrated the loss of steatosis over years as the disease progressed from steatohepatitis with bridging fibrosis or cirrhosis to a stage of bland cirrhosis. The loss of steatosis in the regenerating nodules likely results from altered blood flow from portosystemic shunting [42]. Alternatively, it may result from capillarization of the sinusoids with loss of fenestrations and secondary impairment of lipoprotein delivery. However, a more fundamental alteration in hepatocyte fat metabolism has not been excluded. In both older series of cryptogenic cirrhosis and more recent reports discussed below, females constitute the majority of patients (approximately 60–70%) suggesting an increased risk of disease progression among females.

In histologically assessing cryptogenic cirrhosis, Contos et al. [43] published a useful descriptive scheme

Table 14.4 Classification of cryptogenic cirrhosis. (After Contos *et al.* [43] and Ayata *et al.* [40].)

---

1 Cirrhosis with features of steatohepatitis: scattered steatosis, Mallory bodies and glycogenated nuclei
2 Cirrhosis with features of autoimmune disease: scattered plasma cell or granulomatous inflammation
3 Cirrhosis with features of biliary obstruction: bile ductular proliferation, cholestasis
4 Bland cirrhosis

(Table 14.4). Among 30 liver explants from cryptogenic cirrhosis, six had absence of steatosis but 24 had variable and patchy fatty infiltration (mostly in the mild or 1 + range.) Twenty had Mallory hyaline and 21 had balloon cells. Seventeen of 30 had balloon degeneration, Mallory hyaline and steatosis; 10 more had at least two of these features. Inflammatory changes were mild and mostly limited to the septae. Twenty-six of 30 had glycogenated nuclei (a finding considered corroborative of underlying and antecedent NASH). The high prevalence of risk factors for NASH in these patients and the high recurrence rate following transplantation (nearly 100% by 5 years) supports the assertion that the majority of these cases represented progression of NASH. Based on the description of these explants, cryptogenic cirrhosis patients can be divided broadly into two categories: those with inconclusive but suggestive features of NASH and those with 'bland' cirrhosis.

We reported on a series of 70 consecutive patients with cryptogenic cirrhosis including both transplant and non-transplant candidates [44]. Among these patients, 70% were female and 73% had a history of obesity and/or diabetes. These patients had an average age of 60 years, compared to 50 years for a control group of consecutive NASH patients, suggesting a 10-year interval of disease progression between NASH and cirrhosis. The prevalence of obesity and/or diabetes among the cirrhosis patients was not different from the NASH patients but was significantly greater than that of age-matched patients with cirrhosis from HCV or primary biliary cirrhosis (PBC). In many patients with cryptogenic cirrhosis, a past history of obesity may be hidden because of weight loss associated with either ageing or cirrhosis. A careful history will often reveal the prior existence of long-standing obesity. Another striking finding among the cryptogenic cirrhosis

patients was that over half lacked major symptoms of portal hypertension; the cirrhosis was both cryptogenic and clinically silent.

Also observed in this study was the common presence among both NASH and cryptogenic cirrhosis patients of a family history of unexplained liver disease—an association further supported by two additional publications [45,46]. It was further noted that both among patients with NASH and those with cryptogenic cirrhosis, serum immunoglobulin A (IgA) was commonly elevated out of proportion to IgG. Serum IgA elevation, possibly as a result of lipid peroxidation and neoantigen formation, has long been associated with alcohol-induced steatohepatitis. A histological study has also demonstrated deposition of IgA in liver tissue of both non-alcoholic and alcohol-related steatohepatitis [47]. Further studies are underway to examine serum and liver IgA as a marker of prior NASH in patients with cryptogenic cirrhosis.

A somewhat different approach to associated risks in cryptogenic cirrhosis was taken in examining this issue by Poonwalla *et al.* [48], who published a report of 65 consecutive patients with cryptogenic cirrhosis awaiting liver transplantation. Each patient was compared to two age-matched control subjects with advanced cirrhosis from other aetiologies and awaiting transplantation. The prevalence of obesity (55% versus 24%) and diabetes (47% versus 22%) was twice as high in the cryptogenic group as the control group. Interestingly, the authors found no difference in the prevalence of hypercholesterolaemia between the groups. Ong *et al.* [49] reported on a series of 51 cryptogenic cirrhosis patients undergoing liver transplantation. Similar to other series, the patients were commonly overweight females and one-third had diabetes. Among the 25 patients undergoing post-transplant biopsy, 13 developed NAFLD. Of these, five developed NAFLD type 1 (simple steatosis) and eight developed NAFLD type 3–4 (NASH). Predictors of more severe histology post-orthotopic liver transplantation (OLT) included diabetes, hypertriglyceridaemia and greater BMI. The role of immunosuppression in the course of post-transplant NAFLD remains poorly defined. Possible interactions include the promotion of hepatic steatosis by glucocorticoids and the effects of cyclosporin A on the mitochondrial permeability transition pore.

In these transplant-based studies, cryptogenic cirrhosis patients have typically constituted approximately 10% of the total number of patients listed for transplantation during the study interval. Another perspective on this issue was provided by a report from Nair *et al.* [50], which demonstrated cryptogenic cirrhosis as the second most common cause of cirrhosis (after HCV) among obese patients awaiting transplantation. However, because NASH patients who progress to cirrhosis often are much older (the median age in our series was 63 years) and frequently have comorbid conditions resulting from obesity, diabetes and hyperlipidaemia, their candidacy for transplantation is likely to be compromised. Thus, assessment of the significance of cryptogenic cirrhosis based on transplant lists is probably an underestimation because many such patients are not considered for this intervention.

Prognosis of cryptogenic cirrhosis

As with any form of cirrhosis, a steady rate of attrition to more advanced disease and possibly malignancy can be expected. The prognosis of obesity-related cryptogenic cirrhosis remains somewhat uncertain. However, grounds for increased concern regarding the development of complications of portal hypertension and hepatocellular cancer are slowly emerging. Ratziu *et al.* [51] recently compared the course of 27 overweight patients with cryptogenic cirrhosis to 10 lean patients with cryptogenic cirrhosis and 391 patients with HCV-related cirrhosis in a retrospective follow-up cohort study. The prevalence of diabetes and hyperlipidaemia were significantly higher in the obese cryptogenic group compared to the lean cryptogenic cirrhosis group and the HCV group. This difference persisted even when controlling for BMI in the HCV group. The mean age of the obese cryptogenic cirrhosis group was 62 years compared to 45 years for the lean cryptogenic group.

Most striking in this report was that nine of 27 obese cryptogenic patients were initially diagnosed with cirrhosis at the time of a major complication of portal hypertension, and three more had hepatocellular cancer at or near the time of the initial diagnosis of cirrhosis. This finding, very similar to our own experience, is consistent with the insidious and often silent nature of cirrhosis among obese patients. After a mean follow-up of 22 months, two of the 15 patients presenting only with abnormal liver tests developed major complications of portal hypertension and five developed hepatocellular cancer. While precise rates of progression could not be determined, the overall severity and

risk for either a complication of portal hypertension or hepatocellular cancer were greater compared to the lean cryptogenic cirrhosis group, but were not different from the HCV patients. The authors concluded that obesity-related cirrhosis often diverges from the slow indolent process characteristic of NASH and it may behave as aggressively as HCV-related cirrhosis. The explanation for this observation remains uncertain because loss of an active steatohepatitis would, intuitively, suggest a slowing of the process. Older age or perhaps accelerated parenchymal extinction (a microvascular process) [52] may offer an explanation (see also Chapter 24).

Hepatocellular cancer and NAFLD

Several papers have recently been published linking NAFLD, insulin resistance, cryptogenic cirrhosis and hepatocellular cancer [53]. Obesity itself has been implicated as a risk for various neoplasms [54]. Experimentally, insulin resistance, associated hepatocyte hyperplasia and decreased apoptosis have been implicated as factors in the development of hepatocellular cancer in *ob/ob* mice [55]. Diabetes has also been implicated as a factor in patients with viral hepatitis or alcoholic liver disease [56]. The observations in two recent case reports indicating hepatocellular cancer as a possible natural progression of NASH-related cirrhosis have subsequently been supported by larger studies (in addition to that of Ratziu *et al.* [51] noted above) [57,58]. These two case reports (one male aged 62 years, one female aged 58 years—both with obesity and diabetes) described the development of hepatocellular cancer 6–10 years after the diagnosis of NASH was established by serological evaluation and biopsy.

Following these case reports, Bugianesi *et al.* [59] reported on 23 patients with cryptogenic cirrhosis and hepatocellular cancer and compared this cohort to 115 age-matched controls from a registry of 641 cirrhosis-related hepatocellular cancers. A history of obesity (BMI > 30) was significantly more common in the cryptogenic group (41% versus 16%) as was a history of diabetes (50% versus 20%). The authors did not detect a difference in the duration of disease, the prevalence of genetic markers for haemochromatosis or the character of the tumour (whether multifocal or metastatic). Compared to the overall group of hepatocellular cancer patients ($n = 641$), the cryptogenic cirrhosis group was older, consistent with past reports of cryptogenic cirrhosis largely afflicting an older population. However, in contrast to past series of cryptogenic cirrhosis patients but similar to results found by Ratziu *et al.* [51], there was a preponderance of males, suggesting an increased risk of hepatocellular cancer in males with cryptogenic cirrhosis.

Another report [60] reported the results of a prospective study on cirrhosis-related hepatocellular cancer. Among 105 patients with cirrhosis and hepatocellular cancer, 51% had HCV as the underlying disease but cryptogenic cirrhosis was the second most common association, accounting for 29% of cases. The majority (58%) of these had a history of obesity and six (20%) had documented prior steatohepatitis by biopsy performed an average of 4.5 years before the diagnosis of hepatocellular cancer. In contrast to the patients noted in prior series, these patients were mostly females, the tumours were often more advanced and the patient less likely to have undergone prior screening. In another large UNOS-based study of patients undergoing liver transplantation, Nair *et al.* [50] described obesity as a major risk factor for hepatocellular cancer among alcoholic and cryptogenic cirrhosis patients, but not a factor among other liver diseases including viral disease and autoimmune liver diseases. As discussed in Chapter 1, the role of occult hepatitis B virus infection and alcohol has not always been taken into account as risk factors for hepatocellular cancer in patients with cryptogenic cirrhosis, and the exact risk of this outcome for patients with cirrhosis due to NASH remains unclear.

Conclusions and future directions

In summary, the risk for progression of NAFLD to cirrhosis appears to depend on the initial histology at the time of diagnosis. Because NAFLD types 1 and 2 appear to have a typically long and stable course compared to NAFLD type 3–4 (NASH), it is likely that these broad categories (mild versus severe NAFLD) diverge at an early point after the development of hepatic steatosis. Among those who develop NASH and hence carry the greater risk of disease progression, many factors may influence disease progression to cirrhosis. These factors likely include genetic and nutritional variables as well as age and the use of medications for comorbid conditions. Mortality among these patients

remains, in the majority, a vascular issue but increasingly patients present with complications of cirrhosis in the absence of previously recognized liver disease. This phenomenon is probably a result of the growing epidemic of obesity in industrialized countries. Coupled with the increasing recognition of advanced NASH in younger patients and the often uncertain effects on the liver of medications used for comorbid conditions, these observations indicate a need for greater awareness and study of liver disease in both adult and paediatric patients with the metabolic syndrome. In particular, dietary and pharmacological interventions need to take into account their effects on the fatty liver. Currently, liver biopsy is the only means of accurately staging the disease and assessing the prognosis. However, there may in future be a role for non-invasive tests such as magnetic resonance spectroscopy as a means of widely 'sampling' the liver and determining the effects of various interventions on hepatocyte physiology and patient prognosis.

References

1 Byron D, Minuk GY. Profile of an urban hospital-based practice. *Hepatology* 1996; **24**: 813–5.
2 Mathieson UL, Franzen LE, Fryden A, Foberg U, Bodemar G. The clinical significance of slightly to moderately elevated liver transaminase values in asymptomatic patients. *Scand J Gastroenterol* 1999; **34**: 85–91.
3 Morgan W. *The Liver and its Diseases, Both Functional and Organic: Their History, Anatomy, Chemistry, Pathology, Physiology, and Treatment.* London: Homoeopathic Publishing, 1877: 144. University of Virginia Historical Collection.
4 Bockus HL. Fatty liver disease. In: *Gastro-Enterology,* Ed. HL Bockus. Vol. III, Philadelphia: Saunders, 1946: 385–92.
5 Zelman S. The liver in obesity. *Arch Intern Med* 1958; **90**: 141–56.
6 Faloon WW. Hepatobiliary effects of obesity and weight-reducing surgery. *Semin Liver Dis* 1988; **8**: 229–36.
7 Ludwig J, Viggiano TR, McGill DB, Ott BJ. Non-alcoholic steatohepatitis. *Mayo Clin Proc* 1980; **55**: 434–8.
8 Matteoni CA, Younossi ZM, Gramlich T *et al.* Non-alcoholic fatty liver disease: a spectrum of clinical and pathological severity. *Gastroenterology* 1999; **116**: 1413–9.
9 Saadeh S, Younossi ZM, Remer EM *et al.* The utility of radiological imaging in non-alcoholic fatty liver disease. *Gastroenterology* 2002; **123**: 745–50.

10 Hilden M, Juhl E, Thomsen AC, Christoffersen P. Fatty liver persisting for up to 33 years. *Acta Med Scand* 1973; **194**: 485–9.

11 Teli MR, James OFW, Burt AD, Bennett MK, Day CP. The natural history of non-alcoholic fatty liver: a follow-up study. *Hepatology* 1995; **22**: 1714–9.

12 Andersen T, Gluud C. Liver morphology in morbid obesity: a literature study. *Int J Obesity* 1984; **8**: 97–106.

13 Andersen T, Christoffersen P, Gluud C. The liver in consecutive patients with morbid obesity: a clinical, morphological and biochemical study. *Int J Obesity* 1984; **8**: 107–15.

14 Ratziu V, Giral P, Charlotte F *et al.* Liver fibrosis in overweight patients. *Gastroenterology* 2000; **118**: 1117–23.

15 Garcia-Monzon C, Martin-Perez E, Lo Iacono O *et al.* Characterization of pathogenic and prognostic factors of non-alcoholic steatohepatitis associated with obesity. *J Hepatol* 2000; **33**: 716–24.

16 Braillon A, Capron JP, Herve MA, Degott C, Quenum C. Liver in obesity. *Gut* 1985; **26**: 133–9.

17 Marchesini G, Brizi M, Morselli-Labate AM *et al.* Association of non-alcoholic fatty liver disease with insulin resistance. *Am J Med* 1999; **107**: 450–5.

18 Assy N, Kaita K, Mymin D *et al.* Fatty infiltration of liver in hyperlipidemic patients. *Dig Dis Sci* 2000; **45**: 1929–34.

19 Lee RG. Non-alcoholic steatohepatitis: a study of 49 patients. *Hum Pathol* 1989; **20**: 594–8.

20 Powell EE, Cooksley WG, Hanson R *et al.* The natural history of non-alcoholic steatohepatitis: a follow-up study of 42 patients for up to 21 years. *Hepatology* 1990; **11**: 74–80.

21 Bacon BR, Farahvish MJ, Janney CG, Neuschwander-Tetri BA. Non-alcoholic steatohepatitis: an expanded clinical entity. *Gastroenterology* 1994; **107**: 1103–9.

22 Angulo P, Keach JC, Batts KP, Lindor KD. Independent predictors of liver fibrosis in patients with non-alcoholic steatohepatitis. *Hepatology* 1999; **30**: 1356–62.

23 Nanji AA, French SW, Freeman JB. Serum alanine aminotransferase to aspartate aminotransferase ratio and degree of fatty liver in morbidly obese patients. *Enzyme* 1986; **36**: 266–9.

24 Sorbi D, McGill DB, Thistle JL *et al.* An assessment of the role of liver biopsies in asymptomatic patients with chronic liver test abnormalities. *Am J Gastroenterol* 2000; **95**: 3206–10.

25 Struben VMD, Hespenheide EE, Caldwell SH. Familial patterns of non-alcoholic steatohepatitis (NASH) and cryptogenic cirrhosis. *Am J Med* 2000; **108**: 9–13.

26 Dixon JB, Bathal PS, O'Brien PE. Non-alcoholic fatty liver disease: predictors of non-alcoholic steatohepatitis and liver fibrosis in the severely obese. *Gastroenterology* 2001; **121**: 91–100.

27 Gaede P, Vedel P, Larsen N *et al.* Multifactorial intervention and cardiovascular disease in patients with type 2 diabetes. *N Engl J Med* 2003; **348**: 383–93.

28 Sasaki A, Horiuchi N, Hasegawa K, Uehara M. Mortality and causes of death in type 2 diabetic patients. *Diabetes Res Clin Pract* 1989; **7**: 33–40.

29 Caldwell SH, Hespenheide EE. Subacute liver failure in obese females. *Am J Gastroenterol* 2002; **97**: 2058–62.

30 Caldwell SH, Han K, Hess CE. Thrombocytopenia and unrecognized cirrhosis. *Ann Intern Med* 1997; **127**: 572–3.

31 Sozo A, Arrese M, Glasinovic JC. Evidence of intestinal bacterial overgrowth in patients with NASH. *Gastroenterology* 2001; **120**: A118.

32 Caldwell SH, Swerdlow RH, Khan EM *et al.* Mitochondrial abnormalities in non-alcoholic steatohepatitis. *J Hepatol* 1999; **31**: 430–4.

33 Sanyal AJ, Campbell-Sargent C, Mirshahi F *et al.* Non-alcoholic steatohepatitis: association of insulin resistance and mitochondrial abnormalities. *Gastroenterology* 2001; **120**: 1183–92.

34 Johns DR. Mitochondrial DNA and disease. *N Engl J Med* 1995; **333**: 638–44.

35 Al-Osaimi A, Berg CL, Caldwell SH. Intermittent disconjugate gaze: a novel finding in nonalcoholic steatohepatitis and cryptogenic cirrhosis. *Hepatology* 2002; **36**: 408A.

36 Caldwell SH, Hespenheide EE, Redick JA *et al.* A pilot study of a thiazolidinedione, troglitazone, in non-alcoholic steatohepatitis. *Am J Gastroenterol* 2001; **96**: 519–25.

37 Neuschwander-Tetri BA, Brunt EM, Bacon BR *et al.* Histologic improvement in NASH following increased insulin sensitivity with the PPAR-γ ligand rosiglitazone for 48 weeks. *Hepatology* 2002; **36**: 379A.

38 Acosta RC, Molina EG, O'Brien CB *et al.* The use of pioglitazone in non-alcoholic steatohepatitis [Abstract]. *Gastroenterology* 2001; **120**: A546.

39 Sanyal AJ, Contos MJ, Sargeant C *et al.* A randomized controlled pilot study of pioglitazone and vitamin E versus vitamin E for non-alcoholic steatohepatitis. *Hepatology* 2002; **36**: A382.

40 Horlander JC, Kwo PY, Cummings OW, Koukoulis G. Atorvastatin for the treatment of NASH [Abstract]. *Gastroenterology* 2001; **120**: A544.

41 Ayata G, Gordon FD, Lewis WD *et al.* Cryptogenic cirrhosis: clinicopathologic findings at and after liver transplantation. *Hum Pathol* 2002; **33**: 1098–104.

42 Nosadini R, Avogaro A, Mollo F *et al.* Carbohydrate and lipid metabolism in cirrhosis: evidence that hepatic uptake of gluconeogenic precursors and of free fatty acids depends on effective hepatic flow. *J Clin Endocrinol Metab* 1984; **58**: 1125–32.

43 Contos MJ, Cales W, Sterling RK *et al.* Development of non-alcoholic fatty liver disease after orthotopic liver

transplantation for cryptogenic cirrhosis. *Liver Transpl* 2001; **7**: 363–73.

44 Caldwell SH, Delsner DH, Iezzoni JC *et al.* Cryptogenic cirrhosis: clinical characterization and risk factors for underlying disease. *Hepatology* 1999; **29**: 644–9.

45 Struben VMD, Hespenheide EE, Caldwell SH. Familial patterns of non-alcoholic steatohepatitis (NASH) and cryptogenic cirrhosis. *Am J Med* 2000; **108**: 9–13.

46 Willner IR, Waters B, Patil SR *et al.* Ninety patients with non-alcoholic steatohepatitis: insulin resistance, familial tendency and severity of disease. *Am J Gastroenterol* 2001; **96**: 2957–61.

47 Nagore N, Scheuer PJ. Does a linear pattern of sinusoidal IgA deposition distinguish between alcoholic and diabetic liver disease. *Liver* 1988; **8**: 281–6.

48 Poonawala A, Nair SP, Thuluvath PJ. Prevalence of obesity and diabetes in patients with cryptogenic cirrhosis: a case–control study. *Hepatology* 2000; **32**: 689–92.

49 Ong J, Younossi ZM, Reddy V *et al.* Cryptogenic cirrhosis and post-transplantation non-alcoholic fatty liver disease. *Liver Transpl* 2001; **7**: 797–801.

50 Nair S, Mason A, Eason J, Loss G, Perillo RP. Is obesity an independent risk factor for hepatocellular carcinoma in cirrhosis? *Hepatology* 2002; **36**: 150–5.

51 Ratziu V, Bonhay L, Di Martino V *et al.* Survival, liver failure, and hepatocellular carcinoma in obesity-related cryptogenic cirrhosis. *Hepatology* 2002; **35**: 1485–93.

52 Wanless IR, Wong F, Blendis LM *et al.* Hepatic and portal vein thrombosis in cirrhosis: possible role in the development of parenchymal extinction and portal hypertension. *Hepatology* 1995; **21**: 1238–47.

53 Ong JP, Younossi ZM. Is hepatocellular carcinoma part of the natural history of non-alcoholic steatohepatitis? *Gastroenterology* 2002; **123**: 375–8.

54 Murphy TK, Calle EE, Rodriquez C, Khan HS, Thun MJ. Body mass index and colon cancer mortality in a large prospective study. *Am J Epidemiol* 2000; **152**: 847–54.

55 Yang S, Lin HZ, Hwang J, Chacko VP, Diehl AM. Hepatocyte hyperplasia in non-cirrhotic fatty livers: is obesity-related hepatic steatosis a premalignant condition? *Cancer Res* 2001; **61**: 5016–23.

56 El-Sarag HB, Richardson PA, Everhart JE. The role of diabetes in hepatocellular carcinoma: a case–control study among United States veterans. *Am J Gastroenterol* 2001; **96**: 2462–7.

57 Cotrim HP, Parana R, Braga E, Lyra L. Non-alcoholic steatohepatitis and hepatocellular carcinoma: natural history? *Am J Gastroenterol* 2000; **95**: 3018–9.

58 Zen Y, Katayanagi K, Tsuneyama K *et al.* Hepatocellular carcinoma arising in non-alcoholic steatohepatitis. *Pathol Int* 2001; **51**: 127–31.

59 Bugianasi E, Leone N, Vanni E *et al.* Expanding the natural history of non-alcoholic steatohepatitis from cryptogenic cirrhosis to hepatocellular carcinoma. *Gastroenterology* 2002; **123**: 134–40.

60 Marerro JA, Fontana RJ, Su GL *et al.* NAFLD may be a common underlying liver disease in patients with hepatocellular carcinoma in the US. *Hepatology* 2002; **36**: 1349–54.

15 Practical approach to the diagnosis and management of people with fatty liver diseases

Jacob George & Geoffrey C. Farrell

Key learning points

1 In the appropriate metabolic setting, a primary diagnosis of non-alcoholic fatty liver disease (NAFLD) can be made with relative ease.

2 A complete history (including family history of diabetes) and examination as well as tests to exclude viral hepatitis are part of the initial evaluation of persons with suspected NAFLD.

3 Assessment for other features of the metabolic syndrome (e.g. hypertension, dyslipidaemia, central obesity) is mandatory and helpful as a basis for practical management.

4 Criteria for the diagnosis of obesity and overweight are different across racial groups.

5 Lifestyle intervention with diet and increased physical activity is the cornerstone of management in NAFLD/NASH.

6 Liver biopsy should be considered: (i) in those with warning signs of advanced liver disease; or (ii) in those with clinical features associated with advanced hepatic fibrosis (diabetes, age 45 years, significant overweight or obesity [body mass index ≥ 28 kg/m^2]), particularly if liver tests have failed to normalize after attempts at lifestyle adjustment.

7 Pharmacotherapy, particularly with insulin-sensitizing agents, show great promise but at present application should be limited to clinical trials.

8 In patients with type 2 diabetes and NAFLD, insulin-sensitizing agents could be considered as first-line drug therapy, although further weight gain may be an issue.

Abstract

The spectrum of non-alcoholic fatty liver diseases (NAFLD) encompasses simple hepatic steatosis, steatohepatitis and cirrhosis (Chapters 1 and 2). NAFLD is the hepatic manifestation of the insulin resistance or metabolic syndrome (Chapter 5). Thus, in the appropriate setting, a primary diagnosis of NAFLD can be made with relative ease on the basis of a history, physical examination and a basic panel of biochemical assessments. In persons with liver disease from other causes, the presence of insulin resistance may adversely influence the progression of liver injury (Chapter 24). A liver biopsy is the only method at present that can distinguish simple steatosis from steatohepatitis. The latter represents a progressive form of liver injury that, in a proportion, may lead to advanced hepatic fibrosis. The initial approach to the management of NAFLD is to institute a programme of lifestyle intervention comprising weight-reduction strategies and enhanced physical activity. The simultaneous identification and appropriate treatment of other components of the metabolic syndrome is crucial to reduce hepatic as well as cardiovascular morbidity and mortality. Failure to normalize liver tests after a period of 3–6 months is an indication to consider liver biopsy. To date, no universally accepted algorithms exist to identify persons with a high likelihood of having significant hepatic fibrosis and who may benefit from knowledge of their histopathology. Among the published studies, obesity, older age (over 45 years), the presence of type 2 diabetes, or the presence of warning signs of cirrhosis should prompt serious consideration for biopsy. In those with more advanced stages of disease confirmed by biopsy, aggressive lifestyle intervention strategies and enrolment in clinical trials of pharmacotherapy need to be considered.

Introduction

If current trends continue, primary care physicians and gastroenterologists will need to manage an increasing case-load of persons with NAFLD. Thus, an appreciation of the modes of clinical presentation, the optimal tools for diagnosis and therapeutic options is essential. Given the near epidemic proportions of the problems of diabetes, overnutrition and obesity in industrialized and developing nations, primary care physicians will also bear the brunt for case management. While drug therapies may eventually have a role in management, lifestyle intervention is likely to be more feasible and cost effective for the more than 50% of the population of many countries who are already overweight or obese, as well as specifically for the 10–20% of this group who have concomitant NAFLD/NASH. Thus, up-grading of skills by gastroenterologists, hepatologists and specialist medical societies, of patients, the community and government is a central issue for the prevention and control of NAFLD. The role of the specialist physician is likely to remain the identification and management of patients with NASH as opposed to benign forms of NAFLD (see Chapter 14), and particularly those with advanced hepatic fibrosis. Some patients with NASH may be suitable for pharmacotherapies as well as requiring follow-up for the development of liver-related morbidity and mortality.

This chapter presents a practical approach to diagnosis and management of fatty liver disorders. However, as emphasized thematically throughout the book, NAFLD is the *hepatic* manifestation of the metabolic syndrome, a systemic disorder with many health implications for type 2 diabetes, heart and other vascular disease, and as well as for cirrhosis. A complete metabolic assessment and appropriate therapy of associated conditions is therefore an essential part of individual patient care.

Diagnosis of fatty liver disease

For a more detailed account of the clinical features, investigation and management of persons with NAFLD, the reader is referred to Chapters 13 and 16. The focus of this chapter is a practical road map for clinicians caring for people with fatty liver disorders.

In the past, NAFLD has been primarily recognized in those presenting with abnormal liver tests. It is likely that this bias will continue because physicians are alerted by abnormal pathology results. However, it is now recognized that the full spectrum of NAFLD from steatosis to steatohepatitis, cirrhosis and liver-related morbidity can also occur in those with entirely 'normal' liver enzymes by conventional criteria [1]. This raises an important semantic and practical issue of 'normal' versus 'reference ranges' for liver biochemistry. Two recent publications have assessed the prevalence of elevated aminotransferase (AT) levels in the cohort of subjects from the Third US National Health and Nutrition Survey (NHANES III, 1988–94) (see also Chapter 3). In one report, the data set was evaluated in 15 676 subjects aged 17 years and older and the prevalence of AT elevation (men: aspartate aminotransferase (AST) > 37 IU/L, alanine aminotransferase (ALT) > 40 IU/L; women: AST or ALT > 31 IU/L) was 7.9%. Aminotransferase elevations unrelated to alcohol consumption, hepatitis B and C or haemochromatosis (presumed NAFLD) occurred in 5.4% of the cohort [2]. In contrast, when the data set was subanalysed including only the 8232 participants who had a fasting morning examination, and using the cut-off of ALT > 43 IU/L as elevated, the prevalence of presumed NAFLD after excluding other common causes was 2.8% [3].

To add to the debate, a recent retrospective cohort study from Milan assessed reference ranges for serum ALT levels in 6835 blood donors who were negative for hepatitis B and C markers and HIV. Based on 3927 persons who satisfied the criteria of normal body mass index (BMI), normal serum cholesterol, triglyceride and glucose levels and no concurrent medications, median

Table 15.1 Clinical presentations of patients with NAFLD.

1 Features of the metabolic syndrome*
2 Abnormal liver biochemistry
3 Abnormal hepatic imaging suggestive of fatty infiltration
4 Non-specific symptoms (fatigue, abdominal discomfort)
5 Upper gastrointestinal bleeding (portal hypertension), liver failure or liver cancer

* See Table 15.2.

serum ALT was 11 IU/L, while values were 6, 9, 15 and 26 IU/L for the 5th, 25th, 75th and 95th percentiles, respectively. Based on these data, healthy ranges for serum ALT values, defined as those below the gender-specific 95th percentile, were 30 IU/L for men and 19 IU/L for women [4]. Using the above revised cut-offs for 'abnormal' ALT, Ruhl and Everhart [3] found the prevalence of presumed NAFLD to be 12% for men and 14% for women. Thus, reference ranges for serum AT from many laboratories may not reflect the expected 'normal' values in healthy adults. Physicians therefore need to be alerted to the possibility that significant liver injury may occur in subjects with NAFLD who have AT levels within the 'reference' range, but which are clearly outside the 'normal' range for healthy adults.

With this caveat in mind, patients with NAFLD may present in one of five ways (Table 15.1). NAFLD is now accepted as the hepatic manifestation of the metabolic (or insulin resistance) syndrome (Table 15.2) [5–8] (see also Chapter 5). Thus, while abnormal biochemistry or imaging will alert the physician to follow diag-

nostic pathways for the assessment of liver disease, it is now prudent that all persons presenting with any feature of the metabolic syndrome be assessed for fatty liver disease as well as for other less classic features of the syndrome (as opposed to 'definitional criteria' specified elsewhere in the book) (see Chapter 5); the latter include hyperuricaemia, obstructive sleep apnoea and polycystic ovarian syndrome [9].

In those presenting with abnormal liver biochemistry or imaging suggestive of fatty liver disease, certain clues in the history and physical examination should raise the suspicion of metabolic liver disease (Table 15.3). Of particular importance, questioning regarding recent increases in weight, lifestyle changes and of a family history of NAFLD or type 2 diabetes is mandatory in any patient assessed for abnormal liver biochemistry or a 'bright' liver on ultrasound suggestive of NAFLD. In a recent study of 66 patients with NASH [5], 33 had abnormalities of glucose tolerance, while 13 of 33 (39%) of the remainder had a family history of type 2 diabetes in one or more first-degree relative. In another report [10], 16 of 90 (18%) patients with NASH had a first-degree relative with the condition.

Likewise, an acute phase elevation in serum ferritin that is not associated with increases in transferrin saturation is present in up to 40% of patients with NAFLD; this common finding should therefore alert the physician to the possible diagnosis of NASH [11–15]. Similarly, in patients with non-replicative forms of viral hepatitis, the presence of abnormal liver biochemistry and/or presence of 'rubbery' hepatomegaly should alert the clinician to the presence of NAFLD rather than chronic viral hepatitis. Finally, it is increasingly

Table 15.2 Diagnostic criteria for the insulin resistance syndrome. Modified from the World Health Organization criteria [8].

Component	Definition
Diabetes mellitus, impaired glucose tolerance *and/or* insulin resistance, together with two or more of the following:	
Raised arterial blood pressure	140/90 mmHg, or documented use of antihypertensive therapy
Raised serum triglycerides	≥ 1.7 mmol/L
and/or low serum HDL-cholesterol	< 0.9 mmol/L for men; < 1.0 mmol/L for women
Central obesity	Waist : hip ratio > 0.90 (for men)
	waist : hip ratio > 0.85 (for women)
	or body mass index > 30 kg/m^2
Microalbuminuria	Urinary albumin : creatinine ratio (20 mg/g)
	or urinary albumin excretion rate (20 µg/min)

HDL, high-density lipoprotein.

Table 15.3 Clinical clues to the diagnosis of NAFLD.

Unexplained abnormal liver tests with:

Recent weight gain, expanding waistline, change of lifestyle
(unemployment, retirement, disability)
Type 2 diabetes or impaired glucose tolerance
Family history of type 2 diabetes or NAFLD
Obesity (particularly central [visceral] obesity)
Dyslipidaemia (elevated triglyceride, low high-density
lipoprotein)
Other features of the insulin resistance syndrome or its
complications: arterial hypertension, ischaemic heart
disease, vascular disease
Raised serum ferritin with normal transferrin saturation
Other liver diseases and the presence of 'metabolic' risk
factors
Non-replicative forms of viral hepatitis B or C

recognized that metabolic (fatty) liver disease may be associated with accelerated disease progression in those with liver diseases from any aetiology, including alcoholic liver disease [16] and viral hepatitis [17,18]. Hence, physicians should not be dissuaded from a diagnosis of NAFLD as an additional and modifiable liver disorder in persons with other forms of liver disease and the presence of metabolic risk factors (see Chapters 23 and 24).

The alcohol history must be carefully evaluated in persons with abnormal liver biochemistry. This involves both repeated questioning of the index person, and also of close family members. For clinical research, significant alcohol consumption needs to be excluded. 'Significant' consumption is variously defined as 140 g/ week and 20 g/day in men and 10 g/day in women. In clinical practice, it is likely that there is a large proportion of individuals in whom liver disease may be caused by the combination of toxic levels of alcohol consumption and metabolic fatty liver disease (see also Chapter 2). In these persons, alcohol intake should be reduced to the safe levels suggested above (or discontinued completely if it is unlikely that self-control can limit intake to safe levels), concomitant with other dietary approaches aimed at reducing insulin resistance. The importance of lifetime alcohol exposure (versus recent levels of intake) is discussed in Chapter 24.

Abnormal imaging, typically a hyperechoic liver on an ultrasound performed for another indication, is often the first clue to the presence of NAFLD. Conversely, a 'bright' liver on ultrasound may bring useful confirmatory information in a person with suspected NAFLD. However, it should be emphasized that the presence of fat, fibrosis or elevated hepatic iron stores can have an identical sonographical appearance. The sensitivity of sonography for the detection of hepatic fatty infiltration in a recent study was 67%, specificity was 77% and the positive predictive value was 67% [19]. However, ultrasound had 100% sensitivity for the detection of more extensive hepatic steatosis, as defined by 33% of cells showing steatosis [20].

In NAFLD, presentation with symptomatic liver disease (ascites, variceal bleeding, encephalopathy, hepatocellular cancer) has been infrequent. The large burden of NAFLD in industrialized nations [3], and the fact that NASH-associated cirrhosis has an identical prognosis to cirrhosis from chronic hepatitis C [21] (see also Chapter 3), suggests that there is significant case ascertainment bias in attributing liver disease to end-stage NAFLD.

Recent reports indicate that in patients presenting with cryptogenic or obesity-related cirrhosis, NAFLD is likely to be the underlying aetiological cause in approximately two-thirds of cases (see Chapter 14) [22,23]. Further, in current practice, NASH-associated liver failure may present in the later decades (7th and 8th) in individuals with other comorbid conditions, and is therefore often overlooked. For instance, insulin resistance, diabetes and diabetic metabolic control can be significantly worsened by the presence of advanced hepatic fibrosis or cirrhosis, which impairs insulin clearance. In the future, it is likely that NAFLD-associated liver failure may present in earlier decades, given the epidemics of obesity and diabetes affecting young adults and children (see Chapter 19). Advocacy to improved physician and patient awareness of the hepatic consequences of the metabolic syndrome is therefore important.

Patients with the earlier stages of NAFLD may present with non-specific symptoms (see Chapter 13) including fatigue and right upper quadrant pain. The latter is usually a dull discomfort, sometimes compared to a toothache, and often associated with hepatic tenderness so that the person does not feel comfortable lying on the right side. Rarely, more severe pain may be a clue to hepatic pathology. While fatigue is very common, a thorough psychosocial and medical history, as well as a complete physical examination, is required before attributing it to NAFLD. Other common disorders (depression, anaemia, sleep disorders) need to be considered (see also Chapter 14). Unless liver failure has supervened, the physical examination may be normal or only reveal hepatomegaly; the texture of the liver is firm but not hard ('rubbery'), and this is occasionally associated with some tenderness.

When to diagnose NAFLD

While conventionally considered a disease of exclusion, it is important for physicians to consider a positive diagnosis of NAFLD based on the history and physical examination. Features of the metabolic syndrome in association with abnormal liver biochemistry and serum lipids or a 'bright' liver on ultrasound are present in the vast majority of patients. Often the major clue for considering NAFLD as a diagnostic possibility is the presence of overweight or obesity and, more importantly, central obesity and a family history of diabetes. There is clear evidence that the risk of cardiovascular morbidity and mortality in relation to anthropometric variables differs across ethnic groups. Thus, given the enormous cross-cultural migrations that have taken place to regions such as North America and Australia in recent decades, physicians should be aware of ethno-specific cut-offs for anthropometric criteria (Table 15.4) (see also Chapter 18).

Clearly, a discrete panel of laboratory tests needs to be considered in patients presumed to have NAFLD. Diabetes should be excluded with a fasting blood glucose. Appropriate therapy must be instituted if this is present. Tests of insulin resistance (e.g. the homoeostasis model assessment (fasting glucose [mmol/L] × fasting insulin [units]/22.5) or impaired glucose tolerance based on a glucose tolerance test, while not routinely used in clinical practice, should be strongly considered. This is because NAFLD is rarely if ever present in the absence of insulin resistance (see Chapter 5). Estimation of serum lipids and serology for viral hepatitis B and C is mandatory. In the Anglo-Celtic population, consideration must also be given to the performance of iron studies, as haemochromatosis may occur in up to 1 in 300 of the population and may present with non-specific symptoms. As indicated earlier, serum ferritin is increased in approximately 40%, but haemochromatosis is easily excluded in most cases by the percentage iron saturation of transferrin, together with genetic testing (C282Y, H63D). In those

Table 15.4 Measuring components of adiposity. (After World Health Organization [24] and International Diabetes Institute [25].)

Category	Anthropometric criteria
Overweight	
White	BMI $\geq 25 \, kg/m^2$
Asian	BMI $\geq 23 \, kg/m^2$
Pacific Islander	BMI $\geq 26 \, kg/m^2$
Obese	
White	BMI $\geq 30 \, kg/m^2$
Asian	BMI $\geq 25 \, kg/m^2$
Pacific Islander	BMI $\geq 32 \, kg/m^2$
Central obesity	
White	WC > 102 cm (men)
	WC > 88 cm (women)
Asian	WC $\geq$ 90 cm (men)
	WC $\geq$ 80 cm (women)
Pacific Islander	Not determined

BMI, body mass index; WC, waist circumference.

with pointers in the clinical history or baseline biochemistry (e.g. a positive family history of Wilson's disease or marked elevations in AT levels), other tests may be indicated including tests for autoimmune liver disease, Wilson's disease and coeliac disease (see Chapter 21). Where the clinical history, examination and baseline biochemistry is suggestive of NAFLD, hepatic imaging by ultrasound can be a useful and relatively inexpensive test that will show appearances consistent with steatosis in two-thirds of cases. However, hepatic imaging cannot distinguish steatosis from steatohepatitis and cirrhosis.

A significant conceptual advance in understanding the pathogenesis and progression of chronic liver disease is the knowledge that liver disease of any aetiology can be significantly worsened by the presence of insulin resistance (NAFLD) [17,26,27]. From a clinical perspective, therefore, the assessment of any form of liver disease should include a consideration of modifiable metabolic cofactors, including obesity, insulin resistance, diabetes and features of the metabolic syndrome. Thus, it is incumbent on the physician treating an obese or diabetic patient with chronic hepatitis C or alcoholic liver disease to ensure control of diabetes and lifestyle modification to improve central obesity, lipid disorders and other features of the metabolic syndrome. Control of these factors may contribute to reducing disease progression separately to effective treatment of the underlying liver disease (see also Chapter 24).

When to consider a liver biopsy

While a liver biopsy can ultimately confirm a diagnosis of NAFLD and determine its severity, for the vast majority of patients seen in the primary care setting, biopsy is not required for patient assessment and the institution of appropriate management, at least in the first instance.

The aims of liver biopsy for persons suspected to have NAFLD are threefold. First, a biopsy can confirm the histological diagnosis of fatty liver disease and exclude other disorders. In a recent study of 36 asymptomatic patients with non-specific persistent liver test abnormalities, the presumptive prebiopsy diagnosis was altered in 14% of cases and influenced the frequency of subsequent monitoring in 36% [28]. Likewise, biopsy may help in the diagnosis of surreptitious alcohol abuse by demonstrating 'florid' changes (see Chapter 2) [26].

Secondly, liver biopsy is currently the only available method to distinguish between simple steatosis and steatohepatitis (see Chapter 2). As outlined in Chapters 3, 13 and 14, this distinction is not simply a matter of semantics, as steatohepatitis can progress in a proportion of individuals to advanced hepatic fibrosis, liver failure and, rarely, liver cancer. Finally, a biopsy provides information on the stage of hepatic fibrosis in NASH, the most crucial determinant of long-term outcomes (see Chapter 3). Such information is particularly important in the light of data indicating the difficulty of clinical criteria to identify advanced fibrosis or compensated cirrhosis [21,29–31]. Thus, in a recent study of 23 persons with NASH-associated cirrhosis, only 26% had an AST : ALT > 1 and four were 36 years of age or younger [21].

While there are several cogent reasons for considering liver biopsy in persons with presumed NAFLD/NASH, it is neither feasible nor appropriate to biopsy all patients, except in the setting of a clinical research agenda. To date, no universally accepted algorithms exist to identify patients who have a high likelihood of deriving benefit from the information provided by a liver biopsy (e.g. more aggressive lifestyle intervention, careful monitoring, enrolment in clinical trials). Among the published studies, a few clinical features have consistently suggested an increased likelihood of advanced stages of hepatic fibrosis. These are older age, obesity and type 2 diabetes [15,30,32–34]. Less consistent findings in those with advanced fibrosis include an elevated ALT, hypertriglyceridaemia, hypertension and female gender [11,30,33]. The use of non-invasive markers to predict fibrotic severity of NAFLD/NASH is considered in more detail in Chapter 3, and has been updated (to June 2004) in Chapter 24.

The issue of whether female gender predisposes to advanced hepatic fibrosis is particularly vexed. Currently, it is unclear if this represents case ascertainment bias, the possibility that males with NAFLD die of other disorders, or as yet unknown factors. Until large (more than 300 persons) validated cohort studies are published, it seems prudent to consider liver biopsy in subjects with suspected NAFLD who are 45 years of age or older, diabetic and significantly overweight or obese (BMI ≥ 28 kg/m^2 for white people). The presence of additional features of the metabolic syndrome, including hypertension and hypertriglyceridaemia, should lower the threshold for considering liver biopsy in these individuals. In addition, certain features suggestive of cirrhosis, irrespective of the presence of other criteria, should prompt consideration for early liver biopsy. These include a hard liver edge, an AST : ALT ratio > 1, a low platelet count or serum albumin and imaging findings suggesting portal hypertension (dilated portal vein, hepatofugal blood flow in portal vein, splenomegaly).

While a liver biopsy is being considered in individuals who meet the above criteria, an equally important issue is the timing of the biopsy. Most experts in the field would consider it valuable to embark on or recommend a 3–6 month trial of lifestyle intervention in an attempt to normalize AT levels before proceeding to liver biopsy, unless there are warning signs to suggest advanced hepatic fibrosis (Fig. 15.1). This view is endorsed by the editors.

Management of NAFLD

At present there are no consensus guidelines for the management of patients with NAFLD/NASH. This situation is likely to change over the coming decade with improved understanding of the pathophysiology

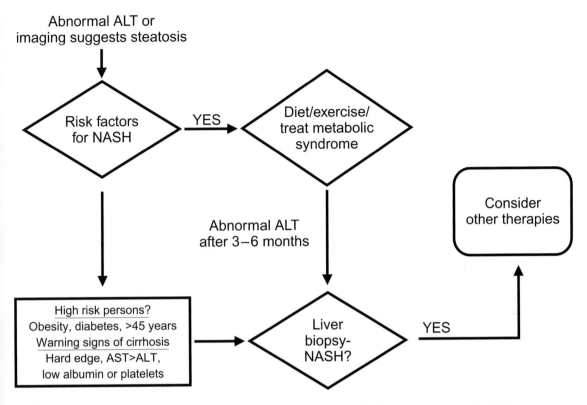

Fig. 15.1 A practical approach to the diagnosis and stepwise therapy of non-alcoholic fatty liver diseases (NAFLD).

of NAFLD and the completion of evidence-based life-style modification and pharmacotherapeutic trials for management of these disorders. In broad terms, therapy should target:

1 Components of the metabolic syndrome

2 Steatohepatitis

3 Advanced liver disease (screening for treatable complications of portal hypertension, e.g. large esophageal varices, gastric arterio-venous ectosia).

Patients with NAFLD are at risk of both liver-related and non-liver-related (particularly vascular) morbidity and mortality. In those with earlier fibrotic stages of NAFLD at diagnosis, non-liver disease-related disease end-points are likely to predominate, while in those with advanced hepatic fibrosis, liver disease-related end-points are likely to have a major impact (see Chapters 3 and 14) [21–23,35,36]. Thus, a thorough assessment for individual components of the metabolic syndrome and appropriate therapy of underlying diabetes, hypertension or dyslipidaemia is warranted.

Because insulin resistance is near universal in persons with NAFLD/NASH, strategies to lower insulin resistance are a logical first step. Given the prevalence of NAFLD in industrialized and developing nations (see Chapters 3, 5 and 18), and the cost and potential untoward adverse effects of drug therapy (Chapter 16), pharmacotherapy is likely to remain a second choice for a disease that is, in large part, lifestyle based [37,38]. As cited in a recent editorial on diabetes prevention, which could apply equally to persons with NAFLD, three types of interventions are possible.

1 Interventions that limit fat accumulation in the body (the reduction of central obesity is associated with less insulin resistance; see Chapter 4)

2 Strategies that uncouple obesity and insulin resistance (reducing insulin resistance and thereby preventing or delaying β-cell failure)

3 Interventions that directly preserve β-cell mass and/or function, thereby preventing or delaying the metabolic consequences of diabetes [39].

Among these, three recent large studies indicate that lifestyle intervention with diet and exercise can reduce the risk of diabetes in high-risk subjects. Further, they are at least as effective as drug therapy with metformin [40–42]. Clearly, therefore, lifestyle intervention can reduce insulin resistance and we believe it should be the first-line treatment of NAFLD/NASH.

In light of the above cogent considerations of pathophysiology, a recent review of the literature found that there are surprisingly few data to support or refute the recommendation for weight reduction as an effective therapy [43]. Among 517 potentially relevant studies, only 15 met the inclusion criteria of reporting histology, serum AT levels or hepatic imaging in obese subjects who had undergone weight reduction. Further, these 15 studies included only one randomized and two randomized controlled trials, and only three included more than 50 persons [43]. Although, all 15 studies reported improvement in liver outcomes (histology, serum AT levels or hepatic imaging), in one study hepatic histology worsened in those with weight loss that exceeded 1.6 kg/week [43,44]. This analysis infers that there is a great need for lifestyle programmes in subjects with NAFLD which include robust markers of liver disease progression, including histology. The results then need to be correlated with potential non-invasive markers, including AT levels, hepatic imaging and potential serum markers suggested as fibrotic markers among persons with hepatitis C [45–47].

Until such evidence-based data are available, it seems prudent to recommend a sustainable programme of diet and exercise aimed at both weight loss and subsequent weight maintenance and increased physical activity. However, rapid weight loss, in excess of 1 kg/week, should be avoided [44]. In order to achieve these goals, a multidisciplinary approach is essential. This could include a dietitian and/or a physical therapist [40–42, 48,49]. Involvement of the family and personal supports of the index case are crucial for establishing long-lasting lifestyle change.

Based on the National Heart Lung and Blood Institute (NHLBI) and the National Institute of Diabetes and Digestive and Kidney Diseases (NIDDK) expert panel guidelines, the initial target for weight loss should be 10% of baseline weight within a period of 6 months (0.5–1 kg/week) [50]. This can be achieved through a variety of strategies. Based on the Diabetes Prevention Programme (DPP) study [51], guidelines include physical activity of moderate intensity (e.g. brisk walking at least 5 days/week, 30 min per occasion, 150 min/week) and a low-energy low-fat diet (less than 30% of energy intake). While the composition of dietary formulations in relation to weight loss and NAFLD have not been examined, it would appear prudent to decrease saturated fats and to increase polyunsaturated fats and antioxidants (particularly vitamin C), and to add complex carbohydrates rich in fibre (e.g. 15 g/day), fruit and vegetables [52]. Guidelines for appropriate diets include the American Heart Association (AHA) heart-healthy diet [53] and for those with diabetes, the American Diabetes Association (ADA) diet [54]. Such interventions and public health promotion programmes should ideally begin in childhood as this group represents the future burden of disease to the community.

Surgical therapies for weight reduction

Absorptive or restrictive (gastric banding) procedures are increasingly being used as therapy for weight reduction (see Chapters 16 and 20). Procedures such as jejuno-ileal bypass are contraindicated in patients with NAFLD/NASH; they may lead to worsening of liver disease and hepatic decompensation. Procedures such as banding are probably safer [33], but significant safety issues remain in those with NAFLD/NASH and hepatic fibrosis, because weight loss of up to 4.5 kg/month can occur and this may be associated with worsening of liver injury [43,44].

Pharmacotherapy of NAFLD

Several small studies of pharmacotherapy in NASH have been completed, and large-scale trials are underway (see Chapters 16 ad 24). Application of pharmacotherapy to NAFLD/NASH may need to be lifelong, thereby incurring a considerable cost to the community and a burden of adverse effects such as weight gain. Thus, a critical issue is the targeting of therapy to patients most likely to benefit in terms of liver-related disease end-points. At present, no algorithms have been prospectively validated for the identification of individuals at high risk for disease progression. Even if such a cohort could be identified, cirrhosis in NASH may be slowly progressive. Hence, to demonstrate cost efficacy (cost per quality year of life saved from liver disease-related morbidity or mortality), long-term

Table 15.5 Potential pharmacotherapeutic agents for use in NAFLD.

Drug class	Examples
Weight loss drugs	Orlistat, phentermine, sibutramine
Insulin-sensitizing medications	
Biguanides	Metformin
PPARγ agonists	Rosiglitazone, pioglitazone
PPARα/γ agonists	Raraglitazone
PPARα agonists	Clofibrate
Lipid-lowering agents	
Triglyceride	Gemfibrozil,* clofibrate, probucol*
HMG CoA reductase inhibitors	Atorvastatin
Antioxidants	Vitamin E, betaine, probucol, N-acetylcysteine
Other hepatoprotective drugs	Ursodeoxycholic acid

* Not available in USA.

studies spanning decades may be required. Given the scope of the epidemic of NAFLD, it is prudent for the clinician to evaluate any new drug treatment study in relation to whether institution of lifelong therapy is likely to alter liver disease end-points, and the associated costs and potential detriments of such treatment. There is a pressing need for clinical studies and consensus guidelines in this field.

A variety of therapeutic strategies have been attempted in patients with NAFLD. These are categorized and discussed in detail in Chapter 16 and summarized in Table 15.5. Of the agents studied, drugs that effect weight loss such as orlistat, in addition to that obtained by diet and exercise, may be of benefit, at least during the weight loss rather than weight maintenance phase of NAFLD/NASH therapy [55,56] (and see Chapter 24). Use of insulin-sensitizing agents hold the most promise; however, large-scale clinical trials are awaited and these agents cannot be recommended, particularly as they facilitate weight gain [57]. Of drugs in this class, metformin reduces hepatic lipid in both animal and human studies [58,59]. It is cheap, has a long history of use in clinical practice, does not cause hypoglycaemia even in non-diabetic persons and has an excellent safety profile in those without advanced liver or renal disease. It is not yet known whether it affects progression of NAFLD.

Peroxisome proliferator activator receptor γ (PPARγ) agonists are potent insulin-sensitizing agents in clinical use for the last decade. The recently published Troglitazone in Prevention of Diabetes (TRIPOD) study [60] clearly demonstrates that in women with impaired glucose tolerance (insulin resistance), diabetes incidence in the treated group was approximately 55% lower than in placebo controls. Further, protection from diabetes was closely related to the degree of reduction in endogenous insulin resistance, and persisted 8 months after study medication was ceased. The results point to the efficacy of this class of compounds to reduce insulin resistance, which is thought to underlie NAFLD. Three small studies of the use of this class of compounds have been reported [57,61–63] (and see Chapter 24). As expected, they showed improvements in serum AT levels, hepatic steatosis, inflammatory scores, ballooning and zone 3 fibrosis. However, adverse effects were reported including elevations in serum ALT and weight gain (67% of subjects). Thus, while PPARγ agonists are likely to be of benefit to patients with NAFLD, their routine use is neither recommended nor licensed. If possible, patients with NAFLD and significant hepatic fibrosis on biopsy should be enrolled into clinical trials. In patients with type 2 diabetes and NAFLD, these agents could be considered as first-line pharmacotherapy, after lifestyle modification. However, even with the newer agents (rosiglitazone, pioglitazone), physicians should remain vigilant to the possibility of rare but sometimes serious hepatotoxicity such as occurred with troglitazone.

While insulin resistance appears to be essential for NAFLD, oxidative stress has been demonstrated both in animal models [64–66] and humans with NAFLD [7,67–70]. It represents either the cause or consequence of liver injury in NAFLD and may be an important determinant of disease progression and inflammatory recruitment [71]. Thus, antioxidants have been studied in small cohorts with NAFLD. Vitamin E perhaps holds the most promise, but again, its routine use awaits large-scale randomized studies (see Chapter 16). While this compound has no significant adverse effects and is cheap, the optimal regimen for clinical use is not known (studies have used 400–1200 IU/day). These compounds may have a role because of their low toxicity profile in children with NAFLD (see Chapter 19).

Management of advanced liver disease in those with NAFLD

This is no different to that for patients with advanced liver disease from other causes who develop ascites, encephalopathy or variceal bleeding. In those with low platelet counts (less than 100×10^9/mL) or other evidence of portal hypertension (see above), endoscopy should be considered and prophylactic β-blocker therapy instituted if large varices are evident. Hepatocellular cancer does occur in subjects with NASH and cirrhosis, but the incidence in obese persons with cirrhosis remains controversial [21,23,34]. Those with multiple risk factors (previous hepatitis B or C virus infection, alcohol, older men) may be at greatest risk. Primary liver tumours in the setting of NASH should be treated by the usual approaches. While patients with NASH and hepatic decompensation need to be considered for hepatic transplantation, the underlying metabolic milieu favours recurrence in the transplanted liver [72]. These matters are discussed in Chapters 2 and 17.

Conclusions

Hepatic steatosis and lipid-mediated liver injury may be primary (NAFLD) or, more commonly, given the prevalence of obesity in our population, a contributing factor to liver disease from other causes (e.g. alcoholic liver disease, viral hepatitis). In both circumstances, steatosis can cause or worsen liver disease. In the appropriate metabolic setting, physicians need to consider NAFLD/NASH or comorbid steatosis in the setting of dual liver disorders as a primary diagnosis. Once a diagnosis of probable NAFLD/NASH has been made on clinical and laboratory grounds, lifestyle inter-

vention incorporating both diet and physical activity should be instituted for a trial period of 3–6 months. In those with warning signs or predictors of advanced liver disease, liver biopsy should be considered, particularly if liver tests fail to normalize. In those with significant fibrosis, more intensive lifestyle intervention and pharmacotherapy can be considered. At this time, the latter can only be endorsed in the setting of clinical trials. After lifestyle intervention, insulin-sensitizing agents should be considered as first-line therapy in those with type 2 diabetes and NAFLD/NASH. An essential role for the physician in the management of NAFLD/NASH remains the identification and appropriate treatment of individual components of the metabolic syndrome that may contribute to hepatic as well as cardiovascular morbidity and mortality.

References

1 Mofrad P, Contos MJ, Haque M *et al.* Clinical and histologic spectrum of non-alcoholic fatty liver disease associated with normal ALT values. *Hepatology* 2003; **37**: 1286–92.

2 Clark JM, Brancati FL, Diehl AM. The prevalence and etiology of elevated aminotransferase levels in the United States. *Am J Gastroenterol* 2003; **98**: 960–7.

3 Ruhl CE, Everhart JE. Relation of elevated serum alanine aminotransferase activity with iron and antioxidant levels in the United States. *Gastroenterology* 2003; **124**: 1821–9.

4 Prati D, Taioli E, Zanella A *et al.* Updated definitions of healthy ranges for serum alanine aminotransferase levels. *Ann Intern Med* 2002; **137**: 1–10.

5 Chitturi S, Abeygunasekera S, Farrell GC *et al.* NASH and insulin resistance: insulin hypersecretion and specific association with the insulin resistance syndrome. *Hepatology* 2002; **35**: 373–9.

6 Pagano G, Pacini G, Musso G *et al.* Non-alcoholic steatohepatitis, insulin resistance, and metabolic syndrome: further evidence for an etiologic association. *Hepatology* 2002; **35**: 367–72.

7 Sanyal AJ, Campbell-Sargent C, Mirshahi F *et al.* Non-alcoholic steatohepatitis: association of insulin resistance and mitochondrial abnormalities. *Gastroenterology* 2001; **120**: 1183–92.

8 World Health Organization. Definition, diagnosis and classification of diabetes and its complications. I. Diagnosis and classification of diabetes. Geneva: World Health Organization, 1999: 20–1.

9 Sir-Petermann T, Angel B, Maliqueo M *et al.* Prevalence of type II diabetes mellitus and insulin resistance in parents of women with polycystic ovary syndrome. *Diabetologia* 2002; **45**: 959–64.

10 Willner IR, Waters B, Patil SR *et al.* Ninety patients with non-alcoholic steatohepatitis: insulin resistance, familial tendency, and severity of disease. *Am J Gastroenterol* 2001; **96**: 2957–61.

11 Chitturi S, Weltman M, Farrell GC *et al.* HFE mutations, hepatic iron, and fibrosis: ethnic-specific association of NASH with C282Y but not with fibrotic severity. *Hepatology* 2002; **36**: 142–9. Erratum in *Hepatology* 2002; **36**: 1307.

12 George DK, Goldwurm S, MacDonald GA *et al.* Increased hepatic iron concentration in non-alcoholic steatohepatitis is associated with increased fibrosis. *Gastroenterology* 1998; **114**: 311–8.

13 Bonkovsky HL, Jawaid Q, Tortorelli K *et al.* Non-alcoholic steatohepatitis and iron: increased prevalence of mutations of the HFE gene in non-alcoholic steatohepatitis. *J Hepatol* 1999; **31**: 421–9.

14 Younossi ZM, Gramlich T, Bacon BR *et al.* Hepatic iron and nonalcoholic fatty liver disease. *Hepatology* 1999; **30**: 847–50.

15 Angulo P, Keach JC, Batts KP, Lindor KD. Independent predictors of liver fibrosis in patients with non-alcoholic steatohepatitis. *Hepatology* 1999; **30**: 1356–62.

16 Raynard B, Balian A, Fallik D *et al.* Risk factors of fibrosis in alcohol-induced liver disease. *Hepatology* 2002; **35**: 635–8.

17 Hui JM, Sud A, Farrell GC *et al.* Insulin resistance is associated with chronic hepatitis C virus infection and fibrosis progression. *Gastroenterology* 2003; **125**: 1695–704.

18 Gordon A, Mclean CA, Pederson JS, Bailey MJ, Roberts SK. Steatosis in chronic hepatitis B and C: predictors, distribution and effect on fibrosis. *Hepatology* 2003; **38**: 268A.

19 Graif M, Yanuka M, Baraz M *et al.* Quantitative estimation of attenuation in ultrasound video images: correlation with histology in diffuse liver disease. *Invest Radiol* 2000; **35**: 319–24.

20 Saadeh S, Younossi ZM, Remer EM *et al.* The utility of radiological imaging in nonalcoholic fatty liver disease. *Gastroenterology* 2002; **123**: 745–50.

21 Hui JM, Kench JG, Chitturi S *et al.* Long-term outcomes of cirrhosis in nonalcoholic steatohepatitis compared with hepatitis C. *Hepatology* 2003; **38**: 420–7.

22 Caldwell SH, Oelsner DH, Iezzoni JC *et al.* Cryptogenic cirrhosis: clinical characterization and risk factors for underlying disease. *Hepatology* 1999; **29**: 664–9.

23 Ratziu V, Bonyhay L, Di Martino V *et al.* Survival, liver failure, and hepatocellular carcinoma in obesity-related cryptogenic cirrhosis. *Hepatology* 2002; **35**: 1485–93.

24 World Health Organization. *Obesity: Preventing and Managing the Global Epidemic.* Geneva: World Health Organization, 1998.

25 International Diabetes Institute. *The Asia–Pacific Perspective: Redefining Obesity and its Treatment.* Health Communications Australia, 2000: 54.

26 Naveau S, Giraud V, Borotto E *et al.* Excess weight risk factor for alcoholic liver disease. *Hepatology* 1997; **25**: 108–11.

27 Sanyal AJ, Contos MJ, Sterling RK *et al.* Non-alcoholic fatty liver disease in patients with hepatitis C is associated with features of the metabolic syndrome. *Am J Gastroenterol* 2003; **98**: 2064–71.

28 Sorbi D, McGill DB, Thistle JL *et al.* An assessment of the role of liver biopsies in asymptomatic patients with chronic liver test abnormalities. *Am J Gastroenterol* 2000; **95**: 3206–10.

29 Pinto HC, Baptista A, Camilo ME *et al.* Non-alcoholic steatohepatitis: clinicopathological comparison with alcoholic hepatitis in ambulatory and hospitalized patients. *Dig Dis Sci* 1996; **41**: 172–9.

30 Ratziu V, Giral P, Charlotte F *et al.* Liver fibrosis in overweight patients. *Gastroenterology* 2000; **118**: 1117–23.

31 Loguercio C, De Girolamo V, de Sio I *et al.* Non-alcoholic fatty liver disease in an area of southern Italy: main clinical, histological, and pathophysiological aspects. *J Hepatol* 2001; **35**: 568–74. Erratum in *J Hepatol* 2002; **36**: 713.

32 Marceau P, Biron S, Hould FS *et al.* Liver pathology and the metabolic syndrome X in severe obesity. *J Clin Endocrinol Metab* 1999; **84**: 1513–7.

33 Dixon JB, Bhathal PS, O'Brien PE. Non-alcoholic fatty liver disease: predictors of non-alcoholic steatohepatitis and liver fibrosis in the severely obese. *Gastroenterology* 2001; **121**: 91–100.

34 Harrison SA, Hayashi P. Clinical factors associated with fibrosis in 102 patients with non-alcoholic steatohepatitis. *Hepatology* 2002; **36**: 412A.

35 Matteoni CA, Younossi ZM, Gramlich T *et al.* Non-alcoholic fatty liver disease: a spectrum of clinical and pathological severity. *Gastroenterology* 1999; **116**: 1413–9.

36 Bugianesi E, Leone N, Vanni E *et al.* Expanding the natural history of nonalcoholic steatohepatitis: from cryptogenic cirrhosis to hepatocellular carcinoma. *Gastroenterology* 2002; **123**: 134–40.

37 Farrell GC. Non-alcoholic steatohepatitis: what is it, and why is it important in the Asia–Pacific region? *J Gastroenterol Hepatol* 2003; **18**: 124–38.

38 Chitturi S, Farrell GC, George J. Non-alcoholic steatohepatitis in the Asia–Pacific region: future shock? *J Gastroenterol Hepatol* 2004; **19**: 368–74.

39 Buchanan TA. Prevention of type 2 diabetes. *Diabetes Care* 2003; **26**: 1306–7.

40 Tuomilehto J, Lindstrom J, Eriksson JG *et al*. Finnish Diabetes Prevention Study Group. Prevention of type 2 diabetes mellitus by changes in lifestyle among subjects with impaired glucose tolerance. *N Engl J Med* 2001; **344**: 1343–50.

41 Knowler WC, Barrett-Connor E, Fowler SE *et al*. Diabetes Prevention Program Research Group. Reduction in the incidence of type 2 diabetes with lifestyle intervention or metformin. *N Engl J Med* 2002; **346**: 393–403.

42 Pan XR, Li GW, Hu YH *et al*. Effects of diet and exercise in preventing NIDDM in people with impaired glucose tolerance. The Da Qing IGT and Diabetes Study. *Diabetes Care* 1997; **20**: 537–44.

43 Wang RT, Koretz RL, Yee HF Jr. Is weight reduction an effective therapy for non-alcoholic fatty liver? A systematic review. *Am J Med* 2003; **115**: 554–9.

44 Andersen T, Gluud C, Franzmann MB, Christoffersen P. Hepatic effects of dietary weight loss in morbidly obese subjects. *J Hepatol* 1991; **12**: 224–9.

45 Imbert-Bismut F, Ratziu V, Pieroni L *et al*. MULTIVIRC Group. Biochemical markers of liver fibrosis in patients with hepatitis C virus infection: a prospective study. *Lancet* 2001; **357**: 1069–75.

46 Forns X, Ampurdanes S, Llovet JM *et al*. Identification of chronic hepatitis C patients without hepatic fibrosis by a simple predictive model. *Hepatology* 2002; **36**: 986–92.

47 Wai CT, Greenson JK, Fontana RJ *et al*. A simple non-invasive index can predict both significant fibrosis and cirrhosis in patients with chronic hepatitis C. *Hepatology* 2003; **38**: 518–26.

48 Hickman IJ, Clouston AD, Macdonald GA *et al*. Effect of weight reduction on liver histology and biochemistry in patients with chronic hepatitis C. *Gut* 2002; **51**: 89–94.

49 Hickman IJ, Jonsson JR, Prins JB *et al*. Benefit of sustained weight loss and exercise in overweight patients with liver disease: indicators for success. *Hepatology* 2003; **34**: 504A.

50 Anonymous. Executive summary of the clinical guidelines on the identification, evaluation and treatment of overweight and obesity in adults. *Arch Intern Med* 1998; **158**: 1855–67.

51 The Diabetes prevention program (DPP) research group. The diabetes prevention program (DPP): description of lifestyle intervention. *Diabetes Care* 2002; **25**: 2165–71.

52 Musso G, Gambino R, De Michieli F *et al*. Dietary habits and their relations to insulin resistance and postprandial lipemia in non-alcoholic steatohepatitis. *Hepatology* 2003; **37**: 909–16.

53 Kraus RM, Eckel RH, Howard B *et al*. AHA dietary guidelines: revision 2000. A statement for health care professionals from the nutrition committee of the American Heart Association. *Stroke* 2000; **31**: 2751–66.

54 Clark MJ Jr, Sterrett JJ, Carson DS. Diabetes guidelines: a summary and comparison of the recommendations of the American Diabetes Association, Veterans Health Administration, and American Association of Clinical Endocrinologists. *Clin Ther* 2000; **22**: 899–910; discussion 898.

55 Assy N, Svalb S, Hussein O. Orlistat (xenical) reverses fatty liver disease and improves hepatic fibrosis in obese patients with NASH. *Hepatology* 2001; **34**: 251A.

56 Harrison SA, Fincke C, Helinski D, Togerson S. Orlistat treatment in obese, non-alcoholic steatohepatitis patients. *Hepatology* 2002; **36**: 406A.

57 Neuschwander-Tetri BA, Brunt EM, Wehmeier KR, Oliver D, Bacon BR. Improved non-alcoholic steatohepatitis after 48 weeks of treatment with the PPAR-gamma ligand rosiglitazone. *Hepatology* 2003; **38**: 1008–17.

58 Lin HZ, Yang SQ, Chuckaree C *et al*. Metformin reverses fatty liver disease in obese, leptin-deficient mice. *Nat Med* 2000; **6**: 998–1003.

59 Marchesini G, Brizi M, Bianchi G *et al*. Metformin in non-alcoholic steatohepatitis. *Lancet* 2001; **358**: 893–4.

60 Buchanan TA, Xiang AH, Peters RK *et al*. Preservation of pancreatic beta-cell function and prevention of type 2 diabetes by pharmacological treatment of insulin resistance in high-risk hispanic women. *Diabetes* 2002; **51**: 2796–803.

61 Neuschwander-Tetri BA, Brunt EM, Wehmeier KR *et al*. Interim results of a pilot study demonstrating the early effects of the PPARγ ligand rosiglitazone on insulin sensitivity, aminotransferases, hepatic steatosis and body weight in patients with non-alcoholic steatohepatitis. *J Hepatol* 2003; **38**: 434–40.

62 Sanyal AJ, Contos MJ, Sargeant C *et al*. A randomised controlled pilot study of pioglitazone and vitamin E versus vitamin E for non-alcoholic steatohepatitis. *Hepatology* 2002; **36**: 382A.

63 Caldwell SH, Hespenheide EE, Redick JA *et al*. A pilot study of a thiazolidinedione, troglitazone, in non-alcoholic steatohepatitis. *Am J Gastroenterol* 2001; **96**: 519–25.

64 Weltman MD, Farrell GC, Liddle C. Increased hepatocyte CYP2E1 expression in a rat nutritional model of hepatic steatosis with inflammation. *Gastroenterology* 1996; **111**: 1645–53.

65 Leclercq IA, Farrell GC, Field J *et al*. CYP2E1 and CYP4A as microsomal catalysts of lipid peroxides in murine nonalcoholic steatohepatitis. *J Clin Invest* 2000; **105**: 1067–75.

66 George J, Pera N, Phung N *et al*. Lipid peroxidation, stellate cell activation and hepatic fibrogenesis in a rat model of chronic steatohepatitis. *J Hepatol* 2003; **39**: 756–64.

67 Weltman MD, Farrell GC, Hall P, Ingelman-Sundberg M, Liddle C. Hepatic cytochrome P450 2E1 is increased in patients with non-alcoholic steatohepatitis. *Hepatology* 1998; **27**: 128–33.

68 Chalasani N, Gorski JC, Asghar MS *et al.* Hepatic cytochrome P450 2E1 activity in non-diabetic patients with non-alcoholic steatohepatitis. *Hepatology* 2003; **37**: 544–50.

69 MacDonald GA, Bridle KR, Ward PJ *et al.* Lipid peroxidation in hepatic steatosis in humans is associated with hepatic fibrosis and occurs predominately in acinar zone 3. *J Gastroenterol Hepatol* 2001; **16**: 599–606.

70 Seki S, Kitada T, Yamada T *et al. In situ* detection of lipid peroxidation and oxidative DNA damage in non-alcoholic fatty liver diseases. *J Hepatol* 2002; **37**: 56–62.

71 Ip E, Farrell, GC, Hall P *et al.* Administration of the potent PPARα against, Wy-14,643, reverses nutritional fibrosis and steatohepatitis in mice. *Hepatology* 2004; **39**: 1286–96.

72 Ong J, Younossi ZM, Reddy V *et al.* Cryptogenic cirrhosis and posttransplantation non-alcoholic fatty liver disease [Abstract]. *Liver Transpl* 2001; **7**: 797–801.

16 Management of NASH: current and future perspectives on treatment

Paul Angulo & Keith D. Lindor

Key learning points

1 In non-alcoholic steatohepatitis (NASH) associated with central obesity, weight reduction may improve liver tests and reduce steatohepatitis, although benefits have been inconsistent. Gradual weight loss should be sought, but total starvation or very low calorie diets may cause worsening of liver histology.

2 While control of hyperglycaemia and hyperlipidaemia is always recommended, this does not always reverse the liver disease.

3 Pharmacological therapy has been assessed only recently, and in short-term pilot studies rather than in definitive randomized controlled trials evaluating fibrotic progression or clinical complications as end-points.

4 Insulin-sensitizing agents (including peroxisome proliferator-activated receptor γ [PPARγ] agonists), lipid-lowering drugs (some with PPARα agonist activity), hepatoprotectants (ursodeoxycholic acid) and antioxidants have all improved liver tests in pilot studies.

5 Appropriate choice and timing of drug therapy, its place in relation to lifestyle intervention and cost efficacy have not been resolved.

6 Empirical therapy is not yet recommended for patients with NAFLD/NASH; any decision to intervene with medical therapy should be aimed at arresting disease progression, and is therefore restricted to those patients with NASH and more advanced fibrosis.

Abstract

Treatment of patients with non-alcoholic steatohepatitis (NASH) has typically been focused on the management of associated conditions such as obesity, diabetes mellitus and hyperlipidaemia. NASH associated with obesity may resolve with weight reduction, although the benefits of weight loss have been inconsistent. Appropriate control of glucose and lipid levels is always recommended, but not always effective in reversing the liver condition. The use of medications that can reduce or reverse liver damage is a reasonable alternative, but pharmacological therapy has only recently been evaluated for patients with NASH. Results of pilot studies evaluating insulin-sensitizing medications (metformin and thiazolidinedione derivatives), lipid-lowering medications (gemfibrozil, atorvastatin, probucol, bezafibrate), hepatoprotective drugs (ursodeoxycholic acid), and medications that improve oxidative stress (betaine, vitamin E or α-tocopherol, vitamin C, N-acetylcysteine), suggest that these medications may be of potential benefit for patients with NASH. The following is a review of the treatment modalities currently available for patients with NASH. Emerging data from clinical trials evaluating promising medications are discussed, as well as possibilities for the future.

Introduction

Non-alcoholic fatty liver disease (NAFLD) is a medical condition that may progress to end-stage liver disease with the consequent development of cirrhosis and liver failure. The spectrum of NAFLD is wide, ranging from simple fat accumulation in hepatocytes (steatosis) without biochemical or histological evidence of inflammation or fibrosis, through fat accumulation plus necroinflammatory activity with or without fibrosis (steatohepatitis or NASH), to the development of advanced liver fibrosis or cirrhosis (cirrhotic stage). All these stages are histologically indistinguishable from those produced by excessive alcohol consumption, but occur in patients who deny alcohol abuse. NASH is a histological diagnosis and represents only a stage within the spectrum of NAFLD. NAFLD should be differentiated from steatosis with or without hepatitis resulting from well-known secondary causes of fatty liver as they have distinctly different pathogeneses and outcomes; these disorders are listed in Chapter 1 (Table 1.2) and discussed in Chapter 21. The terms 'NAFLD' and 'NASH' are currently reserved for those patients in whom none of the known single causes of fatty liver disease are responsible for the liver condition. Other liver diseases that may present with a component of steatosis such as viral or autoimmune hepatitis and metabolic/hereditary liver diseases should be appropriately excluded. These other liver diseases may themselves be associated with steatosis, and individuals suffering from these other liver diseases may also have risk factors for NAFLD (see Chapter 23) [1].

Obesity, type 2 (non-insulin dependent) diabetes mellitus and hypertriglyceridaemia, common features of the insulin resistance (metabolic) syndrome (IRS) (see Chapter 5), are the most common risk factors or co-existent conditions associated with NAFLD/NASH. Given the common occurrence and increasing prevalence of these comorbidities in the general population (see Chapter 3), NAFLD seems to be the most prevalent liver disease in the USA and many other countries. Although the pathogenesis of NAFLD remains unknown, insulin resistance represents the most reproducible predisposing factor for this liver condition (see Chapters 4 and 5) [2].

The natural history of NAFLD at its different stages remains incompletely studied (see Chapters 3 and 14), but it is clear that some patients, particularly those with simple steatosis, follow a relatively benign course. Simple steatosis usually remains stable for many years, and will probably never progress in most patients [3]. Thus patients who develop problems from NAFLD usually have NASH with advanced fibrosis, at least as we currently understand this condition (see Chapters 1, 2 and 14). Hence, the decision to intervene with medical therapy should be aimed at arresting disease progression and, ideally, be restricted to those patients at risk of developing advanced liver disease (NASH patients and those with more advanced fibrosis).

In this chapter, we review existing medical therapy for patients with NASH, the emerging data from clinical trials evaluating potentially useful medications, and the potential therapeutic implications of recent studies on the pathogenesis of this liver disease.

Treatment of associated conditions

A large body of clinical and epidemiological data gathered during the last three decades indicates that obesity, type 2 diabetes mellitus and hyperlipidaemia are major associated conditions or predisposing factors leading to the development of NAFLD. Hence, it is reasonable to believe that the prevention or appropriate management of these conditions would lead to improvement or arrest of the liver disease.

NAFLD associated with obesity

Effects of weight loss
Weight loss improves insulin sensitivity (see Chapter 4), and NAFLD may resolve with weight reduction (see Chapter 15), but there are no randomized clinical trials of weight control as treatment for this liver condition. An early report describes two patients whose biopsy showed steatosis, necroinflammation and fibrosis which significantly improved following 11 and 20 kg weight loss, respectively over 1 year [4]. In another report, five obese patients stopped eating for some time and lost 14–30 kg within 1 month. Serum levels of liver enzymes appeared to be unaffected by starvation. The hepatic fat content decreased in three of them, but fibrosis became more prominent in four of the five patients [5]. In another series [6], 10 obese patients

who were treated with prolonged fasting for a mean of 71 days lost a mean of 41 kg and had a marked reduction in fatty infiltration. However, areas of focal necrosis were more numerous and some patients developed bile stasis. Similar effects were noted in seven obese subjects who experienced a mean weight reduction of 60 kg during a mean period of 5 months after treatment with a diet of 500 kcal/day. In this same series, 14 patients maintained a mean weight loss of approximately 65 kg for 1.5 years, and in nine of them the liver biopsy findings normalized; there were only rare areas of focal necrosis in the remaining five patients [6].

Another case series of 39 obese patients reported marked biochemical improvement, particularly in those patients who lost more than 10% of body weight [7]. Liver biopsies were not performed in any of these patients. In another series [8], 41 morbidly obese patients with different stages of NAFLD had a median weight loss of 34 kg during treatment with a very low energy diet (388 kcal/day). The degree of fat infiltration improved significantly. However, one-fifth of patients, particularly those patients with more pronounced reduction of fatty changes and faster weight loss, developed slight portal inflammation or fibrosis. None of the patients losing less than 230 g/day or approximately 1.6 kg/week developed fibrosis. A significant improvement in liver test results was noted regardless of the histological changes.

In a more recent study [9], liver biochemistries and the degree of fatty infiltration improved significantly in 15 obese patients with different stages of NAFLD who were treated with a restricted diet (25 cal/kg/day) plus exercise for 3 months. Improvement in the degree of inflammation and fibrosis also occurred in some patients.

Weight reduction in obese children

Information regarding the effect of weight loss in obese children with NAFLD is sparse (see Chapter 19). In one case series [10], seven of nine obese children with NAFLD who adhered to treatment with energy restricting diet and increased exercise lost approximately 500 g/week. This led to improvement in serum aminotransferase (AT) levels and degree of hepatic steatosis evaluated by ultrasonography. Post-treatment liver histology normalized in the only child who underwent liver biopsy.

In a more recent series [11], 33 obese children with abnormal liver tests resulting from NAFLD underwent 6 months of treatment with a moderately energy restrictive diet (mean 35 cal/kg/day; carbohydrates 65%, protein 12%, fat 23%) plus aerobic exercise (≥ 6 h/week) to achieve a weight loss of approximately 500 g/week. Liver tests became normal in all children who lost weight, whereas the degree of steatosis evaluated by ultrasonography improved significantly or normalized in all children who lost ≤ 10% of body weight. In another report [12], six obese children with NAFLD had improvement in serum AT with weight loss after a mean follow-up of 18 months.

Optimal rate and extent of weight loss

Based on the analysis of these studies [4–12], it is clear that weight loss, particularly if gradual, may lead to improvement in liver histology. However, the rate and degree of weight loss required for normalization of liver histology have not been established. It seems that the means by which or how fast weight loss is achieved is important, and may have a critical role in determining whether improvement or more severe liver damage results. In patients with very extensive fatty infiltration, pronounced reduction of fatty change and fast weight loss may promote portal inflammation and fibrosis. Similarly, starvation or total fasting may lead to development of pericellular and portal fibrosis, bile stasis and focal necrosis [5,8]. This paradoxical effect seen in some patients may be caused by increased circulating free fatty acid levels derived from fat mobilization and thus a greater rate of exposure of the liver to an unusually high concentration of free fatty acids. Increased intrahepatic levels of fatty acids favour oxidative stress, lipid peroxidation and cytokine induction, leading to a worsening of liver damage (see Chapters 7–10). Furthermore, serum AT levels almost always improve or normalize with weight loss, but they are poor predictors of worsening of liver histology despite of or resulting from weight loss.

The National Heart, Lung and Blood Institute (NHLBI) and National Institute of Diabetes and Digestive and Kidney Diseases (NIDDK) expert panel clinical guidelines for weight loss recommend that the initial target for weight loss should be 10% of baseline weight within a period of 6 months [13]. This can be achieved by losing approximately 0.45–0.90 kg/week (1–2 lb/week). Following initial success, further weight loss can be attempted, if indicated, through further assessment. The panel recommends weight loss using multiple interventions and strategies, including diet modifications, physical activity, behavioural therapy, pharmacotherapy and surgery, or a combination of these treatment modalities. The recommendation for a particular treatment modality or combination should be individualized, taking into consideration the body mass index and presence of concomitant risk factors and other diseases. The panel does not make specific recommendations for the subgroup of patients with NAFLD. However, given the lack of clinical trials in this area, the overall panel recommendations may be a useful and safe first step for obese patients with NAFLD. Similarly, no specific recommendations were made for monitoring of liver tests during weight loss. However, measuring serum AT once a month during weight loss seems appropriate.

Composition of dietary prescriptions

Different dietary energy restrictions have been used. However, further studies are necessary to determine the most appropriate content of the formula to be recommended for obese and/or diabetic patients with NAFLD/NASH. In the absence of well-controlled clinical trials in patients with NAFLD, it may be tempting to recommend a heart-healthy diet as recommended by the American Heart Association (AHA) for those without diabetes [14], and a diabetic diet as recommended by the American Diabetes Association (ADA) for those with diabetes [15]. Dietary supplementation with n-3 polyunsaturated and monounsaturated fatty acids may improve insulin sensitivity and prevent liver damage [16]. Saturated fatty acids worsen insulin resistance whereas dietary fibre can improve it. Nevertheless, the effect of such dietary modifications on the underlying liver disease in patients with NAFLD remains to be established. Diet to produce weight loss should always be prescribed on an individual basis and taking into consideration the patient's overall health. Patients who have other obesity-related diseases such as diabetes mellitus, hyperlipidaemia, hypertension or cardiovascular disease will require close medical supervision during weight loss to adjust the medication dosage as needed.

Medications to reduce weight

Medications used to reduce body weight currently approved by the Food and Drug Administration include orlistat, phentermine and sibutramine. Their use results in weight reduction in many patients, but their effects on the liver disease remain undefined. Two small case series [17,18] suggest that weight loss achieved during treatment with the gastrointestinal lipase inhibitor orlistat may improve liver disease in obese patients. However, orlistat has been associated with cases of hepatotoxicity [19], and it therefore remains to be proven whether the risk : benefit ratio of orlistat or other weight-reducing medications justifies their use for the treatment of NAFLD.

Surgical approaches to weight reduction

Malabsorptive procedures (jejuno-ileal bypass, biliopancreatic diversions), popular weight-reducing surgical procedures in the 1960s and 1970s, have been virtually abandoned, mainly because of the high frequency of severe postoperative complications including worsening of liver disease (see Chapter 20) [20]. The development and worsening of NAFLD in obese patients undergoing bariatric surgery may be caused by a combination of additive factors including protein or calorie malnutrition, increased fluxes and liver exposure to free fatty acids, and bacterial overgrowth in the defunctionalized intestinal segment. In this regard, enteral and parenteral supplementation of amino acids and proteins may be of benefit [21]. In a series of 33 obese patients undergoing intestinal bypass [22], metronidazole given at random intervals after surgery led to a significant improvement or normalization in the degree of steatosis.

Restrictive procedures to achieve weight loss (gastric bypass, gastroplasty) are safer than malabsorptive procedures. In 1999, the US Food and Drug Administration approved adjustable gastric banding as a weight-reducing procedure. The adjustable gastric band seems to be safer for liver disease because of the more gradual weight loss achieved (approximately 2.7–4.5 kg/month [6–10 lb/month]) [23].

Parenteral nutrition

Patients receiving long-term total parenteral nutrition may develop fatty liver (see Chapter 21), partially because of choline deficiency. Choline supplementation has been reported to improve or revert hepatic steatosis [24,25]. Similarly, bacterial overgrowth in the resting intestine along with the lack of enteral stimulation has been implicated in the genesis of liver damage, including NAFLD, in patients on long-term total parenteral nutrition. Polymyxin B, a non-absorbable antibiotic that specifically binds to the lipid A-core region of lipopolysaccharide [26] and metronidazole [27] has been shown to significantly improve the degree of fatty infiltration and reduce the production of tumour necrosis factor (TNF), a key molecule in the development of insulin resistance in rats receiving total parenteral nutrition.

NAFLD/NASH associated with diabetes mellitus and hyperlipidaemia

Obese patients with diabetes mellitus and/or hyperlipidaemia should be enrolled in a weight control programme. The NHLBI/National Institutes of Health (NIH) [13], AHA [14] and ADA [15] expert panel recommendations may be useful for these patients (see above). However, the effect of such recommendations on liver disease in diabetic or hyperlipidaemic patients have not been studied systematically. Furthermore, the appropriate control of glucose and lipid levels in patients with diabetes and hyperlipidaemia is not always effective in reversing NAFLD.

In obese *ob/ob* mice, an animal model of steatosis that develops insulin resistance, diabetes and hyperlipidaemia [28], metformin, an oral antidiabetic medication, led to improvement in liver tests and degree of steatosis. Based on these findings, metformin and other insulin-sensitizing medications are being evaluated in humans with NAFLD (see later section and Chapter 24). Patients with type 1 (insulin-dependent) diabetes mellitus and hepatomegaly show improvement in symptoms of hepatomegaly when appropriate control of hyperglycaemia is achieved. Hypertriglyceridaemia, rather than hypercholesterolaemia, is a risk factor for NAFLD (see Chapters 1 and 3). In this regard, gemfibrozil, atorvastatin and probucol but not clofibrate may improve the liver condition (see p. 201 and Chapter 24).

NAFLD 'without' risk factors

A subgroup of patients with liver biopsy-proven NAFLD/NASH have normal body mass index and normal waist : hip ratio as well as normal glucose tolerance and normal lipid profile. These NAFLD patients who lack the most common associated risk factors are candidates for other treatment modalities such as pharmacological therapy. Also, although further work is necessary, this subset of patients with NAFLD may still be insulin resistant, and so improving insulin sensitivity through changing diet composition as opposed to caloric restriction, as well as increasing physical activity, may improve insulin sensitivity and lead to improvement of the liver disease.

Drugs and hepatotoxins

Several drugs and environmental exposure to some hepatotoxins have been recognized as potential causes of fatty liver, steatosis, steatohepatitis and even cirrhosis (see Chapter 21) [29]. The liver conditions resulting from these secondary causes differ to some extent from NAFLD in pathogenesis, pathology and outcomes. However, a drug cause should always be sought in patients with NAFLD because withdrawal of a causative agent, when possible, can often lead to resolution of the liver disease.

Pharmacological therapy

Because rapid weight loss may worsen NAFLD/NASH, and weight control is a difficult task to accomplish for most obese patients, use of medications that can directly reduce the severity of liver damage independent of weight loss is a logical alternative. Pharmacological therapy may also benefit those patients who lack the most common risk factors or associated conditions, although it is becoming highly questionable whether such individuals, in the absence of central obesity or insulin resistance, have significant NASH (see Chapters 3, 5 and 15). The decision to intervene with pharmacological therapy aimed at the underlying liver disease is based on the anticipated risk of progression to severe liver disease. However, pharmacological therapy directed specifically at the liver disease has only recently been evaluated in patients with NAFLD. Most of these studies have been uncontrolled, open-label and lasting 1 year or less, and only a few of them have evaluated the effect of treatment on liver histology. Several studies are currently in progress, but some preliminary results have been reported (updated information is presented in Chapter 24).

Insulin-sensitizing medications (Table 16.1)

Type 2 diabetes mellitus and truncal (central) obesity are well-known conditions associated with resistance to normal peripheral actions of insulin. Indeed, insulin resistance represents the most reproducible predisposing factor for NAFLD, being present in more than 95% of cases, with more than 85% having other manifestations of the insulin-resistance (metabolic) syndrome (see Chapter 5). Hence, it is reasonable to speculate that the use of medications that improve insulin sensitivity

Table 16.1 Insulin-sensitizing medications evaluated in the treatment of non-alcoholic fatty liver disease.

Study [Reference]	Drug	No. of patients	Type of study	Compared with	Duration of treatment (months)	Aminotransferases	Histology
Caldwell *et al.* (2001) [30]	Troglitazone	10	Open-label	Baseline	3–6	Improved	Improved
Acosta *et al.* (2001) [34]	Pioglitazone	8	Open-label	Baseline	2–12	Improved	ND
Marchesini *et al.* (2001) [37]	Metformin	14	Open-label	Baseline	4	Improved	ND
Nair *et al.* (2002) [38]	Metformin	25	Open-label	Baseline	6	Improved	ND
Neuschwander-Tetri *et al.* (2002) [32,33]†	Rosiglitazone	25	Open-label	Baseline	12	Improved	Improved
Loguercio *et al.* (2002) [59]	Probiotics	10	Open-label	Baseline	2	Improved	ND
Sanyal *et al.* (2002) [35]	Pioglitazone + vitamin E	21	Randomized (open-label)	Baseline; vitamin E alone	6	Improved*	Improved*
Promrat *et al.* (2003) [36]	Pioglitazone	9	Open-label	Baseline	12	Improved	Improved

ND, not done

* Aminotransferases and liver histology (steatosis, hepatocyte ballooning, Mallory hyaline) improved in both groups, but greater histological improvement occurred with combination therapy.

† An updated account of this important study is given in Chapter 24.

may benefit the liver disease of patients with associated insulin-resistance conditions. Thiazolidinediones, more commonly termed glitazones (troglitazone, rosiglitazone, pioglitazone), are a new class of antidiabetic drugs that act as PPARγ agonists, thereby selectively enhancing or partially mimicking certain actions of insulin. The resultant beneficial effects include an antihyperglycaemic effect, frequently accompanied by a reduction in circulating concentrations of insulin, triglycerides and non-sterified (free) fatty acids.

Troglitazone

Troglitazone (400 mg/day) was given to 10 patients with liver biopsy-proven NASH for 3–6 months [30]. Alanine aminotransferase (ALT) levels normalized in seven patients and, although features of NASH remained in the post-treatment liver biopsy, the grade of necro-inflammation improved in four parients. Troglitazone proved to be hepatotoxic and was withdrawn from the market after the report of several dozen deaths or cases of severe hepatic failure requiring liver transplantation [31]. There is little evidence to indicate underlying liver disease in those who experienced troglitazone-induced liver failure [31].

Rosiglitazone

Rosiglitazone (4 mg twice daily) was given to 25 patients

with liver biopsy-proven NASH for 1 year [32,33]. Liver enzymes including aspartate aminotransferase (AST), alkaline phosphatase and γ-glutamyl transpeptidase (GGT) improved significantly as well as the degree of insulin sensitivity as determined by quantitative insulin-sensitive check index (QUICKI). Post-treatment liver biopsies were performed and showed a significant improvement in the degree of centrilobular fibrosis [33] (and see Chapter 24). In this study, one patient experienced an abrupt rise in AT levels possibly related to rosiglitazone, and some cases of possible drug-induced liver injury related to rosiglitazone have been reported [31]. Hence, not only the efficacy, but also the safety of rosiglitazone in patients with NAFLD needs to be evaluated in larger placebo-controlled trials with extended follow-up.

Pioglitazone

Pioglitazone has been evaluated in three pilot studies, and the preliminary results reported in abstracts [34–36] (and see Chapter 24). In one study [34], pioglitazone was given to eight patients with NASH for a mean of 28 weeks (range 8–48 weeks); normalization of AT occurred in five patients, with decrease to approximately 50% of the baseline value in two others. Steatosis improved in the only patient who had post-treatment liver biopsy performed.

In another pilot study [35], 10 patients with NASH were treated with pioglitazone (30 mg/day) plus vitamin E (400 IU/day) and compared to 11 patients treated with the same regimen of vitamin E alone. After 6 months of therapy, ALT decreased in both groups as well as the degree of steatosis, ballooning of hepatocytes and Mallory hyaline. However, the histological improvement was more marked in the combination group. In this study [35], one patient in the combination group had a worsening of liver enzymes, possibly related to pioglitazone, and had to be withdrawn. Some cases of possible drug-induced liver injury have been reported with pioglitazone [31].

Pioglitazone (30 mg/day) was given to nine patients with NASH for 1 year in an open-label pilot study [36]. Improvement or normalization of AT as well as improvement in the degree of insulin resistance occurred at the end of treatment. Also, a significant improvement in severity of steatosis, necroinflammation and Mallory hyaline was noted on liver biopsies performed at the end of treatment. Pioglitazone was well tolerated, but there was a significant gain in body weight and total body fat. The promising results of these three pilot studies along with the long-term safety of pioglitazone in patients with NASH need to be evaluated in well-controlled clinical trials.

Metformin

Metformin is an antidiabetic medication that improves insulin sensitivity. In *ob/ob* mice, an animal model of fatty liver, metformin reversed hepatomegaly as well as steatosis and AT abnormalities [28]. These beneficial effects of metformin seemed to be through inhibiting hepatic expression of TNF and TNF-inducible factors that promote hepatic lipid accumulation, such as steroid regulatory element binding protein-1 (SREBP-1), and factors promoting hepatic adenosine triphosphate (ATP) depletion, such as uncoupling protein-2 (UCP-2) [28]. Based on these results, a regimen of metformin 500 mg three times daily was given for 4 months to 14 patients with NASH [37]. Metformin therapy was associated with a significant improvement in liver tests and glucose disposal, an index of insulin sensitivity, as well as a significant decrease in hepatic volume and body mass index.

In another pilot study [38], 25 patients were treated with metformin (20 mg/kg/day). At 6 months of therapy, patients had a significant decrease in body weight and AT levels. Unfortunately, the effect on liver histology has not been evaluated in any study. Metformin was well tolerated in these studies, but it should be noted that although no patient developed lactic acidosis, serum lactic acid levels did rise [37]. Thus, larger controlled trials are needed to determine the safety and efficacy of metformin in the treatment of NAFLD.

Antioxidants

In patients with NAFLD, antioxidant therapy may be potentially useful in preventing progression from steatosis to steatohepatitis and fibrosis (see Chapters 7–10). Antioxidants that have been evaluated in patients with NAFLD include vitamin E (α-tocopherol), vitamin C, betaine, N-acetylcysteine and iron depletion (Table 16.2). Vitamin E, a potent antioxidant that is particularly effective against membrane lipid peroxidation, suppresses expression of TNF, interleukin 1 (IL-1), IL-6 and IL-8 by monocytes and/or Kupffer cells, and inhibits liver collagen-α1(I) gene expression.

Vitamin E (α-tocopherol)

A recent study reported the results of treatment with α-tocopherol in 11 children with a clinical diagnosis of NAFLD [39]. Vitamin E (400–1200 IU/day orally) was given for 4–10 months and led to a significant improvement in liver tests. In another study [40], α-tocopherol in a regimen of 300 mg/day was given for 1 year to 12 patients with liver biopsy-proven NASH, and 10 patients with a clinical diagnosis of NAFLD. Liver tests improved significantly compared to baseline, whereas the degree of steatosis, inflammation and fibrosis improved or remained unchanged in the nine patients with NASH who had post-treatment liver biopsy performed. Plasma levels of transforming growth factor-β1 (TGF-β1) in patients with NASH were reduced significantly with α-tocopherol treatment [40].

In another study [41], 45 patients with NASH were randomized to treatment with the combination of vitamin E (1000 IU/day) plus vitamin C (1000 IU/day), or an identical placebo for 6 months. At the end of therapy, 48% of patients in the vitamin group and 41% in the placebo group showed improvement in at least one stage of fibrosis. Although the score for stage of fibrosis was statistically lower post-treatment compared to baseline in the vitamin group, changes post-treatment were not statistically different between the vitamin and placebo groups. Also, liver enzymes and the degree of steatosis and necroinflammatory activity

Table 16.2 Antioxidant medications evaluated in the treatment of non-alcoholic fatty liver disease.

Study [Reference]	Drug	No. of patients	Type of study	Compared with	Duration of treatment (months)	Aminotransferases	Histology
Miglio et al. (2000) [43]	Betaine + diethanolamine + nicotinamide	191	Randomized	Placebo	2	Improved*	ND
Abdelmalek et al. (2001) [42]	Betaine	8	Open-label	Baseline	12	Improved	Improved
Gulbahar et al. (2000) [44]	N-acetylcysteine	11	Open-label	Baseline	3	Improved	ND
Lavine (2000) [39]†	Vitamin E	11	Open-label	Baseline	4–10	Improved	ND
Hasegawa et al. (2001) [40]	Vitamin E	22	Open-label	Baseline; diet	12	Improved	Improved‡
Harrison et al. (2003) [41]	Vitamins E + C	45‡	Randomized (double blind)	Placebo	6	Not mentioned	Improved§

ND, not done

* Improvement in abdominal discomfort, hepatomegaly and degree of fat infiltration determined by ultrasonography was noted in the betaine–diethanolamine–nicotinamide combination group compared to placebo.

† Study performed in children.

‡ Liver biopsy performed in nine patients post-treatment.

§ Improvement in degree of fibrosis.

were not significantly affected by treatment. Thus, 6 months of therapy with the combination of vitamin E plus vitamin C was not better than placebo at improving the liver disease in patients with NASH. However, given the high proportion of patients in the placebo group who appeared to improve fibrosis stage at 6 months, the study [41] did not have enough power to detect a benefit from treatment with these vitamins. It is concluded that larger controlled trials are still warranted to better define the potential efficacy of vitamin E for patients with NAFLD.

Betaine

Betaine, a normal component of the metabolic cycle of methionine, increases *S*-adenosylmethionine levels, which in turn protects the liver from ethanol-induced triglyceride deposition in rats. In a recent study [42], betaine 20 mg/day was given to eight patients with NASH. After 1 year of treatment, a significant improvement or normalization of serum AT levels was noted, whereas the degree of steatosis, necroinflammatory activity and fibrosis improved or remained unchanged in all patients. Based on these results, a larger placebo-controlled trial is now in progress.

In another study [43], 191 patients with a clinical diagnosis of NAFLD were randomized to treatment with betaine glucuronate (300 mg/day) in combination with diethanolamine glucuronate and nicotinamide ascorbate (96 patients), or placebo (95 patients); they were treated for 8 weeks. A significant improvement in right upper quadrant abdominal discomfort, liver enzymes, hepatomegaly and the degree of steatosis evaluated by ultrasonography was noted at the end of treatment with combination therapy; such changes did not occur in the placebo group. Unfortunately, because liver biopsies were not performed and the treatment period was too short, it is difficult to derive meaningful conclusions from this study.

N-acetylcysteine

N-acetylcysteine is a glutathione prodrug that increases glutathione levels in hepatocytes. In turn, this counters hepatocyte production of reactive oxygen species (ROS) and hence prevents the development of oxidative stress in liver cells. In a pilot study [44], 11 patients with NASH were treated with N-acetylcysteine (1 g/day) for 3 months. A significant improvement in AT levels occurred at the end of treatment, but unfortunately liver histology was not evaluated.

Phlebotomy

Although the role of iron in the pathogenesis and development of more severe liver injury in patients with NAFLD remains controversial (see Chapters 1, 2,

5 and 7), iron has been hypothesized to induce oxidative stress by catalysing production of ROS. Two pilot studies involving a total of 30 patients with NASH have been reported [45,46]. Quantitative phlebotomy was performed to induce iron depletion to a level of near-iron deficiency. The two studies reported a significant improvement in AT levels.

In another recent study [47], 17 carbohydrate-intolerant patients with the clinical diagnosis of NAFLD were treated with quantitative phlebotomy to induce iron depletion to a level of near-iron deficiency. Serum ALT levels improved to near normal and there was also improvement in insulin sensitivity, unfortunately, liver biopsy was not performed in any of these studies, and thus, the effect of iron depletion on liver histology in patients with NAFLD remains uncertain.

Lipid-lowering medications

Clofibrate

Clofibrate is a lipid-lowering drug that decreases the hepatic triglyceride content in rats with ethanol-induced hepatic steatosis [48]. Based on this, a pilot study was performed to evaluate the usefulness of clofibrate (2 g/day) in the treatment of patients with NASH [49]. After 1 year of treatment, no significant changes in liver tests or histological features were noted.

Gemfibrozil

In a recent report [50], 46 patients with NASH were randomized to treatment with gemfibrozil 600 mg/day for 4 weeks or no treatment. A significant improvement in AT levels was noted with gemfibrozil compared to baseline values, and this did not occur in the untreated patients. Body weight remained unchanged during treatment, and improvement in liver tests seemed to be independent of baseline triglyceride levels.

Atorvastatin

In another pilot study [51], seven patients with NASH and hyperlipidaemia were treated with atorvastatin (10–30 mg/day) for up to 12 months. At the end of therapy, there was a significant improvement in serum lipid levels as well as the degree of hepatic inflammation, ballooning and Mallory hyaline on liver biopsy. These positive results need to be reproduced in a placebo-controlled trial.

Probucol

Probucol is another lipid-lowering medication that has insulin-sensitizing properties. Thirty patients with NASH were randomized to therapy with probucol (500 mg/day) or an identical placebo and treated for 6 months [52]. Improvement or normalization of AT levels was significantly greater or more common in the probucol than the placebo group and this was independent of changes in body weight or serum lipid levels. Post-treatment liver biopsy was not performed. It is therefore uncertain whether probucol improves liver histology. Probucol may cause severe, sometimes fatal cardiac arrhythmias and was withdrawn from the market in the USA in 1995; as a consequence, there is little enthusiasm in evaluating probucol in a larger trial.

Ursodeoxycholic acid

Ursodeoxycholic acid (UDCA) is the non-hepatotoxic epimer of chenodeoxycholic acid. During UDCA treatment, UCDA replaces endogenous bile acids, which are dose-dependent hepatotoxins. UDCA has membrane stabilizing or cytoprotective effects exerted on mitochondria, as well as immunological effects. Hydrophobic bile acids increase cellular damage and oxidative stress in steatotic hepatocytes. By decreasing hydrophobic bile acids, UDCA could protect against hepatocyte injury and decrease oxidative stress in patients with NAFLD. Also, treatment with UDCA leads to less production of TNF, which, in turn, may improve insulin sensitivity. UDCA has been used in the treatment of some hepatobiliary diseases for approximately two decades. Thus, unlike other medications evaluated for patients with NAFLD, there are abundant data on the safety of long-term use of UDCA in patients with liver disease.

Four open-label pilot studies have evaluated the therapeutic benefits of UDCA in adults with NASH. In one of these studies [49], 24 patients received UDCA in a regimen of 13–15 mg/kg/day for 12 months. This led to a significant improvement in liver tests and the degree of hepatic steatosis compared to baseline. In another study [53], liver tests normalized or significantly improved after 6 months of treatment with UDCA (10 mg/kg/day) in 13 patients with NASH. Similarly, among 31 patients with NASH randomized to UDCA (10 mg/kg/day) plus low-fat diet or low-fat diet alone for 6 months, normalization of liver tests was significantly more common among those treated with UDCA plus diet than with diet alone [54]. In the most recent study [55], UDCA (250 mg three times daily) given for 6–12 months improved AT levels in 24 patients with

NASH; UDCA therapy also improved several serum markers of fibrogenesis.

Based on these results, we developed a large-scale multicentric placebo-controlled trial of UDCA in patients with NASH. A total of 168 patients were enrolled and randomized to UDCA (13–15 g/kg/day) or identical placebo and treated for 2 years. The study has recently been completed and the results will soon be analysed and reported (see Chapter 24).

Future directions

In order to develop effective medical therapy for patients with NAFLD, further work is clearly needed to enhance our understanding of the pathogenesis and natural history of this condition (see Chapters 3, 7–12 and 14). Some lines of evidence, albeit still inconclusive, indicate that oxidative stress/lipid peroxidation, bacterial toxins, overproduction of TNF, alteration of hepatocyte ATP stores and CYP2E1 and 4A enzyme activity may have a role in the genesis and progression of NAFLD.

Regardless of the cause, acute or chronic hepatic steatosis is associated with lipid peroxidation; this seems to increase with the severity of steatosis [56] and with NASH versus steatosis (see Chapter 12); the end-products of lipid peroxidation stimulate collagen production and fibrogenesis. Further studies should focus on increasing antioxidant defences through dietary and/or pharmacological manipulations.

Because metronidazole and polymyxin B may prevent the development of NAFLD in obese patients undergoing intestinal bypass, as well as in rats receiving total parenteral nutrition [22,26,27], a role of endotoxin- and/or cytokine-mediated injury has been suggested as a contributing factor for the development of NAFLD (see Chapter 10). Furthermore, it has been shown that genetically obese mice are very sensitive to the effect of lipopolysaccharide in developing inflammation in the setting of steatosis [57].

More recently, treatment with probiotics or anti-TNF antibodies improved liver steatosis and inflammation and decreased ALT levels in obese leptin-deficient *ob/ob* mice [58]. The treated animals had decreased hepatic expression of TNF messenger RNA, reduced activity of Jun N-terminal kinase (a TNF-regulated kinase that promotes insulin resistance) and decreased DNA binding activity of nuclear factor κB (NF-κB),

the target of inhibitor of κB kinase β (IKK-β), another enzyme that causes insulin resistance (Chapters 5 and 10). In a recent case series [59], 10 patients with NASH who were treated for 2 months with a mixture of different bacteria strains showed a significant improvement in liver enzymes, serum levels of TNF and end-products of lipid peroxidation when compared to baseline, but post-treatment liver biopsies were not performed. Hence, if this concept is valid, the potential benefit of intestinal decontamination or modification of the intestine microflora with probiotics, the administration of soluble cytokine receptors and neutralizing anticytokine antibodies as well as biopharmaceuticals with anti-TNF activity may warrant further evaluation as therapies for patients with NAFLD.

Hepatocyte ATP stores in patients with NASH seem vulnerable to depletion compared to lean controls [60]. Hence, treatment efforts primarily directed toward protecting hepatocyte ATP stores might potentially benefit patients with NAFLD. Similarly, CYP2E1 and 4A activity may contribute to hepatotoxicity in mice and humans with NAFLD [61–63]. Treatment strategies to limit its activity, such as dietary modifications (fat-reduced diet), may be beneficial.

Patients with NAFLD may develop advanced liver fibrosis and progress to end-stage liver disease. Fibrosis represents the most worrisome feature on liver biopsy in patients with NAFLD, indicating a more severe and potentially progressive form of liver injury. The development of antifibrotic therapies aimed at the underlying liver disease is an attractive yet unaccomplished goal. However, substantial advances on our understanding of the molecular mechanisms of liver fibrosis made in the last decade have led to the development of new agents that inhibit stellate cell and/or myofibroblast proliferation and collagen synthesis [64,65]. Many of these agents have proved antifibrogenic in *in vitro* studies, but only a few agents are tolerable or effective in suitable animal models *in vivo*. Agents with antifibrotic effects that may hold promise for patients with NAFLD/NASH are silymarin (a mixture of flavonoids that also have antioxidant properties), pentoxifylline (a phosphodiesterase inhibitor) and pentifylline (a more potent pentoxifylline derivative), LU135252 (an oral inhibitor of the endothelin A-receptor), angiotensin I receptor antagonists or angiotensin-converting enzymes inhibitors, and profibrogenic cytokines antagonists (soluble TGF-β1 receptor antagonists or adenoviral TGF-β1 blocking constructs).

Table 16.3 Lipid-lowering medications evaluated in the treatment of non-alcoholic fatty liver disease.

Study [Reference]	Drug	No. of patients	Type of study	Compared with	Duration of treatment (months)	Aminotransferases	Histology
Laurin et al. (1996) [49]	Clofibrate	16	Open-label	Baseline	12	No improvement	No improvement
Basaranoglu et al. (1999) [50]	Gemfibrozil	46	Randomized (open-label)	No treatment Baseline	1	Improved	ND
Horlander et al. (2001) [51]	Atorvastatin	7	Open-label	Baseline	Up to 12	No improvement	Improved*
Merat et al. (2003) [52]	Probucol	30	Randomized (double blind)	Placebo	6	Improvement	ND

ND, not done

* Improvement in the inflammation, ballooning, Mallory hyaline and total histological score.

Table 16.4 Ursodeoxycholic acid for the treatment of non-alcoholic fatty liver disease.

Study [Reference]	Drug	No. of patients	Type of study	Compared with	Duration of treatment (months)	Aminotransferases	Histology
Laurin et al. (1996) [49]	UDCA	24	Open-label	Baseline	12	Improved	Improved
Guma et al. (1997) [53]	UDCA + diet	24	Randomized (open-label)	Baseline Diet alone	6	Improved†	ND
Ceriani et al. (1998) [54]†	UDCA + diet	31	Open-label	Baseline Diet alone	6	Improved†	ND
Holoman et al. (2000) [55]	UDCA	24	Open-label	Baseline	6–12	Improved	ND

ND, not done

UDCA, ursodeoxycholic acid.

† Greater biochemical improvement with UDCA + diet.

The encouraging results of pilot studies with insulin-sensitizing drugs, antioxidants, lipid-lowering and hepatoprotective medications (Tables 16.1–16.4) warrant their further evaluation in clinical trials. However, in order to make solid recommendations of routine administration of any of the previously evaluated (or other) medications in the treatment of patients with NAFLD/NASH, further well-controlled clinical trials are clearly necessary. These studies must have enough power, adequate duration of follow-up, and should also include clinically relevant end-points. In particular, simple improvement or normalization of liver tests and/or the degree of steatosis on imaging studies, as used in most of the pilot studies reported to date, do not necessarily imply that these agents will have a real effect on the natural history (fibrotic progression) of this liver disease. Similarly, although improvement of liver histology may possibly be a more accurate surrogate

marker of a better long-term prognosis, a beneficial medication for patients with NAFLD should be not only safe and well tolerated, but also prove beneficial in improving health-related quality of life [66,67]. It should also be cost-effective, bearing in mind the other morbidity of at-risk patients (obesity, type 2 diabetes, hyperlipidaemia, arterial hypertension), and the unknown cost-efficacy of lifestyle interventions.

Although an ideal end-point in clinical trials would be a delay in developing liver-related complications and improvement of long-term survival, such end-points may not be practical given the slowly progressive nature of this condition. Because NAFLD progresses slowly over many years, hundreds of patients with this condition would need to be enrolled in prospective clinical trials and followed-up for a number of years, perhaps decades, in order to see a real effect of a medication on long-term survival. It may be unrealistic to believe that such a study is both feasible for the patients and affordable. Better identification of those patients with NAFLD/NASH who are at risk of progressing to end-stage liver disease may allow selective enrolment in therapeutic trials of those 'high-risk' patients who, in theory, would be expected to derive the most benefit from medical therapy. Although this still has to be proven in population-based studies, those patients with NAFLD at high risk for disease progression seem to be those with necroinflammatory activity (NASH) on liver biopsy as well as those patients with more advanced fibrosis (see Chapters 3 and 14). Thus, until further work is carried out, we believe that further clinical trials should focus on patients with liver biopsy-proven NASH and those with more advanced fibrosis.

Conclusions

Management of associated conditions or risk factors for NAFLD, including obesity, diabetes mellitus and hyperlipidaemia, may improve the liver disease. Gradual weight loss should be sought, particularly with the combination of diet and increased physical activity. Total starvation or very low-energy diets may cause worsening of liver histology, and should be avoided. Improvement in liver test results, particularly AT, is almost universal in obese children and adults after weight reduction, but liver test results are poor indicators of worsening of liver histology after weight loss. Emerging data from small pilot studies suggest that several insulin-sensitizing, antioxidant, lipid-lowering and hepatoprotective medications may be of benefit. However, such agents must now to be evaluated in well-controlled clinical trials with extended follow-up and clinically relevant end-points, particularly fibrosis progression. Improved understanding of the pathogenesis and natural history of NAFLD, along with recent advances in the understanding of molecular mechanisms involved in liver fibrosis, should lead to development of new medical therapies targeted to patients at 'high risk' for disease progression.

References

1 Angulo P. Non-alcoholic fatty liver disease. *N Engl J Med* 2002; **346**: 1221–31.

2 Angulo P, Lindor KD. Insulin resistance and mitochondrial abnormalities in NASH: a cool look into a burning issue. *Gastroenterology* 2001; **120**: 1281–5.

3 Teli M, Oliver FW, Burt AD *et al*. The natural history of non-alcoholic fatty liver: a follow-up study. *Hepatology* 1995; **22**: 1714–7.

4 Eriksson S, Eriksson KF, Bondesson L. Non-alcoholic steatohepatitis in obesity: a reversible condition. *Acta Med Scand* 1986; **220**: 83–8.

5 Rozental P, Biava C, Spencer H, Zimmerman HJ. Liver morphology and function tests in obesity and during total starvation. *Am J Dig Dis* 1967; **12**: 198–208.

6 Drenick EJ, Simmons F, Murphy J. Effect on hepatic morphology of treatment of obesity by fasting, reducing diets, and small bowel bypass. *N Engl J Med* 1970; **282**: 829–34.

7 Palmer M, Schaffner F. Effect of weight reduction on hepatic abnormalities in overweight patients. *Gastroenterology* 1990; **99**: 1408–13.

8 Andersen T, Gluud C, Franzmann MB, Christoffersen P. Hepatic effects of dietary weight loss in morbidly obese patients. *J Hepatol* 1991; **12**: 224–9.

9 Ueno T, Sugawara H, Sujaku K *et al*. Therapeutic effects of restricted diet and exercise in obese patients with fatty liver. *J Hepatol* 1997; **27**: 103–7.

10 Vajro P, Fontanella A, Perna C *et al*. Persistent hyper-aminotransferasemia resolving after weight reduction in obese children. *J Pediatr* 1994; **125**: 239–41.

11 Franzese A, Vajro P, Argenziano A *et al*. Liver involvement in obese children: ultrasonography and liver enzyme levels at diagnosis and during follow-up in an Italian population. *Dig Dis Sci* 1997; **42**: 1428–32.

12 Rashid M, Roberts E. Non-alcoholic steatohepatitis in children. *J Pediatr Gastroenterol Nutr* 2000; **30**: 48–53.

13 Anonymous. Executive summary of the clinical guidelines on the identification, evaluation, and treatment of overweight and obesity in adults. *Arch Intern Med* 1998; **158**: 1855–67.

14 Kraus RM, Eckel RH, Howard B *et al*. AHA dietary guidelines: revision 2000. A statement for health care professionals from the nutrition committee of the American Heart Association. *Stroke* 2000; **31**: 2751–66.

15 Clark MJ Jr, Sterrett JJ, Carson DS. Diabetes guidelines: a summary and comparison of the recommendations of the American Diabetes Association, Veterans Health Administration, and American Association of Clinical Endocrinologists. *Clin Ther* 2000; **22**: 899–910; discussion 898.

16 Fernandez MI, Torres MI, Rios A. Steatosis and collagen content in experimental liver cirrhosis are affected by dietary monounsaturated and polyunsaturated fatty acids. *Scand J Gastroenterol* 1997; **32**: 350–6.

17 Assy N, Svalb S, Hussein O. Orlistat (xenical) reverses fatty liver disease and improve hepatic fibrosis in obese

patients with NASH [Abstract]. *Hepatology* 2001; **34**: 251.

18 Harrison SA, Fincke C, Helinski D, Torgerson S. Orlistat treatment in obese, non-alcoholic steatohepatitis patients [Abstract]. *Hepatology* 2002; **36**: 406.

19 Lau G, Chan CL. Massive hepatocellular [correction of hepatocullular] necrosis: was it caused by Orlistat? *Med Sci Law* 2002; **42**: 309–12.

20 Campbell JM, Hung TK, Karam JH, Forsham PH. Jejunoileal bypass as a treatment of morbid obesity. *Arch Intern Med* 1977; **137**: 602–10.

21 Ackerman NB. Protein supplementation in the management of degenerating liver function after jejunoileal bypass. *Surg Gynecol Obstetr* 1979; **149**: 8–14.

22 Drenick EJ, Fisler J, Johnson D. Hepatic steatosis after intestinal bypass: prevention and reversal by metronidazole, irrespective of protein-calorie malnutrition. *Gastroenterology* 1982; **82**: 535–48.

23 Weiner R, Blanco-Engert R, Weiner S *et al.* Outcome after laparoscopic adjustable gastric banding: 8 years' experience. *Obes Surg* 2003; **13**: 427–34.

24 Buchman AL, Dubin M, Jenden D *et al.* Lecithin increases plasma free choline and decreases hepatic steatosis in long-term total parenteral nutrition in rats. *Gastroenterology* 1992; **102**: 1363–70.

25 Buchman AL, Dubin MD, Moukarzel AA *et al.* Choline deficiency: a cause of hepatic steatosis during parenteral nutrition that can be reversed with intravenous choline supplementation. *Hepatology* 1995; **22**: 1390–403.

26 Pappo I, Becovier H, Berry EM, Freud HR. Polymyxin B reduces cecal flora, TNF production and hepatic steatosis during total parenteral nutrition in rat. *J Surg Res* 1991; **51**: 106–12.

27 Freud HR, Muggia-Sullan M, Lafrance R *et al.* A possible beneficial effect of metronidazole in reducing TPN-associated liver function derangements. *J Surg Res* 1985; **38**: 356–63.

28 Lin HZ, Yang SQ, Chuckaree C *et al.* Metformin reverses fatty liver disease in obese, leptin-deficient mice. *Nat Med* 2000; **6**: 998–1003.

29 Farrell GC. Drugs and steatohepatitis. *Semin Liver Dis* 2002; **22**: 185–94.

30 Caldwell SH, Hespenheiden EE, Redick JA *et al.* A pilot study of thiazolidinedione, troglitazone, in non-alcoholic steatohepatitis. *Am J Gastroenterol* 2001; **96**: 519–25.

31 Chitturi S, George J. Hepatotoxicity of commonly used drugs: non-steroidal anti-inflammatory drugs, antihypertensives, antidiabetic agents, anticonvulsivants, lipid-lowering agents, psychotropic drugs. *Semin Liver Dis* 2002; **22**: 169–83.

32 Neuschwander-Tetri BA, Sponseller C, Hamptom KK *et al.* Rosiglitazone improves insulin sensitivity, ALT and hepatic steatosis in patients with non-alcoholic steatohep-

atitis [Abstract]. *Gastroenterology* 2002; **122** (Suppl.): 622.

33 Neuschwander-Tetri BA, Brunt EM, Bacon BR *et al.* Histological improvement in NASH following reduction of insulin resistance with 48-week treatment with the PPAPγ agonist rosiglitazone [Abstract]. *Hepatology* 2002; **36**: 379.

34 Acosta RC, Molina EG, O'Brien CB *et al.* The use of pioglitazone in non-alcoholic steatohepatitis [Abstract]. *Gastroenterology* 2001; **120** (Suppl.): 2778.

35 Sanyal AJ, Contos MJ, Sargeant C *et al.* A randomized controlled pilot study or pioglitazone and vitamin E versus vitamin E for non-alcoholic steatohepatitis [Abstract]. *Hepatology* 2002; **36**: 382.

36 Pomrat K, Lutchman G, Kleiner DE *et al.* Pilot study of pioglitazone in non-alcoholic steatohepatitis [Abstract]. *Gastroenterology* 2003; **124** (Suppl 1.): 708.

37 Marchesini G, Brizi M, Bianchi G *et al.* Metformin in non-alcoholic steatohepatitis. *Lancet* 2001; **358**: 893–4.

38 Nair S, Diehl AM, Perrillo R. Metformin in non-alcoholic steatohepatitis (NASH): efficacy and safety—a preliminary report [Abstract]. *Gastroenterology* 2002; **122** (Suppl.): 4.

39 Lavine JE. Vitamin E treatment of non-alcoholic steatohepatitis in children: a pilot study. *J Pediatr* 2000; **136**: 734–8.

40 Hasegawa T, Yoneda M, Nakamura K, Makino I, Terano A. Plasma transforming growth factor-β1 level and efficacy of α-tocopherol in patients with non-alcoholic steatohepatitis: a pilot study. *Aliment Pharmacol Ther* 2001; **15**: 1667–72.

41 Harrison SA, Torgerson S, Hayashi P, Ward J, Schenker S. Vitamin E and vitamin C treatment improves fibrosis in patients with non-alcoholic steatohepatitis. *Am J Gastroenterol* 2003; **98**: 2485–90.

42 Abdelmalek M, Angulo P, Jorgensen RA, Sylvestre P, Lindor KD. Betaine, a promising new agent for patients with non-alcoholic steatohepatitis: results of a pilot study. *Am J Gastroenterol* 2001; **96**: 2711–7.

43 Miglio F, Rovati LC, Santoro A, Setkikar I. Efficacy and safety of oral betaine glucurontae in non-alcoholic steatohepatitis. *Arzneimittelforschung/Drug Res* 2000; **50** (II): 722–7.

44 Gulbahar O, Karasu ZA, Ersoz G, Akarca US, Musoglu A. Treatment of non-alcoholic steatohepatitis with *N*-acetylcysteine [Abstract]. *Gastroenterology* 2000; **118** (Part 2 Suppl.): 6550.

45 Desai TK. Phlebotomy reduces transaminase levels in patients with non-alcoholic steatohepatitis [Abstract]. *Gastroenterology* 2000; **118** (Part 1, Suppl. 2): 1071.

46 Nitecki J, Jackson FW, Allen ML, Farr VL, Jackson FW. Effect of phlebotomy on non-alcoholic steatohepatitis (NASH) [Abstract]. *Gastroenterology* 2000; **118** (Part 2, Suppl. 2): 6679.

47 Facchini FS, Hua NW, Stoohs RA. Effect of iron depletion in carbohydrate-intolerant patients with clinical evidence of non-alcoholic fatty liver disease. *Gastroenterology* 2002; **122**: 931–9.

48 Rawat AK. Effect of clofibrate on cholesterol and lipid metabolism in ethanol-treated mice. *Res Commun Chem Pathol Pharmacol* 1975; **10**: 501–10.

49 Laurin J, Lindor KD, Crippin JS *et al.* Ursodeoxycholic acid or clofibrate in the treatment of non-alcohol-induced steatohepatitis: a pilot study. *Hepatology* 1996; **23**: 1464–7.

50 Basaranoglu M, Acbay O, Sonsuz A. A controlled trial of gemfibrozil in the treatment of patients with non-alcoholic steatohepatitis. *J Hepatol* 1999; **31**: 384.

51 Horlander JC, Kwo PY, Cummings OW, Koukoulis G. Atorvastatin for the treatment of NASH [Abstract]. *Gastroenterology* 2001; **120** (Suppl.): 2767.

52 Merat S, Malekzadeh R, Sohrabi MR *et al.* Probucol in the treatment of non-alcoholic steatohepatitis: a double-blind randomized controlled study. *J Hepatol* 2003; **38**: 414–8.

53 Guma C, Viola L, Thome M, Galdame O, Alvarez E. Ursodeoxycholic acid in the treatment of non-alcoholic steatohepatitis: results of a prospective clinical controlled trial [Abstract]. *Hepatology* 1997; **26** (Part 2 Suppl.): 1036.

54 Ceriani R, Bunati S, Morini L, Sacchi E, Colombo G. Effect of ursodeoxycholic acid plus diet in patients with non-alcoholic steatohepatitis [Abstract]. *Hepatology* 1998; **28** (Part 2 Suppl.): 894.

55 Holoman J, Glasa J, Kasar J *et al.* Serum markers of liver fibrosis in patients with non-alcoholic steatohepatitis (NASH): correlation to liver morphology and effect of therapy [Abstract]. *J Hepatol* 2000; **32** (Suppl 2): 210.

56 Letterson P, Fromenty B, Terris B, Degott C, Passayre D. Acute and chronic hepatic steatosis lead to *in vivo* lipid peroxidation in mice. *J Hepatol* 1996; **24**: 200–8.

57 Yang SS, Lin HZ, Lane MD, Clemens M, Diehl AM. Obesity increases sensitivity to endotoxin liver injury: implications for the pathogenesis of steatohepatitis. *Proc Natl Acad Sci USA* 1997; **94**: 2557–62.

58 Li Z, Yang S, Lin H *et al.* Probiotics and antibodies to TNF inhibit inflammatory activity and improve non-alcoholic fatty liver disease. *Hepatology* 2003; **37**: 343–50.

59 Loguercio C, De Simone T, Federico A *et al.* Gut-liver axis: a new point of attack to treat chronic liver damage? *Am J Gastroenterol* 2002; **97**: 2144–6.

60 Cortez-Pinto H, Chatham J, Chacko VP *et al.* Alterations in liver ATP homeostasis in human non-alcoholic steato-heaptitis: a pilot study. *J Am Med Assoc* 1999; **282**: 1659–64.

61 Weltman MD, Farrell GC, Liddle C. Increased hepatocyte CYP2E1 expression in a rat nutritional model of hepatic steatosis with inflammation. *Gastroenterology* 1996; **111**: 1645–53.

62 Weltman MD, Farrell GC, Hall P, Ingelman-Sundberg M, Liddle C. Hepatic cytochrome P450 2E1 is increased in patients with non-alcoholic steatohepatitis. *Hepatology* 1998; **27**: 128–33.

63 Leclercq IA, Farrell GC, Field J *et al.* CYP2E1 and CYP4A as microsomal catalysts of lipid peroxides in murine non-alcoholic steatohepatitis. *J Clin Invest* 2000; **105**: 1067–75.

64 Friedman SL. Molecular regulation of hepatic fibrosis: an integrated cellular response to tissue injury. *J Biol Chem* 2000; **275**: 2247–50.

65 Bataller R, Brenner DA. Stellate cells as a target for treatment of liver fibrosis. *Semin Liver Dis* 2001; **21**: 437–52.

66 Talwalkar J, Keach J, Angulo P, Lindor KD. Health-related quality of life assessment in non-alcoholic steatohepatitis [Abstract]. *Hepatology* 2001; **34** (Suppl): 309.

67 Talwalkar AJ, Donlinger JJ, Gossard AA, Lindor KD. Health state preferences among patients with non-alcoholic steatohepatitis [Abstract]. *Hepatology* 2002; **36** (Suppl): 382.

17 NAFLD, NASH and orthotopic liver transplantation

Anne Burke & Michael R. Lucey

Key learning points

1 NASH cirrhosis and NASH associated cryptogenic cirrhosis now account for 5–10% of the liver transplantation performed in the United States.
2 The degree of steatosis (macrovesicular more so than microvesicular) of the donor liver is directly related to primary non-function and graft survival post-transplant. Potential donor livers containing more than 30–50% fat are usually not accepted.
3 NASH and cryptogenic cirrhosis frequently recur or develop *de novo* post-transplant independently from the immunosuppressive drugs used post-transplant.
4 Transplant physicians need to recognize the clinical importance of hepatic steatosis and the metabolic syndrome both before and after liver transplantion.

Abstract

Non-alcoholic fatty liver disease (NAFLD) and non-alcoholic steatohepatitis (NASH)—a severe form of NAFLD—has produced an ironic combination of adverse effects for orthotopic liver transplantation (OLT), in that NAFLD has increased the need for donor livers at the same time as decreasing the number of donors available. Increasing evidence indicates that NASH cirrhosis and NASH-related cryptogenic cirrhosis can progress to end-stage liver disease, now accounting for as many as 10% of patients undergoing OLT.

Unfortunately, the high prevalence of NAFLD (associated with the epidemic of obesity and diabetes) in the population has decreased the donor pool. Because livers with steatosis (macrovesicular more so than microvesicular) result in poor post-OLTx outcomes, including primary graft non-function and decreased patient and graft survival, livers containing more than 30–50% of fat are usually not accepted as donors. The mechanism that these fatty livers perform poorly is related to a combination of diminished blood flow, poor membrane function, impaired energy production and oxidative stress. These issues affect both cadaver and living donor livers.

Hepatic steatosis is also common and affects other forms of end-stage liver disease, in particular patients with hepatitis C virus (HCV) infection. Fatty liver and related fibrosis may occur post-transplant in patients who had NASH or cryptogenic cirrhosis prior to the liver transplant or it can occur *de novo* and adversely affect outcomes. It is now clear that hepatic steatosis and its comorbidities associated with the insulin resistance syndrome (obesity, diabetes, hypertension and dyslipidaemias) impact the clinical outcomes and management issues of these patients. Therefore it is important for transplant physicians to be aware of the clinical relevance of fatty liver and its relationship with the insulin resistance syndrome and its comorbidities while performing patient selection and formulating targeted therapeutic strategies in these patients.

Introduction

NAFLD and NASH are becoming increasingly common in the population. We discuss here the impact of these conditions on OLT. In particular, we review the literature regarding the use of steatotic donor livers; NAFLD as a cause of end-stage liver disease requiring liver transplantation and the evaluation of NAFLD patients for OLT; recurrence or *de novo* NAFLD post-OLT; and the management of NAFLD both pre- and post-OLT.

Use of steatotic livers for liver transplantation

The demand for OLT continues to outstrip the supply of available cadaveric donor livers and each year many patients with end-stage liver disease die for lack of a suitable donor liver. Every year more than 1000 patients on the waiting list die without a liver transplant [1]. Steatosis of the donor liver is associated with an increased risk of primary non-function in the allograft, which may result in mortality or requirement for retransplantation [2]. Thus, a tension exists between the wish to put every potential donor liver to use and the wish to avoid primary non-function.

Primary non-function

Primary non-function (PNF) is defined as allograft failure within 7 days of OLT in the absence of technical problems such as hepatic artery thrombosis, biliary obstruction or dehiscence of the bile duct anastamosis. PNF is accompanied by increasing coagulopathy, rising bilirubin and the excretion of thin pale bile. The latter observation can be made in those recipients with a biliary drainage cannula. PNF has a high mortality and usually requires relisting and emergent retransplantation. Outcomes for retransplantation are less favourable than for primary transplantation (69% versus 87% 1-year survival) [1].

Poor early graft function is a variant of PNF in which hepatic function fails to advance as expected, albeit with more modest derangement of coagulation and biliary excretion. Poor early graft function may resolve with careful medical management, but it increases the cost by extending ICU stay and sometimes necessitates retransplantation.

Prevalence of NAFLD/NASH in donors

Steatosis is typically non-uniform and is difficult to assess accurately, particularly when it is less severe. In a review of more than 500 consecutive medicolegal autopsies following road traffic accidents, 24% of cadavers were found to have a fatty liver [3,4]. According to the estimates of 94 liver transplant surgeons from the UK and USA, the degree of steatosis ranged from 20% to 40% in approximately half of all retrieved livers, and a further 14–19% donor livers showed 40–60% steatosis [5]. The diagnosis of steatosis of the donor liver was often based on clinical impression. For example, in the survey cited above, 12 of 94 surgeons declared that they undertook a liver biopsy in every potential donor, but eight of 94 said that they never took a biopsy to determine fat content in any donor. There remained 70 of 94 who said that they took one or more biopsies whenever they were concerned about the appearance of the liver or the donor had risk factors for steatosis.

Outcomes after transplantation using steatotic donor livers

There is evidence to support the belief that macrovesicular steatosis is associated with increased rates of PNF and poorer outcome. For example, the outcomes of 59 patients receiving livers with up to 30% macrovesicular steatosis were worse than those observed in 57 patients receiving livers without fatty infiltration. The recipients of the steatotic livers had higher rates of PNF (5.1% compared to 1.8%) and worse 2-year patient survival (77% compared to 91%) and graft survival (70% compared to 82%) [6]. A retrospective study of 443 patients showed that increasing donor steatosis grade was associated with 1-month but not 3- or 12-month allograft loss [7]. In both of these studies, recipient status was similarly distributed between the varying grades of steatosis, refuting the concern that poorer outcomes among recipients of fatty livers are confounded by greater severity of illness pre-OLT.

In contrast, microvesicular steatosis does not seem to carry the same risk of PNF as does macrovesicular steatosis. In a single centre study from the USA, 40 of 426 liver transplants involved donor livers with at least 30% microvesicular steatosis were compared to the 386 livers without steatosis [8]. The rates of PNF (5.0% and 5.1%) were identical irrespective of allograft microvesicular fatty deposition, although there was a tendency for more prolonged postoperative 'early poor graft function' in the study group. One-year patient survival (80% compared to 79.8%) and graft survival (72.5% compared to 68.4%) were similar in both groups.

Donor selection in relation to donor liver fat content

There is no consistent threshold of estimated macrovesicular fat deposition above which liver transplantation is precluded. Practices regarding acceptance of donor livers with fat accumulation vary considerably between surgeons. In the study of the attitudes of liver transplant surgeons to donor liver fat content cited above, 27% of surgeons surveyed would automatically reject a liver with an estimated 30% steatosis. Seventy-six per cent of surgeons would decline the offered liver that was thought to contain greater than 50% steatosis [5]. Interestingly, 50% of the surveyed surgeons considered microvesicular steatosis to be a risk factor for PNF in the allograft (see above).

Risk factors such as diabetes mellitus in the donor or poor health in the recipient may influence the outcome of transplantation. Thus, whereas livers with more than 60% macrosteatosis should probably be excluded automatically, livers with more moderate steatosis (30–60%) may be utilized in the absence of additional risk factors in the donor or recipient, or when the recipient's circumstances are judged to be sufficiently critical to justify the risk [9].

Mechanisms of primary non-function or poor early graft function

The mechanisms whereby steatosis of the donor organ leads to PNF are not understood completely, but several have been proposed [9,10]:

1 *Diminished portal blood flow.* In animal studies, hepatocytes ballooned with macrovesicular steatosis distort the sinusoidal lumen and lead to increased hepatic portal resistance, reduced blood flow and secondary ischaemia.

2 *Inefficient anaerobic metabolism.* Fatty livers have a relative increase in uncoupling protein levels with decreased mitochondrial adenosine triphosphate (ATP) production [11]. This is compounded during the anaerobic phase of warm ischaemia and cold preservation. The energy level within the hepatocyte has been shown to correlate with the eventual outcome after transplantation [12].

3 *Physical properties of lipid.* Some studies suggest that the sinusoids of steatotic livers have altered plasma membrane fluidity, leaving them prone to increased Kupffer cell adhesion and activation on reperfusion [13]. Alternatively, it has been hypothesized that the lipid solidifies during cold preservation, causing physical disruption to the hepatocytes.

4 *Oxidative stress.* The steatotic liver is believed to be prone to oxidative stress at baseline [14]. Oxidative stress is a key component to reperfusion injury of the newly perfused graft. One could speculate that a steatotic liver already predisposed to oxidative stress would suffer greater injury at reperfusion than a non-steatotic liver which is more able to maintain redox balance. Indeed, administration of tocopherol, an oxygen radical scavenger, improves survival of Zucker rats exposed to ischaemia and reperfusion injury [15].

Living donor liver transplantation

In recent years, living donor liver transplantation both from adult to child, and from adult to adult has been adopted as a means to avoid death on the liver transplant waiting list and to improve overall outcomes [16]. Given the small graft size, the need for rapid regeneration of liver volume in both the donor and recipient and the importance of avoiding morbidity in the donor, most centers aim to select donors with less than 10% steatosis and are reluctant to use livers with more than 20% steatosis [17,18]. Many centers exclude potential donors with a body mass index (BMI) > 28. MRI is becoming the preferred method of detecting steatosis as it allows for estimation of the quantity of fat present [19]. Alternatively, an unenhanced computerized tomography (CT) scan of the liver showing the attenuation of the liver to be at least 10 Hounsfield units less than the spleen is highly suggestive of fatty liver [19]. Thus, potential donors with these findings can be excluded from liver donation without being exposed to the risk of liver biopsy.

Table 17.1 Prevalence of obesity and diabetes in patients with cryptogenic cirrhosis awaiting liver transplantation.

Study reference	Cases	Controls*	Prevalence of obesity (%)†			Diabetes (%)‡		
			Cases	Controls	Gen pop	Cases	Controls	Gen pop
Caldwell *et al.* [26]	70	72	47	8	12	53	21	6
Poonawala *et al.* [25]	65	98	47	24	12	47	22	6

* Controls for Caldwell *et al.* [26] exclude those with diagnosis of NASH.
† Obesity defined as BMI > 31.1 (males), > 32.3 (females) (Caldwell *et al.* [26]), BMI > 30 (Poonawala *et al.* [26]).
‡ Overall prevalence of diabetes in USA is 6.2%, but 20% in those over 65 years of age [27].

NAFLD and NASH as causes of end-stage liver disease leading to transplantation

It has been recognized for some time that obesity is an independent risk factor for end-stage liver disease and for cirrhosis in patients with HCV infection [20] or alcoholic liver disease [21,22]. Furthermore, obesity may accelerate the progression to liver failure in a broad spectrum of liver disease patients. Thus, 54% of patients undergoing liver transplantation in one North American series were overweight or obese [23]. Although a minority of these recipients were morbidly obese, short- and long-term morbidity and mortality were increased significantly in the obese group. Much of the increased late mortality is caused by increased cardiovascular death.

The prevalence of NAFLD or NASH among patients with cirrhosis leading to liver failure in the absence of chronic viral hepatitis, alcoholism or other definable cause (cryptogenic cirrhosis) has been studied only recently. Nevertheless, although circumstantial, an ever-increasing body of evidence suggests that NASH can progress to end-stage liver disease. A single center study [24] noted that 2.9% of their primary liver transplants were performed for NASH. However, they did not include patients who carried the diagnosis of cryptogenic cirrhosis. In 2002, approximately 7% of US patients undergoing OLT had cryptogenic cirrhosis as the aetiology of their liver disease [1]. Recent studies suggest that up to 50% of cases identified as cryptogenic cirrhosis may in fact have arisen from NASH [25,26]. The prevalence of the insulin resistance syndrome (also known as the metabolic syndrome) is increased in patients given the diagnosis of cryptogenic cirrhosis. In two case–control studies of 70 [26] and 65 [25] patients, respectively, obesity (defined as BMI > 31 [26] or BMI > 30 [25]) and diabetes were considerably more common among patients with cryptogenic cirrhosis than among cirrhotic controls or the general population (Table 17.1).

Impact of the insulin resistance or metabolic syndrome on selection of liver transplant candidates

It is likely that many potential transplant candidates with cryptogenic cirrhosis are excluded because of the comorbid impact of the insulin resistance syndrome [28]. Nevertheless, drawing from available data, one can make some estimates of the potential contribution of NASH to the pool of patients in need of liver transplantation in the next few years. We start with the presumption that 3% of the normal population and 20% of the obese population have NASH [29–31]. We then conservatively estimate that 15% of these persons are likely to progress to cirrhosis [32]. The Centers for Disease Control (CDC) estimate that the prevalence of overweight and obesity will increase to 65% and 30% respectively in the next 20 years, which would translate to a prevalence of 25 million patients with NASH and 3.7 million with cirrhosis. This prevalence would exceed by 10-fold the current USA prevalence of HCV of 2.7 million and approximately 400 000 cases of HCV-related cirrhosis.

Impact of the insulin resistance syndrome on morbidity and mortality after liver transplantation

There are no data directly addressing the impact of the insulin resistance syndrome on outcome after liver transplantation; at most, we can look at the impact of some of its component features. For example, diabetes is an independent risk factor for 'poor outcome' after liver transplantation. Shields *et al.* [33] reported on survival in more than 1000 patients with a median follow-up of 15 months. They compared patients with and without diabetes (defined according to the World Health Organization criteria: fasting blood glucose level > 7.8 mmol/L, or the preoperative requirement for insulin therapy or oral antidiabetic drugs). They found survival of only 64% in recipients who were diabetic prior to transplant, although only one death could be directly attributed to diabetes. In contrast, 91% of recipients who did not demonstrate insulin-requiring or tablet-controlled diabetes prior to transplant survived [33].

Data on morbidity and mortality after liver transplantation among obese subjects are mixed. Data from single transplant series suggest that obese patients are not at increased risk [34,35]. In contrast, Nair *et al.* [23] reviewed the United Network for Organ Sharing (UNOS) database and described the recorded outcomes in 2966 patients with a BMI > 30. This study showed a higher prevalence of cryptogenic cirrhosis in the obese recipients. Survival at all time points (immediate to 5 years post-OLT) was significantly reduced in obese subjects, largely as a result of cardiovascular events.

The above data suggest that although the prevalence of NASH and insulin resistance is high and may be increasing, it has infrequently led to OLT up to now [24]. In addition, obesity probably increases the morbidity and mortality of OLT. One approach to these data might be to conclude that NASH is a relatively benign condition, at least in relation to the risk of end-stage liver disease sufficient to require transplantation. An alternative hypothesis is that of competing risk. Liver transplant recipients constitute a carefully selected group. They must demonstrate severe liver disease, albeit without comorbid conditions that would preclude OLT. In at least one study, OLT recipients whose underlying liver disease was attributed to NASH were younger than those in the control groups [26]. Furthermore, the observation that liver-related mortality, but not overall mortality, is increased in some single centre series [28] may be a reflection of the increased all cause mortality of these patients. In other words, NASH patients do not often come to transplantation because premature non-liver death or comorbid conditions prevent OLT.

Evaluation for OLT of patients with NASH or cryptogenic cirrhosis

Assessment of severity of liver disease

Evaluation of patients with NASH or cryptogenic cirrhosis for OLT should follow the same guidelines as that of patients with other forms of liver disease. In each case, their liver disease should be of such severity so as to warrant OLT. In general, this means that they should manifest decompensated cirrhosis [36]. Compensated cirrhosis in general has a better 1-year prognosis than liver transplantation, whereas decompensated cirrhosis has a worse 1-year prognosis than OLT [36]. In addition, the patient should be free of comorbidities that would mitigate against a good outcome.

The evaluation of the potential OLT candidate should include an assessment of cardiovascular risk factors, remembering that obesity is associated with an increased risk of cardiovascular disease. Most commonly, evaluation involves history and physical examination, electrocardiogram, echocardiogram and dobutamine stress echo. Important findings include cardiac risk factors (smoking, hypertension, diabetes, hypercholesterolaemia, family history of heart disease), chest discomfort or undue dyspnoea on exertion. A poor functional capacity (e.g. inability to walk up a flight of stairs) has been shown to predict increased perioperative and long-term risk [37]. Physical examination may reveal cardiac murmurs and/or left ventricular heave (often difficult to ascertain in the obese). Repolarization defects on electrocardiography, and segmental wall motion abnormalities and decreased ejection fraction on echocardiography should be noted. Given that cirrhotic patients tend to have peripheral vasodilation and afterload reduction, a decreased ejection fraction is of concern. Those patients with significant findings on the above screening should undergo cardiac catheterization.

Pulmonary evaluation should include screening for pulmonary hypertension. Through its links with obstructive sleep apnoea, restrictive lung disease and thromboembolic disease, obesity is a risk factor for pulmonary hypertension, independent of the porto-pulmonary hypertensive syndrome. Pulmonary hypertension leads to right ventricular overload and failure. Pulmonary hypertension in cirrhotic patients is often asymptomatic until severe (e.g. pulmonary artery pressures > 60 mmHg). Likely findings are a history of dyspnoea on exertion and a loud pulmonary heart sound on auscultation. However, 'moderate' pulmonary hypertension is silent and is noted only on echocardiogram [38]. Pulmonary hypertension leads to an increased risk of perioperative mortality in the setting of liver transplantation. At the time of reperfusion, even with careful rinsing, the venous drainage from the newly perfused liver tends to be cold, acidic and hyperkalaemic, all of which have negative inotropic and arrhythmogenic effects. This in turn causes acute right heart failure, circulatory collapse and underperfusion and ischaemia of the engrafted liver. Even when patients with severe pulmonary hypertension survive the liver transplant operation, ongoing right ventricular failure may ensue, with approximately 50% 1-year mortality [39]. Thus, a mean pulmonary artery pressure of 50 mmHg, although considered 'moderate' by the pulmonologists, is a contraindication to OLT [40].

Obese patients should also be screened for obstructive sleep apnoea. Not only can obstructive sleep apnoea promote pulmonary hypertension, but also the associated daytime somnolence may be mistaken for hepatic encephalopathy. The typical findings are interrupted sleep with loud snoring and excessive daytime somnolence.

The morbidly obese liver transplant candidate may suffer from restrictive lung disease and increased work of breathing, resulting from decreased chest wall compliance and increased pressure from the abdomen [41]. Morbid obesity also increases gastric pressure and the risk of gastroesophageal reflux and aspiration [42,43]. Again history and physical examination is vital: history may reveal undue dyspnoea on exertion and/or heartburn; physical examination is often non-specific. Spirometry may reveal decreased total lung capacity, functional residual capacity and vital capacity [41].

Previously unrecognized diabetes mellitus should be ruled out and, if found, screening for diabetic complications (vasculopathy, nephropathy, neuropathy and retinopathy) is warranted. Finally, in the postoperative state, vigilance should be maintained for thromboembolism and wound infection [42].

Fatty liver disease following liver transplantation

There are now several case reports of NASH developing *de novo* or recurring in the OLT recipient [44–46]. Steatosis has been seen within 6 months of transplantation, with fibrosis and cirrhosis being recognized at 2 and 6 years, respectively [44,47].

Recurrence

NASH with fibrosis has been documented following OLT for cryptogenic cirrhosis [34]. In one descriptive series from a single centre, 27 of 30 patients transplanted for cryptogenic cirrhosis or NASH were followed for at least 1 year, and had follow-up liver. Fourteen of 25 (56%) demonstrated steatosis albeit mild, with only three patients having steatosis involving more than 50% of the hepatocytes. This is in contrast to age- and sex-matched control patients who were transplanted for cholestatic or alcoholic liver disease, of whom only 25% developed steatosis. Although the majority of cases of steatosis arose within 12 months of OLT, the probability of being free of steatosis continued to decline with the duration of follow-up. The authors commented that the majority had not progressed to end-stage liver disease, albeit after a relatively short follow-up of 3.5 years. Garcia *et al.* [46] described four patients who developed NASH post-OLT. All subjects were at risk of post-OLT NASH. Two were transplanted for cryptogenic cirrhosis and had diabetes (one obese). One had hyperlipidaemia and one was obese with post-OLT hypertriglyceridaemia. Although all four patients were alive without graft failure 5 years post-OLT, two had developed cirrhosis at 44 and 84 months, respectively. Taken together, these data suggest that the post-liver transplant state may promote fatty reaccumulation in the allograft.

De novo post-OLT NASH

This has not been studied systematically but the immunosuppressive medications used may predispose to the development of NAFLD. Prednisone is used particularly in the early post-OLT period and boluses of corticosteroids are used to treat episodes of acute cellular rejection. Prednisone is a risk factor for fatty liver. Tacrolimus may be more diabetogenic than cyclosporin A in liver transplant recipients [48]. Both corticosteroids and calcineurin inhibitors promote hypertension and hypercholesterolaemia.

These observations should be considered in the context of the more general risk for component features of

Table 17.2 Risk factors for insulin resistance syndrome/fatty liver disease following liver transplantation and in the general population. (Modified from Burke [57].)

Risk factor	Prevalence post-transplant (%) [49–54]	Rate in US population (%) [55,56]
Hypertension (BP > 140/90 mmHg)	41–81	15.7
Hypercholesterolaemia (> 240 mgdl)	20–66	14.9
HDL (< 35 mgdl)	52	12
Diabetes mellitus	21–32	6.2
Obesity (BMI > 30)	39–43	16.1

the insulin resistance syndrome in solid organ transplant recipients (Table 17.2).

Environmental factors leading to NAFLD/NASH after liver transplantation

The rates of obesity, hypercholesterolaemia, diabetes mellitus and hypertension—all features of the insulin resistance syndrome—are increased after liver transplantation (Table 17.2) [57]. In addition, only a minority (24%) of long-term liver transplant survivors achieve the level of physical activity recommended by the surgeon general [58], although these data merely mimic the sedentary habits of the US population (26.2%). Physical fitness has been shown to be as powerful a modulator of insulin resistance as body weight, each independently accounting for approximately 25% of the differences in insulin-mediated glucose disposal in non-diabetic individuals [59,60].

Mechanisms for NAFLD/NASH in the transplanted liver

The two-hit hypothesis for the development of NASH proposed by Day and James [61] proposed that steatosis and oxidative stress, rather than just hepatic steatosis, are required to develop NASH. The metabolic aberrations described in Table 17.2 are associated with steatosis. Hypercholesterolaemia and diabetes mellitus have been associated with increased oxidative stress [62,63]. In addition, we have shown that markers of oxidative stress are markedly elevated in during liver transplantation, and remain elevated throughout the first postoperative year (Fig. 17.1) [64]. The rapid progression from pristine allograft to steatosis and fibrosis described in the foregoing account is very consistent with the Day–James hypothesis.

NASH and hepatitis C virus in liver allografts

Almost 50% of liver transplants are performed for HCV infection. HCV infection is associated with an increased prevalence of diabetes mellitus [65], steatosis [66,67] (although this has been disputed [68]) and oxidative stress [69]. Furthermore, HCV infection of the graft is almost universal in HCV-positive OLT recipients. However, for reasons of definition, as with excessive alcohol consumption, the presence of HCV precludes the diagnosis of NAFLD, thus these patients are not included among those with post-OLT NASH. It seems likely, none the less, that HCV acts in concert with NASH and insulin resistance to promote oxidative injury in the transplanted liver.

Management of the metabolic syndrome after liver transplantation

Remarkably little has been written on the management of the insulin resistance or metabolic syndrome after OLT. De novo research on the topic is almost non-existent. However, with 3-year survival of approximately 80% and increasing recognition of the long-term medical problems of the liver transplant recipient there is need for research in this area.

Fatigue is a major limitation in functional capacity for patients with end-stage liver disease and after liver transplantation. The sedentary lifestyle of many liver transplant recipients has been commented on in earlier sections of this chapter. Liver transplant recipients need to be encouraged to return to regular physical activity. Exercise has been shown to be associated with better blood glucose, blood pressure and lipid levels and decreased cardiovascular mortality in the non-transplant population. Physical exercise has also been shown to maintain bone mass—another problem post-liver trans-

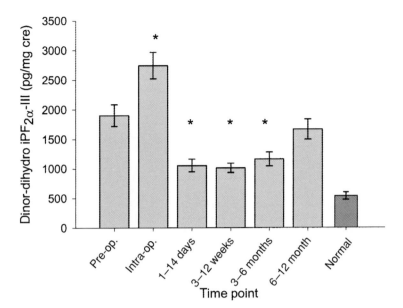

Fig. 17.1 Urinary dinor-dihydro $iPF_{2\alpha}$-III per mg creatinine excretion in OLT recipients and healthy volunteers. $iPF_{2\alpha}$-III levels in OLT subjects at all time points significantly different to healthy volunteers (dark grey bar). Levels at 6–12 months post-OLT not significantly different to pre-OLT levels. * Significantly different to preoperative levels; $P < 0.05$.

plant. It has been suggested that the metabolic benefits of exercise are related to overall energy expenditure rather than intensity of exercise and can occur without significant changes in cardiovascular fitness [70,71]. Diet and exercise has also been shown to decrease weight and improve transaminases in non-OLT patients with NASH.

Return to work after liver transplantation is related not only to physical status but also to marital status and to duration of pretransplant illness and the interval without work prior to transplantation [72]. Consequently, the capacity of the successful liver transplant recipient to undertake adequate physical activity may be determined by more than just their physical ability. Although it is intuitive that early application of a physical exercise programme in conjunction with a calorie controlled nutritionally adequate diet would decrease the rates of post-OLT hypertension, diabetes, obesity and hypercholesterolaemia, it is not known how best to achieve these aims nor how effective they might be. It is unlikely that lifestyle measures alone will be sufficient for control of the insulin resistance syndrome post-OLT but should be combined with antihypertensive and lipid-lowering medications, glycaemic control and smoking cessation. Treatment of the insulin resistance syndrome in non-transplant patients has been reviewed in Chapters 4, 15 and 16. The role of these therapeutic modalities in the transplant setting remains to be investigated.

References

1 Liver transplant waiting list. UNOS database, 2000.
2 Todo S, DeMetris AJ, Makowka L *et al.* Primary non-function of hepatic allografts with pre-existing fatty infiltration. *Transplantation* 1989; **47**: 903–5.
3 Hilden M, Christoffersen P, Juhl E, Dalgaard JB. Liver histology in a 'normal' population: examinations of 503 consecutive fatal traffic casualties. *Scand J Gastroenterol* 1977; **12**: 593–7.
4 Ostrom M, Eriksson A. Single-vehicle crashes and alcohol: a retrospective study of passenger car fatalities in northern Sweden. *Accid Anal Prev* 1993; **25**: 171–6.
5 Imber CJ, St Peter SD, Lopez I, Guiver L, Friend PJ. Current practice regarding the use of fatty livers: a trans-Atlantic survey. *Liver Transpl* 2002; **8**: 545–9.
6 Marsman WA, Wiesner RH, Rodriguez L *et al.* Use of fatty donor liver is associated with diminished early patient and graft survival. *Transplantation* 1996; **62**: 1246–51.
7 Verran D, Kusyk T, Painter D *et al.* Clinical experience gained from the use of 120 steatotic donor livers for orthotopic liver transplantation. *Liver Transpl* 2003; **9**: 500–5.
8 Fishbein TM, Fiel IM, Emre S *et al.* Use of livers with microvesicular fat safely expands the donor pool. *Transplantation* 1997; **64**: 248–51.
9 Urena MA, Moreno GE, Romero CJ, Ruiz-Delgado FC, Moreno SC. An approach to the rational use of steatotic

donor livers in liver transplantation [Review]. *Hepato-gastroenterology* 1999; **46**: 1164–73.

10 Imber CJ, St Peter SD, Handa A, Friend PJ. Hepatic steatosis and its relationship to transplantation. *Liver Transpl* 2002; **8**: 415–23.

11 Cortez-Pinto H, Lin HZ, Yang SQ, Da Costa SO, Diehl AM. Lipids upregulate uncoupling protein 2 expression in rat hepatocytes. *Gastroenterology* 1999; **116**: 1184–93.

12 Cisneros C, Guillen F, Gomez R *et al.* Analysis of warm ischaemia time for prediction of primary non-function of the hepatic graft. *Transplant Proc* 1991; **23**: 1976.

13 Fukumori T, Ohkohchi N, Tsukamoto S, Satomi S. The mechanisms of injury in a steatotic liver graft during cold preservation. *Transplantation* 1999; **67**: 195–200.

14 Seki S, Kitada T, Yamada T *et al. In situ* detection of lipid peroxidation and oxidative DNA damage in non-alcoholic fatty liver diseases. *J Hepatol* 2002; **37**: 56–62.

15 Soltyl K, Dikdan G, Koneru B. Oxidative stress in fatty livers of obese Zucker rats: rapid amelioration and improved tolerance to warm ischemia with tocopherol. *Hepatology* 2003; **34**: 13–8.

16 Brown RS, Russo MW, Lai M *et al.* A survey of liver transplantation from living adult donors in the United States. *N Engl J Med* 2003; **348**: 818–25.

17 Rinella ME, Alonso E, Rao S *et al.* Body mass index as a predictor of hepatitic steatosis in living liver donors. *Liver Transpl* 2001; **7**: 409–14.

18 Trotter JF. Thin chance for fat people to become living donors. *Liver Transpl* 2001; **7**: 415–7.

19 Siegelman I, Rosen MA. Imaging of hepatic steatosis. *Semin Liver Dis* 2001; **21**: 71.

20 Ortiz V, Berenguer M, Rayon JM, Carrasco D, Berenguer J. Contribution of obesity to hepatitis C-related fibrosis progression. *Am J Gastroenterol* 2002; **97**: 2408–14.

21 Raynard B, Balian A, Falik D *et al.* Risk factors of fibrosis in alcohol-induced liver disease. *Hepatology* 2002; **35**: 635–58.

22 Naveau S, Giraud V, Borotto E *et al.* Excess weight risk factor for alcoholic liver disease. *Hepatology* 1997; **25**: 108–11.

23 Nair SP, Verma S, Thuluvath PJ. Obesity and its effect on survival in patients undergoing orthotopic liver transplantation in the United States. *Hepatology* 2002; **35**: 105–9.

24 Charlton M, Kasparova P, Weston S *et al.* Frequency of non-alcoholic steatohepatitis as a cause of advanced liver disease. *Liver Transpl* 2001; **7**: 608–14.

25 Poonawala A, Nair SP, Thuluvath PJ. Prevalence of obesity and diabetes in patients with cryptogenic cirrhosis: a case–control study. *Hepatology* 2000; **32**: 689–92.

26 Caldwell SH, Oelsner DH, Iezzoni JC *et al.* Cryptogenic cirrhosis: clinical characterization and risk factors for underlying disease. *Hepatology* 1999; **29**: 664–9.

27 National Diabetes Fact Sheet, 2002. Centers for Disease Control, 2002.

28 Matteoni CA, Younossi ZM, Gramlich T *et al.* Non-alcoholic fatty liver disease: a spectrum of clinical and pathological severity. *Hepatology* 1999; **116**: 1413–9.

29 Wanless IR, Lentz JS. Fatty liver hepatitis (steatohepatitis) and obesity: an autopsy study with analysis of risk factors. *Hepatology* 1990; **12**: 1106–10.

30 Sheth SG, Gordon FD, Chopra S. Non-alcoholic steato-hepatitis. *Ann Intern Med* 1997; **126**: 137–45.

31 Propst A, Propst T, Judmaier G, Vogel W. Prognosis in non-alcoholic steatohepatitis. *Gastroenterology* 1995; **108**: 1607.

32 Angulo P, Keach JC, Batts K, Lindor KD. Independent predictors of liver fibrosis in patients with non-alcoholic steatohepatitis. *Hepatology* 1999; **30**: 1356–62.

33 Shields PL, Tang H, Neuberger JM *et al.* Poor outcome in patients with diabetes mellitus undergoing liver transplantation. *Transplantation* 1999; **68**: 530–5.

34 Contos MJ, Cales W, Sterling RK *et al.* Development of non-alcoholic fatty liver disease after orthotopic liver transplantation for cryptogenic cirrhosis. *Liver Transpl* 2001; **7**: 363–73.

35 Sawyer RG, Pelletier SJ, Pruett TL. Increased early morbidity and mortality with acceptable long-term function in severely obese patients undergoing liver transplantation. *Clin Transplant* 1999; **13** (part 2): 126–40.

36 Lucey MR, Browne KA, Everson GT *et al.* Minimal criteria for placement of adults on the liver transplant waiting list: a report of a national conference organized by the American Society of Transplant Physicians and the American Association for the Study of Liver Diseases. *Liver Transplant Surg* 1997; **3**: 628–37.

37 Morris CK, Ueshima K, Kawaguchi T *et al.* The prognostic value of exercise capacity: a review of the literature. *Am Heart J* 1991; **122**: 1423–31.

38 Colle IO, Moreau R, Godinho E *et al.* Diagnosis for portopulmonary hypertension in candidates for liver transplantation: a prospective study. *Hepatology* 2003; **37**: 401–9.

39 Ramsay MAE, Simpson BR, Nguyen A-T *et al.* Severe pulmonary hypertension in liver transplant candidates. *Liver Transplant Surg* 1997; **3**: 494–500.

40 Krowka MJ, Plevak DJ, Findlay JY *et al.* Pulmonary hemodynamics and perioperative cardiopulmonary-related mortality in patients with portopulmonary hypertension undergoing liver transplantation. *Liver Transpl* 2000; **6**: 443–50.

41 Ray CS, Sue DY, Bray G, Hansen JE, Wasserman K. Effects of obesity on respiratory function. *Am Rev Respir Dis* 1983; **128**: 501–6.

42 Marik P, Varon J. The obese patient in the ICU. *Chest* 1998; **113**: 492–8.

43 Rose DK, Cohen MM, Wigglesworth DF, DeBoer DP. Critical respiratory events in the post-anesthesia care unit: patient, surgical and anesthetic factors. *Anesthesiology* 1994; **81**: 410–8.

44 Cauble MS, Gilroy R, Sorrell MF *et al.* Lipoatrophic diabetes and end-stage liver disease secondary to non-alcoholic steatohepatitis with recurrence after liver transplantation. *Transplantation* 2001; **71**: 892–5.

45 Duchini A, Brunson ME. Rous-en-Y gastric bypass for recurrent non-alcoholic steatohepatitis in liver transplant recipients with morbid obesity. *Transplantation* 2001; **72**: 156–71.

46 Garcia RF, Morales E, Garcia CE *et al.* Recurrent and *de novo* non-alcoholic steatohepatitis following orthotopic liver transplantation. *Arq Gastroenterol* 2001; **38**: 247–53.

47 Molloy RM, Komorowski R, Varma RR. Recurrent non-alcoholic steatohepatitis and cirrhosis after liver transplantation. *Liver Transplant Surg* 1997; **3**: 117–78.

48 Tacrolimus versus microemulsified ciclosporin in liver transplantation: the TMC randomized controlled trial. *Lancet* 2002; **360**: 1119–25.

49 Guckelberger O, Langrehr JM, Bechstein WO *et al.* Does the choice of primary immunosuppression influence the prevalence of cardiovascular risk factors after liver transplantation. *Transplant Proc* 1996; **28**: 3173–4.

50 Ali A, Befeler AS, Bacon BR *et al.* Hyperhomocysteinemia in liver transplant recipients [Abstract]. *Transplantation* 2000; **68** (Suppl.): S391.

51 Canzanello VJ, Schwartz L, Taler SJ *et al.* Evolution of cardiovascular risk after liver transplantation: a comparison of cyclosporin A and tacrolimus (FK506). *Liver Transplant Surg* 1997; **3**: 1–9.

52 Monsour HP, Wood RP, Dyer CH *et al.* Renal insufficiency and hypertension as long-term complications in liver transplantation. *Semin Liver Dis* 1995; **15**: 123–32.

53 Bismuth M, Pageaux G-P, Onea D *et al.* Follow-up of patients surviving more than 5 years after liver transplantation [Abstract]. *Hepatology* 2000; **32**: 255A.

54 Sanchez EQ, Marubashi S, Jung GJ *et al.* De novo tumours after liver transplantation occur in a set timeline [Abstract]. *Transplantation* 2000; **69**: S392.

55 Greenlee RT, Hill-Harmon MB, Murray T, Thun M. Cancer statistics, 2001. *CA Cancer J Clin* 2001; **51**: 15–36.

56 Jones CA, McQuillan GM, Kusek JW *et al.* Serum creatinine levels in the US population: third National Health and Nutrition Examination Survey. *Am J Kidney Dis* 1998; **32**: 992–9.

57 Burke A. Medical management of the liver transplant patient. In: Lucey MR, Shaked A, Neuberger JM, eds. *Liver Transplantation*. Texas: Landes Bioscience, 2003.

58 Painter P, Krasnoff J, Paul SM, Ascher NL. Physical activity and health-related quality of life in liver transplant recipients. *Liver Transpl* 2001; **7**: 213–9.

59 Reaven GM. Importance of identifying the overweight patient who will benefit the most by losing weight. *Ann Intern Med* 2003; **138**: 420–3.

60 Bogardus C, Lillioja S, Mott DM, Hollenbeck C, Reaven GM. Relationship between degree of obesity and *in vivo* insulin action in man. *Am J Physiol* 2003; **248** (part 1): E286–91.

61 Day CP, James OFW. Hepatic steatosis: innocent bystander or guilty party. *Hepatology* 1998; **27**: 1463–6.

62 Free radicals, and other reactive species and disease. In: Halliwell B, Gutteridge JMC, eds. *Free Radicals in Biology and Medicine*. Oxford: Oxford University Press, 1999: 617.

63 Reilly M, Pratico D, Delanty N *et al.* Increased formation of distinct F_2 isoprostanes in hypercholesterolemia. *Circulation* 1998; **98**: 2822–8.

64 Burke A, FitzGerald GA, Lucey MR. A prospective analysis of oxidative stress and liver transplantation. *Transplantation* 2002; **74**: 217–21.

65 Mehta SH, Brancati FL, Sulkowski MS *et al.* Prevalence of type 2 diabetes mellitus among persons with hepatitis C virus infection in the United States. *Ann Intern Med* 2000; **133**: 592–9.

66 Monto A. Hepatitis C and steatosis. *Semin Gastrointest Dis* 2002; **13**: 40–6.

67 Fujie H, Yotsuyanagi H, Moriya K *et al.* Steatosis and intrahepatic hepatitis C virus in chronic hepatitis. *J Med Virol* 1999; **59**: 141–5.

68 Fiore G, Fera G, Vella F, Schiraldi O. Liver steatosis and chronic hepatitis C: a spurious association? *Gastroenterol Hepatol* 1996; **8**: 125–9.

69 Jain SK, Pemberton PW, Smith A *et al.* Oxidative stress in chronic hepatitis C: not just a feature of late stage disease. *J Hepatol* 2002; **36**: 805–11.

70 Després J-P, Lamarche B. Effects of diet and physical activity on adiposity and body fat distribution: implications for the prevention of cardiovascular disease. *Nutr Res Rev* 1993; **6**: 137–59.

71 Després J-P. Visceral obestiy, insulin resistance, and dyslipidaemia: contribution of endurance exercise training to the treatment of the plurimetabolic syndrome. *Exerc Sport Sci Rev* 1997; **25**: 271–300.

72 Nicholas JJ, Oleske D, Robinson LR, Switala JA, Tarter RE. The quality of life after orthotopic liver transplantation: an analysis of 166 cases. *Arch Phys Med Rehabil* 1994; **75**: 431–7.

18 NAFLD/NASH is not just a 'Western' problem: some perspectives on NAFLD/NASH from the East

Shivakumar Chitturi & Jacob George

Key learning points

1 Non-alcoholic fatty liver disease (NAFLD) should be regarded as a global health problem of increasing dimensions.

2 More data are required on the prevalence of NAFLD in Asia and from the Pacific Rim countries.

3 Clinical and metabolic profiles of Asian patients are broadly similar to Western patients with NAFLD.

4 Cut-off for body mass index is lower than in Western populations. Assessment of central adiposity is critical in 'lean' patients.

5 Diet and exercise should probably be the initial options for management in the Asian context. The role of pharmacological therapy is not clearly defined.

6 Public health initiatives are imperative to halt or reverse the 'diabesity' epidemic, the underlying basis of NAFLD.

Abstract

Non-alcoholic fatty liver disease (NAFLD), as conventionally recognized, is a metabolic disorder largely confined to residents of affluent industrialized Western countries. However, insulin resistance, the common substrate of NAFLD, is not restricted to the West, as witnessed by its increasingly universal distribution. In particular, there has been an upsurge in insulin resistance-associated disease states in the Asia–Pacific region. In light of this, we provide a regional perspective of NAFLD, reviewing existing data and examine the epidemiological basis for its anticipated increase. Other than for Japan (10–15%) and Taiwan (36.9%), little is known about the prevalence rates of NAFLD in this region. However, changing demographic trends, especially the epidemic of 'diabesity', are expected to profoundly increase the future incidence and prevalence

rates of NAFLD. While the clinical profiles of NAFLD in Asian patients are broadly similar to those described in Western case series, there are critical differences with respect to the extent of adiposity. Because Asian patients with NAFLD generally have a lower body mass index (BMI), regional guidelines for anthropometric measurements should be adhered to. With the accrual of many 'lean' patients with NAFLD, the importance of body fat distribution, especially central obesity, and the necessity for girth measurements are now well appreciated. Although existing case series have not included many patients with overt decompensated liver disease, this apparently benign nature of NAFLD may be related to the short duration of follow-up rather than to true biological differences. Preliminary evidence presented so far support the concept of insulin resistance and involvement of oxidative stress-related liver injury in the pathogenesis of NAFLD in

Asian patients. Diet and exercise remain the cornerstone of managing individual cases of NAFLD. However, robust regional interventional studies need to be initiated. Pharmacotherapy-based treatment protocols may be successful but for practical reasons are less likely to succeed than public health initiatives that promote healthy lifestyle activities.

Introduction

NAFLD can be regarded as a disorder of our times. There is a clear relationship to affluence and, not surprisingly, NAFLD has emerged as the principal cause of abnormal liver tests in industrialized Western nations. However, as a result of this focus on affluence, NAFLD has been overlooked in a global context. This has become apparent from the results of national health surveys such as the National Health and Nutritional Examination (NHANES III) survey in the USA [1]. Contrary to expectations, Mexican-Americans and African-Americans were more likely to have NAFLD than white persons, a group usually over-represented in NAFLD reports [1]. These ethnic differences raise similar questions about the prevalence and spectrum of NAFLD in Eastern populations ('the East'), which in this discussion include Asia and countries from the Pacific Rim. Data from countries with European populations (Australia, New Zealand) are not discussed.

The case for studying NAFLD in the East

There are several compelling reasons for evaluating

non-alcoholic steatohepatitis (NASH) in the Eastern hemisphere (Table 18.1). First, although NAFLD represents only a small proportion of symptomatic liver disease, *actual* patient numbers are likely to exceed those in the West. High population growth rates and density coupled with changing demographic trends, such as the precipitous rise in obesity and diabetes, are likely to contribute. Second, regional differences exist in the profile of NAFLD and should be taken into account while assessing patients from this region. For example, hepatic steatosis can occur in Asian subjects at levels of adiposity much lower than traditionally defined Western standards [2]. Finally, awareness of NAFLD and its spectrum is critical both for health care evaluation and also for resource allocation. Even though viral hepatitis predominates in much of this region and should not be overlooked, the converse is also true. A diagnosis of NAFLD has to be considered in patients with non-replicating forms of chronic viral hepatitis presenting with abnormal liver tests, particularly if other metabolic risk factors are present. While NAFLD may not command much resource allocation at present, this policy will change if the anticipated increase in insulin resistance-related disorders (including NASH) becomes more perceptible, as it already has for cardiovascular disease.

Prevalence of NAFLD in the East

Up to 20% of persons living in the West will have liver test abnormalities attributable to NAFLD [3]. Between 2% and 3% will have NAFLD [3]. Similar data are yet to be compiled for much of Asia and are completely lacking for the Pacific Rim countries.

Table 18.1 The case for studying non-alcoholic fatty liver disease (NAFLD) in Eastern countries.

Demographic trends in Eastern countries	Implications
High population growth rates and density	More regional cases of NAFLD can be anticipated than in the West
Epidemic of obesity and diabetes	Increasing prevalence of the insulin resistance syndrome and also NAFLD, the hepatic manifestation of the syndrome
Development of NAFLD at lower levels of body mass index	Different anthropometric criteria need to be used
Heterogeneous nature of populations between and within individual countries	Insight into genetic/environmental factors involved in pathogenesis

Table 18.2 Prevalence of NAFLD in surveys from Japan and Taiwan.

Study location	Year of study	Number	Participants	Proportion with fatty liver	Reference
Okinawa, Japan	1988	2574	Community survey	14%	5
Tokyo, Japan	1991	715	Non manual workers undergoing annual medical evaluation	15%	6
Nagasaki, Japan	1990–92	2083	Community survey of elderly residents	21.6% in obese men,* 18.8% in obese women; 3.3% in non-obese men, 3.8% in non-obese women	7
Nagasaki, Japan	2000	3579	Self-referral by employees to a hospital for shipyard and heavy industry workers	22% overall; 9% in those with alcohol intake < 20 g/day and 4.1% in non-overweight non-alcoholic individuals	8
Taichung city, Taiwan	2000	1012	Periodic health examination of persons visiting a teaching hospital department of family medicine	36.9%	9

* Obesity was defined as a body mass index $\geq 26 \, kg/m^2$.

Asian data on NAFLD

Thirty per cent of persons screened by ultrasound in an Indonesian centre had NAFLD [4]. Other than this report, prevailing Asian data on NAFLD are largely derived from Japanese surveys, which reveal a prevalence of 14–22% (Table 18.2) [5–8]. However, these earlier studies have not stratified patients by alcohol intake. When patients with significant alcohol intake were excluded, prevalence levels of NAFLD have been under 10% [8]. As expected, non-obese and elderly subjects have lower rates of NAFLD [7].

Taiwan has recorded the highest prevalence (36.9%) of NAFLD in the region [9]. The reasons for this extraordinarily high prevalence are unknown. When the obvious risk factors are sought (obesity or type 2 diabetes), no clues are forthcoming; only 17% had a BMI of more than 28 kg/m^2 and 17% had fasting blood glucose levels above 110 mg/dL (6.1 mmol/L). Because this was a hospital-based study, these results could reflect ascertainment bias, with more affluent individuals seeking medical attention. However, another explanation could be the differences in anthropometric criteria used. Although subjects with a BMI cut-off of 28 kg/m^2 are classified as being overweight in the West, they would be categorized as frankly obese in Asia, accounting for the high prevalence rates [10]. While NAFLD

data from the rest of the region are awaited, the recent publication of several small case series from other Asian countries emphasizes the growing interest in this disorder (Table 18.3) [11–15].

Increasing prevalence of NAFLD in the East: fact or fiction?

Is there a real increase in NAFLD or merely better case ascertainment because of greater awareness? To an extent, annual medical screening examinations may have contributed to detecting NAFLD, with the initial visit prompted by an abnormality in abdominal sonography or serum transaminases. However, there are some pointers to a genuine increase in the incidence and hence prevalence of NAFLD. Fundamental among these trends are the rising prevalence of obesity and type 2 diabetes mellitus ('diabesity') in both adults and children. Some pertinent data are summarized below.

Obesity

Only 2–3% of Asians are classified as obese by current Western criteria (BMI of more than 30 kg/m^2). However, it is now recognized that obesity-related metabolic

Table 18.3 Studies on NAFLD in other Asian countries.

Region	Number	Male : female	Mean age (years)	Obesity	Type 2 diabetes	Dyslipidaemia	Severe liver fibrosis	Reference
North Asia								
China (Hong Kong)	30	NA	NA	65%	10%; IGT (60%)	Present		11
South Asia								
India (New Delhi)	52	24 : 28		12%	IGT (8%)	28%	Bridging fibrosis 12%	12
India (Mumbai)	13	9 : 4	55	33%	33%	15%	Cirrhosis 7%	13
South Korea (Seoul)	39	30 : 9	32	NA	NA	NA		14
Sri Lanka (Kelaniya)	34	27 : 7	38*	44%	35%	41%		15

NA, data not available; DM, type 2 diabetes mellitus; IGT, impaired glucose tolerance.
* Median.

disorders commence at much lower levels of BMI in Asians. In Japan, a BMI ≥ 25 kg/m^2 was associated with type 2 diabetes, hypertension and raised triglycerides (odds ratio > 2.0 for each disorder) [10]. Similar data were obtained from the Korean annual health examination survey (1994–97) where a BMI as low as 25 kg/m^2 was associated with fatty liver (odds ratio 1.3) [10]. In Taiwan, 83% of those with fatty liver had a BMI lower than 28 kg/m^2 [9].

Recognizing these metabolic health risk correlates, the World Health Organization defines obesity in Asians as a BMI ≥ 25 kg/m^2 (Table 18.4) [10]. Conversely, a much higher BMI is suggested for the large-built Pacific Islanders. Applying these new criteria presents a very different picture on the prevalence of obesity in Asia, which is summarized as follows: China (12% in men, 14% in women); Japan (24%, 20%); Malaysia (24%, 18%); Philippines (13%, 15%); Taiwan (18%,

16%); and Thailand (17%, 20%) [10]. The prevalence of NAFLD in obese Asians is unknown. However, extrapolating autopsy data from the West, where approximately 20% of obese individuals have NASH [16], it becomes clear that a forthcoming increase in NAFLD is inevitable in Asia.

Central obesity

Central obesity is relevant to NAFLD because it provides an explanation for the development of NASH in lean patients [17]. When so-called 'lean' patients undergo bioimpedance analysis, some may actually have a higher percentage of body fat than anticipated [8]. This is attributable to unrecognized central obesity in these individuals. Central obesity is a correlate of visceral adiposity and is more closely linked to insulin resistance (the central event in NASH) than generalized

Table 18.4 Measuring adiposity in patients from the Asia–Pacific. (Modified from the Asia–Pacific guidelines published by the World Health Organization [10].)

	Measurement	Anthropometric criteria
Obesity	Body mass index	≥ 25 kg/m^2 (Asians); ≥ 32 kg/m^2 (Pacific Islanders)
Central obesity	Waist*	Men ≥ 90 cm; women ≥ 80 cm
	Waist : hip ratio†	Men ≥ 0.90; women ≥ 0.85

* Measured with the subject standing. Reading taken anteriorly at a point midway between the lower border of the last rib above and the upper border of the iliac crest below.
† Hip measurements are taken at the point of maximal protrusion of the buttocks.

obesity [18]. This point is well illustrated in a Japanese survey of over 2500 men, subdivided by BMI and waist/height measurements [2]. These four groups were as follows:

1 Normal weight, not centrally obese
2 Normal weight, centrally obese
3 General obesity, not centrally obese
4 General and central obesity.

With group 1 as reference, the odds ratio for fatty liver for the other groups was 1.89, 2.57 and 5.64, respectively. Therefore, fatty liver can occur in 'lean' but centrally obese individuals (group 2) and its prevalence rises with further degrees of obesity (especially central obesity) [2]. An important observation was that persons from groups 2 and 4 ('the centrally obese') had much lower levels of exercise activity than the others, underscoring the importance of lifestyle in contributing to this epidemic of obesity [2]. Ethnic differences in central adiposity are well recognized. South Asians, particularly those from the Indian Subcontinent, have high prevalence levels of central obesity, suggesting that they may be at an increased risk of NAFLD [19].

Type 2 diabetes mellitus

Of the 10 leading countries with type 2 diabetes mellitus, five are in Asia (India, China, Pakistan, Indonesia and Japan). By 2025, nearly 130 of the 300 million cases of type 2 diabetes mellitus worldwide are anticipated in these five countries alone [20]. A increase in the prevalence of type 2 diabetes mellitus across the region is expected, with early trends already visible. For example, in Japan the prevalence of type 2 diabetes mellitus has increased two- to fourfold over the last 20 years [21]. Likewise, traditional hunter–gatherer populations (Australian Aborigines, Nauruan fishermen) have also witnessed a profound upsurge in the prevalence of type 2 diabetes mellitus [22]. It is worth recalling that type 2 diabetes mellitus was unheard of in Nauru 40 years ago. Epidemiological studies have registered high prevalence rates among migrant Asian–Pacific populations living in the West [23]. The prevalence rates of type 2 diabetes in these migrants has not only exceeded those found in residents of their currently domiciled countries but also in comparison with data drawn from populations in their native countries.

Because population profiles of insulin resistance are lacking, the prevalence of type 2 diabetes mellitus has to be relied upon as a surrogate marker of insulin resist-

ance. Even if only 5% (a very conservative estimate) of persons with diabetes should develop NASH, a regional escalation in its prevalence is foreseeable. Further, because diabetes is an independent risk factor for severe liver hepatic fibrosis [24], an increase in NASH-related end-stage liver disease may also be predicted.

Obesity and diabetes in children and young adults

The previous section focused on the 'diabesity' epidemic in adults. Unfortunately, the outlook for the future seems gloomy, with figures mounting for childhood obesity and also type 2 diabetes mellitus. Currently, nearly 10% of Japanese school children are obese [25]. Likewise, the increase in type 2 diabetes mellitus among teenagers and young adults is striking. In Japan, over the last 2 decades, the prevalence of diabetes among school children has increased 36-fold from 0.2 in 100 000 children/year to 7.3 in 100 000 children/year [26]. Although data on NAFLD in Asian children with diabetes are not available, NAFLD is now well recognized in obese children. A Japanese survey of 810 children (aged 4–12 years) found that 2.6% had fatty liver (3.4% in boys, 1.8% in girls) [27]. NAFLD can begin early in life, with children as young as 6 years of age showing the changes of fatty liver. In another study enrolling only obese children, up to one-quarter had NAFLD [28].

Pathogenesis of NAFLD in the Asian population

Experimental models and detailed pathogenetic studies of NAFLD in Asia are lacking. Preliminary Asian data on NASH are consistent with the involvement of insulin resistance and oxidative stress but the significance of cytokine alterations, hyperleptinaemia and the interplay of genetic and environmental factors is not well understood.

Insulin resistance

Although studies of insulin resistance in Asian patients are lacking, there is indirect evidence that insulin resistance may underlie the development of NAFLD in these individuals. Insulin resistance-associated metabolic disorders such as obesity, impaired glucose tolerance or type 2 diabetes mellitus and hypertriglyceridaemia often coexist in Asian patients with NAFLD (Table 18.3). Hyperinsulinaemia (a correlate of insulin resistance) has been observed in at least two studies. Further, in one of these reports, which involved 228 obese Japanese children with fatty liver (aged 6–15 years), serum insulin levels correlated with the serum alanine aminotransferase (ALT), accounting for 24.1% of the variance in serum ALT [28].

Hyperinsulinaemia has been also reported in Sri Lankan patients with NASH; one-third of patients with NASH in this study had raised serum insulin levels [15].

Leptin

Hyperleptinaemia occurs in NASH, representing either an adaptation to visceral lipid increase (lipotoxicity) or as a correlate of insulin resistance [29]. Increased serum leptin concentrations have been reported in Japanese male adolescents [30]. Interestingly, the serum leptin concentration correlated with serum ALT ($r = 0.518$; $P < 0.0005$) and was found to be a risk factor for fatty liver, independent of the BMI and percentage of body fat. However, another Japanese study did not find an independent relationship of serum leptin with fatty liver in women, although there was a trend in men (odds ratio 1.75; $P = 0.051$) [31].

Oxidative stress

Several lines of evidence confirm the involvement of oxidative stress with liver cell injury and fibrosis in NAFLD. First, markers of oxidative stress were assessed in liver biopsies from Japanese patients with NAFLD and controls [32]. Hepatic expression of 4-hydroxy-2′-nonenal (HNE), a marker of lipid peroxidation, was examined by immunohistochemical staining. HNE adducts were observed predominantly within zone 3 of hepatocytes (the usual locus of injury in NASH) in all cases of NAFLD. Further, the HNE index correlated with the grade of hepatic necroinflammation and fibrosis.

Measuring serum thioredoxin (TRX) levels provides further evidence for the role of oxidative stress in NASH. TRX is a thiol-containing protein, inducible by many forms of oxidative stress. TRX controls the activity of NF-κB, a nuclear transcription factor directing inflammatory cytokine expression. Further, extracellular TRX itself has cytokine-like activities [33]. Sumida *et al.* from Kyoto, Japan [33] tested the hypothesis that if oxidative stress were operational in NASH, then serum TRX levels should be increased. Serum TRX was measured in 25 patients with NASH, 15 with simple steatosis and 17 healthy volunteers. As expected, serum TRX levels were significantly higher in the NASH group (median 60.3 ng/mL) than in those with simple steatosis (24.6 ng/mL) or controls (23.5 ng/mL). Like the HNE index above, serum TRX levels also correlated with the grade of inflammation and the stage of fibrosis.

Administration of vitamin E, an antioxidant, has been beneficial in some patients with NASH in reducing serum markers of hepatic necroinflammation (ALT) [34]. It is unclear whether this effect can be explained entirely by its antioxidant properties and not because of its other possible effects (e.g. on hepatic fibrosis).

Genetic factors

NAFLD may be viewed as the end expression of an imbalance between pro- and antisteatotic mechanisms across several metabolic pathways. Genes involved in the regulation of body weight, insulin signalling, lipid metabolism and export, oxidative stress and cytokine expression are therefore all potential candidate genes in NAFLD/NASH (for a more detailed discussion see Chapter 6). Only preliminary data are available on genetic influences in NAFLD in the Asian population. Polymorphisms of the β_2-adrenergic receptor gene were studied in Japan [35]. Mutations in this gene have been previously described in association with insulin resistance in Japanese subjects. Heterozygotes with the Gln27Glu variant had higher serum triglycerides levels and a slightly increased prevalence of fatty liver (12%) than those without this mutation (7%; $P = 0.047$). However, by multivariate analysis, the presence of this variant was not found to be an independent predictor of fatty liver.

Impaired apolipoprotein B synthesis, leading to impaired hepatic lipid export and steatosis, has been reported in Western patients [36]. Although similar data are not available, the association with apolipoprotein E, another related protein, has been examined [37]. Frequencies of three isoforms of the apoE gene (ε 2, 3 and 4) were assessed in 116 Korean patients with NAFLD and 50 controls. However, no significant differences were found. These results suggest that apoE gene polymorphisms are not directly involved in NAFLD.

Cytokines

Detailed cytokine profiling in Asian patients has yet to be carried out. Data obtained so far suggest similar profiles as in the West. Park *et al.* [38] from Seoul, South Korea studied Kupffer cell (CD14 staining), endotoxin-activated Kupffer cell (CD68 staining), tumour necrosis factor-α (TNF-α) and uncoupling protein-2 expression (UCP-2) expression in liver biopsies from five patients with NASH. Increased CD14, TNF-α and UCP-2 expression were observed but not for CD68, suggesting that endotoxin-mediated Kupffer cell activation may not be involved [38].

Clinical features of NAFLD in Asian cohorts

Most patients with NAFLD have been identified by incidental liver test and/or liver sonographical abnormalities or by non-specific symptoms such as right upper quadrant discomfort or lassitude. Although stigmata of portal hypertension such as oesophageal varices, ascites and splenomegaly have been recorded, signs of decompensated liver disease have not been conspicuous. However, cases of advanced hepatic fibrosis including cirrhosis are now recognized (Table 18.3). It is hoped that better definition of risk factors will aid in the selection of patients for liver biopsy. Hepatocellular carcinoma has been reported from Japan [39]. Implications of this finding are not clear at present. Long-term data on liver-related mortality in Asians are lacking and the apparently benign outcome is probably attributable to the relatively short duration of follow-up.

Risk factors for advanced hepatic fibrosis

Independent risk factors for severe hepatic fibrosis in NASH were assessed in a Japanese study [40]. As expected, prebiopsy cirrhosis-related variables such as low platelet count and AST : ALT ratio > 1 were selected as independent determinants. All four patients with a low platelet count had cirrhosis. On the other hand, an AST : ALT ratio > 1 was less specific, seven of 19 patients with a ratio > 1 had only mild hepatic fibrosis. However, among those with stage 3 or 4 hepatic fibrosis, 52% had an AST : ALT ratio > 1. When data were reanalysed to exclude variables that were a consequence of cirrhosis, age and absence of

hyperlipidaemia were identified as independent predictors. In agreement with Western studies [24,41], patients with severe hepatic fibrosis were older than those with milder disease (mean ages, 64 and 50 years, respectively).

Although female gender and diabetes mellitus were not selected, women (65%) and patients with diabetes mellitus (48%) predominated among those with severe fibrosis in comparison with those with mild fibrosis (45% and 24%, respectively). The non-association of BMI with severe liver fibrosis, in contrast to Western reports [24,41] may be related to differences in defining BMI. In this study, obesity was defined as a BMI > 25 kg/m^2 in contrast to BMI of up to 37 kg/m^2 in Western studies [24]. In agreement with recent reports [42], hepatic siderosis was observed only in 10% of these patients. The degree of iron overload was mild and did not correlate with hepatic fibrosis [40].

Hepatocellular carcinoma

Of all the sequelae ascribable to NASH, the association with hepatocellular carcinoma (HCC) is perhaps the most controversial. Several issues merit consideration [43]. First, the evidence of an association with NASH is at best indirect. Most HCC cases have occurred in patients with cryptogenic cirrhosis (CC), a disorder with metabolic risk factors allied to NASH [44] and therefore considered to represent 'burnt out' NASH. While CC could be an end-result of NASH in the West, this association has not been verified in other parts of the world where viral hepatitis predominates. For example, the involvement of carcinogens such as aflatoxin cannot always be established. Similarly, viral hepatitis B as a cause of HCC cannot be completely discounted by the mere absence of hepatitis B surface antigenaemia. Second, no prospective data are available. There have been only two case reports documenting HCC 4–10 years after the diagnosis of NASH [45,46]. Third, the argument that all persons with cirrhosis irrespective of aetiology are at risk of HCC belies the subtle differences between the individual liver disorders; the risks of developing HCC in chronic hepatitis B and C, alcoholic liver disease and haemochromatosis considerably exceed that in patients with Wilson's disease. This implies that disease-specific factors may be important. Finally, because NASH is such a frequent abnormality in many populations (including Japan), such a relationship of these two disorders may be coincidental rather than representing cause and effect. Therefore, it is important to define the risks of HCC associated with NASH before committing patients to long-term intense surveillance.

East–West comparisons of NAFLD

The clinical profiles of Asian patients with NAFLD resemble their Western counterparts with respect to age at presentation, prevalence of diabetes and hyperlipidaemia. The differences in the prevalence of obesity are probably related to the criteria used to define BMI. Males predominate in most Eastern series, possibly because of the greater prevalence of central obesity. Whether this is also because males are probably more likely to seek medical attention in this region is unclear. To date, only a few cases of cirrhosis have been reported. It will be interesting to see whether the gender differences reported in Western series (the majority are women) also hold true in Asia. Finally, as expected, short-term reports generally attest to the apparently benign prognosis of NAFLD, leading to a somewhat cavalier attitude to this disorder. The long-term outcome of NAFLD can only be answered by studies with adequate follow-up (at least 5–10 years), particularly in the subgroup with severe hepatic fibrosis.

Treatment of NAFLD/NASH

Managing NAFLD in Asia remains contentious. The present approach of extrapolating the results of Western pharmacological intervention studies cannot be recommended outside clinical trials. Such a strategy fails to take into account lifestyle differences and also perhaps insulin sensitivity between these populations. From an Eastern perspective, diet and exercise take precedence over pharmacotherapy for several reasons. First, financial constraints and cultural barriers will restrict access to and use of drugs in large sections of the region. Part of the reluctance to treat may also reflect the attitudes of primary care physicians, and also specialists, who may not be cognizant of the liver-related morbidity resulting from NAFLD. Second, although only limited regional data are available, the impact of strict diet and exercise protocols has been encouraging in small non-randomized controlled trials (Table 18.5) [33,47–49].

Ultimately, a lifestyle-related disorder of near epidemic proportions can be managed only by public health initiatives and not by small-scale interventional weight or activity studies. Population-wide strategies appear more likely to be effective in reducing disease burden than small-scale high-cost intervention programmes such as the diabetes prevention programme research study [50]. A case in point is the positive impact of mass hepatitis B vaccination on reducing the incidence of childhood HCC in Taiwan. Prevailing attitudes to obesity need to be revised. In one survey in Malaysia, 15% of men and 23% of women considered obesity as a normal state and even desirable [51]!

Future directions

The epidemiological transition being witnessed in the Asia–Pacific region offers a unique opportunity to study the evolution of previously described 'First' world diseases. Thus, future studies should continue to focus both on the similarities and highlight differences in the regional presentation of NAFLD. Although it is likely that there will be reconfirmation of many global themes, such as insulin resistance or oxidative stress, there is every likelihood that this may lead to a better understanding of the environment and its potential interaction with genetic factors. While the focus of this chapter has been on the Asia–Pacific region, there is a paucity of NAFLD data from other emerging or reorganized industrialized economies such as the Latin American countries, regions of the former Soviet Union and the Middle East. Because demographic changes are similar in many respects to those observed in the East, increases in prevalence rates of diabetes and obesity and, as a consequence, NAFLD, are also anticipated in these regions.

A perspective of NAFLD beyond its hepatic consequences is also needed. Because NAFLD is now a recognized manifestation of the insulin resistance syndrome, a known risk factor for coronary artery disease, its extrahepatic associations need to be studied. For example, are persons with NAFLD at a greater risk of coronary artery disease? There has been a perceptible shift in focus from pathogen (hepatitis virus) to what may be termed 'NAFLD-plus' disorders. The latter refers to histological changes of NAFLD in association with other liver disorders, a relationship shown to confer risk of increased disease severity (e.g. advanced liver fibrosis)

Table 18.5 Therapeutic trials of NAFLD in Asia.

Number	Country	Treatment protocol	Results	Reference
25 obese patients with NAFLD	Japan	Treatment group ($N = 15$), dietary restriction (25 kcal/kg) with exercise for 3 months Untreated group ($N = 10$), no diet or lifestyle restrictions	Reduction in ALT, liver steatosis grade. Trend towards improvement of hepatic fibrosis. No significant changes in ALT or liver histology in the untreated group	47
12 patients with NASH and 10 with steatosis	Japan	Two phase trial. An initial 6-month dietary intervention phase followed by vitamin E 100 mg three times daily for 1 year	NASH group- ALT reduced only with vitamin E. Reduced steatosis in 6 of 9 and fibrosis in 5 of 9 patients with post-treatment liver biopsies Steatosis group-steatosis improved with diet but not with vitamin E	34
25 patients with NAFLD	Korea	Group 1: weight reduction for 1 year Group 2: no weight reduction	Reduction in ALT only in group 1	48
110 obese children with NAFLD	Japan	Group 1 ($N = 73$): raised serum ALT, AST Group 2 ($N = 37$): normal serum ALT, AST Both groups put on a weight-reducing diet	Reduction in serum ALT, AST in those achieving more than 5% weight loss	49

ALT, serum alanine aminotransferase; AST, serum aspartate aminotransferase; NASH, non-alcoholic steatohepatitis; NAFLD, non-alcoholic fatty liver disease.

[52]. This interaction is particularly relevant to a region with a massive backlog of viral hepatitis now confronting a novel lifestyle-related disorder (see Chapter 23).

Conclusions

NAFLD should be regarded as a global problem, with Asian countries likely to harbour a significant reservoir of disease. The clinical and metabolic profile of NAFLD in Asia is broadly similar to that in the West, although the 'cut-off' BMI for overweight and obesity is lower than that in Western populations. Assessment of central adiposity is critical in so-called 'lean' patients. Studies in Asia have reported severe hepatic fibrosis and also cirrhosis, but natural history studies are not as yet available. The relationship of NAFLD with HCC merits further study. In the Asian context, public health initiatives that encourage diet and exercise to promote a healthy lifestyle are particularly crucial to prevent a massive burden of disease.

References

1 Clark JM, Brancati FL, Diehl AM. Non-alcoholic fatty liver disease. *Gastroenterology* 2002; **122**: 1649–57.
2 Hsieh SD, Yoshinaga H, Muto T, Sakurai Y, Kosaka K. Health risks among Japanese men with moderate body mass index. *Int J Obese Relat Metab Disord* 2000; **24**: 358–62.
3 Younossi ZM, Diehl AM, Ong JP. Non-alcoholic fatty liver disease: an agenda for clinical research. *Hepatology* 2002; **35**: 746–52.
4 Hasan I, Gani RA, Machmud R *et al.* Prevalence and risk factors for non-alcoholic fatty liver in Indonesia. *J Gastroenterol Hepatol* 2002; **17** (Suppl.): A30.
5 Nomura H, Kashiwagi S, Hayashi J *et al.* Prevalence of fatty liver in a general population of Okinawa, Japan. *Jpn J Med* 1988; **27**: 142–9.
6 Oshibuchi M, Nishi F, Sato M, Ohtake H, Okuda K. Frequency of abnormalities detected by abdominal ultrasound among Japanese adults. *J Gastroenterol Hepatol* 1991; **6**: 165–8.
7 Akahoshi M, Amasaki Y, Soda M *et al.* Correlation between fatty liver and coronary risk factors: a population

study of elderly men and women in Nagasaki, Japan. *Hypertens Res* 2001; **24**: 337–43.

8 Omagari KH, Kadokawa Y, Masuda J *et al*. Fatty liver in non-alcoholic non-overweight Japanese adults: incidence and clinical characteristics. *J Gastroenterol Hepatol* 2002; **17**: 1089–105.

9 Lai SW, Tan CK, Ng KC. Epidemiology of fatty liver in a hospital-based study in Taiwan. *South Med J* 2002; **95**: 1288–92.

10 International Diabetes Institute. The Asia–Pacific perspective: redefining obesity and its treatment. Health Communications Australia, 2000.

11 Leung NWY, Tsang TWC, Liew CT, Tomlinson B. Non-alcoholic steatohepatitis (NASH) in Hong Kong: role of hepatologist in the diagnosis of diabetes mellitus. Abstracts of World Congress of Gastroenterology, Vienna, 1998.

12 Agarwal SR, Malhotra V, Sakhuja P, Sarin SK. Clinical, biochemical and histological profile of non-alcoholic steatohepatitis. *Indian J Gastroenterol* 2001; **20**: 183–6.

13 Amarapurkar DN, Amarapurkar AD. Non-alcoholic steatohepatitis: clinicopathological profile. *J Assoc Physicians India* 2000; **48**: 311–3.

14 Park J, Kim MK, Kim SJ *et al*. Clinical predictors reflecting the pathologic grade of non-alcoholic steatohepatitis in patients with non-alcoholic fatty liver: Korean cases different from western patients. *Hepatology* 2000; **32**: 419A.

15 Janaki S, Hewavisenthi S. Profile of non-alcoholic steatohepatitis in a Sri Lankan population. *J Gastroenterol Hepatol* 2001; **16** (Suppl.): A81.

16 Wanless IR, Lentz JS. Fatty liver hepatitis (steatohepatitis) and obesity: an autopsy study with analysis of risk factors. *Hepatology* 1990; **12**: 1106–10.

17 Chitturi S, Abeygunasekera S, Farrell GC *et al*. NASH and insulin resistance: insulin hypersecretion and specific association with the insulin resistance syndrome. *Hepatology* 2002; **35**: 373–9.

18 Farrell GC. Non-alcoholic steatohepatitis: what is it, and why is it important in the Asia–Pacific region? *J Gastroenterol Hepatol* 2003; **18**: 124–38.

19 Fall CHD. Non-industrialised countries and affluence. *J R Soc Med* 2001; **60**: 33–50.

20 King H, Aubert R, Herman W. Global burden of diabetes, 1995–2025: prevalence, numerical estimates and projections. *Diabetes Care* 1998; **21**: 1414–31.

21 Sekikawa A, Tominaga M, Takahashi K *et al*. Prevalence of diabetes and impaired glucose tolerance in Funagata area, Japan. *Diabetes Care* 1993; **16**: 570–4.

22 Zimmet P, Alberti KG, Shaw J. Global and societal implications of the diabetes epidemic. *Nature* 2001; **414**: 782–7.

23 Hara H, Egusa G, Yamakido M, Kawate R. The high prevalence of diabetes mellitus and hyperinsulinemia among the Japanese-Americans living in Hawaii and Los Angeles. *Diabetes Res Clin Pract* 1994; **24** (Suppl.): S37–42.

24 Angulo P, Keach JC, Batts KP, Lindor KD. Independent predictors of liver fibrosis in patients with non-alcoholic steatohepatitis. *Hepatology* 1999; **30**: 1356–62.

25 Shirai K, Shinomiya M, Saito Y *et al*. Incidence of childhood obesity over the last 10 years in Japan. *Diabetes Res Clin Pract* 1990; **10** (Suppl. 1): S65–70.

26 Kitagawa T, Owada M, Urakami T, Yamauchi K. Increased incidence of non-insulin dependent diabetes mellitus among Japanese schoolchildren correlates with an increased intake of animal protein and fat. *Clin Pediatr (Phila)* 1998; **37**: 111–5.

27 Tominaga K, Kurata JH, Chen YK *et al*. Prevalence of fatty liver in Japanese children and relationship to obesity: an epidemiological ultrasonographic survey. *Dig Dis Sci* 1995; **40**: 2002–9.

28 Kawasaki T, Hashimoto N, Kikuchi T, Takahashi H, Uchiyama M. The relationship between fatty liver and hyperinsulinemia in obese Japanese children. *J Pediatr Gastroenterol Nutr* 1997; **24**: 317–21.

29 Chitturi S, Farrell GC, Frost L *et al*. Serum leptin in NASH correlates with hepatic steatosis but not fibrosis: a manifestation of lipotoxicity? *Hepatology* 2002; **36**: 403–9.

30 Tobe K, Ogura T, Tsukamoto C *et al*. Relationship between serum leptin and fatty liver in Japanese male adolescent university students. *Am J Gastroenterol* 1999; **94**: 3328–35.

31 Nakao K, Nakata K, Ohtsubo N *et al*. Association between non-alcoholic fatty liver, markers of obesity, and serum leptin level in young adults. *Am J Gastroenterol* 2002; **97**: 1796–801.

32 Seki S, Kitada T, Yamada T *et al*. *In situ* detection of lipid peroxidation and oxidative DNA damage in non-alcoholic fatty liver diseases. *J Hepatol* 2002; **37**: 56–62.

33 Sumida Y, Nakashima T, Yoh T *et al*. Serum thioredoxin levels as a predictor of steatohepatitis in patients with non-alcoholic fatty liver disease. *J Hepatol* 2003; **38**: 32–8.

34 Hasegawa T, Yoneda M, Nakamura K, Makino I, Terano A. Plasma transforming growth factor-β1 level and efficacy of α-tocopherol in patients with non-alcoholic steatohepatitis: a pilot study. *Aliment Pharmacol Ther* 2001; **15**: 1667–72.

35 Iwamoto N, Ogawa Y, Kajihara S *et al*. Gln27Glu β2-adrenergic receptor variant is associated with hypertriglyceridemia and the development of fatty liver. *Clin Chim Acta* 2001; **314**: 85–91.

36 Charlton M, Sreekumar R, Rasmussen D, Lindor K, Nair KS. Apolipoprotein synthesis in non-alcoholic steatohepatitis. *Hepatology* 2002; **35**: 898–904.

37 Lee DM, Mun BS, Ahn HS *et al*. Relation of apolipo-protein E polymorphism to clinically diagnosed fatty liver disease [in Korean]. *Taehan Kan Hakhoe Chi* 2002; **8**: 355–62.

38 Park J, Kim MK, Jung G *et al*. Expression of Kupffer cells and uncoupling protein 2 in the liver of patients with non-alcoholic steatohepatitis: difference and similarity to alcoholic hepatitis. *Hepatology* 2000; **34**: 423A.

39 Shimada M, Hashimoto E, Taniai M *et al*. Hepatocellular carcinoma in patients with non-alcoholic steatohepatitis. *J Hepatol* 2002; **37**: 154–60.

40 Shimada M, Hashimoto E, Kaneda H, Noguchi S, Hayashi N. Non-alcoholic steatohepatitis: risk factors for liver fibrosis. *Hepatology Res* 2002; **24**: 429–38.

41 Ratziu V, Giral P, Charlotte F *et al*. Liver fibrosis in over-weight patients. *Gastroenterology* 2000; **118**: 1117–23.

42 Chitturi C, Weltman M, Farrell GC *et al*. HFE mutations, hepatic iron, and fibrosis: ethnic-specific associations of NASH with C282Y but not with fibrotic severity. *Hepatology* 2002; **36**: 142–8.

43 Ong JP, Younossi ZM. Is hepatocellular carcinoma part of the natural history of non-alcoholic steatohepatitis? *Gastroenterology* 2002; **123**: 375–8.

44 Caldwell SH, Oelsner DH, Iezzoni JC *et al*. Cryptogenic cirrhosis: clinical characterization and risk factors for underlying disease. *Hepatology* 1999; **29**: 664–9.

45 Cotrim HP, Parana R, Braga E, Lyra L. Non-alcoholic steatohepatitis and hepatocellular carcinoma: natural history? *Am J Gastroenterol* 2000; **95**: 3018–9.

46 Zen Y, Katayanagi K, Tsuneyama K *et al*. Hepatocellular carcinoma arising in non-alcoholic steatohepatitis. *Pathol Int* 2001; **51**: 127–31.

47 Ueno T, Sugawara H, Sujaku K *et al*. Therapeutic effects of restricted diet and exercise in obese patients with fatty liver. *J Hepatol* 1997; **27**: 103–7.

48 Park HS, Kim MW, Shin ES. Effect of weight control on hepatic abnormalities in obese patients with fatty liver. *J Korean Med Sci* 1995; **10**: 414–21.

49 Tazawa Y, Noguchi H, Nishinomiya F, Takada G. Effect of weight changes on serum transaminase activities in obese children. *Acta Paediatr Jpn* 1997; **39**: 210–4.

50 Diabetes Prevention Program Research Group. Reduction in the incidence of type 2 diabetes with lifestyle intervention or metformin. *N Engl J Med* 2002; **346**: 393–403.

51 Jackson A, Cole C, Esquiro J, Edwards M. Obesity in primary care patients in Kelantan, Malaysia: prevalence, and patients' knowledge and attitudes. *Southeast Asian J Trop Med Public Health* 1996; **27**: 776–9.

52 Hwang SJ, Luo JC, Chu CW *et al*. Hepatic steatosis in chronic hepatitis C virus infection: prevalence and clinical correlation. *J Gastroenterol Hepatol* 2001; **16**: 190–5.

19 NAFLD/NASH in children

Joel E. Lavine & Jeffrey B. Schwimmer

Key learning points

1 Paediatric non-alcoholic steatohepatitis (NASH) is a global and increasingly prevalent form of chronic liver disease found mainly in obese insulin-resistant pre-adolescents and adolescents.

2 Paediatric NASH differs histologically from that found in adults with respect to the extent of fat and the location of fibrosis and inflammation.

3 Vigorous exercise, diet change and weight loss is the most desirable therapy. If this is unsuccessful, either oral vitamin E or metformin may be beneficial. Confirmation of efficacy is required in controlled randomized masked trials with clinically relevant end-points.

Abstract

Non-alcoholic steatohepatitis (NASH) is an increasingly prevalent and global problem in both children and adults. NASH is a subset of non-alcoholic fatty liver disease (NAFLD), likely to be the most common chronic liver condition in industialized nations. The diagnosis is predicated on the finding of macrovesicular steatosis with accompanying inflammation, hepatocellular injury and fibrosis. Important differences exist between adult and paediatric NASH in terms of the extent, quality and location of the inflammatory and fibrotic process. Conditions such as Wilson's disease, alcoholic steatohepatitis or hepatitis C virus infection may mimic these findings and need to be excluded. All paediatric clinical series report that NASH is more frequently found in boys than girls, and that the usual age at presentation is approximately 12 years. The vast majority of patients are obese, and usually present incidentally with elevated serum aminotransferases. Physical examination often reveals hepatomegaly and acanthosis nigricans. Clinical evaluation usually reveals modest elevation of serum alanine aminotransferase (ALT) (greater than aspartate aminotransferase [AST]) along with evidence of hyperlipidaemia. Recent studies demonstrate that affected individuals are insulin resistant, and certain clinical parameters in children are predictive in retrospective analyses of histological findings. Promising but yet unproven therapies for children include diet and exercise, or treatment with vitamin E or metformin.

Introduction

NASH is part of the clinical spectrum of NAFLD. NAFLD demonstrates a range of severity from the most benign (simple steatosis) to NASH that may result in cirrhosis. Initially recognized histologically as a complication of weight loss surgery involving jejunal bypass, Ludwig *et al.* [1] later recognized the condition in obese non-alcoholic middle-aged adults, and coined the term 'non-alcoholic steatohepatitis'. Moran *et al.* [2] first described the condition in children. The three reported children, two boys and one girl, were obese and without any other identifiable cause of chronic liver disease. The biopsies from these children were similar to adults with NASH, and the children demonstrated biochemical improvement of their serum aminotransferases with weight loss. Subsequent reports of children with biopsy-proven NASH have appeared from Japan [3], USA [4,5], Canada [6], Australia [7] and Italy [8]. Reports now document the presence or progression to cirrhosis in children with NASH [6,9]. This chapter summarizes what is known about fatty liver disease in children, how this condition compares and contrasts to that in adults, and where attention needs to be focused in basic and clinical sciences to improve understanding and treatment of this problem in children.

Terminology

Steatohepatitis, the histological entity of fatty liver with inflammation and potential fibrosis, can result from a variety of metabolic, infectious, nutritional or toxic insults. Many of these aetiologies are listed below. When steatohepatitis fits certain histological criteria, in the context of insulin resistance or the metabolic syndrome, the entity is termed NASH. In adults, NASH staging and grading has been developed [10]. Recently, a large analysis of NASH histology in children was performed, detailing the histological features of paediatric NASH using the criteria developed for adults [11]. Adult NASH histology differs from paediatric NASH histology, particularly with regard to the extent and location of hepatic inflammation and fibrosis. For the purposes of this chapter, we define paediatric NASH as a biopsy-proven diagnosis of predominantly macrovesicular steatosis with evidence of either lobular or portal inflammation, evidence of cellular injury and either portal or pericellular fibrosis. Lipogranulomas are considered sufficient evidence of cellular injury, as the adult features of hepatocellular ballooning or Mallory hyaline is infrequent in children.

Differential diagnosis

NASH is by definition a histological diagnosis. Conditions that mimic NASH (Table 19.1) must be excluded by careful history, physical and clinical evaluation. These

Table 19.1 Differential diagnosis of paediatric steatohepatitis.

Alcoholic steatohepatitis

Infectious (hepatitis C)

Drug-induced
Glucocorticoids
Valproic acid
Amiodarone
L-asparaginase
Vitamin A

Metabolic
Wilson's disease
Cystic fibrosis
Glycogen storage disease
Carnitine deficiency
Fatty oxidation defects
Urea cycle defects
Lipid storage disorders
α_1-Antitrypsin deficiency

Nutritional
Total parenteral nutrition
Rapid weight loss
Kwashiorkor
Diabetes mellitus

Syndromes with/without obesity disorders
Bardet–Biedl
Alström
Polycystic ovary
Turner
Prader–Willi
Lipodystrophy

Other/surgical
Jejuno-ileal bypass
Liver transplantation
Autoimmune hepatitis

aetiologies may be toxic, drug-induced, infectious, metabolic, nutritional, autoimmune, surgically induced or syndrome associated. In adults, exclusion of alcohol as a cause for steatohepatitis may be difficult because of the distinction between social and problem drinking. The young age at which paediatric NASH patients present makes this possibility less concerning, although the possibility of ethanol abuse needs to be excluded. History also reveals whether drugs such as valproic acid, amiodarone or glucocorticoids are being administered. Health care providers need to enquire about a history of supplemental parenteral nutrition, rapid weight loss, or biliary or intestinal surgery. Hepatitis C virus infection needs to be excluded by serum tests for antibodies to the virus.

A variety of inborn errors of metabolism may cause fat accumulation within the liver. Many of these metabolic errors may be asymptomatic or mild enough to cause few symptoms. Wilson's disease shares many of the histological features of paediatric NASH, with portal inflammation and fibrosis. Wilson's disease, although relatively rare, is usually asymptomatic in young children so serum ceruloplasmin should be checked. Errors in fatty acid oxidation, amino acid metabolism, glycogen storage and the urea cycle may be excluded with a urine screen for organic acids and a serum amino acid profile. Children younger than 6 years with steatohepatitis should be examined more carefully for inborn metabolic errors.

Certain childhood syndromes may be associated with obesity and/or insulin resistance. These syndromes include Bardet–Biedl, Alström, Turner, Prader–Willi and lipodystrophy. Associations such as deafness, retinal dystrophy, renal dysgenesis, neurodevelopmental delay, hypotonia, short stature or dysmorphic facies should prompt a dysmorphology referral.

Prevalence

The prevalence of NASH in the paediatric population is not known. Determination of prevalence is derailed by the requirement for examination of liver histology to make a diagnosis. Estimates of prevalence can be inferred from data on the prevalence of childhood obesity, the frequency of 'bright' liver on ultrasound in obese children, the frequency of abnormal ALT tests in obese children with echogenic liver, and the frequency of NASH versus simple steatosis in obese children with echogenic livers who undergo biopsy.

The prevalence of child and adolescent obesity has risen dramatically over the past 20–30 years. Recent data from the National Health and Nutrition Examination Survey (NHANES) from 1999–2000 shows that 14–16% of boys and girls between 6 and 19 years of age are obese, with obesity defined as being greater than the 95th percentile for body mass index (BMI) adjusted for age [12]. This is a dramatic increase from

the approximate 5% prevalence reference population found in the Second and Third National Health Examination Surveys in 1963–1965. The prevalence has increased with every survey since the 1960s in the USA, with no promise of a plateau (Fig. 19.1). The increased prevalence of obesity is blamed on a multitude of changes in US lifestyle, such as increased sedentary activities and increased caloric intake of high-fat foods and soda with refined sugars.

Given that more than 85% of children with NAFLD are obese, the next question is how many of them have imaging studies by ultrasound or magnetic resonance imaging (MRI) consistent with fatty infiltration? Franzese et al. [13] performed ultrasonographical examinations on 72 consecutive, otherwise healthy, obese children with a mean age 9.5 years. Fifty-three per cent of these children exhibited a 'bright' liver consistent with steatosis. If the prevalence of obesity in Italy were the same as in the USA, one would calculate that 8% of the paediatric population were obese with an echogenic liver. In Japan, an epidemiological ultrasonographical survey was performed on 810 school children aged 4–12 years. No children were found with echogenic liver under the age of 4 years, but the overall incidence of presumed fatty liver ranged from 1.8% in girls to 3.4% in boys (2.6% overall). The likelihood of fatty liver was best predicted by measurement of subcutaneous fat thickness [14]. Because ultrasound imaging is insensitive for demonstration of hepatic fat, these two studies hint that a minimum of 2.6–8% of children have NAFLD. Using the more sensitive technique of hepatic MRI for fat quantitation, Fishbein et al. [15] found that 21 of 22 obese children aged 6–18 years with modest hepatomegaly demonstrated elevated fat fractions. Data from this study, in conjunction with current NHANES data, suggest that as many as 16% of US children have NAFLD.

A number of investigators performed studies of fatty liver prevalence using serum ALT as a screening tool [3,8,16]. Whether ALT is a sensitive enough measure to evaluate NASH or NAFLD is not known, as recent evidence in adults provides ample evidence that 'normal ALT NASH' occurs [17]. Further complicating interpretation is the realization that elevated ALT may not be caused by fatty liver in some cases. Realizing that the requirement for abnormal ALT in obese children likely underestimates the prevalence of NASH, it appears that 10–25% of obese children have abnormal ALT in these studies. Using US data for obesity prevalence,

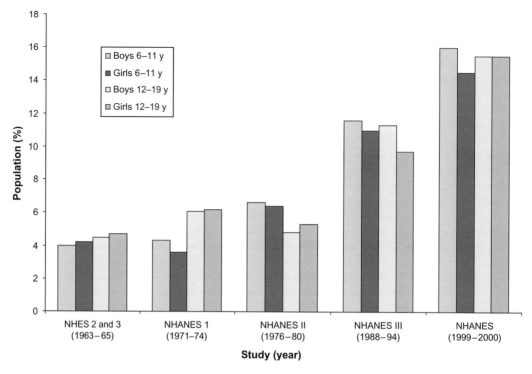

Fig. 19.1 Increasing prevalence of obesity correlates with increasing recognition of non-alcoholic steatohepatitis (NASH). Data from studies monitoring the prevalence of overweight children in the USA is summarized, demonstrating a fourfold rise in prevalence over the past 40 years [12]. NHES, National Health and Examination Survey; NHANES, National Health and Nutrition Examination Survey.

this would indicate that at least 1.6–4% of children have NAFLD.

Demographics

Publications describing paediatric NASH over the past 20 years demonstrate remarkable concordance for gender and age (Table 19.2). In all series, boys are reported twice as often as girls. The mean age at diagnosis in all series ranges between 11.6 and 13.5 years. It is not known why boys may be predisposed to NASH or why NASH appears at this age. Puberty is associated with dynamic changes in body composition and hormone levels. Children experience a stage of physiological insulin resistance beginning at the onset of puberty. While prepubertal children and postpubertal young adults are equally sensitive to insulin, adolescents are insulin-resistant compared with either of these groups. An intriguing question about pathogenesis involves the potential role of pubertal development and sex hormones, which may promote (in boys) or protect against (in girls) liver injury in susceptible individuals. Insulin resistance is reported to change at various stages of pubertal development, independent of changes in body composition with pubertal stage [18,19]. Recently, we are noting increasing numbers of children as young as 8 years presenting with NASH in our clinics. These children are still prepubertal Tanner stage I. This observation may indicate that earlier and more severe obesity may abrogate the need for puberty-related 'promoters'. Alternatively, the remarkable concordance among series in age and gender may reflect uniform selection bias.

The series in Table 19.2 reflect populations of children in Asia, Australia, North America and Europe. Races or ethnicities most often reported are Asian, white Hispanics and white non-Hispanics. Whether some races or ethnicities are more prone to develop NASH, given a particular BMI, is unknown. Body fat distribution varies by race. In San Diego, we diagnose

Table 19.2 Demographic comparisons between studies on paediatric NASH. Six published studies on paediatric NASH are compared. All patients had liver biopsies to confirm the diagnosis of NASH. In some reports that identified children with simple steatosis (no inflammation or fibrosis), the cases were excluded for this compilation.

Study (year) [Reference]	Location	Boys/girls	Age (mean) (years)	Ethnicity
Moran *et al.* (1983) [2]	USA	2/1	12.6	White non-Hispanic (all)
Kinugasa *et al.* (1984) [3]	Japan	6/2	11.8	Asian (all)
Baldridge *et al.* (1995) [4]	USA	10/4	13.5	NS
Rashid & Roberts (2000) [6]*	Canada	21/15	12	NS
Manton *et al.* (2000) [7]	Australia	8/4	11.6	NS
Schwimmer *et al.* (2003) [5]	USA	30/13	12.4	White non-Hispanic 25% White Hispanic 53% Black non-Hispanic 5% Other 17%

* Includes six cases of simple steatosis from the total cases reported.

NASH in Mexican American children three times as often as in other children, despite the fact that only 24% of the children in San Diego are Hispanic. Studies have demonstrated that when adjusted for body size, Hispanic male children have significantly higher body fat and percentage fat than white or black males [20]. Obese Hispanic peripubertal children are reported to have an increased risk for the development of type 2 diabetes, indicative of severe insulin resistance [21]. The increased fat in Hispanic males for a given BMI along with the increased insulin resistance in this population coincident with puberty may explain why we observe proportionally larger numbers of Hispanic males in our NASH population.

Clinical presentation

Most children with NAFLD are asymptomatic and identified incidentally. Many paediatricians and family practice physicians are unfamiliar with NASH in children. How children present is subject to selection bias reporting by centres. Asymptomatic children are usually identified because of persistently elevated serum aminotransferases, or an echogenic liver detected on ultrasound of the abdomen. In our general paediatric gastroenterology clinic in San Diego, we screen obese children older than 6 years for NASH, irrespective of the reason for referral. Clearly, most children found with NASH with this approach will differ from those identified elsewhere.

Children presenting with symptoms generally complain of either diffuse or right upper quadrant abdominal pain in 42–67% of reported series (Table 19.3). Those with right upper quadrant pain often have tenderness of the liver margin exacerbated by inspiratory effort. Occasionally, those complaining of right upper quadrant pain may be found to have gallstones, particularly frequent in obese Hispanic girls with associated hypercholesterolaemia.

On physical examination, the most common findings are obesity, hepatomegaly and acanthosis nigricans (Table 19.3). Comparing published studies on biopsy-confirmed NASH, 83–100% of paediatric patients are obese, 29–51% demonstrate hepatomegaly and 36–49% exhibit acanthosis nigricans. Most patients are more than 120% of ideal body weight or have a BMI greater than 30 kg/m^2. Hepatomegaly may be difficult to appreciate by palpation or percussion because of overlying fat. On occasion, particularly in those complaining of right upper quadrant pain, the liver edge may be tender to palpation and exacerbated by palpation during inspiration. Acanthosis nigricans is a prominent discoloration, usually presenting on the posterior neck folds, extending variable degrees anteriorly with increasing severity of insulin resistance. Hypertension may also be present, and comparison must be made for age-appropriate norms. Rarely, normal weight patients present with paediatric NASH. These patients have insulin resistance, often type 2 diabetes. These patients should be carefully examined for congenital or acquired lipodystrophies. Patients with NAFLD generally do not

Table 19.3 Comparisons of clinical findings in paediatric NASH. The definition of obesity varies between studies so comparisons are approximate. Rashid and Roberts' study [6] includes two patients with Bardet–Biedl syndrome, and the study by Manton *et al.* [7] includes one with Alström syndrome.

Study (year) [Reference]	Obesity		Acanthosis nigricans (%)	IDDM (%)	Hepatomegaly (%)	Presenting symptoms (%)
	(%)	BMI or % IBW				
Moran *et al.* (1983) [2]	100	30.1 kg/m^2	NS	0	33	Abdominal pain (67%)
Kinugasa *et al.* (1984) [3]	100	144% IBW	NS	13	NS	Obesity clinic (all)
Baldridge *et al.* (1995) [4]	100	159% IBW	NS	0	29	Abdominal pain (64%)
Rashid & Roberts (2000) [6]*	83	147% IBW	36	11	44	Abdominal pain 'most patients'
Manton *et al.* (2000) [7]	94	147% IBW	NS	0	47	Abdominal pain (59%)
Schwimmer *et al.* (2003) [5]	88	31.3 kg/m^2	49	14	51	Abdominal pain (42%)

IBW, ideal body weight; IDDM, insulin-dependent diabetes mellitus; NS, not stated.

* Includes six patients with simple steatosis.

have ascites, caput medusae or jaundice. Those rare patients with cirrhosis may demonstrate physical findings such as ascites, splenomegaly or palmar erythema.

Clinical evaluation

In all series of biopsy-proven paediatric NAFLD, patients uniformly demonstrate elevated serum aminotransferases. Generally, children with NAFLD have serum ALT anywhere from the upper limit of normal to 10 times the upper limit of normal. Children with normal ALT may also have NAFLD, but because of lack of referral of children with normal enzymes (detection bias), and reluctance of paediatric hepatologists to biopsy children with normal enzymes, we know little about 'normal-ALT NAFLD'. This entity has recently been described in adults [17]. At our centre, we have a biopsy-proven example of normal-ALT NASH, obtained in the context of performing a computerized tomography (CT) guided liver biopsy for an unrelated focal lesion. In many centres it appears that the upper limit of normal for the normal range of serum aminotransferases has been creeping up over the years. Certain centres periodically sample a 'normal healthy population', which includes overweight or obese individuals who skew the upper end of 'normal'. Other centres use historical norms and report lower normal ranges. Thus, many children with higher ALT may be erroneously reported as having normal ALT. In paediatric series

of biopsy-proven NASH, serum ALT values range from 100 to 200 IU, and AST values range from 60 to 100 IU. As in adults, the ALT : AST ratio is > 1, with remarkable concordance between paediatric series reporting the ratio ranging from 1.5 to 1.7. This contrasts with a ratio generally < 1 in alcoholic steatohepatitis. In series reporting serum gamma-glutamyl transpeptinase (GGT) or alkaline phosphatase, the values are mildly abnormal. Other significantly elevated serum tests include fasting cholesterol and triglycerides. Interpretation of these results requires comparison to age- and gender-specific norms. Total and direct bilirubin should be normal.

Pathogenesis

There is strong evidence of an association between NAFLD and conditions known to be associated with insulin resistance in adults [22]. These conditions include type 2 diabetes, obesity and hyperlipidaemia. Studies have demonstrated insulin resistance in adult patients with NASH [23]. A recent retrospective study in children ($N = 43$) was performed to determine clinicopathological predictors of paediatric NASH. Criteria for insulin resistance were met by 95% of the subjects. Fasting insulin levels were also strongly predictive on univariate regression analysis for portal inflammation and perisinusoidal fibrosis [5]. Thus, in both adult and paediatric NASH, it appears that insulin resistance and accumulation of fat in the liver is a prerequisite first insult. The mechanism by which insulin resistance leads to steatosis is usually attributed to the action of insulin in increasing peripheral lipolysis, delivery of free fatty acid to the liver, inhibition of free fatty acid release from the liver and induction of hepatic gluco-neogenesis [22]. Apparently, secondary mechanisms are required for provoking inflammation and fibrosis in susceptible fat livers, because many individuals exhibit insulin resistance with simple steatosis only. In this 'two-hit' hypothesis [24], the second hit results from oxidative stress and generation of increased reactive oxygen species (ROS). Hypothetically, increased ROS can result from particular genetic predispositions (such as polymorphisms in pro-inflammatory cytokine genes or cytochrome detoxification genes) or environmental induction (such as diet, medications, bacterial flora in the colon). Nothing is known about secondary mechanisms contributing to paediatric NASH.

Imaging

Imaging has a limited role in the diagnosis of NAFLD because of the variation in the sensitivity of the techniques, the inability of all modalities to discriminate simple steatosis from NASH and the lack of general availability. The most commonly used imaging medium is ultrasonography. Livers infiltrated with fat are hyper-echogenic or 'bright'. Detection of bright liver with milder degrees of fatty infiltration becomes relatively subjective, with modest sensitivity. The brightness of the liver echo is compared to either the kidney, spleen, intrahepatic portal veins, or fall in echo intensity with increasing depth from the transducer [25]. For the detection of fat, a more sensitive technique is CT scanning. Estimates of the degree of fatty infiltration is reported in Hounsfield units. Neither CT nor ultrasonography can distinguish between NASH and simple steatosis.

The most sensitive technique for detecting and quantitating hepatic fat is fast MRI or magnetic resonance spectroscopy. The fat fraction is derived from signal differences in in-phase and out-of-phase signals between fat and water [26]. Using this technique, Fishbein et al. [15] recently demonstrated a correlation between the quantity of hepatic fat and serum ALT in obese children with hepatomegaly.

Histology

Steatohepatitis is a morphological pattern of liver injury that results from a wide number of aetiological insults. The histopathological features of steatohepatitis can result from alcoholism, drug toxicity, type 2 diabetes and a variety of inborn metabolic errors. NASH is a diagnosis requiring liver tissue examination as well as exclusion of other causes of steatohepatitis. Adult NASH is generally considered to include macrovesicular steatosis, mixed acute and chronic lobular inflammation with evidence of cellular injury, and zone 3 perisinusoidal fibrosis. Recently, attempts have been made to establish a grading and staging system for adult NASH. The purpose of grading and staging is to standardize diagnosis, establish criteria associated with presumed progression and arrive at a 'score' that can be useful in the design of treatment or natural history trials. Brunt et al. [10] established a grade for necroinflammatory activity and a stage for the extent of fibrosis with or without architectural remodelling. The necroinflammatory grade is derived from a combination of features of hepatocellular steatosis, cell ballooning and inflammation. The staging of fibrosis reflects the pattern as well as the extent of fibrosis.

Paediatric NASH demonstrates striking differences and some similarities to the adult NASH findings (Table 19.4). By definition, paediatric NASH includes hepatocellular steatosis and inflammation with evidence

Table 19.4 Histological differences between paediatric and adult NASH.

Quality	Paediatric NASH	Adult NASH
Steatosis	Marked	Less pronounced
Inflammation	Portal more common	Lobular more common
Ballooning	Rare	Frequent
Fibrosis	Portal more common	Lobular more common
Cirrhosis	Infrequent	More frequent

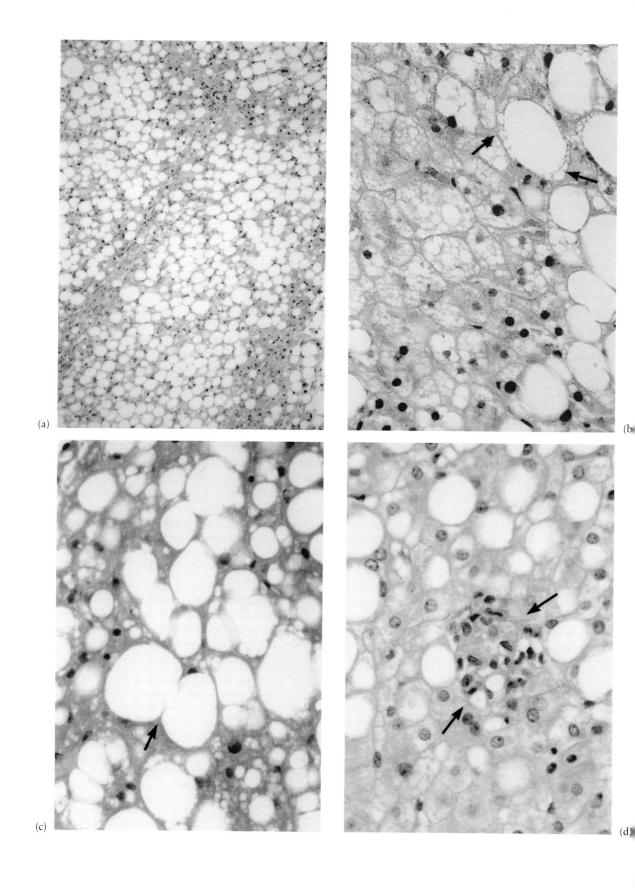

(a)

(b)

(c)

(d)

of cellular injury [3,4,6,7]. These reports highlight the usually moderate to severe steatosis (Fig. 19.2a–c), mild mixed portal tract inflammation and megamitochondria (Plate 5 (a),(b), facing 22), increased glycogen, occasional lipogranulomas (Fig. 19.2d) and mild lipofuscinosis. Presence of fibrosis in the portal and pericellular space is also found (Plate 5 (c),(d)). However, none have attempted to grade or stage the findings. Recently, we sought to grade and stage our patients with paediatric NASH. Forty-three patients under 18 years were identified with NAFLD from a computerized database at the Children's Hospital, San Diego, from 1999–2002. Two independent board-certified pathologists reviewed slides of tissue stained with haematoxylin and eosin (H&E), trichrome, periodic acid–Schiff (PAS) and oil red O. Slides were assessed for the percentage of hepatocytes with fat, presence or absence of hepatocellular ballooning, mixed acute and chronic lobular inflammation, Mallory hyaline, lipid granulomas, megamitochondria, lipofuscin and perisinusoidal fibrosis. Steatosis was moderate to severe in 96% of the cases. In contrast to adults' data, signs of liver injury such as ballooning, lobular inflammation and Mallory hyaline were found in less than 5% of the cases. Glycogen nuclei and lipogranulomas were found in the majority. In contrast to adults, portal inflammation was common but lobular inflammation was infrequent. Also in contrast, mild portal inflammation was common but perisinusoidal fibrosis was only found in 19%. Using the criteria of Brunt et al. [10], no biopsies were stage 3 or 4. Seventy per cent of the biopsies with portal fibrosis lacked findings of pericellular or perisinusoidal fibrosis [11]. Thus, significant differences are appreciated between paediatric and adult NASH (Table 19.4).

Albeit rare, cirrhosis occurs in children with NASH [3,6,9]. In our experience, cirrhosis with NASH is more common in children with precedent or other concurrent precipitants of liver injury, such as hepatitis C virus infection or alcoholism. In adults, cryptogenic cirrhosis is thought to often result from 'burned-out NASH' [27]. Cryptogenic cirrhosis occurs in adults generally susceptible to NASH, and is found in some individuals with precedent biopsies demonstrating NASH. Why the characteristic hallmark of steatosis disappears in those with cryptogenic cirrhosis is unknown. No cases of cryptogenic cirrhosis from paediatric NASH are described.

Treatment

Rational treatment strategies require informed knowledge of pathogenesis. As proposed by Oliver and Day [24], NASH may require two 'hits': the first is fat accumulation within the liver, the second may involve excessive production or concentration of free radicals with increased oxidative stress. Increased oxidative stress to the liver can be generated by environmental or genetic factors. Treatment strategies are mainly geared towards diminishing hepatic fat or reducing oxidative stress. Because NASH is a component of the metabolic syndrome, a rational therapy to treat NASH along with other comorbidities of the metabolic syndrome is to encourage steady and sustainable weight loss. Weight loss can be achieved by either decreasing caloric intake relative to needs or increasing caloric expenditure. Thus, a few trials in children have examined the role of diet in conjunction with exercise to treat NASH (Table 19.5). In both open-label trials of weight loss, obese children with a 'bright' liver on ultrasound were provided with instruction on diet and exercise and encouraged to lose more than 10% of their body weight. Vajro et al. [28] found that in seven of nine patients who were able to lose this much weight, a decrease in the intensity of the liver echogenicity was found and serum ALT became normal. A subsequent weight loss trial in 28 children treated for 3–6 months demonstrated resolution (24 patients) or improvement (four patients) in liver echogenicity with this degree of weight loss. Whether or not all subjects in these trials had NASH or NAFLD was not ascertained, and follow-up liver biopsies were not performed. Many health care providers to adults and children alike find it difficult to motivate or maintain patients with lifestyle habits that promote sustained weight loss. While this strategy is most appealing, how

Fig. 19.2 (*opposite*) Prominent steatosis in paediatric NASH. (a) Diffuse macro- and microvesicular neutral fat deposition within the cytoplasm of hepatocytes. (b) Higher magnification showing microvesicular (left) and macrovesicular (right) steatosis; transition cells with coalescence of fat vesicles into large vacuoles are indicated by arrows. Large vacuoles displace nuclei to the cytoplasmic periphery. (c) Microcystic change with disruption of hepatocytic cytoplasmic membranes (arrow). (d) Lipogranuloma (between arrows) formed by a discrete aggregate of epithelioid histiocytes, fat droplets and few inflammatory cells.

Table 19.5 Paediatric treatment trials in NASH.

Intervention	Reference	Sample size	Entry criteria	Treatment duration (months)	Outcome
Vitamin E	[29]	11	Obese, US bright, > ALT	4–10	Normal ALT, same BMI
Metformin	[32]	10	Biopsy, > ALT	6	Decreased ALT, decreased hepatic fat on MRI, decreased insulin resistance
UDCA	[28]	7	Obese, > ALT	4	Unchanged ALT, unchanged US
Weight loss 1	[8]	7	Obese, > ALT	2–6	Normal ALT, decreased 'bright' liver on US
Weight loss 2 (> 10% loss of ideal body weight)	[13]	28	Obese, 'bright' liver on US	3–6	Bright liver resolved (N = 24) or improved (N = 4) on US

ALT, alanine aminotransferase; BMI, body mass index; MRI, magnetic resonance imaging; UDCA, ursodeoxycholic acid; US, ultrasound.

to help patients succeed stymies providers of health care everywhere.

A second treatment strategy is to decrease oxidative stress by providing supplemental antioxidants. Obese children studied in NHANES III were found to have a relative deficiency of serum α-tocopherol relative to normal-weight controls. An open-label treatment trial of oral vitamin E in 11 obese children with elevated serum ALT and echogenic livers demonstrated normalized serum ALT in all patients [29]. In this pilot trial, treatment consisted of escalating dosage of vitamin E 400–1200 IU once daily. These patients did not have liver biopsies to confirm diagnosis or histological response. How diminution of serum ALT corresponds with clinically relevant outcomes is uncertain, and future paediatric studies with vitamin E or other antioxidants should have baseline and follow-up liver biopsies after an appropriate duration of therapy. A non-randomized treatment trial using vitamin E 300 mg/day for 1 year in Japanese adults with biopsy-proven NASH (N = 12) demonstrated significant reduction in serum ALT and improvement in histological findings including steatosis, inflammation and fibrosis [30]. A subsequent randomized masked trial of vitamin E 400 IU/day for NASH in adults was performed with biopsies at the start and end of the therapeutic trial. After 6 months, patients demonstrated normalization of serum ALT and improvement in the degree of hepatic steatosis (A. Sanyal, personal communication).

Another target for treatment in NASH is reduction of insulin resistance [23]. Insulin resistance is pres-

ent in over 95% of paediatric NAFLD cases, and the degree of resistance significantly predicts the presence of inflammation and fibrosis present in the liver [5]. Adults with NASH demonstrate significant improvement in serum ALT after completing a 4-month trial of treatment with metformin, an insulin-sensitizing reagent [31]. Recently, an open-label pilot trial of metformin for biopsy-proven paediatric NASH was completed. Ten patients were treated for 6 months with metformin 500 mg orally twice daily. Significant improvement was noted in serum ALT, hepatic steatosis (by MRI quantitation) and insulin resistance [32]. Median serum ALT decreased from 149 to 51 IU, median liver fat from 41% to 32% and paediatric quality of life increased from a score of 69 to 81. Thiazolidinediones, another class of insulin-sensitizing drugs, are being tested for their safety and efficacy in adult NASH. However, severe cholestatic hepatitis has been reported in an adult NASH patient treated with troglitazone [33], and inadequate experience using other thiazolidinediones in children with or without pre-existing liver disease warrants caution in considering its use in paediatric clinical trials of NASH.

Research agenda

While NASH studies in adults are informative, enough differences exist between adult and paediatric cases to warrant distinct studies. Although some epidemiological studies have been performed using hepatic imaging modalities and serum ALT, the prevalence of NASH is still not known. As we develop other non-invasive predictive markers of liver fibrosis and inflammation, we may be in a position to estimate the prevalence of NASH from population-based studies. There have been no longitudinal studies of NASH in children. Given that this is arguably the most common cause of chronic liver disease in children, we need to know what happens to affected children as they age and become young adults. Studies need to address what factors are involved in the progression of simple steatosis to NASH. In children, there have been no reports on genetic or environmental factors that may aggravate or protect against injury in vulnerable fatty livers. Studies of genetic polymorphisms within kindreds may be very informative, as will studies on environmental factors such as diet composition and energy expenditure. In order to learn more about prevalence, natural history and treatment response, validated non-invasive imaging and serum biomarkers are needed to assess hepatic steatosis and fibrosis. Finally, well-designed clinical trials (randomized, controlled, adequately powered and blinded) are required to assess which interventions or combinations of interventions demonstrate efficacy and safety in altering clinically relevant outcomes.

Conclusions

The metabolic syndrome, also known as syndrome X, encompasses a constellation of problems associated with insulin resistance. It is generally associated with abdominal obesity, hyperinsulinaemia, dyslipidaemia and essential hypertension. Children with NASH also demonstrate insulin resistance, hyperinsulinaemia and hyperlipidaemia. Thus, paediatric NASH should be considered to be the hepatic manifestation of the metabolic syndrome. The increasing prevalence of NASH in children appears to be a result of the concurrent rise in paediatric obesity prevalence in industrialized nations. The majority of NASH patients are asymptomatic, so efforts must be made by health care providers to identify patients at risk and screen them appropriately. Safe and effective interventions to treat NASH are under investigation. While we await results of well-designed trials, reasonable therapies include regular and sustained aerobic exercise, appropriate diet with antioxidant-laden foods and moderate caloric restriction. Treatments with supplemental oral antioxidants or insulin-sensitizing agents demonstrate promise in pilot trials.

References

1 Ludwig J, Viggiano TR, McGill DB, Oh BJ. Non-alcoholic steatohepatitis: Mayo Clinic experiences with a hitherto unnamed disease. *Mayo Clin Proc* 1980; **55**: 434–8.

2 Moran JR, Ghishan FK, Halter SA, Greene HL. Steatohepatitis in obese children: a cause of chronic liver dysfunction. *Am J Gastroenterol* 1983; **78**: 374–7.

3 Kinugasa A, Tsunamoto K, Furukawa N *et al*. Fatty liver and its fibrous changes found in simple obesity of children. *J Pediatr Gastroenterol Nutr* 1984; **3**: 408–14.

4 Baldridge AD, Perez-Atayde AR, Graeme-Cook F, Higgins L, Lavine JE. Idiopathic steatohepatitis in childhood: a multicenter retrospective study. *J Pediatr* 1995; **127**: 700–4.

5 Schwimmer JB, Deustch R, Behling C *et al*. Obesity, insulin resistance, and other clinicopathological correlations of pediatric non-alcoholic fatty liver disease. *J Pediatr* 2003; **143**: 500–6.

6 Rashid M, Roberts EA. Non-alcoholic steatohepatitis in children. *J Pediatr Gastroenterol Nutr* 2000; **30**: 48–53.

7 Manton ND, Lipsett J, Moore DJ *et al*. Non-alcoholic steatohepatitis in children and adolescents. *Med J Aust* 2000; **173**: 476–9.

8 Vajro PFA, Perna C, Orso G, Tedesco M, De Vincenzo A. Persistent hyperaminotransferasemia resolving after weight reduction in obese children. *J Pediatr* 1994; **125**: 239–41.

9 Molleston JP, White F, Teckman J, Fitzgerald JF. Obese children with steatohepatitis can develop cirrhosis in childhood. *Am J Gastroenterol* 2002; **97**: 2460–2.

10 Brunt EM, Janney CG, Di Bisceglie AM, Neuschwander-Tetri BA, Bacon BR. Non-alcoholic steatohepatitis: a proposal for grading and staging the histological lesions. *Am J Gastroenterol* 1999; **94**: 2467–74.

11 Schwimmer JB, Behling C, Newbury R *et al*. The histological features of pediatric non-alcoholic fatty liver disease (NAFLD) [Abstract]. *Hepatology* 2002; **36**: 412A.

12 Ogden CL FK, Carroll MD, Johnson CL. Prevalence and trends in overweight among US children and adolescents. *J Am Med Assoc* 2002; **288**: 1728–32.

13 Franzese A, Vajro P, Argenziano A *et al*. Liver involvement in obese children: ultrasonography and liver enzyme levels at diagnosis and during follow-up in an Italian population. *Dig Dis Sci* 1997; **42**: 1428–32.

14 Tominaga K, Kurata JH, Chen YH *et al*. Prevalence of fatty liver in Japanese children and relationship to obesity: an epidemiological ultrasonographic survey. *Dig Dis Sci* 1995; **40**: 2002–9.

15 Fishbein MH, Miner M, Mogren C, Chalckson J. The spectrum of fatty liver in obese children and the relationship of serum aminotransferases to severity of steatosis. *J Pediatr Gastroenterol Nutr* 2003; **36**: 54–61.

16 Bergomi A, Lughetti L, Corciulo N. Italian multicenter study on liver damage in pediatric obesity [Abstract]. *Int J Obes Relat Metab Disord* 1998; **22**: S22.

17 Mofrad P, Contos MJ, Haque M *et al*. Clinical and histologic spectrum of non-alcoholic fatty liver disease associated with normal ALT values. *Hepatology* 2003; **37**: 1286–92.

18 Cook JS. Effects of maturational stage on insulin sensitivity during puberty. *J Clin Endocrinol Metab* 1993; **77**: 725–30.

19 Bloch CA, Clemens P, Sperling MA. Puberty decreases insulin sensitivity. *J Pediatr* 1987; **110**: 481–7.

20 Ellis KJ. Body composition of a young, multiethnic, male population. *Am J Clin Nutr* 1997; **1997**: 1323–31.

21 Goran MI, Ball GD, Cruz ML. Obesity and risk of type 2 diabetes and cardiovascular disease in children and adolescents. *J Clin Endocrinol Metab* 2003; **88**: 1417–27.

22 Haque M, Sanyal A. The metabolic abnormalities associated with non-alcoholic fatty liver disease. *Best Pract Res Clin Gastroenterol* 2002; **16**: 709–31.

23 Sanyal AJ, Campbell-Sargent C, Mirshahi F *et al*. Non-alcoholic steatohepatitis: association of insulin resistance and mitochondrial abnormalities. *Gastroenterology* 2001; **120**: 1183–92.

24 Day CP, James OF. Steatohepatitis: a tale of two 'hits'? *Gastroenterology* 1998; **114**: 842–5.

25 Saverymuttu SH, Joseph AE, Maxwell JD. Ultrasound scanning in the detection of hepatic fibrosis and steatosis. *Br Med J* 1986; **292**: 13–5.

26 Fishbein MH, Stevens WR. Rapid MRI using a modified Dixon technique: a non-invasive and effective method for detection and monitoring of fatty metamorphosis of the liver. *Pediatr Radiol* 2001; **31**: 806–9.

27 Matteoni CA, Younossi ZM, Gramlich T *et al*. Non-alcoholic fatty liver disease: a spectrum of clinical and pathological severity. *Gastroenterology* 1999; **116**: 1413–9.

28 Vajro PFA, Vlaerio G, Iannucci MP, Aragione N. Lack of efficacy of ursodeoxycholic acid for the treatment of liver abnormalities in obese children. *J Pediatr* 2000; **136**: 739–43.

29 Lavine JE. Vitamin E treatment of non-alcoholic steatohepatitis in children: a pilot study. *J Pediatr* 2000; **136**: 734–8.

30 Hasegawa T, Yoneda M, Nakamura K, Makino I, Terano A. Plasma transforming growth factor-β1 level and efficacy of α-tocopherol in patients with non-alcoholic steatohepatitis: a pilot study. *Aliment Pharmacol Ther* 2001; **15**: 1667–72.

31 Marchesini G, Brizi M, Bianchi G *et al*. Metformin in non-alcoholic steatohepatitis. *Lancet* 2001; **358**: 893–4.

32 Schwimmer JB, Middleton M, Deutsch R, Lavine JE. Metformin as a treatment for non-diabetic NASH. *J Pediatr Gastroenterol Nutr* 2003; **37**: 342.

33 Menon KVN, Angulo P, Lindor KD. Severe cholestatic hepatitis from troglitazone in a patient with non-alcoholic steatohepatitis and diabetes mellitus. *Am J Gastroenterol* 2001; **96**: 1631–4.

20 Steatohepatitis resulting from intestinal bypass

Christiane Bode & J. Christian Bode

Key learning points

1 Jejuno-ileal bypass, which was used to treat morbid obesity, was associated with a multitude of serious acute and chronic complications, and was replaced by other operative procedures in the early 1980s.
2 One of the most important complications was liver injury—severe forms of fatty liver and steatohepatitis that led to both acute liver failure and cirrhosis.
3 A variety of mechanisms including protein malnutrition and gut-derived endotoxins and other bacterial toxins contribute to the genesis of post-bypass liver disease.

Abstract

Jejuno-ileal bypass (JIB) became popular as a treatment for morbid obesity in the 1970s. Unfortunately, this operation resulted in numerous postoperative complications, the most serious of which was the development of acute liver failure or hepatic fibrosis and cirrhosis. The pathological spectrum of liver disease following JIB has included increase in steatosis, non-alcoholic steatohepatitis (NASH), fibrosis and cirrhosis. The incidence of these types of liver disease published by different groups varies distinctly. Important factors implicated in the pathogenesis of liver injury after JIB are intestinal bacterial overgrowth in the excluded segment of the small intestine and protein and amino acid malnutrition. The bacterial overgrowth leads to mucosal injury and increased gut permeability to bacterial toxins, especially endotoxins. Endotoxins absorbed into the portal vein may then induce overproduction of pro-inflammatory mediators, such as certain cytokines (e.g. tumour necrosis factor-α [TNF-α] and interleukin 1 [IL-1]) and reactive oxygen species (ROS), which are capable of causing influx of leukocytes and hepatocellular damage. In accordance with the aforementioned hypothesis is the observation that hepatic dysfunction and liver injury after JIB in humans and experimental animals could be prevented by antibiotic treatment.

Introduction

JIB is a surgical procedure of small bowel exclusion, which was performed frequently during the 1960s to early 1980s, as a treatment of morbid obesity in patients who failed to lose weight by other means. More than 25 000 patients in the USA have undergone JIB surgery [1,2]. Although significant weight lost (30–35% of the pre-operative weight) and decrease of several obesity-related health risk factors were achieved, it soon became apparent that numerous side-effects could occur, including some serious and possibly fatal complications (Table 20.1) [1–6]. The prevalence of these side-effects varies markedly from series to series.

241

Table 20.1 Morbidity after jejuno-ileal bypass (JIB) in humans [1–4,7–9].

Gastrointestinal complications
Diarrhoea (E > L)
Bypass enteropathy
Abdominal bloating (E > L)
Fluid and electrolyte deficiencies: hypokalaemia, hypomagnesaemia, hypocalcaemia (E > L)
Vitamin deficiency, predominantly vitamin B_{12} and folate (E > L)

Hepatobiliary complications
Acute liver failure (E > L)
Steatosis (E > L)
Steatohepatitis (E = L)
Fibrosis, cirrhosis (E < L)
Biliary calculi (E < L)

Renal complications
Renal calculi (E < L)
Renal failure

Polyarthralgia and polymygalgia (E > L)

E, predominantly early complication; L, predominantly late complication.

Factors that may contribute to the variable frequency of early and late complications of JIB are differences in the technique of the operation (end-to-side jejuno-ileostomy; end-to-end jejuno-ileostomy with drainage of the excluded small bowel into the colon or sigmoid), in the selection of patients such as age, sex, body mass index (BMI), the length of follow-up and the incidence of reversal of the bypass [1–8].

Hepatic injury following jejuno-ileal bypass in humans

Of the many complications described following JIB, one of the most important is the development of progressive liver disease resulting either in acute liver failure or hepatic fibrosis and cirrhosis [1,6–9]. When discussing the clinical and morphological spectrum and the pathogenesis of JIB-induced liver disease, it should be realized that the liver injury is, in most instances, part of complex functional disturbances and multiorgan injury (Table 20.1).

Pathological spectrum of jejuno-ileal bypass-induced liver disease

The morphological spectrum of liver disease following JIB includes hepatic steatosis [2,5,9–12], NASH [2,8,10,12,13], hepatic fibrosis [2,8,10,11,14] and cirrhosis [1,2,6,8,10,11] (see Chapter 2. The incidence of the various patterns of liver injury reported by different groups varies widely (Tables 20.2 & 20.3). These differences may be explained in part by differences in the study population, the type of JIB operation and the length of follow-up. In some studies, the inter-

Table 20.2 Effect of JIB on hepatic steatosis in subjects with morbid obesity.

Follow-up (years)	N	Type of JIB*	Hepatic steatosis	Reference
1	132	EE + ES	Worse 55.3% Improved 31%	[6]
2	103		Worse 44.7% Improved 31%	[6]
1	88	EE	Before 68% After 94%	[11]
2	27	ES	Before 92% After 100%	[12]
7.5	40	EE + ES	Before 65% After 28%	[13]
12.6	43	ES	No change	[9]

* Type of JIB: EE, end-to-end anastomosis; ES, end-to-side anastomosis.

Table 20.3 Incidence of hepatic fibrosis and cirrhosis after JIB operation.

Follow-up (years)	N	Type of JIB*	Cirrhosis	Fibrosis			Reference
				Portal (P)	Central (C)	C–P bridging	
	132	EE	4.5	ND**	ND	ND	[5]
2	103		6.5	ND	ND	ND	[5]
1	88	EE	3.4	9.8%[b] → 32%[a]	8.6%[b] → 48%[a]	6.4%	[10]
2	27	ES	4%[b] → 26%[a]	80%[b] → 93%[a]	26%[b] → 59%[a]	ND	[11]
4.8	180	ES	0	In a subgroup no change			[7]
5	453	ES	3.2%	ND	ND	ND	[1]
10			6.1%				
15			8.1%				
12.6	43	ES	7%	C or C–P: 4.8% → 38% [8]			
11.4	23	ES	0	P + C mild 18.2% → 22.7%			[13]
				P + C moderate 0 → 9%			

* Type of JIB: EE, end-to-end anastomosis; ES, end-to-side anastomosis.
Histology: b, before JIB; a, after JIB.
ND, no data.

pretation of the results is hampered by the fact that no details are given for the method of histological evaluation [1,5,7].

Steatosis
Some degree of hepatic steatosis is found in 60–90% of morbidly obese patients prior to JIB [2,15]. An increased hepatic fat content following JIB has repeatedly been reported (Table 20.2) [2,9]. Fat accumulation was reported to be maximal in the first year postoperatively, frequently subsiding to pre-operative levels 2–3 years after surgery [2,9]. Most studies on hepatic steatosis in obese patients before and after JIB have used histological assessment, which provides only an approximate guide to total liver fat. A significant correlation of histological assessment of hepatic steatosis with chemical lipid accumulation was only observed in cases of marked fat accumulation; histological differences between mild and moderate steatosis were judged to be meaningless for practical purposes [9]. Chemical estimates showed a lipid accumulation of three times or more the pre-operative values 1 year after JIB [9].

Inflammation and necrosis
Prior to JIB, mild portal inflammation was present in 20–32% in three reports [10,12,13] and 59% in another study [8]. The type of inflammation was described to

be lymphocytic infiltration of portal tracts in two of the studies [8,10] and not specified in the other reports [12,13].

In follow-up liver biopsies, variable results regarding inflammatory infiltrates have been published. Ten years or more after JIB, portal inflammation was reported to be mild and unchanged [14] or decreased in amount [8]. Similar results were seen in liver biopsies taken more than 7 years following JIB [12].

Patchy hepatocellular necrosis and polymorphonuclear inflammatory infiltrates have also been described in some patients [2,10,11,14]. These more serious histological abnormalities, which have been found to be combined with central 'hyaline sclerosis' and/or cirrhosis, were described to be indistinguishable from changes characteristic of alcoholic steatonecrosis (alcoholic hepatitis) [16]. However, in the majority of patients in whom the histological changes after JIB have been described in detail, the diagnosis of 'steatohepatitis' was equivalent to the 'literal definition' of NASH [15].

Hepatic fibrosis and cirrhosis
Mild degrees of hepatic fibrosis have been reported to be present in severe obesity (Table 20.3) [15]. Advanced stages of fibrosis and cirrhosis are distinctly less frequent (Table 20.3).

There is good evidence that fibrosis may develop *de novo* or progress after JIB (Table 20.3) [2,9]. The incidence of cirrhosis after JIB varies markedly (Table 20.3). In some studies, the risk of developing cirrhosis increases with the period of follow-up [1,5], while in other studies the development of cirrhosis has not been observed during a mean follow-up of nearly 5 years [7] or even more than 11 years [14]. The early type of elective jejuno-colic anastomosis proved to have the most serious complications and was therefore soon abandoned [2].

Clinical course of jejuno-ileal bypass-associated liver disease

Apart from the complications after JIB described above (Table 20.1), in most patients in whom progressive liver abnormalities were documented in follow-up liver biopsies, no clinical symptoms of acute or chronic liver failure and no hospital admissions for liver-related problems were reported [1,2,5–8]. Mild to moderate elevation of activities of liver enzymes in the serum (aspartate aminotransferase [AST], alanine aminotransferase [ALT], alkaline phosphatase) were common in the first postoperative year but in most cases had largely returned to normal by the end of that period [2,5].

One of the most severe complications of JIB was acute liver failure. In several reports including at least 100 patients, acute liver failure occurred in 1.2–11% [1,5–7]. However, in several small series including less than 50 patients, no acute liver failure was reported [11–13]. JIB reversal has been an effective therapy in some patients with this life-threatening complication [1,9]. The intravenous infusion of aminoacids improved liver function in several cases [17] and allowed safer reversal of the JIB [1]. Oral supplements of all essential aminoacids, however, were ineffective in preventing this complication [18]. Improvement of severe hepatic steatosis after JIB was also brought about by metronidazole treatment [19].

Progressive liver disease following JIB may become evident only in the stage of decompensated cirrhosis with jaundice, ascites, hepatic encephalopathy and variceal haemorrhage. In this situation, JIB reversal has little impact on the disease and the perioperative mortality is high [1]. Under such circumstances liver transplantation has been a successful therapy [20].

Experimental studies of jejuno-ileal bypass-induced hepatic dysfunction and liver injury

In studies conducted to evaluate the rat as a model for JIB-induced liver injury, various biochemical changes and indicators of hepatic dysfunction were reported, but steatosis, inflammation and fibrosis comparable to that seen in humans after JIB were not observed [21–25]. Steatosis and inflammatory infiltrates in the liver were observed only when the distal end of the excluded part of the small intestine was anastomosed end-to-side into the caecum [26].

When rats subjected to an end-to-side JIB were fed an alcohol-containing liquid diet they developed marked steatosis (macro- and microvesicular), focal ballooning of hepatocytes, single-cell necrosis, focal clustering of necrosis, and on review some apoptosis, disarray of the trabecular structure, inflammatory cell infiltrates (mainly mononuclear cells), 'hyalin inclusions' resembling megamitochondria and increased numbers of mitotic figures. These features were similar to those seen in human alcoholic liver disease [24]. Neither the control animals without a JIB receiving the alcohol-containing liquid diet nor controls with a JIB that received the liquid diet without alcohol exhibited any histological evidence of liver injury [24]. The alcohol-induced liver injury after JIB in rats could be almost completely prevented by supplementation of the diet with high doses of methionine [27]. On the other hand, low methionine content of the diet distinctly enhanced the susceptibility of rats to liver damage after JIB.

Pathogenesis of liver injury after jejuno-ileal bypass

Most studies of the pathogenesis of liver injury after JIB were performed in the 1970s and early 1980s [22–31]. Once JIB was replaced by other surgical procedures, such as gastroplasty, interest in further research in this field declined abruptly. This explains why the pathogenesis of steatohepatitis, including the role of intestinal bacteria and bacterial toxins, proinflammatory cytokines and other mediators from macrophages, and oxidative stress [28,29], has not been further studied in animal models after JIB.

Non jejuno-ileal bypass-related factors

Alcohol

In some cases, alcohol abuse has been reported to be an important aetiological factor in the development of post-bypass cirrhosis [1,2,5]. In most studies on liver injury after JIB, no detailed information on alcohol consumption was given [5–8,10–12]. In an extensive meta-analysis, even moderate amounts of ethanol (25 g/day) have been shown to be associated with a 2.5-fold increase in risk to develop cirrhosis [30], so alcohol consumption might have contributed to liver injury after JIB in a significant portion of cases [1].

Viral hepatitis B and C infection

In cases where inflammatory infiltrates were present before JIB, chronic viral hepatitis may also have contributed to progression of liver disease after JIB. The type and pattern of the inflammatory infiltrates, and other abnormal findings in the liver biopsies, would have been compatible with chronic viral hepatitis [1,5,7,10,11]. Tests to detect hepatitis C virus (HCV) infection were not available until 1989 and in most published studies information on hepatitis B virus (HBV) infection prevalence is lacking [1,3,5–8,10–14].

Other contributing factors

In the aforementioned studies on post-bypass liver injury, no information is given on other potentially confounding types of chronic liver disease, such as autoimmune hepatitis and inherited metabolic disorders. Despite the uncertainties regarding other contributing factors, there is good evidence that liver disease after JIB is predominantly a genuine complication of this operation [2,3,9].

Nutritional deficiency

Protein-calorie malnutrition occurs in nearly all patients after JIB. The similarity to the marked hepatic steatosis seen in kwashiorkor leads to the suggestion that protein deficiency might account for the perpetuation or increase in lipid accumulation in the liver after JIB [2,9]. This hypothesis is supported by the observation of reversal of massive hepatic steatosis in JIB patients by intravenous infusion of calorie-free amino acid solutions [1,17]. The relevance of deficiency of essential amino acids for the development of liver injury and dysfunction after JIB is further supported by the results of a recent experimental study in which marked hepatic steatosis developed when the casein in the diet (17.7% of total calories) was the only source of methionine [27]. Methionine supplementation completely prevented the histological abnormalities and functional disturbances in the liver. On the other hand, oral amino acid supplementation failed to alter postoperative deterioration of hepatic steatosis and function [18], and metronidazole treatment in patients after JIB decreased hepatic steatosis despite developing malnutrition [19].

Malabsorption of other nutritional factors, such as essential fatty acids and lipotropes, have also been implicated in liver damage. However, animals with experimental resection of the small intestine, comparable to the excluded segment after bypass, did not develop liver dysfunction although the degree of malabsorption did not differ [2]. Protein-amino acid deficiency may contribute to steatosis and liver dysfunction after JIB but it is unlikely to cause the more significant changes of hepatocellular necrosis, inflammation or fibrosis [2,9].

Intestinal bacteria (bacterial toxins) and increased gut permeability

The observation that various types of liver dysfunction follow experimental JIB, but are not seen after equivalent intestinal resection [2], leads to the recognition of the importance of the excluded segment of the small intestine for the development of post-bypass liver damage. Further evidence for the importance of the excluded segment for many of the systemic complications after JIB including liver injury came from patients who developed signs of acute intestinal obstruction. Surgical exploration demonstrated a marked inflammatory process involving the excluded loops with non-obstructive ileus [4]. When the bacterial flora was studied in a subgroup of patients, the proximal excluded segment harboured the quantitative and qualitative equivalent of faecal flora [4]. The most persuasive evidence implicating small intestinal bacterial overgrowth in the production of post-bypass liver damage came from trials with antibiotics. Hepatic dysfunction after JIB in dogs could be prevented by doxycycline [32]. Similar beneficial effects of antibiotic administration on liver function after JIB were observed in rats [23]. More importantly, metronidazole treatment prevented

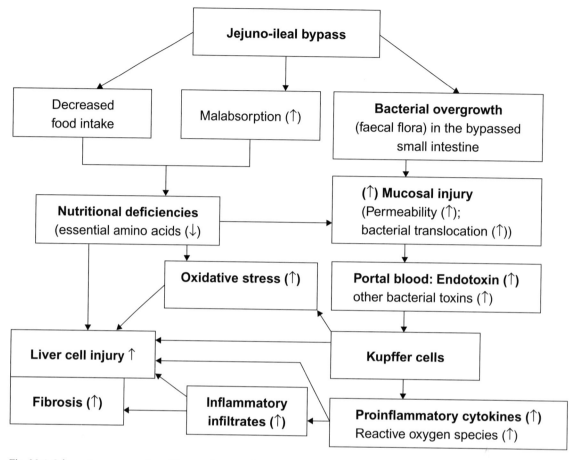

Fig. 20.1 Schematic representation of factors that contribute to the pathogenesis of liver injury after jejuno-ileal bypass (JIB) [1,2,28,29].

and reversed hepatic steatosis after JIB in humans, irrespective of protein-calorie malnutrition [19].

Bacterial toxins, especially endotoxins, absorbed via the portal vein to the liver are likely candidates for causing liver injury and dysfunction [2,19]. The results of research performed in the last two decades on the role of gut-derived bacterial toxins, especially endotoxins, in the pathogenesis of alcoholic hepatitis [29,33] and NASH [28,33] suggest the sequence of factors schematically summarized in Fig. 20.1. The bacterial overgrowth with faecal flora in the excluded blind group leads, by direct and indirect toxic effects, to mucosal injury. The mucosal injury promotes an increase in gut permeability for macromolecules, enhancing the translocation of endotoxins and other bacterial toxins from the gut lumen to the portal blood and/or the lymphatics.

The resulting endotoxaemia stimulates Kupffer cells and other macrophages, thereby increasing the release of proinflammatory cytokines, such as TNF-α, IL-1, IL-6 and other potentially toxic mediators, and ROS. Chronic overproduction of such mediators may induce the accumulation and activation of polymorphs, endothelial lesions, increased permeability of sinusoids, disturbed microcirculation and other damaging events that finally lead to necrosis or apoptosis of hepatocytes, inflammatory infiltrates and deposition of collagen (further details are reviewed elsewhere [28,29,33,34]). Malnutrition, especially protein-amino acid deficiency, has been shown to increase gut permeability [35] and even bacterial translocation [36], and may contribute to the damage of the mucosal barrier in the excluded segment after JIB.

Conclusions

JIB was introduced in the 1960s for treating morbid obesity that failed non-operative management. When it became evident that JIB was associated with a multitude of serious acute and chronic complications it was substituted by other operative procedures in the early 1980s. Among the prominent complications were severe forms of fatty liver and steatohepatitis that led to both acute liver failure and cirrhosis. The pathogenic mechanisms of post-bypass liver injury have not been not completely clarified. A variety of mechanisms, which include protein malnutrition and gut-derived endotoxins and other bacterial toxins, contribute to the genesis of post-bypass liver disease.

References

1 Requarth JA, Burchard KW, Colacchio TA *et al*. Long-term morbidity following jejuno-ileal bypass: the continuing potential need for surgical reversal. *Arch Surg* 1995; **130**: 318–25.

2 Maxwell JD, McGouran RC. Jejuno-ileal bypass: clinical and experimental aspects. *Scand J Gastroenterol* 1982; **74** (Suppl): 129–47.

3 Bray GA, Benfield JR. Intestinal bypass for obesity a summary and perspective. *Am J Clin Nutr* 1977; **30**: 121–7.

4 Drenick ED, Ament ME, Finegold SM *et al*. Bypass enteropathy: an inflammatory process in the excluded segment with systemic complications. *Am J Clin Nutr* 1977; **30**: 76–89.

5 Baddeley RM. The management of gross refractory obesity by jejuno-ileal bypass. *Br J Surg* 1979; **66**: 525–32.

6 Hocking MP, Duerson MC, O'Leary JP *et al*. Jejuno-ileal bypass for morbid obesity: late follow-up in 100 cases. *N Engl J Med* 1983; **308**: 995–9.

7 McFarland RJ, Gazet JC, Pilkington TR. A 13-year review of jejuno-ileal bypass. *Br J Surg* 1985; **72**: 81–7.

8 Hocking MP, Davis GL, Franzini DA *et al*. Long-term consequences after jejuno-ileal bypass for morbid obesity. *Dig Dis Sci* 1998; **43**: 2493–9.

9 Holzbach RT. Hepatic effects of jejuno-ileal bypass for morbid obesity. *Am J Clin Nutr* 1977; **30**: 43–52.

10 Marubbio AT, Buchwald, H, Schwartz MZ *et al*. Hepatic lesions of central pericellular fibrosis in morbid obesity, and after jejuno-ileal bypass. *Am J Clin Pathol* 1976; **66**: 684–91.

11 Haines NW, Baker, AL, Boyer JL. Prognostic indicators of hepatic injury following jejuno-ileal bypass performed for refractory obesity: a prospective study. *Hepatology* 1981; **1**: 161–7.

12 Kaminski, DL, Herrmann, VM, Martin S. Late effects of jejuno-ileal bypass operations on hepatic inflammation, fibrosis and lipid content. *Hepatogastroenterology* 1985; **32**: 159–62.

13 Peters RL, Gay T, Reynolds TB. Post-jejunoileal-bypass hepatic disease: its similarity to alcoholic hepatic disease. *Am J Clin Pathol* 1975; **63**: 318–31.

14 Boon AP, Thompson H, Baddeley RM. Use of histological examination to assess ultrastructure of liver in patients with long-standing jejuno-ileal bypass for morbid obesity. *J Clin Pathol* 1988; **41**: 1281–7.

15 McCullough AJ. Non-alcoholic liver disease: natural history. In: Leuschner U, James OFW, Dancygier H, eds. *Steatohepatitis (NASH and ASH)*. Dordrecht: Kluwer Academic, 2001: 11–20.

16 Hall P. Pathological spectrum of alcoholic liver disease. In: Hall P, ed. *Alcoholic Liver Disease*. London: Edward Arnold, 1995: 41–68.

17 Heimburger SL, Steiger E, Gerfo PL *et al*. Reversal of severe fatty hepatic infiltration after intestinal bypass for morbid obesity by calorie-free amino acid infusion. *Am J Surg* 1975; **129**: 229–35.

18 Lockwood DH, Amatruda J-M, Moxley RT *et al*. Effect of oral amino acid supplementation on liver disease after jejuno-ileal bypass for morbid obesity. *Am J Clin Nutr* 1977; **30**: 58–63.

19 Drenick EJ, Fisler J, Johnson D. Hepatic steatosis after intestinal bypass-prevention and reversal by metronidazole, irrespective of protein-calorie malnutrition. *Gastroenterology* 1982; **82**: 535–48.

20 Lowell JA, Shenoy S, Ghalib R *et al*. Liver transplantation after jejuno-ileal bypass for morbid obesity. *J Am Coll Surg* 1997; **185**: 123–7.

21 Grenier JF, Marescaux J, Stock C *et al*. BSP clearance as the most reliable criterion of hepatic dysfunction after jejuno-ileal bypass in the rat: arguments in favor of the existence of a pathogenetic mechanism involving a transient malnutrition state. *Dig Dis Sci* 1981; **26**: 334–41.

22 Baker H, Vanderhoof JA, Tuma DJ *et al*. A jejuno-ileal bypass rat model for rapid study of the effects of vitamin malabsorption. *Int J Vitam Nutr Res* 1992; **62**: 43–60.

23 Vanderhoof JA, Tuma DJ, Antonson DL *et al*. Effect of antibiotics in the prevention of jejuno-ileal bypass-induced liver dysfunction. *Digestion* 1982; **23**: 9–15.

24 Bode C, Gast J, Zelder O *et al*. Alcohol-induced liver injury after jejuno-ileal bypass operation in rats. *J Hepatol* 1987; **5**: 75–84.

25 Viddal KO, Nygaard K. Intestinal bypass: a comparison between two different bypass operations and resection of the small intestine in rats. *Scand J Gastroenterol* 1977; **12**: 465–72.

247

26 Serbource-Goguel Seta N, Borel B, Dodeur M *et al.* Endocytosis and binding of asialo-orosomucoid by hepatocytes from rats with jejunoileal bypass. *Hepatology* 1985; **5**: 220–30.

27 Parlesak A, Bode C, Bode JC. Free methionine supplementation limits alcohol-induced liver damage in rats. *Alcohol Clin Exp Res* 1998; **22**: 352–80.

28 Lands WE. Cellular signals in alcohol-induced liver injury: a review. *Alcohol Clin Exp Res* 1995; **19**: 928–38.

29 Bode JC, Parlesak A, Bode C. Gut-derived bacterial toxins (endotoxin) and alcoholic liver disease. In: Agarwal DP, Seitz HK, eds. *Alcohol in Health and Disease*. New York: Marcel Dekker, 2001: 369–86.

30 Corrao G, Arico S. Independent and combined action of hepatitis C virus infection and alcohol consumption on the risk of symptomatic liver cirrhosis. *Hepatology* 1998; **27**: 914–9.

31 Vanderhoof JA, Tuma DJ, Sorrell MF. Role of defunctionalized bowel in jejunoileal bypass-induced liver disease in rats. *Dig Dis Sci* 1979; **24**: 916–200.

32 Hollenbeck JI, O'Leary JP, Maher JW *et al.* An etiologic basis for fatty liver after jejuno-ileal bypass. *J Surg Res* 1975; **18**: 83–9.

33 Bode C, Schäfer C, Bode JC. The role of gut-derived bacterial toxins (endotoxin) for the development of alcoholic liver disease in man. In: Blum HE, Bode C, Bode JC, Sartor RB, eds. *Gut and the Liver*. Dordrecht: Kluwer Academic, 1998: 281–98.

34 Tilg H, Diehl AM. Cytokines in alcoholic and non-alcoholic steatohepatitis. *N Engl J Med* 2000; **343**: 1467–76.

35 De Blaauw I, Deutz NE, van der Hulst RR *et al.* Glutamine depletion and increased gut permeability in non-anorectic, non-weight-losing tumor-bearing rats. *Gastroenterology* 1997; **112**: 118–26.

36 Casafont F, Sanchez E, Martin L *et al.* Influence of malnutrition on the prevalence of bacterial translocation and spontaneous bacterial peritonitis in experimental cirrhosis in rats. *Hepatology* 1997; **25**: 1334–70.

21 Specific disorders associated with NAFLD

Geraldine M. Grant, Vikas Chandhoke & Zobair M. Younossi

Key learning points

1 In addition to obesity and type 2 diabetes, a number of other conditions and drugs have been associated with the development of hepatic steatosis and steatohepatitis.
2 The pathways involved in pathogenesis of these conditions overlap, but in some cases involve specific metabolic defects or toxicity. Further study may provide insight into the pathogenesis and progression of more common 'idiopathic' forms of non-alcoholic fatty liver disease (NAFLD)/non-alcoholic steatohepatitis (NASH).
3 The natural history of drug-induced steatohepatitis may differ from typical NAFLD and NASH, with some drug reactions leading to rapid onset of cirrhosis and liver failure.
4 In adults, total parenteral nutrition can lead to liver disease related to steatosis.
5 Congenital and acquired lipodystrophies are associated with insulin resistance, and some case studies have indicated a high rate of potentially progressive NAFLD/NASH.
6 Polycystic ovary syndrome is commonly associated with insulin resistance and glucose intolerance, but studies of the frequency and severity of resultant NAFLD are lacking.

Abstract

A number of conditions related to insulin-resistance syndrome (obesity, type 2 diabetes and hyperlipidaemia) are associated with non-alcoholic fatty liver disease (NAFLD) and non-alcoholic steatohepatitis (NASH). In addition, several other genetic and acquired conditions can mimic the clinical and pathological features of NAFLD and present with hepatic steatosis or NASH. The pathogenesis of these conditions may be quite different from NAFLD that results from metabolic causes, but they may also share a number of potential pathogenic mechanisms. This chapter discusses and summarizes conditions that can present with hepatic manifestations of steatosis or steatohepatitis. Insights into pathogenic mechanisms that could be informative of 'idiopathic' or 'primary' NAFLD/NASH are considered, together with brief comments on diagnosis and management.

Introduction

The spectrum of non-alcoholic fatty liver disease

As discussed in earlier chapters, NAFLD represents a spectrum of clinicopathological conditions characterized by significant lipid deposition in the liver parenchyma of patients without a history of excessive alcohol ingestion. At one end of this spectrum is steatosis alone. Many cases of cirrhosis associated with metabolic factors may lie at the other end of the spectrum, and pivotal between them is steatohepatitis or NASH. NASH is a metabolic (non-alcoholic) form of liver disease characterized by steatosis, hepatocyte ballooning degeneration, and Mallory hyaline and/or perisinusoidal fibrosis most prominent in acinar zone 3 (see Chapter 2). Although NASH can progress to cirrhosis, such progression is difficult to predict [1–9].

Estimates of the prevalence of NAFLD are high and expected to increase with the epidemic of obesity and type 2 diabetes in the USA and all other affluent societies around the world (see Chapter 3). Several recent studies show that cirrhosis can occur in up to 26% of clinical patients with NASH. Although only 2.6% of liver transplants are related to NASH cirrhosis, a large number of patients undergoing liver transplantation for cryptogenic cirrhosis may actually have 'burned-out' NASH.

Insulin resistance and NAFLD

The metabolic disorders that comprise the insulin resistance syndrome (IRS) include impaired glucose tolerance, dyslipidaemia, arterial hypertension, visceral or truncal adiposity, hyperuricaemia, the polycystic ovary syndrome (PCOS) and impaired fibrinolysis. These conditions share insulin resistance (IR) as a common defect. PCOS is a special, but common cause of IR, in which the underlying metabolic defect may be overlooked in favour of the implications for fertility or physical appearance; PCOS is discussed later in this review. A variety of genetic and acquired defects can lead to IR, including lipodystrophy syndromes, which are also considered here.

There is a strong association between IR and NASH (see Chapter 4). The frequency of IR among patients with NASH can be as high as 87% and 98% (see Chapter 5). Further, the clinical variables associated with a more progressive course in NAFLD/NASH, such as type 2 diabetes, obesity and increasing age, are those associated with insulin resistance (see Chapter 4).

Acquired disorders associated with NAFLD and NASH

The acquired disorders associated with NAFLD/NASH are summarized in Table 21.1.

Table 21.1 Conditions associated with non-alcoholic fatty liver disease (NAFLD).

Conditions	Associated metabolic syndrome	Associated hepatic disorders
IRS	Impaired glucose tolerance, obesity and diabetes	NAFLD/NASH
TPN	IR	Elevated ALT, cholestasis, steatosis, hepatic fibrosis, cirrhosis
Malnutrition	Impaired glucose and lipid metabolism	Steatosis, Mallory bodies
Acquired LD	IR and IRS	NAFLD/NASH
Familial lipodystrophies CGL	IRS and acanthosis nigricans	NAFLD, cirrhosis
Familial partial lipodystrophies	Acanthosis nigricans	NAFLD
MAD	IR	NAFLD
PCOS	IR, hyperandrogenism, dyslipidaemia	?NAFLD/NASH
Wilson's disease	Copper accumulation and toxicity	Steatosis, hepatitis, cirrhosis, hepatic failure
A-β-lipoproteinaemia	IR	NAFLD/NASH
Coeliac disease	Malabsorption/malnutrition	Elevated ALT, steatosis, chronic hepatitis, septal fibrosis, cirrhosis
Drug-induced	Variable	NAFLD, NASH, cirrhosis

ALT, alanine aminotransferase; CGL, congenital generalized lipodystrophies; IR, insulin resistance; IRS, insulin resistance syndrome; LD, lipodystophies; MAD, mandibuloacral dysplasia; NASH, non-alcoholic steatohepatitis; PCOS, polycystic ovarian syndrome; TPN, total parenteral nutrition.

Total parental nutrition

Total parental nutrition (TPN) is associated with a number of hepatic abnormalities, which occur in approximately 15% of patients depending on age, duration and formulation of TPN [10]. The duration of TPN influences the progression and severity of TPN-induced liver disease [10–14]. The hepatic disorders attributed to long-term TPN include increased serum alanine aminotransferase (ALT) levels, cholestasis, steatosis, hepatic fibrosis and cirrhosis. Biliary diseases related to TPN include biliary sludge, acalculous cholecystitis and cholelithiasis. Furthermore, hyperinsulinaemia and IR, similar to type 2 diabetes, have also been observed [14,15]. Histological abnormalities include macrovesicular steatosis with a varying degree of portal and periportal fibrosis [16]. The importance of TPN-induced hepatic abnormalities is demonstrated by a study involving 90 patients receiving long-term TPN. Among these, 26% developed liver disease at 2 years, 50% at 6 years and 6.6% of patients died from the complications of liver disease, some instances of which were attributed to steatosis [16]. Potential causes of steatosis in patients receiving TPN are summarized in Table 21.2.

In adults, steatosis is the most common manifestation of TPN-induced liver disease. It appears within the first few weeks of TPN, with biochemical abnormalities (ALT elevations) presenting after approximately 3 months of continuous TPN. Steatosis usually has a benign and reversible course after nutritional treatment is terminated. However, for patients requiring long-term TPN, these issues become more problematic [11,13,15]. Steatosis should be suspected in long-term TPN patients with elevated ALT in the absence of biliary disease or viral hepatitis [22].

In contrast, the dominant manifestation of TPN-induced liver disease in young children is cholestasis; this can also potentially lead to progressive liver disease and death from complications of cirrhosis.

Prevention and treatment options for TPN-induced liver disease include reformulation of TPN. Excessive carbohydrates can lead to an increase in lipogenesis, which may not be counterbalanced by the export mechanism of the liver such as formation of very-low-density lipoprotein (VLDL) (see Chapter 9). This mechanism can be overwhelmed, resulting in accumulation of lipid in the liver and development of steatosis [14,15]. The addition of 2.5% lipid in combination with 25% or 17% dextrose can prevent steatosis elevation by correcting portal insulin : glucagon (I : R) ratio [23]. Additionally, increasing the lipid concentration can reduce the excessive contribution of the carbohydrate dextrose and decrease the portal I : R [15,23].

In animal studies, supplementation with glucagon appears to prevent steatosis, and may also help reverse the progression of TPN-induced hepatic steatosis [24–26]. Although supplementation with L-glutamine may be another option, there is much debate about its

Table 21.2 Potential causes of TPN-induced steatosis.

Putative cause	Effect	Corrective response	Result
Excessive carbohydrate, such as high dextrose infusions	Steatosis	Increase lipid ratio in formulation	Decreased hepatic lipid accumulation Decreased hepatic acetyl-CoA carboxylase activity [18]
Elevated insulin : glucagon ratio	Steatosis	Addition of glucagon	Decrease in steatosis [19]
Essential fatty acid deficiency	Decreased lipoprotein formation	Supplementation of essential fatty acids	Decrease in steatosis [14,15]
Choline deficiency	Steatosis decreased lipoprotein formation	Addition of choline	Reversal of fatty liver [14,15]
Carnitine deficiency	Steatosis	Addition of carnitine	No obvious effect, but normalizes plasma carnitine levels [14,15]
Drug metabolizing enzyme deficiencies, GSH, P450	Steatosis and NASH	Addition of glutamine	May induce P450s, increases [GSH] [20,21]

effectiveness [27,28]. This debate is interesting considering the contribution of glutamine in the production of glutathione, the substrate for glutathione-*S*-transferases, and a major intracellular antioxidant. In addition to its potential antioxidant activity, glutathione may also aid in protecting the integrity of intestinal mucosa, reducing the possibility of intestinal bacterial translocation. Both oxidative stress and bacterial endotoxins have been suggested as potential pathways for progressive NAFLD [20,21,29,30].

Deficiency in other nutrients such as carnitine, choline and essential amino acids may result from the formulation, poor delivery and degradation of TPN components [14]. Carnitine deficiency has been documented in long-term TPN patients. Carnitine can negatively impact the mitochondrial fatty acid shuttling system (see Chapters 9 and 11). Mobilization of long-chain fatty acids into the mitochondria for β-oxidation cannot occur without this shuttling system, resulting in an increase of free fatty acids (FFA) and the development of hepatic steatosis. Supplementing TPN with carnitine can decrease fat deposition in animal experiments. However, human studies with carnitine supplements have failed to confirm this finding and show no substantial benefit [14,15,32,33].

Choline participates in the production of lipoproteins (especially VLDL), which are required for the export of fatty acids from the liver. This export mechanism is compromised in the absence of choline, further contributing to TPN-induced steatosis. A number of studies have shown that addition of choline to TPN can reduce the incidence of hepatic steatosis [14,15,34,35].

In addition to specific supplementation, cyclic TPN infusion (stopping delivery for 8 h/day) simulates natural nutrition and aids in reducing hepatic steatosis [14,22].

In summary, several factors are likely to contribute to TPN-induced steatosis. TPN reformulation and adjusting the delivery schedule appear to help in some instances. However, prompt return to a normal nutritional state is the most advisable strategy.

Malnutrition

Severe malnutrition can be caused by a number of environmental, social and medical circumstances including famine, poverty, poor dietary habits, obesity, surgery and coeliac disease [14,15,36]. Under normal circumstances, increased FFA levels induce the production of insulin [14,37,38], which inhibits hormone-sensitive lipase and prevents the mobilization of fatty acids from adipose tissue (see Chapter 4). The mechanisms of malnutrition becomes more complicated under circumstances of extreme starvation and depletion of carbohydrate stores (e.g. kwashiorkor and marasmus) [14,39].

Kwashiorkor results from severe protein malnutrition and excessive carbohydrate nutrition. The presenting biochemical features are elevated circulating FFA levels accompanied by hepatic steatosis [14]. Although glucose intolerance and impaired insulin secretion are evident, unlike obesity-related IR, the levels of circulating insulin tend to be low in kwashiorkor. The defect is believed to involve post-receptor binding [14,40–42]; this may be an adaptation that prevents hypoglycaemia [43]. Additionally, studies of high-carbohydrate and fat-free diets report gene induction associated with lipogenesis, increased fatty acid synthetase transcription and an increase in hepatic triglycerides [44,45]. Carnitine deficiency can also result from the high circulating levels of triglycerides in kwashiorkor, and this results in a reduction in carnitine-mediated long-chain fatty acids and mobilization across the outer mitochondrial membrane for the process of β-oxidation (discussed in more detail in Chapter 11). The body attempts to compensate for hepatic FFA accumulation by producing VLDL to package and export the excess triglycerides. However, when this adaptive mechanism is overwhelmed, increases in the circulating level of serum triglycerides can occur. The increases in plasma triglycerides and FFA, as well as hyperinsulinaemia, can further promote fat deposition in the liver and contribute to the subsequent development of hepatic steatosis [14,15].

Despite the apparent link between kwashiorkor and fatty liver, the link between marasmus and steatosis seems to be more complex. In marasmus, or total nutritional deprivation, all groups of nutrients are absent, so that fat deposition should not occur [14]. However, a study of 55 children documented radiological evidence of apparent hepatic steatosis by ultrasonography. Subjects were divided into four groups:

1 Marasmus
2 Marasmic kwashiorkor
3 Kwashiorkor
4 Undernutrition.

All groups exhibited ultrasonographical evidence of steatosis (see Chapter 13) [39].

Although they have not been extensively studied, the histological patterns of steatosis in kwashiorkor and marasmus may differ. In kwashiorkor, there is macrovesicular steatosis, usually involving acinar zones 1 and 2. Initially, small fat droplets are deposited in the periportal hepatocytes; these droplets then merge to form macrovesicles. Kwashiorkor-induced steatosis does not generally progress, but Mallory bodies have occasionally been identified. On the other hand, steatosis in marasmus is uncommon and tends to be mild and focal with no particular acinar distribution [17].

Causes of malnutrition and NAFLD related to obesity surgery and coeliac disease are covered elsewhere in this book (see Chapter 20).

In summary, hepatic steatosis can occur in response to a number of medical and environmental conditions such as generalized malnutrition, kwashiorkor, marasmus, 'fad' diets, anorexia, cachexia (e.g. bulimia and systemic malignancy) and massive weight loss associated with obesity surgery [38]. Despite these reports, a systematic assessment of histological findings in such patients is currently lacking.

Acquired lipodystrophies

Lipodystrophies are characterized by selective loss of adipose tissue from distinct regions of the body and severe alterations in lipid and carbohydrate metabolism [46]. Lipodystrophies are classified as familial (inherited) or acquired. These conditions are usually associated with the IRS (or metabolic syndrome, syndrome X) and, as such, present a risk for the development of NAFLD [47,48]. In fact, NASH has commonly been reported in patients with lipodystrophy [49]. The degree of fat loss in lipodystrophy appears to predicate the severity of hepatic steatosis and development of NASH [49].

Acquired generalized lipodystrophy (AGL), or Lawrence syndrome, develops in late childhood or early adolescence. Patients present with generalized absence of fat, IR or overt diabetes mellitus, absence of ketosis, elevated metabolic rate, hyperlipidaemia with low high-density lipoprotein (HDL), and hepatomegaly [50]. The disease may appear after an acute infection such as measles, diphtheria, osteomyelitis or pneumonia [46,48]. A recently published report by Misra and Garg [50] on 16 AGL patients described hepatomegaly and serum ALT elevation resulting from hepatic steatosis or NASH. Hepatic fibrosis, steatosis and complications of cirrhosis (portal hypertension, hepatocellular carcinoma) have also been reported. Metabolic complications of AGL require management with high doses of insulin and thiazolidinediones.

Genetic disorders: familial lipodystrophies

Familial lipodystrophies include a number of genetic conditions presenting as generalized or partial lipodystropies, as summarized below. These conditions are also associated with IR and may be associated with NAFLD.

Congenital generalized lipodystrophy or Beradinelli–Seip syndrome

Congenital generalized lipodystrophy (CGL), also known as the Beradinelli–Seip syndrome, is an autosomal recessive disorder that presents with near complete absence of body fat, extreme IR and muscularity from birth. In this condition, metabolically active adipose tissue is absent but mechanical adipose tissue is well preserved. CGL may result from a failure of pre-adipocytes to differentiate or the failure of differentiated adipocytes to correctly synthesize or store triglycerides [46]. The condition is associated with the 1-acylglycerol-3-phosphate O-acyltransferase (*AGPAT2*) gene located on chromosome 9q34, which encodes for a key enzyme in the biosynthetic pathway of triacylglycerol and glycerophospholipids from glycerol-3-phospate [49].

Common presentations of CGL include hypertriglyceridaemia and premature diabetes. The disorder is associated with low serum HDL cholesterol concentrations, acanthosis nigricans and acromegaloid appearance. As expected by its strong association with IR, progressive fatty liver leading to cirrhosis has also been reported [46,48].

Familial partial lipodystrophy

The Dunnigan variety of familial partial lipodystrophy (FPLD) usually occurs in female patients [47]. This is a monogenic autosomal dominant disease with a missense mutation in lamins A and C (*LMNA*) gene [51]. This gene is situated on chromosome 1q21-22 and encodes nuclear lamin proteins A and C. This protein interacts with sterol regulatory element-binding proteins (SREBP) 1 and 2 (see Chapter 4 for further discussion of this insulin receptor regulated pathway). Mutations in

253

LMNA gene may negatively impact pre-adipocyte proliferation and differentiation of adipocytes [47]. The disease presents at puberty with a loss of subcutaneous fat from limbs and trunk, with the accumulation of fat in the neck, face and shoulders. Other features include acanthosis nigricans, menstrual abnormalities and hirsuitism. Patients with FPLD also present with glucose intolerance, diabetes and hepatic steatosis [51]. Management of FPLD is again focused on treatment of IRS with diet and medication [52].

Köbberling syndrome

Köbberling syndrome is a partial lipodystrophy that is characterized by a loss of fat from limbs, with excess subcutaneous truncal fat and normal facial distribution. This is a rare syndrome that usually affects female patients. Herbst *et al.* [53] reported a series of 13 patients who demonstrated clinical evidence of metabolic syndrome, including central obesity, diabetes and hypertriglyceridaemia. One patient also had acanthosis nigricans and others presented with evidence of IR. Although not extensively studied, given its strong association with IR, prevalence of NAFLD in these patients is expected to be high. Systematic liver biopsy studies are required.

Mandibuloacral dysplasia

Mandibuloacral dysplasia (MAD) is an autosomal recessive disorder with regional distribution of fat loss similar to Köbberling syndrome. In this condition, patients also present with mandibular and clavicular hypoplasia, dental abnormalities, acro-osteolysis, stiff joints and loss of fat from the limbs. Missense mutations in the *LMNA* gene have been reported in nine patients [54]. These patients also demonstrated IR, which responded to rosiglitazone therapy. Although extensive evaluation of liver disease is not available, like other lipodystrophies, hepatic steatosis and NAFLD are probably common in this disorder. Future investigation of NAFLD in patients with MAD will be important.

Other metabolic disorders associated with steatosis

A number of other metabolic disorders have also been associated with insulin resistance and hepatic steatosis (Table 21.1). These include the polycystic ovarian syndrome (PCOS), inborn errors of metabolism such as a-β-lipoproteinaemia and Weber–Christian syndrome, and possibly coeliac disease.

Polycystic ovarian syndrome

PCOS is a common endocrinopathy affecting approximately 6–10% of white women [55], including 4–7% during their reproductive years [56,57]. Patients present with reproductive, endocrine and metabolic abnormalities, including hyperandrogenism, chronic anovulation, oligomenorrhoea, hirsutism and infertility [58]. Metabolic disorders in these patients include IR, obesity and dyslipidaemia. More recently, the requirements for clinical definition of PCOS have been debated, as half of the patients lack one or more of these clinical manifestations [59,60].

The metabolic abnormality of patients with PCOS is primarily related to IR. An association between hyperandrogenism and disordered carbohydrate metabolism was reported as early as 1921 by Achard and Thiers [61]. In 1980, Burghen *et al.* [62] documented both basal and glucose-induced hyperinsulinaemia in women with PCOS. Post-menopausal women with PCOS have a high incidence of diabetes mellitus, with rates exceeding 20–40% among obese patients. Although the severity of IR may vary in women with chronic anovulation [56], both obese and lean women with PCOS have evidence of IR.

In general, hyperinsulinaemia can result from increased insulin synthesis, reduced hepatic insulin clearance, or both. IR results from negative regulation of glucose transport and antilipolysis in adipocytes, leading to hyperinsulinaemia [63]. The resultant elevated serum insulin levels can affect the regulation of hepatic and peripheral lipid metabolism.

Although IR in lean women with PCOS appears to be intrinsic, IR in obese PCOS patients is further compounded by adiposity [64]. A number of mechanisms for IR have been described in PCOS. Most women with PCOS develop IR as a consequence of increased phosphorylation of insulin receptor serine residues, with correspondingly diminished autophosphorylation of tyrosine residues; this is the same mechanism that governs IR in obesity and type 2 diabetes (see Chapter 4). Serine phosphorylation may also be involved in increasing androgen synthesis. Thus, a mutation in the insulin receptor may also affect androgen metabolism.

As for other patients with IR (see Chapter 4), patients with PCOS may eventually develop pancreatic islet β-cell dysfunction, leading to or exacerbating glucose intolerance and diabetes mellitus.

It is important to recognize that in PCOS, hyperinsulinaemia and IR may be linked to obesity; 40–50% of women affected by PCOS are also obese [56]. Obesity is associated with IR and hyperlipidaemia, thereby contributing to worsening IR and increased risk of cardiovascular disease in patients with PCOS (see Chapters 4 and 5).

In addition to diabetes, lipid abnormalities observed in women with PCOS include hypertriglyceridaemia, and hypercholesterolaemia with high low-density lipoprotein (LDL) and low HDL (mostly HDL-2) [65]. These changes are usually attributable to IR rather than elevated serum androgens. Women with PCOS also have evidence of impaired fibronolytic activity with increased circulating levels of plasminogen activator inhibitor I (PA-I). Such elevated PA-I levels have been associated with IR and with an increased risk of cardiovascular disease. Despite the high prevalence of obesity, leptin levels in PCOS patients do not appear to be significantly different from control women [66].

The strong familial linkage association of hyperandrogenism and IR in PCOS patients suggests a polygenic disorder, which may involve genes regulating steroid hormone synthesis and glucose metabolism. IR in women with PCOS can be attributed to serine phosphorylation in insulin receptors, which may in turn regulate P450c17 (an enzyme involved in androgen biosynthesis). Studies using theca interna cells on mutations of *CYP17* (encodes P450c17) gene are inconclusive [67]. A comprehensive understanding of the regulation of androgen biosynthesis and glucose homoeostasis in patients with PCOS is still lacking.

IR and obesity have an important role in the pathogenesis of both NAFLD and PCOS, suggesting an association between NAFLD and PCOS. However, the published literature currently offers little regarding the frequency and nature of liver diseases, including NAFLD, in patients with PCOS. At present there appear to be no systematic evaluations of the prevalence, incidence and natural history of NAFLD in patients with this disorder.

Finally, four main targets for treatment of PCOS include the management of obesity, hyperandrogenism, infertility and cardiovascular disease [58]. Weight loss and the maintenance of an ideal weight represent the primary approach to PCOS-associated hyperinsulinaemia. Insulin levels may also be regulated pharmacologically. Metformin and troglitzone (a now discontinued thiazolidinedione; see Chapter 16 for discussion of currently used analogous agents) [55] both alleviate IR. Any therapeutic modality that could adversely affect IR, such as oral contraceptive steroids and glucocorticoids, need to be avoided.

In summary, PCOS has been linked to the IRS through the presence of hyperinsulinaemia, glucose intolerance and dyslipidaemia. Together, the high prevalence of NAFLD and the potential for NASH progression in patients with the IRS (see Chapter 5) suggest that an association between progressive forms of NAFLD/NASH and PCOS is likely; clarifying this issue should become a priority for future research.

Wilson's disease

Wilson's disease is an autosomal recessive disorder affecting 1 in 30 000 individuals [68]. It results from a number of mutations in the copper-transporting ATPase (ATP7B) located at the hepatocyte canalicular membrane. Hepatic involvement in Wilson's disease ranges from hepatic steatosis, chronic hepatitis and cirrhosis, to fulminant hepatic failure (Wilsonian crisis). Primary hepatic lesions in Wilson's disease include steatosis in hepatocytes, followed by nuclear glycogen deposits and major mitochondrial aberrations, contributing to oxidative damage [22]. Because Wilson's disease may be associated with steatosis, it may be mistaken for NAFLD in the absence of appropriate diagnostic tests for Wilson's disease (e.g. copper studies, serum ceruloplasmin, Kayser–Fleischer rings by slit lamp examination of cornea) [69–71]. Wilson's disease is not a primary cause of fatty liver disease, it only masquerades as NAFLD. Treatment for Wilson's disease is not directed against hepatic steatosis, it involves copper chelation, or liver transplantation for the end-stage liver disease.

A-β-lipoproteinaemia

Apolipoprotein B1 is a transport protein that forms VLDL complexes with triglycerides, cholesterol and phospholipids. This complex is the mechanism by which lipids are transported from the liver to the peripheral tissues. A-β-lipoproteinaemia (ABL) may result from advancing liver disease or from a rare autosomal recessive disorder of lipoprotein metabolism in which a lack of apolipoprotein B1 impairs VLDL secretion into plasma [72–74]. The absence of apolipoprotein B1 secretion by hepatocytes effects lipid transport in other tissues, causing neurological disturbances, retinitis pigmentosa, abnormal erythrocyte morphology and malnutrition; the latter leads to weight loss and other symptoms resembling coeliac disease [75].

Hepatic apolipoprotein B1 synthesis is partly regulated by insulin, which provides a link between ABL and the IRS [76]. Furthermore, microsomal triglyceride transport protein (MTP), another protein present in the endoplasmic reticulum of liver and intestine, is responsible for intracellular transport of apolipoproteins. MTP has also been implicated in the manifestation of ABL [77] and is frequently absent in patients with ABL. This defect results in poor VLDL assembly, low or absent plasma VLDL and chylomicrons, and lipid droplet deposition in the intestinal mucosa and the hepatic parenchyma with resultant hepatic steatosis [72,73,75].

The diagnosis of ABL is suggested by plasma lipid profiles demonstrating a reduction in total triglycerides, cholesterol and VLDL, but the primary diagnostic features are serum cholesterol levels less than 0.5–1.3 mmol/L accompanied by neuropathy, retinopathy, or both [78]. In the presence of these changes, ABL can lead to malabsorption of fat-soluble vitamins and consequent reductions in vitamin A, D, E and K, which contributes to the pathophysiology of the disease. For example, vitamin E deficiency contributes to hepatic, neurological and retinal manifestation of ABL because of reduced protection against oxidative damage.

Patients with ABL can present with hepatic steatosis. In such instances, steatosis is the result of impaired lipoprotein assembly, which prevents the secretion of excess lipid through the normal intracellular network, thereby leading to accumulation of fat in the cytoplasm of hepatocytes [75,76,79]. The association of ABL with abnormal lipid metabolism and the IRS indicates a high risk for developing NAFLD/NASH. However, while case reports confirm a possible association between ABL and NAFLD [75,76,78], strong evidence for this relationship is currently lacking.

Symptoms associated with a-β-proteinaemia can be alleviated by dietary control of fat intake, particularly saturated fats, and supplementation with vitamins A, K and E. Vitamins K and E can easily be replaced through oral consumption as their absorption and trans-port to the liver are independent of lipoproteins [78]. Neurological symptoms can also be ameliorated by vitamin E administration [78]. Although deficiency of vitamin D is possible, its absorption is independent of lipoprotein, and vitamin D deficiency is not a major contributor to ABL symptoms [75,78].

Coeliac disease

Coeliac disease is an autoimmune disorder in which villus atrophy of the intestinal mucosa is caused by exposure to dietary gluten. Classic symptoms result from malabsorption, leading to weight loss, diarrhoea, steatorrhoea and malnutrition. Silent (subclinical) forms of coeliac disease may present later in life as asymptomatic mild elevations of ALT and iron-deficiency anaemia [80–82]. Several cases of liver dysfunction in association with coeliac disease have been reported over the past decade [80,83–86]. A mild form of hepatic dysfunction that manifests as elevated ALT, may respond to a gluten-free diet [87]. Silent coeliac disease may also lead to vitamin deficiencies and malabsorptions of the nutrients, leading to the development of hepatic steatosis [11,88,89].

Several studies report patients with coeliac disease and elevated ALT in which a spectrum of histological findings was found, ranging from mild to moderate chronic hepatitis, steatosis, septal fibrosis and cirrhosis [85,86,90–93]. In one study of 30 patients with NASH, four patients (13%) were diagnosed with coeliac disease and responded to a gluten-free diet [80]. Unlike patients with IR, patients with steatosis and coeliac disease are often underweight (BMI < 22 kg/m²). Despite these case reports, the association between NAFLD and coeliac disease remains controversial [31,94,95].

Drug-induced steatosis

Drug-induced steatosis is rare; it appeared to be implicated in less than 2% of the reported cases of steatosis diagnosed in liver clinics [97]. The link between pharmacological agents and steatosis can be difficult to establish, but is strongly suggested by a reduction in symptoms and liver test abnormalities when a drug is discontinued, and the return of steatosis when therapy is reinstated. A large number of drugs have been associated with hepatic steatosis [97–100]. A few of the more important agents are discussed in more detail below.

Synthetic oestrogens and oestrogen receptor agonists and antagonists

Tamoxifen is one of the most commonly used non-steroidal anti-oestrogen anticancer agents. Serious side-effects are few, but tamoxifen may induce diffuse hepatic fatty infiltration [101]. A recent report indicated that more than 30% of breast cancer patients who were receiving tamoxifen had hepatic steatosis [102]. This number was reduced to 7.7% by replacing tamoxifen with its analogue, toremifene [103].

The mechanism of tamoxifen-induced hepatic steatosis is not clear. However, there is evidence from animal studies that both tamoxifen and its 4-hydroxy metabolite can cause mitochondrial uncoupling with resultant inhibition of electron transport [104]. In this situation, steatosis can be reduced by discontinuing therapy or combining this drug with peroxisome proliferator-activated receptor-α (PPARα) agonist (see Chapter 16) [38,105,106].

Nucleotide and nucleoside analogues

Several nucleoside and nucleotide inhibitors are currently used to treat human immunodeficiency virus (HIV) and other viral diseases. These drugs clearly lead to macro- and microvesicular steatosis [100]. Nucleotide analogues such as zidovudine, didanosine and stavudine are used to manage patients with HIV infection, usually in combination with other drugs in highly active anti-retroviral therapy (HAART). The mechanism of hepatic steatosis related to these drugs is probably multifaceted. These drugs block HIV reverse transcriptase by being incorporated into growing chains of DNA, thereby terminating DNA replication. As such, they can also block mitochondrial DNA (mtDNA) replication (mitochondrial DNA polymerase γ) [97] and cause mtDNA depletion. Mitochondrial damage can lead to severe steatosis in these patients. Long-term use of these drugs in HAART has been associated with hepatic steatosis, myopathy and, in some instances, lactic acidosis [107,108]. Additionally, these drugs increase hepatic triglyceride synthesis inducing hepatic steatosis and hypertriglyceridaemia. Terminating nucleoside analogue therapy reduces steatosis and returns liver enzymes to normal [107].

HIV patients on HAART also demonstrate lipodystrophy (LD) syndrome. Nearly half of the HIV patients on HAART regimens develop LD within 12–18 months [109], with loss of subcutaneous fat in the face and periphery [110]. Furthermore, such LD is associated with secondary and other metabolic abnormalities [111]. LD in patients on HAART is believed to be induced by adipocyte-specific mtDNA depletion [110,112]. Although a direct link between HAART and NAFLD is difficult to establish, the association of IR and LD in patients receiving HAART, as well as direct mitochondrial toxicity of those drugs, suggests a strong possibility of high prevalence of NAFLD in these patients [97].

Amiodarone

Amiodarone is a cardiac anti-arrhythmic agent used to treat resistant tachyarrhythmias. Amiodarone accumulates in the liver of approximately 25% of patients, potentially causing mild to moderate elevation of serum ALT and chronic liver disease [97]. Clinical presentations of amiodarone hepatotoxicity range from severe cholestasis and hepatitis to acute liver failure [97,100]. Long-term usage of this drug may result in fibrosis and cirrhosis, also leading to liver failure. Histological findings of amiodarone hepatotoxity include phospholipidosis, steatosis, focal necrosis with Mallory's hyaline, infiltration with polymorphonuclear neutrophils, pericellular fibrosis and cirrhosis [97]. The presence of lysosomal myeloid bodies in the hepatocytes of patients with amiodarone-induced steatohepatitis distinguishes this condition from 'idiopathic' NASH.

The pathophysiology of amiodarone-induced liver disease is probably related to the protonated form of this drug. Amiodarone protonation occurs readily, and is believed to be driven across the inner mitochondrial membrane where it accumulates. This protonated form of amiodarone seems to inhibit β-oxidation of carnitine palmitoyltransferase 1 and acyl-coenzyme A dehydrogenase, affecting mitochondrial respiration and contributing to hepatic steatosis. Hepatotoxic effects of amiodarone can be reversed by dosage reduction or removal. However, because of the long half-lives of both the drug and its main metabolite (desethylamiodarone), reversal may take months, with ongoing hepatic injury and worsening liver failure despite discontinuation [113].

Perhexiline maleate

Perhexiline maleate, previously used to treat angina pectoris, was associated with severe hepatic steatosis and severe complications such as portal hypertension leading to death in over 50% of cases. This form of drug-induced steatohepatitis could present with characteristic Mallory bodies and pericellular fibrosis. It has been suggested that a polymorphism in *CYP2D6* may decrease the rate of perhexiline clearance, ultimately leading to a longer exposure time and drug accumulation, causing mitochondrial damage and inhibition of β-oxidation [38,97,114]. This drug is currently not available for clinical use.

Glucocorticoids

Although corticosteroids can be associated with fatty liver, the development of chronic liver disease related to glucocorticoids is rare, and its mechanism is not entirely clear. The reported cases of chronic liver disease related to glucocorticoids have been problematic because of a number of potential confounders that were not systematically excluded [115,116]. Most importantly, glucocorticoids cause central obesity, IR and type 2 diabetes, conditions that are strongly associated with NAFLD/NASH. This issue may be especially important in patients receiving long-term corticosteroids, such as those with autoimmune hepatitis and after liver transplantation.

Conclusions

Over the past decade, the spectrum of NAFLD/NASH has received increasing attention as one of the most common causes of chronic liver disease in the world. IR related to the metabolic syndrome is strongly implicated in these disorders. In addition to obesity and type 2 diabetes, a number of other conditions and drugs have been associated with the development of hepatic steatosis and steatohepatitis. Several pathways may be involved in the pathogenesis of these conditions, some in common with primarily metabolic forms of NAFLD/NASH, and others invoking specific metabolic defects or toxicity. Hence, it is not surprising that the natural history of these conditions may differ from the course of typical NAFLD and NASH. Common disorders related to IR, particularly the PCOS and HAART, require further study to elucidate the prevalence, pathogenic mechanisms and clinical importance of fatty liver diseases. The molecular mechanisms underlying these and some genetic conditions that manifest as hepatic steatosis may provide clues to the pathogenesis of 'idiopathic' NAFLD, and may elucidate other molecular abnormalities that can lead to the development of NAFLD and facilitate its progression.

References

1 Younossi ZM, Diehl AM, Ong JP. Non-alcoholic fatty liver disease: an agenda for clinical research. *Hepatology* 2002; **35**: 746–52.

2 Mulhall BP, Ong JP, Younossi ZM. Non-alcoholic fatty liver disease: an overview. *J Gastroenterol Hepatol* 2002; **17**: 1136–43.

3 Matteoni CA, Younossi ZM, Gramlich T *et al.* Non-alcoholic fatty liver disease: a spectrum of clinical and pathological severity. *Gastroenterology* 1999; **116**: 1413–9.

4 Lee RG. Non-alcoholic steatohepatitis: a study of 49 patients. *Hum Pathol* 1989; **20**: 594–8.

5 Powell EE, Cooksley WG, Hanson R *et al.* The natural history of non-alcoholic steatohepatitis: a follow-up study of forty-two patients for up to 21 years. *Hepatology* 1990; **11**: 74–80.

6 Bacon BR, Farahvash MJ, Janney CG, Neuschwander-Tetri BA. Non-alcoholic steatohepatitis: an expanded clinical entity. *Gastroenterology* 1994; **107**: 1103–9.

7 Ratziu V, Bonyhay L, Di Martino V *et al.* Survival, liver failure, and hepatocellular carcinoma in obesity-related cryptogenic cirrhosis. *Hepatology* 2002; **35**: 1485–93.

8 Harrison SA, Kadakia S, Lang KA, Schenker S. Non-alcoholic steatohepatitis: what we know in the new millennium. *Am J Gastroenterol* 2002; **97**: 2714–24.

9 Le Roith D, Zick Y. Recent advances in our understanding of insulin action and insulin resistance. *Diabetes Care* 2001; **24**: 588–97.

10 Muller MJ. [Hepatic complications in parenteral nutrition]. *Z Gastroenterol* 1996; **34**: 36–40.

11 Nehra V, Angulo P, Buchman AL, Lindor KD. Nutritional and metabolic considerations in the etiology of non-alcoholic steatohepatitis. *Dig Dis Sci* 2001; **46**: 2347–52.

12 Saadeh S, Younossi ZM. The spectrum of non-alcoholic fatty liver disease: from steatosis to non-alcoholic steatohepatitis. *Cleve Clin J Med* 2000; **67**: 96–7, 101–4.

13 Fisher RL. Hepatobiliary abnormalities associated with total parenteral nutrition. *Gastroenterol Clin North Am* 1989; **18**: 645–66.

14 Fong DG, Nehra V, Lindor KD, Buchman AL. Metabolic and nutritional considerations in non-alcoholic fatty liver. *Hepatology* 2000; **32**: 3–10.

15 Allard JP. Other disease associations with non-alcoholic fatty liver disease (NAFLD). *Best Pract Res Clin Gastroenterol* 2002; **16**: 783–95.

16 Macsween R, Burt A. Liver pathology associated with diseases of other organs. In: Macsween R, Anthony P, Scheuer P, Burt A, BC P, eds. *Pathology of Liver disease*, 3rd edn. Churchill Livingstone, 1997: 713–64.

17 Cavicchi M, Beau P, Crenn P, Degott C, Messing B. Prevalence of liver disease and contributing factors in patients receiving home parenteral nutrition for permanent intestinal failure. *Ann Intern Med* 2000; **132**: 525–32.

18 Hall RI, Grant JP, Ross LH *et al*. Pathogenesis of hepatic steatosis in the parenterally fed rat. *J Clin Invest* 1984; **74**: 1658–68.

19 Nussbaum MS, Fischer JE. Pathogenesis of hepatic steatosis during total parenteral nutrition. *Surg Annu* 1991; **23** (Part 2): 1–11.

20 Shaw AA, Hall SD, Franklin MR, Galinsky RE. The influence of L-glutamine on the depression of hepatic cytochrome P450 activity in male rats caused by total parenteral nutrition. *Drug Metab Dispos* 2002; **30**: 177–82.

21 Denno R, Rounds JD, Faris R, Holejko LB, Wilmore DW. Glutamine-enriched total parenteral nutrition enhances plasma glutathione in the resting state. *J Surg Res* 1996; **61**: 35–8.

22 Sandhu IS, Jarvis C, Everson GT. Total parenteral nutrition and cholestasis. *Clin Liver Dis* 1999; **3**: 489–508, viii.

23 Nussbaum MS, Li S, Bower RH *et al*. Addition of lipid to total parenteral nutrition prevents hepatic steatosis in rats by lowering the portal venous insulin/glucagon ratio. *J Parenter Enteral Nutr* 1992; **16**: 106–9.

24 Li S, Nussbaum MS, Teague D *et al*. Increasing dextrose concentrations in total parenteral nutrition (TPN) causes alterations in hepatic morphology and plasma levels of insulin and glucagon in rats. *J Surg Res* 1988; **44**: 639–48.

25 Li SJ, Nussbaum MS, McFadden DW *et al*. Addition of glucagon to total parenteral nutrition (TPN) prevents hepatic steatosis in rats. *Surgery* 1988; **104**: 350–7.

26 Li SJ, Nussbaum MS, McFadden DW, Dayal R, Fischer JE. Reversal of hepatic steatosis in rats by addition of glucagon to total parenteral nutrition (TPN). *J Surg Res* 1989; **46**: 557–66.

27 Li SJ, Nussbaum MS, McFadden DW *et al*. Addition of L-glutamine to total parenteral nutrition and its effects on portal insulin and glucagon and the development of hepatic steatosis in rats. *J Surg Res* 1990; **48**: 421–6.

28 Yeh SL, Chen WJ, Huang PC. Effects of L-glutamine on induced hepatosteatosis in rats receiving total parenteral nutrition. *J Formos Med Assoc* 1995; **94**: 593–9.

29 Sokol RJ, Taylor SF, Devereaux MW *et al*. Hepatic oxidant injury and glutathione depletion during total parenteral nutrition in weanling rats. *Am J Physiol* 1996; **270**: G691–700.

30 Dzakovic A, Kaviani A, Eshach-Adiv O *et al*. Trophic enteral nutrition increases hepatic glutathione and protects against peroxidative damage after exposure to endotoxin. *J Pediatr Surg* 2003; **38**: 844–7.

31 Liang LJ, Yin XY, Luo SM *et al*. A study of the ameliorating effects of carnitine on hepatic steatosis induced by total parenteral nutrition in rats. *World J Gastroenterol* 1999; **5**: 312–5.

32 Bowyer BA, Miles JM, Haymond MW, Fleming CR. L-carnitine therapy in home parenteral nutrition patients with abnormal liver tests and low plasma carnitine concentrations. *Gastroenterology* 1988; **94**: 434–8.

33 Buchman AL, Dubin MD, Moukarzel AA *et al*. Choline deficiency: a cause of hepatic steatosis during parenteral nutrition that can be reversed with intravenous choline supplementation. *Hepatology* 1995; **22**: 1399–403.

34 Hall RI, Ross LH, Bozovic MG, Grant JP. The effect of choline supplementation on hepatic steatosis in the parenterally fed rat. *J Parenter Enteral Nutr* 1985; **9**: 597–9.

35 Gopalan S. Malnutrition: causes, consequences, and solutions. *Nutrition* 2000; **16**: 556–8.

36 Jorquera F, Culebras JM, Gonzalez-Gallego J. Influence of nutrition on liver oxidative metabolism. *Nutrition* 1996; **12**: 442–7.

37 Chitturi S, Farrell GC. Etiopathogenesis of non-alcoholic steatohepatitis. *Semin Liver Dis* 2001; **21**: 27–41.

38 Doherty JF, Adam EJ, Griffin GE, Golden MH. Ultrasonographic assessment of the extent of hepatic steatosis in severe malnutrition. *Arch Dis Child* 1992; **67**: 1348–2.

39 Agbedana EO, Johnson AO, Taylor GO. Studies on hepatic and extrahepatic lipoprotein lipases in protein-calorie malnutrition. *Am J Clin Nutr* 1979; **32**: 292–8.

40 Vajreswari A, Narayanareddy K, Rao PS. Fatty acid composition of erythrocyte membrane lipid obtained from children suffering from kwashiorkor and marasmus. *Metabolism* 1990; **39**: 779–82.

41 McLaren DS, Bitar JG, Nassar VH. Protein-calorie malnutrition and the liver. *Prog Liver Dis* 1972; **4**: 527–36.

42 Sims EA, Horton ES. Endocrine and metabolic adaptation to obesity and starvation. *Am J Clin Nutr* 1968; **21**: 1455–70.

43 Kim TS, Freake HC. High carbohydrate diet and starvation regulate lipogenic mRNA in rats in a tissue-specific manner. *J Nutr* 1996; **126**: 611–7.

44 Iritani N, Nishimoto N, Katsurada A, Fukuda H. Regulation of hepatic lipogenic enzyme gene expression by diet quantity in rats fed a fat-free, high carbohydrate diet. *J Nutr* 1992; **122**: 28–36.

45 Garg A. Lipodystrophies. *Am J Med* 2000; **108**: 143–52.

46 Bhayana S, Hegele RA. The molecular basis of genetic lipodystrophies. *Clin Biochem* 2002; **35**: 171–7.

47 Cauble MS, Gilroy R, Sorrell MF *et al.* Lipoatrophic diabetes and end-stage liver disease secondary to non-alcoholic steatohepatitis with recurrence after liver transplantation. *Transplantation* 2001; **71**: 892–5.

48 Garg A, Misra A. Hepatic steatosis, insulin resistance, and adipose tissue disorders. *J Clin Endocrinol Metab* 2002; **87**: 3019–22.

49 Misra A, Garg A. Clinical features and metabolic derangements in acquired generalized lipodystrophy: case reports and review of the literature. *Medicine (Baltimore)* 2003; **82**: 129–46.

50 Haque WA, Oral EA, Dietz K *et al.* Risk factors for diabetes in familial partial lipodystrophy, dunnigan variety. *Diabetes Care* 2003; **26**: 1350–5.

51 Caux F, Dubosclard E, Lascols O *et al.* A new clinical condition linked to a novel mutation in lamins A and C with generalized lipoatrophy, insulin-resistant diabetes, disseminated leukomelanodermic papules, liver steatosis, and cardiomyopathy. *J Clin Endocrinol Metab* 2003; **88**: 1006–13.

52 Herbst KL, Tannock LR, Deeb SS *et al.* Köbberling type of familial partial lipodystrophy: an underrecognized syndrome. *Diabetes Care* 2003; **26**: 1819–24.

53 Sbraccia P, D'Adamo M, Massimo F *et al.* Rosiglitazone treatment improves insulin sensitivity and increases production in lipodystrophic patients with mandibuloacral dysplasic. *Diabetes* 2003; **52**.

54 Norman RJ. Obesity, polycystic ovary syndrome and anovulation: how are they interrelated? *Curr Opin Obstet Gynecol* 2001; **13**: 323–7.

55 Lobo RA, Carmina E. The importance of diagnosing the polycystic ovary syndrome. *Ann Intern Med* 2000; **132**: 989–93.

56 Pirwany IR, Fleming R, Greer IA, Packard CJ, Sattar N. Lipids and lipoprotein subfractions in women with PCOS: relationship to metabolic and endocrine parameters. *Clin Endocrinol (Oxf)* 2001; **54**: 447–53.

57 Davidson MB. Clinical implications of insulin resistance syndromes. *Am J Med* 1995; **99**: 420–6.

58 Baumann E, Rosenfield R. Polycystic ovary syndrome in adolescence. *Endocrinologist* 2002; **12**: 333–48.

59 Balen A, Michelmore K. What is polycystic ovary syndrome? Are national views important? *Hum Reprod* 2002; **17**: 2219–27.

60 Achard C, Thiers J. Le virilisme pailaire et son association a l'insuffisance glycolytique (diabete des femmes a barb). *Bull Acad Natl Med* 1921; **86**: 51–64.

61 Burghen GA, Givens JR, Kitabchi AE. Correlation of hyperandrogenism with hyperinsulinism in polycystic ovarian disease. *J Clin Endocrinol Metab* 1980; **50**: 113–6.

62 Ovalle F, Azziz R. Insulin resistance, polycystic ovary syndrome, and type 2 diabetes mellitus. *Fertil Steril* 2002; **77**: 1095–105.

63 Baillargeon JP, Iuorno MJ, Nestler JE. Insulin sensitizers for polycystic ovary syndrome. *Clin Obstet Gynecol* 2003; **46**: 325–40.

64 Robinson S, Henderson AD, Gelding SV *et al.* Dyslipidaemia is associated with insulin resistance in women with polycystic ovaries. *Clin Endocrinol (Oxf)* 1996; **44**: 277–84.

65 Dunaif A. Insulin resistance and the polycystic ovary syndrome: mechanism and implications for pathogenesis. *Endocr Rev* 1997; **18**: 774–800.

66 Wickenheisser J, Strauss J, McAllister J. Steroidogenic abnormalities in ovarian theca cells in polycystic ovary syndrome. *Curr Opin Endocrinol Diabetes* 2002; **9**: 486–91.

67 Palsson R, Jonasson JG, Kristjansson M *et al.* Genotype–phenotype interactions in Wilson's disease: insight from an Icelandic mutation. *Eur J Gastroenterol Hepatol* 2001; **13**: 433–6.

68 Pfeil SA, Lynn DJ. Wilson's disease: copper unfettered. *J Clin Gastroenterol* 1999; **29**: 22–31.

69 Gu M, Cooper JM, Butler P *et al.* Oxidative-phosphorylation defects in liver of patients with Wilson's disease. *Lancet* 2000; **356**: 469–74.

70 Mansouri A, Gaou I, Fromenty B *et al.* Premature oxidative aging of hepatic mitochondrial DNA in Wilson's disease. *Gastroenterology* 1997; **113**: 599–605

71 Shah SS, Desai HG. Fatty liver and elevated transaminases with heterozygous apolipoprotein B deficiency. *J Assoc Physicians India* 2001; **49**: 284–5.

72 Tarugi P, Lonardo A, Ballarini G *et al.* A study of fatty liver disease and plasma lipoproteins in a kindred with familial hypobetalipoproteinemia due to a novel truncated form of apolipoprotein B (APO B-54.5). *J Hepatol* 2000; **33**: 361–70.

73 Black DD, Hay RV, Rohwer-Nutter PL *et al.* Intestinal and hepatic apolipoprotein B gene expression in abetalipoproteinemia. *Gastroenterology* 1991; **101**: 520–8.

74 Triantafillidis JK, Kottaras G, Sgourous S *et al.* A-β-lipoproteinemia: clinical and laboratory features, therapeutic manipulations, and follow-up study of three members of a Greek family. *J Clin Gastroenterol* 1998; **26**: 207–11.

75 Charlton M, Sreekumar R, Rasmussen D, Lindor K, Nair KS. Apolipoprotein synthesis in non-alcoholic steatohepatitis. *Hepatology* 2002; **35**: 898–904.

76 Lin MC, Gordon D, Wetterau JR. Microsomal triglyceride transfer protein (MTP) regulation in HepG2 cells: insulin negatively regulates *MTP* gene expression. *J Lipid Res* 1995; **36**: 1073–81.

77 Rader DJ, Brewer HB Jr. Abetalipoproteinemia: new insights into lipoprotein assembly and vitamin E metabolism from a rare genetic disease. *J Am Med Assoc* 1993; **270**: 865–9.

78 Avigan MI, Ishak KG, Gregg RE, Hoofnagle JH. Morphologic features of the liver in abetalipoproteinemia. *Hepatology* 1984; **4**: 1223–6.

79 Grieco A, Miele L, Pignatoro G *et al.* Is coeliac disease a confounding factor in the diagnosis of NASH? *Gut* 2001; **49**: 596.

80 Bottaro G, Cataldo F, Rotolo N, Spina M, Corazza GR. The clinical pattern of subclinical/silent celiac disease: an analysis on 1026 consecutive cases. *Am J Gastroenterol* 1999; **94**: 691–6.

81 Riestra S, Dominguez F, Rodrigo L. Nodular regenerative hyperplasia of the liver in a patient with celiac disease. *J Clin Gastroenterol* 2001; **33**: 323–6.

82 Franzese A, Iannucci MP, Valerio G *et al.* Atypical celiac disease presenting as obesity-related liver dysfunction. *J Pediatr Gastroenterol Nutr* 2001; **33**: 329–32.

83 Shamir R, Koren I, Rosenbach Y *et al.* Celiac, fatty liver, and pancreatic insufficiency. *J Pediatr Gastroenterol Nutr* 2001; **32**: 490–2.

84 Capron JP, Sevenet F, Quenum C *et al.* [Massive hepatic steatosis disclosing adult coeliac disease: study of a case and review of the literature]. *Gastroenterol Clin Biol* 1983; **7**: 256–60.

85 Christl SU, Muller JG. [Fatty liver in adult coeliac disease]. *Dtsch Med Wochenschr* 1999; **124**: 691–4.

86 Davison S. Coeliac disease and liver dysfunction. *Arch Dis Child* 2002; **87**: 293–6.

87 Gonzalez-Abraldes J, Sanchez-Fueyo A, Bessa X *et al.* Persistent hypertransaminasemia as the presenting feature of celiac disease. *Am J Gastroenterol* 1999; **94**: 1095–7.

88 Angulo P. Non-alcoholic fatty liver disease. *N Engl J Med* 2002; **346**: 1221–31.

89 Novacek G, Miehsler W, Wrba F *et al.* Prevalence and clinical importance of hypertransaminasaemia in coeliac disease. *Eur J Gastroenterol Hepatol* 1999; **11**: 283–8.

90 Morillas MJ, Gaspar E, Moles JR *et al.* [Adult coeliac disease and hepatopathy]. *Rev Esp Enferm Dig* 1991; **79**: 197–200.

91 Mitchison HC, Record CO, Bateson MC, Cobden I. Hepatic abnormalities in coeliac disease: three cases of delayed diagnosis. *Postgrad Med J* 1989; **65**: 920–2.

92 Naschitz JE, Yeshurun D, Zuckerman E, Arad E, Boss JH. Massive hepatic steatosis complicating adult celiac disease: report of a case and review of the literature. *Am J Gastroenterol* 1987; **82**: 1186–9.

93 Angulo P, Lindor KD. Non-alcoholic fatty liver disease. *J Gastroenterol Hepatol* 2002; **17** (Suppl.): S186–90.

94 Marignani M, Angeletti S. Non-alcoholic fatty liver disease. *N Engl J Med* 2002; **347**: 768–9; author reply 768–9.

95 Robertson G, Leclercq I, Farrell GC. Non-alcoholic steatosis and steatohepatitis. II. Cytochrome P450 enzymes and oxidative stress. *Am J Physiol Gastrointest Liver Physiol* 2001; **281**: G1135–9.

96 Farrell GC. Drugs and steatohepatitis. *Semin Liver Dis* 2002; **22**: 185–94.

97 Novak D, Lewis J. Drug-induced liver disease. *Curr Opin Gastroenterol* 2003; **19**: 203–15.

98 Lewis J. Drug-induced liver disease. *Curr Opin Gastroenterol* 2002; **18**: 307–13.

99 Stravitz RT, Sanyal AJ. Drug-induced steatohepatitis. *Clin Liver Dis* 2003; **7**: 435–51.

100 Cai Q, Bensen M, Greene R, Kirchner J. Tamoxifen-induced transient multifocal hepatic fatty infiltration. *Am J Gastroenterol* 2000; **95**: 277–9.

101 Coskun U, Toruner FB, Gunel N. Tamoxifen therapy and hepatic steatosis. *Neoplasma* 2002; **49**: 61–4.

102 Hamada N, Ogawa Y, Saibara T *et al.* Toremifene-induced fatty liver and NASH in breast cancer patients with breast-conservation treatment. *Int J Oncol* 2000; **17**: 1119–23.

103 Tuquet C, Dupont J, Mesneau A, Roussaux J. Effects of tamoxifen on the electron transport chain of isolated rat liver mitochondria. *Cell Biol Toxicol* 2000; **16**: 207–19.

104 Steindl P, Ferenci P, Dienes HP *et al.* Wilson's disease in patients presenting with liver disease: a diagnostic challenge. *Gastroenterology* 1997; **113**: 212–8.

105 Saibara T, Onishi S. [Non-alcoholic steatohepatitis (NASH)]. *Nippon Shokakibyo Gakkai Zasshi* 2002; **99**: 570–6.

106 Chariot P, Drogou I, de Lacroix-Szmania I *et al.* Zidovudine-induced mitochondrial disorder with massive liver steatosis, myopathy, lactic acidosis, and mitochondrial DNA depletion. *J Hepatol* 1999; **30**: 156–60.

107 Brivet FG, Nion I, Megarbane B *et al.* Fatal lactic acidosis and liver steatosis associated with didanosine and stavudine treatment: a respiratory chain dysfunction? *J Hepatol* 2000; **32**: 364–5.

108 Yki-Jarvinen H, Sutinen J, Silveira A *et al.* Regulation of plasma PAI-1 concentrations in HAART-associated lipodystrophy during rosiglitazone therapy. *Arterioscler Thromb Vasc Biol* 2003; **23**: 688–94.

109 Nolan D, Hammond EAM, Taylor L *et al.* Mitochondrial DNA depletion and morphologic changes inadipocytes associated with nucleoside reverse transcriptase inhibitor therapy. *AIDS* 2003; **17**: 1329–38.

110 Vigouroux C, Maachi M, Nguyen TH *et al.* Serum adipocytokines are related to lipodystrophy and metabolic

disorders in HIV-infected men under antiretroviral therapy. *AIDS* 2003; **17**: 1503–11.

111 Brinkman K, Smeitink JA, Romijn JA, Reiss P. Mitochondrial toxicity induced by nucleoside-analogue reverse-transcriptase inhibitors is a key factor in the pathogenesis of antiretroviral-therapy-related lipodystrophy. *Lancet* 1999; **354**: 1112–5.

112 Simon C, Schlienger JL, Cherfan J *et al.* [Efficacy of dexamethasone in the treatment of hyperthyroidism caused by amiodarone]. *Presse Med* 1984; **13**: 2767.

113 Pessayre D, Mansouri A, Fromenty B. Non-alcoholic steatosis and steatohepatitis. V. Mitochondrial dysfunction in steatohepatitis. *Am J Physiol Gastrointest Liver Physiol* 2002; **282**: G193–9.

114 Dourakis SP, Sevastianos VA, Kaliopi P. Acute severe steatohepatitis related to prednisolone therapy. *Am J Gastroenterol* 2002; **97**: 1074–5.

115 Nanki T, Koike R, Miyasaka N. Subacute severe steatohepatitis during prednisolone therapy for systemic lupus erythematosis. *Am J Gastroenterol* 1999; **94**: 3379.

22 Hepatocellular carcinoma in NAFLD

Vlad Ratziu & Thierry Poynard

Key learning points

1 Hepatocellular carcinoma (HCC) can occur in patients with NASH-related cirrhosis. Future studies need to assess its incidence in comparison to cirrhosis from other aetiologies.
2 In most cases of 'NASH-associated' HCC, the underlying cirrhosis was undiagnosed despite a long-standing history of abnormal liver tests and obesity and/or diabetes.
3 Most patients with 'NASH-associated' HCC are not eligible for curative treatment as a result of the delay in diagnosis.
4 An increased risk for HCC has been demonstrated in both obese and diabetic subjects. This risk is most likely independent of alcohol consumption, viral hepatitis or a known history of cirrhosis.
5 Experimental data demonstrated the existence of preneoplastic changes in the steatotic liver prior to the occurrence of inflammation and cirrhosis.

Abstract

Large cohort and case–control studies have shown an increased risk of liver cancer, mainly hepatocellular carcinoma (HCC), in obese and diabetic persons. While concomitant hepatic viral infections or alcohol consumption could explain part of this association, a variable but significant number of cases of HCC still occur in the absence of any epidemiologically linked carcinogenic associations. As obesity and diabetes predispose to non-alcoholic steatohepatitis (NASH), the carcinogenic potential of this condition has come under focus. Several case series have documented the occurrence of HCC in NASH-associated cirrhosis. A salient feature of these observations is that diagnosis was often made at an advanced stage. Indeed, HCC and the underlying liver disease were often diagnosed simultaneously, despite a known but long overlooked elevation in liver tests. In most cases, this hampered efforts for curative therapy. To date, no cases of HCC have been described in patients with NASH without cirrhosis nor in subjects with steatosis but no NASH. A significant body of evidence has accumulated pointing to alterations in various hormonal axes and cytokines during obesity and/or diabetes that carry a carcinogenic potential and which might explain the increased prevalence of cancer at various organ sites. Fatty liver itself displays increased basal hepatocyte proliferative activity and decreased apoptosis, suggesting that conditions for neoplastic transformation are present before the stage of cirrhosis. Careful correlation of these experimental data with prospective clinical observations are required for a better understanding of the full spectrum of non-alcoholic fatty liver disease (NAFLD) -induced liver damage in humans.

Table 22.1 Studies reporting hepatocellular carcinoma (HCC) in patients with non-alcoholic steatohepatitis (NASH)-associated cirrhosis.

Author [Reference]	N*	Sex (M/F)	Age at HCC diagnosis (median, range)	Obesity; diabetes (n/N*)	NASH diagnosed at cirrhotic stage (n/N*)	Time interval between diagnosis of cirrhosis and HCC (yr)	Known prior history of abnormal LFT	Single nodule at diagnosis (n/N*)	Evolution	Suitability for curative treatment upon presentation† (n/N*)
Cotrim et al. [14]	1	1/0	66	1/1; 1/1	1/1	4	1/1	1/1	Multinodular/ metastasis	1/1
Zen et al. [15]	1	0/1	72	NA; 1/1	1/1	6	1/1	1/1	Multinodular	1/1
Shimada et al. [13]	6	3/3	68 (56–72)	3/6; 3/6	6/6	0 in three; 0.5–2.5 in three	5/6	4/6	Multinodular 3/4; metastasis 2/6	5/6
Ratziu et al. [11]	8	7/1	68 (52–75)	8/8; 6/8	NA	0 in five; 1.8–5.8 years in three	6/8	2/8; 4/8	Multinodular; portal thrombosis	2/8

LFT, liver function tests; NA, not available.
* N, total number of patients.
† Liver transplantation or hepatectomy.

Introduction

A spectacular rise in the incidence of obesity and diabetes has occurred over the past few decades in both industrialized and developing countries. As a consequence, the incidence of NAFLD, which is the form of liver injury associated with these conditions, has soared to become one of the top three causes of chronic liver enzyme elevation. While this unquestionably establishes NAFLD as a very frequent form of liver injury, its severity is a matter of debate. Steatosis (pure fatty liver) is considered to be non-progressive [1,2], and steatohepatitis (NASH) to be slowly evolving in the majority of patients. However, recent data have challenged the view of NASH as a disease with a mostly indolent course. Significant fibrosis including cirrhosis can be present at diagnosis [2,3] and fibrotic progression has been demonstrated on serial liver biopsies [2,4–6]. A significant proportion of cases with cryptogenic cirrhosis could result from the end-stage evolution of NASH [7], and NASH-related cryptogenic cirrhosis may result in liver failure, warranting liver transplantation [8,9] or, in its absence, increased liver-related mortality [10,11]. Although evidence of a wide spectrum of severity for this condition continues to accumulate, significant limitations pertaining to the quality of these data—all retrospective and subject to referral bias—have become evident, feeding further controversy.

The most unambiguous demonstration of the potential severity of a chronic liver disease is when it can induce liver cancer. Among all tumours, HCC is especially worrisome for two reasons: a rising incidence [12] and a heavy toll in terms of mortality because curative treatment is limited by multifocal development and late diagnosis. For the same reasons, the prospect of an association between NASH and HCC is particularly alarming. First, the number of future cases of NASH-associated HCC might constitute a real public health concern considering the rising frequency of NASH in the general population, even if the probability of neoplastic occurrence in a given individual may be low. Secondly, in many patients with NASH-associated HCC, curative treatments such as liver transplantation will probably not be feasible because of the delay in the diagnosis of NASH-induced cirrhosis and the presence of comorbid conditions, such as morbid obesity or diabetes and its vascular complications.

The identification and description of HCC cases among patients with NASH is difficult because of the current lack of a serological, biochemical or genetic marker of NASH and the reliance on liver biopsy, an obviously unsuitable diagnostic tool for large cohort studies. The few case series of HCC in patients with previously diagnosed NASH provide the most relevant information but such observation is the tip of the iceberg. Assuming that a significant proportion of patients with obesity and/or diabetes develop NASH, valuable data on the magnitude of the association can be gained from descriptive studies of the prevalence of HCC in large cohorts of obese or diabetic individuals.

NASH and hepatocellular carcinoma

Several studies have documented the occurrence of HCC in patients diagnosed with NASH. Others have identified a subset of HCC patients in whom the underlying liver disease was probably NASH-associated cirrhosis.

The occurrence of HCC in NASH has been mostly documented through case series of less than 10 patients. The proportion (of HCC) among cirrhotic patients with NASH ranges from 30% in Asian series [13] to 37% in a European one [11], which is surprisingly close, although a meaningful prevalence estimate would require much larger numbers. Although studies are limited (Table 22.1), certain similarities are striking. All cases of HCC occurred in cirrhotic individuals. Although most cases were identified in men, a significant proportion occurred in women (31%, 5 of 16). This is of interest considering the male predominance of this neoplasm in cirrhosis from aetiologies other than NASH, as well as the fact that most recent NASH series have not identified female gender to be a risk factor either for NASH occurrence or for the progression of NASH to cirrhosis. This raises speculation about specific interactions between steatosis or insulin resistance and sex hormones with regard to neoplastic transformation. At this point, however, relevant experimental or epidemiological data are lacking.

Another striking feature of reports is the delay before a diagnosis was established. In most instances, the diagnosis of NASH was only made once cirrhosis had supervened, even though liver test elevations had been noted for several years. Moreover, cirrhosis itself was ignored until HCC was discovered in half of the patients, thus precluding any effort at early HCC detection through regular surveillance. From the small amount of available data, it is not clear if this delay in diagnosis resulted in more advanced neoplastic disease at presentation compared to patients with HCC occurring in other liver diseases. However, local or metastatic spread was detected in most cases during short follow-up.

Cohort studies of patients with HCC provide an alternative view. In these reports, patients with cryptogenic cirrhosis and HCC were screened for past or present exposure to risk factors for NAFLD, with the assumption that if these were present then cirrhosis was the result of end-stage NASH. This concept, first developed by Caldwell et al. [7], not only fully established NASH as a cause of cirrhosis beyond anecdotal reports available from case series, but also acknowledged the magnitude of this association. A crude estimate was that as many as half of the cases of cryptogenic cirrhosis could represent the final stage of fibrotic progression in NASH. Fine-tuning of this epidemiological link is to be expected if specific biochemical or genetic markers of NASH are discovered. Indeed, not all patients exposed to NAFLD risk factors go on to develop NASH, just as NASH can develop in the absence of overt obesity, diabetes or dyslipidaemia [6].

Keeping in mind these limitations, the studies by Bugianesi et al. [16] and Marrero et al. [17] nevertheless provide valuable data. Among all HCC patients, the proportion of those who developed from cryptogenic cirrhosis was much lower in the large Italian study (4%) than in the US one (30%), the latter being conducted in an area of high prevalence of obesity and obesity-related metabolic complications. The fact that differences in obesity prevalence translate into grossly proportional differences in the occurrence of HCC strongly reinforces the concept of NASH being a cause of cirrhosis and ultimately liver cancer.

As already anticipated from earlier studies of cryptogenic cirrhosis [7] and end-stage liver disease [8], patients with HCC and cryptogenic cirrhosis have a higher prevalence of clinical features associated with the dysmetabolic syndrome and of biological markers of insulin resistance [16]. This was not explained by the older mean age in the cryptogenic group, as this association was independent of age in multivariate analysis. For the reasons discussed above, the true proportion of NASH-related HCC among those with cryptogenic cirrhosis is unknown, although in the study by Marrero et al. [17] 47% of cryptogenic cases were considered to have NASH, based on exposure to risk factors or compatible histological lesions in non-tumorous liver sections. Even with this lower-end estimate, NASH was among the leading causes of HCC in US patients, second only to hepatitis C virus (HCV) infection, and accounted for the same proportion (13%) of cases as alcoholic liver disease with or without HCV infection, and a higher proportion than chronic hepatitis B virus infection.

However, the main lesson to be learned from the US study is that the diagnosis of NASH-related HCC is often made too late. Indeed, patients with cryptogenic cirrhosis were less likely to undergo HCC surveillance than those with cirrhosis of other well-established aetiologies (23% versus 61%). Considering the commonly accepted recommendation for HCC surveillance in cirrhotic patients, such a low prevalence of HCC detection through surveillance most likely reflects the lack of full recognition and diagnosis of NASH-induced cirrhosis and/or of its carcinogenic potential. This has resulted in the detection of larger tumours at diagnosis and consequently, a lower proportion of patients eligible for curative therapy [17]. The straightforward conclusion from these data is that it is time for a greater effort to be made to educate health care providers, especially those outside the field of liver disease, about the risk of liver injury in obese and/or diabetic patients, including serious lesions such as cirrhosis and liver cancer.

Diabetes and hepatocellular carcinoma

There is some evidence of an excessive risk of HCC in diabetic patients (Table 22.2). Some of this is based on large population-based cohorts, while most is provided by case–control studies. All but one study [19] demonstrated an increased risk for HCC in diabetics. In one Veterans study, however, the association was significant only in the presence of another risk factor such as alcoholic cirrhosis or viral hepatitis [26]. The magnitude of the risk is variable, depending on the prevalence of other risk factors for HCC in the population examined. However, it is closer to or even higher than that for alcohol exposure [18,28] (with some studies demonstrating a synergism between alcohol consumption and diabetes), while modest compared with the one for viral hepatitis. The association between diabetes and HCC was similar in men and women, consistent between various age groups and persisted even after allowance for a number of relevant confounding

Table 22.2 Studies evaluating the relative risk of HCC in patients with diabetes.

Author [Reference]	Country, time period	Type of study	Cases (cohort)/ controls	Assessment of viral hepatitis	Relative risk for HCC*	P
Adami et al. [18]	Sweden 1965–83	Population-based cohort	153 852	Discharge diagnosis	4.1 (3.8–4.5)†	< 0.001
Lawson et al. [19]	Scotland 1977–81	Case–control‡	105/105+105§	No	4.9 (1.9–13.5)	< 0.001
Wideroff et al. [20]	Denmark 1977–89	Population-based cohort	109 581	No?	4 (3.5–4.6)† (in males)	NP
Lu et al. [21]	Taiwan 1985	Case–control‡	131/207	Discharge diagnosis	NP	NS
Yu et al. [22]	Los Angeles County 1984–90	Case–control‡	74/162	Serology	3.3 (1.5–7.2)	NP
La Vecchia et al. [23]	Italy 1984–96	Case–control	428/1502	Discharge diagnosis	2.1 (1.4–3.2)	NP
Hassan et al. [24]	Texas 1994–96	Case–control‡	115/230	Serology	4.3 (1.9–9.9)	NP
Lagiou et al. [25]	Greece 1995–99	Case–control‡	333/360	Serology	1.86 (1–3.5)	NP
El-Serag et al. [26]	Texas 1997–99	Case–control	823/3459	Discharge diagnosis	1.27 (1.02–1.57)	0.03
Nair et al. [27]	USA 1991–2000	UNOS (liver transplant) cohort¶	19 271	Serology	1.48 (1.07–2.03)	0.007

NS, not significant; NP, not provided.
* Multivariate analysis after adjustment for relevant covariates (risk factors)
† Standardized incidence ratios.
‡ Controls matched on age and sex with cases.
§ 105 patients with colon cancer and another 105 admitted for fractures were used as controls.
¶ Pathological diagnosis of HCC on explanted liver specimens.

variables. The risk seems to be similarly increased for both type 1 and type 2 diabetes [24]. More importantly, this statistical association is probably clinically and epidemiologically significant. Most studies of patients with HCC failed to identify any of the major risk factors for HCC in 15–50% of cases [29].

As can be expected from the time period during which these studies were conducted (Table 22.2), they contain a number of methodological flaws. Of particular concern in some is the possibility of undiagnosed

viral hepatitis (especially HCV), haemochromatosis or cirrhosis. In most reports, however, the diagnosis of diabetes was made several years before that of HCC, thus making it improbable that clinical diabetes merely resulted from the neoplastic process or from advanced underlying liver disease. In fact, the association remained significant even in subjects without a history of hepatitis or cirrhosis [22,23]. Arguably, an overestimation of the risk of HCC in diabetics could also result from the strong epidemiological association between haemochromatosis and diabetes [30]. However, even after taking into account this possible under-ascertainment bias, there was still a twofold increased risk of HCC in diabetics [31]. As for viral hepatitis, only a few studies allowed for systematic serological screening in cases and controls. However, this did not change the significance of the association.

As a whole, the data suggest that patients with diabetes have a significantly increased risk of developing HCC as a result of diabetes *per se*. In regions of the world with both high and low prevalence of viral hepatitis, 10–20% of cases of HCC could be attributable to diabetes alone [24,32]. As this finding may be of tremendous importance on a public health level, given the expected rise in incidence of diabetes in the years to come, more studies are needed to clarify important aspects. The confounding impact of viral hepatitis [33] should be ruled out through exhaustive serological testing, and that of alcoholic cirrhosis through rigorous assessment of past and present alcohol consumption. Whether the link between diabetes and HCC relies solely on the presence of NASH-associated cirrhosis is currently not known, although this seems probable. An equally relevant issue is whether the risk of liver cancer is different between patients with

type 2 diabetes mellitus and those with type 1 diabetes mellitus, and whether it is affected by the type of diabetes treatment. Finally, longitudinal follow-up studies are warranted in order to rule out the possibility that diabetes is secondary to cirrhosis of an unrelated cause, which in turn predisposes to HCC.

Obesity and hepatocellular carcinoma

Several studies in obese individuals have uniformly documented an increased incidence of HCC [27,34,35], while another has shown an increase in mortality from liver cancer (Table 22.3) [37]. Although the risk is low compared to established procarcinogenic conditions such as viral hepatitis or alcoholic cirrhosis, it may have a considerable impact in terms of public health because of the current high prevalence of obesity. In most instances, the association of HCC incidence was significant for a body mass index (BMI) higher than $30 \, kg/m^2$ (which defines obesity), and was even higher in severe obesity (BMI > $35 \, kg/m^2$) [27,36]. Although predictably weaker, an excessive risk in the overweight has not been specifically assessed and therefore cannot be ruled out. Whatever the magnitude of the

Table 22.3 Studies evaluating the relative risk of HCC in obese patients.

Author [Reference]	Country, time period	Type of study	N	Assessment of confounding variables	Excess risk for HCC	P
Wolk *et al.* [34]	Sweden 1965–93	Population-based cohort	28 129	Diabetes and alcoholism (discharge diagnosis)	3.6 (2–6)* (in men only)	NA
Moller *et al.* [35]	Denmark 1977–87	Population-based cohort	37 957	No	1.9 (1.5–2.5)	NA
Calle *et al.* [36]	USA 1982–98	Prospective population-based cohort	900 053	Alcoholism	4.52 (2.94–6.94)† (in men only)	< 0.001
Nair *et al.* [27]	USA 1991–2000	UNOS (liver transplant) cohort‡	19 271	Viral hepatitis, diabetes, alcohol	1.65 (1.22–2.22)	0.002

NA, not available.
* Standardized incidence ratios.
† Denotes excess risk of mortality from liver cancer and not HCC incidence.
‡ Pathological diagnosis of HCC on explanted liver specimens.
§ Multivariate analysis after adjustment for relevant covariates (risk factors).

risk associated with obesity, this only becomes significant in the context of ageing. In the single study where the association was tested across different age groups, obesity on its own increased the risk of HCC only in patients over 50 years of age [27]. As this study was performed exclusively in patients with cirrhosis, this finding does not simply reflect the delay that is necessary for the development of obesity-related cirrhosis, a premalignant state. It is more probable, although at this point speculative, that complex interactions exist between ageing and putative procarcinogenic mechanisms associated with obesity, which might fully operate only in the context of senescence.

The contribution of obesity *per se* to an added risk for HCC is hard to delineate. Factors epidemiologically linked to obesity might confound the relationship, as they are not always thoroughly accounted for in large epidemiological surveys. For instance, two studies have shown an increased risk in men but not in women [34,36]. Although male gender is an independent risk factor for liver cancer whatever the underlying liver disease, this alone might not explain a sex-related difference as large as the one documented by Calle *et al.* [36]. A possible confounding factor for liver carcinogenesis could be alcohol consumption, a behaviour more frequent in men than women. High alcohol consumption as a source of extra calories could contribute to obesity and there is a correlation between abdominal obesity and alcohol consumption [38]. This raises the possibility that drinkers are over-represented in the cohort of obese individuals. When specifically addressing this issue, Wolk *et al.* [34] demonstrated a much lower odds ratio for HCC in obese non-drinkers than in obese drinkers (two versus 12) (Fig. 22.1). Another example is diabetes because, in the same study, subjects who were obese but not diabetic failed to show an increased risk of HCC, whereas those who were both obese and diabetic had a relative risk of 6.3 (Fig. 22.1). Undoubtedly, a small proportion of HCC cases (21% of cases in the above mentioned study [34]) are associated with obesity alone, in the absence of either alcoholism or diabetes. In most instances, however, the association of HCC appears to be stronger with diabetes than with obesity. This suggests that obesity is a surrogate marker of an underlying condition common to the two processes, such as insulin resistance, and possibly casually related to neoplastic transformation.

These large cohort studies are highly powered for detecting small but significantly increased risks associated with individual risk factors that are easy to identify

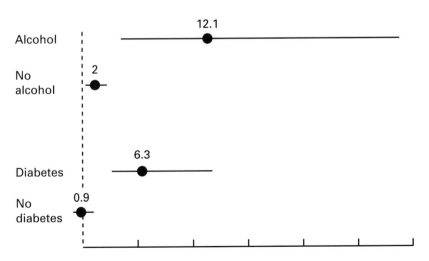

Fig. 22.1 Standardized incidence ratios with 95% confidence intervals for hepatocellular carcinoma (HCC) among obese patients with and without a diagnosis of alcoholism or diabetes mellitus. (Adapted with permission from Wolk *et al.* [34].)

from hospital discharge diagnosis or crude clinical assessment. However, they are not suited to analysing intricate associations of epidemiologically linked pathological conditions. None of these studies can determine the differential effect of different types of obesity, in particular central obesity. They all rely upon a diagnosis of obesity made at one point in time, at study entry, which ignores the dynamics of weight change throughout the usual long follow-up. Perhaps even more relevant is the difficulty of diagnosing asymptomatic diabetes or assessing the impact of treated versus poorly controlled diabetes. Finally, the assessment of alcohol consumption in terms of 'ever/never' is insufficient for evaluating its impact on the development of chronic liver disease and liver cancer. None the less, the studies document a significant epidemiological link that justifies further investigation aimed at carving out more precisely the role of obesity or diabetes as independent procarcinogenic conditions for liver cancer.

Potential mechanisms of carcinogenesis in NAFLD

The current paradigm in human hepatocarcinogenesis holds that cirrhosis is a preneoplastic lesion and that hepatocellular carcinoma emerges from a cirrhotic liver. While this is true in most instances, it does not entirely describe the progression of liver damage from the initial liver disease to the eventual occurrence of HCC. Indeed, this neoplasm develops in a non-cirrhotic liver in at least 10% of cases. Moreover, the risk of liver cancer is not the same in cirrhosis of different aetiologies.

The clinical and epidemiological data summarized above on HCC occurrence in case series of NASH and from large cohorts of obese and diabetic subjects leave important questions unresolved, especially on the relationship between NASH or its metabolic predisposing conditions and HCC occurrence. Is cirrhosis an obligatory prerequisite for HCC emergence, as it appears from the reported case series, or do predisposing conditions for NASH favour neoplastic transformation independent of cirrhosis, as can be anticipated from large cohort series? Is the epidemiological association between obesity and diabetes and HCC confounded by common risk factors without a direct causative link or are there discernable mechanisms of neoplastic transformation operating specifically in the context of insulin resistance and a fatty liver?

Several lines of evidence suggest that these mechanisms exist and could explain the emergence of neoplastic clones before the liver becomes cirrhotic. They could also explain the overall increased prevalence of cancer of numerous extrahepatic sites documented in obese or diabetic patients [37]. Some of the evidence is provided from animal models of steatosis, others from *in vitro* experiments with hepatoma cell lines. Most relevant to human cancer are those concerning hyperinsulinaemia; disturbance of the insulin growth factor (IGF) axis; alterations in proliferation and apoptosis encountered in a fatty liver; and cellular fatty acid toxicity and peroxisome proliferator activator receptor-α (PPARα) activation.

Insulin and hepatocarcinogenesis

Insulin resistance and compensatory hyperinsulinaemia are cardinal features of obesity and diabetes. It has been hypothesized that conditions creating a state of hyperinsulinaemia predispose to cancer development in a number of organs [39–41]. Interestingly, type 2 diabetes is characterized by a long period of hyperinsulinaemia preceding the appearance of overt clinical symptoms. Liver cells are therefore exposed, directly from the portal blood, to high circulating levels of insulin for prolonged periods.

Insulin signals through both the insulin receptor (IR) and the insulin growth factor-1 receptor (IGF-1R), although selective insulin action on IGF-1R can occur in insulin-resistant states [42]. Although not a primary mitogen for normal hepatocytes [43], insulin is a potent activator of hepatocyte proliferation through its signalling pathways [44,45]. In contrast, both insulin and IGF-1 act as dominant cellular mitogens for different tumour types including HCC in humans [46]. Upon binding to the IR, insulin activates antiapoptotic mediators such as nuclear factor-κB (NF-κB) and tumour necrosis factor α (TNF-α), thus reducing loss of cells by apoptosis especially in preneoplastic lesions [47,48]. In experimental models of chemical carcinogenesis there is a correlation between insulinaemia and the development of liver tumours [49]. Direct exposure to insulin through hepatic implants of insulin-producing islet cells causes proliferative lesions in surrounding parenchyma, very reminiscent of preneoplastic lesions caused by chemical carcinogens, and eventually tumours [50]. Finally, a key molecule involved in insulin signalling, insulin receptor substrate-1 (IRS-1), is overexpressed in HCC cell lines and tumour tissue [51] and may have transforming properties [52]. Inactivation of IRS-1 by a dominant negative mutant reverses the malignant phenotype of HCC cells mainly by inhibiting insulin–IGF-1 mediated signal transduction pathways [53].

Insulin growth factor axis and hepatocarcinogenesis

Patients with type 2 diabetes display elevated levels of IGF [54] that sometimes precede the onset of overt diabetes by many years [55]. Moreover, in the context of insulin resistance, IGF-1 action at the tissue level may be amplified by alterations of serum concentrations of IGF-1 binding proteins [40].

The IGF axis has important autocrine, paracrine and endocrine roles in the promotion of growth [56,57]. IGF-1 stimulates hepatic cell proliferation [58], including in preneoplastic foci [60]. It is also known to inhibit apoptosis [59,60]. IGF-2 overexpression is associated with the development of multiple cancers including liver cancer [61], while inhibition of IGF-2 expression through antisense oligonucleotides is associated with decreased cell proliferative activity [62].

IGF-1R, whose main ligands are insulin and IGF-1, is also involved in the process of malignant transformation [63]. A number of cancers, including HCC, as well as several hepatoma cell lines, have been shown to express elevated levels of IGF-1R. IGF-1R is required for optimal growth [64] and is key to the establishment and maintenance of the transformed phenotype [65]. The transforming capacity of IGF-1R is further demonstrated by its dose-dependent inhibition of apoptosis and the quantitative correlation between the fraction of surviving cells and the induction of tumorigenesis [66].

Fatty liver as a premalignant condition

Animal models of steatosis, such as the *ob/ob* mice, provide a unique opportunity to study preneoplastic changes occurring in the fatty liver without the confounding effect of overt hepatic inflammation or cirrhosis. Fatty livers from *ob/ob* mice have higher hepatic DNA content than normal livers and display induction of cell cycle associated genes such as c-*jun*, *cyclin D1* and *cyclin A* [67]. An activation of signalling pathways involved in hepatocyte proliferation and the induction of several antiapoptotic mechanisms have also been observed [67]. These data suggest that fat-laden hepa-

tocytes display an increased proliferative activity and decreased apoptosis. The chronic disruption of the balance between cell growth and cell loss in these obese mice might set the stage for neoplastic transformation, as ageing *ob/ob* mice are known to develop hepatic tumours [68].

The precise mechanisms driving increased proliferation and inhibition of apoptosis in steatotic hepatocytes have not yet been identified but free radical production may be an important factor. Hepatic mitochondrial production of reactive oxygen species (ROS) is increased significantly in *ob/ob* mice [67,69] and excessive oxidative stress is a universal finding in animal [70,71] and human models of steatohepatitis [72,73]. Interestingly, hepatic tumours have also been described in animal models of steatosis unrelated to insulin resistance but characterized by increased oxidative stress [74]. The disruption of the methionine adenosyltransferase-1A (*MAT-1A*) gene results in increased liver weight, steatosis and steatohepatitis in mice fed a normal diet [75]. Eventually, these mice spontaneously develop HCC [74]. Decreased *MAT-1A* and induction of *MAT-2A* gene, as seen in *MAT-1A* knockout mice, change the normal pattern of hepatic gene expression and result in metabolic complications such as increased hepatic triglyceride content and hyperglycaemia, similar to that seen in human NASH. This is accompanied by increased levels of oxidative stress and the induction of genes involved in cell proliferation [74,76]. The relevance to human HCC has been recently proven by the demonstration that the β catalytic subunit of the *MAT-2* gene encoded by *MAT-2A* is expressed in HCC and stimulates cell proliferation of in liver cancer cell lines [77].

Fatty acids cellular toxicity, PPARα activation and carcinogenesis

It is tempting to speculate about a role for chronic PPARα activation in hepatic carcinogenesis. Noting that hepatic metabolism of long-chain fatty acids results in increased oxidative stress, which in turn induces DNA damage and an altered profile of expression of key genes involved in cell proliferation (*fos, jun, NF-κB* and *p53*), Ockner *et al.* [78] first hypothesized that alterations in fatty acid metabolism could be implicated in hepatic carcinogenesis. Subsequently, it has been recognized that peroxisome proliferators induce liver cancers through the activation of PPARα [79], that PPARα can activate growth regulatory genes resulting in neoplastic transformation and that PPARα null mice are not able to develop liver tumours upon treatment with peroxisome proliferators [80,81]. The observation that long-chain fatty acids are natural ligands and activators of PPARα provided a possible link with human diseases. It has been therefore proposed that in obesity and diabetes, increased fatty acid flux and fat overload might reproduce PPARα activation seen with long-chain and very-long-chain fatty acids. This could result in chronic PPARα induction and activation, which could ultimately lead to hepatocarcinogenesis [82].

Animal models provide a perfect framework to examine this hypothesis. Mice that are deficient for acylCoA oxidase, the first and rate-limiting enzymatic step of peroxisomal oxidation of fatty acids, develop steatosis by intrahepatic accumulation of long-chain fatty acids which then results in steatohepatitis and ultimately liver tumours [83]. This model, however appealing, has not yet proven to be transposable to humans. Although human PPARs share numerous functional characteristics with their rodent counterparts, there is an obvious lack of human susceptibility to per-oxisome proliferator-induced hepatocarcinogenesis as long-term exposure to fibrates does not result in liver cancers in humans. These species differences might result from quantitative differences in gene expression as PPARα is less abundant in human than in rodent liver [84]. Nevertheless, the relevance to liver carcinogenesis of a mild physiological activation of PPARα in response to human insulin resistance states cannot be discarded because, as Bass wisely stated, 'what can take months in a mouse may take decades in a human' [82].

Conclusions

NAFLD is a complex entity. It encompasses benign forms of liver injury as well as progressively evolving conditions that in a minority of patients can be life-threatening. The true prevalence of severe forms outside specialized tertiary care referral centres needs to be prospectively assessed. Clearly, HCC can complicate the course of cirrhotic NASH and its population prevalence that is probably similar to that for viral or alcoholic cirrhosis, although incidence estimates are not available. Particularly worrisome is the description of an excessive risk of liver cancer in large cohorts of diabetic or obese individuals. Although the respective contribution of epidemiologically linked cofactors for carcinogenesis has not been systematically delineated, it is probable that even in their absence the risk remains significant. Exciting new data show that steatosis is a remarkably adaptive state of the liver to insulin resistant conditions, but this may come at the price of increased vulnerability to liver injury and the activation of procarcinogenic pathways in the steatotic liver, well before cirrhosis or even inflammation is present. Considering the dire prognosis of this tumour, a major effort needs to be made towards the detection of severe forms of liver injury in patients exposed to NASH risk factors, mainly obesity and diabetes.

Acknowledgments

The authors thank the Association pour la Recherche sur le Cancer for grant support and Janet Ratziu for manuscript revision.

References

1 Teli MR, James OFW, Burt D et al. The natural history of non-alcoholic fatty liver: a follow-up study. *Hepatology* 1995; **22**: 1714–9.
2 Ratziu V, Giral P, Charlotte F et al. Liver fibrosis in overweight patients. *Gastroenterology* 2000; **118**: 1117–23.
3 Angulo P, Keach JC, Batts KP et al. Independent predictors of liver fibrosis in patients with non-alcoholic steatohepatitis. *Hepatology* 1999; **30**: 1356–62.
4 Powell EE, Cooksley WGE, Hanson R et al. The natural history of non-alcoholic steatohepatitis: a follow-up study of forty-two patients for up to 21 years. *Hepatology* 1990; **11**: 74–80.
5 Lee RG. Non-alcoholic steatohepatitis: a study of 49 patients. *Hum Pathol* 1989; **20**: 594–8.
6 Bacon BR, Farahvash MJ, Janney CG et al. Non-alcoholic steatohepatitis: an expanded clinical entity. *Gastroenterology* 1994; **107**: 1103–9.
7 Caldwell SH, Oelsner DH, Iezzoni JC et al. Cryptogenic cirrhosis: clinical characterization and risk factors for underlying disease. *Hepatology* 1999; **29**: 664–9.
8 Poonawala A, Nair SP, Thuluvath PJ. Prevalence of obesity and diabetes in patients with cryptogenic cirrhosis: a case–control study. *Hepatology* 2000; **32**: 689–92.
9 Nair S, Verma S, Thuluvath PJ. Obesity and its effect on survival in patients undergoing orthotopic liver transplantation in the United States. *Hepatology* 2002; **35**: 105–9.

10 Matteoni CA, Younossi ZM, Gramlich T *et al.* Non-alcoholic fatty liver disease: a spectrum of clinical and pathological severity. *Gastroenterology* 1999; **116**: 1413–9.

11 Ratziu V, Bonyhay L, Di Martino V *et al.* Survival, liver failure, and hepatocellular carcinoma in obesity-related cryptogenic cirrhosis. *Hepatology* 2002; **35**: 1485–93.

12 El-Serag H, Mason A. Rising incidence of hepatocellular carcinoma in the United States. *N Engl J Med* 1999; **340**: 745–50.

13 Shimada M, Hashimoto E, Taniai M *et al.* Hepatocellular carcinoma in patients with non-alcoholic steatohepatitis. *J Hepatol* 2002; **37**: 154–60.

14 Cotrim HP, Parana R, Braga E *et al.* Non-alcoholic steatohepatitis and hepatocellular carcinoma: natural history? *Am J Gastroenterol.* 2000; **95**: 3018–9.

15 Zen Y, Katayanagi K, Tsuneyama K *et al.* Hepatocellular carcinoma arising in non-alcoholic steatohepatitis. *Pathol Int* 2001; **51**: 127–31.

16 Bugianesi E, Leone N, Vanni E *et al.* Expanding the natural history of non-alcoholic steatohepatitis: from cryptogenic cirrhosis to hepatocellular carcinoma. *Gastroenterology* 2002; **123**: 134–40.

17 Marrero JA, Fontana RJ, Su GL *et al.* NAFLD may be a common underlying liver disease in patients with hepatocellular carcinoma in the United States. *Hepatology* 2002; **36**: 1349–54.

18 Adami HO, Chow WH, Nyren O *et al.* Excess risk of primary liver cancer in patients with diabetes mellitus. *J Natl Cancer Inst* 1996; **88**: 1472–7.

19 Lawson DH, Gray JM, McKillop C *et al.* Diabetes mellitus and primary hepatocellular carcinoma. *Q J Med* 1986; **61**: 945–55.

20 Wideroff L, Gridley G, Mellemkjaer L *et al.* Cancer incidence in a population-based cohort of patients hospitalized with diabetes mellitus in Denmark. *J Natl Cancer Inst* 1997; **89**: 1360–5.

21 Lu SN, Lin TM, Chen CJ *et al.* A case–control study of primary hepatocellular carcinoma in Taiwan. *Cancer* 1988; **62**: 2051–5.

22 Yu MC, Tong MJ, Govindarajan S *et al.* Non-viral risk factors for hepatocellular carcinoma in a low-risk population, the non-Asians of Los Angeles County, California. *J Natl Cancer Inst* 1991; **83**: 1820–6.

23 La Vecchia C, Negri E, Decarli A *et al.* Diabetes mellitus and the risk of primary liver cancer. *Int J Cancer* 1997; **73**: 204–7.

24 Hassan MM, Hwang LY, Hatten CJ *et al.* Risk factors for hepatocellular carcinoma: synergism of alcohol with viral hepatitis and diabetes mellitus. *Hepatology* 2002; **36**: 1206–13.

25 Lagiou P, Kuper H, Stuver SO *et al.* Role of diabetes mellitus in the etiology of hepatocellular carcinoma. *J Natl Cancer Inst* 2000; **92**: 1096–9.

26 El-Serag HB, Richardson PA, Everhart JE. The role of diabetes in hepatocellular carcinoma: a case–control study among United States Veterans. *Am J Gastroenterol* 2001; **96**: 2462–7.

27 Nair S, Mason A, Eason J *et al.* Is obesity an independent risk factor for hepatocellular carcinoma in cirrhosis? *Hepatology* 2002; **36**: 150–5.

28 Adami HO, McLaughlin JK, Hsing AW *et al.* Alcoholism and cancer risk: a population-based cohort study. *Cancer Causes Control* 1992; **3**: 419–25.

29 Di Bisceglie AM, Carithers RL Jr, Gores GJ. Hepatocellular carcinoma. *Hepatology* 1998; **28**: 1161–5.

30 Ellervik C, Mandrup-Poulsen T, Nordestgaard BG *et al.* Prevalence of hereditary haemochromatosis in late-onset type 1 diabetes mellitus: a retrospective study. *Lancet* 2001; **358**: 1405–9.

31 Nelson R, Persky V, Davis F *et al.* Re: excess risk of primary liver cancer in patients with diabetes mellitus. *J Natl Cancer Inst* 1997; **89**: 327–8.

32 Braga C, La Vecchia C, Negri E *et al.* Attributable risks for hepatocellular carcinoma in northern Italy. *Eur J Cancer* 1997; **33**: 629–34.

33 Mehta SH, Brancati FL, Sulkowski MS *et al.* Prevalence of type 2 diabetes mellitus among persons with hepatitis C virus infection in the United States. *Ann Intern Med* 2000; **133**: 592–9.

34 Wolk A, Gridley G, Svensson M *et al.* A prospective study of obesity and cancer risk (Sweden). *Cancer Causes Control* 2001; **12**: 13–21.

35 Moller H, Mellemgaard A, Lindvig K *et al.* Obesity and cancer risk: a Danish record-linkage study. *Eur J Cancer* 1994; **30A**: 344–50.

36 Calle EE, Rodriguez C, Walker-Thurmond K *et al.* Overweight, obesity, and mortality from cancer in a prospectively studied cohort of US adults. *N Engl J Med* 2003; **348**: 1625–38.

37 Moore MA, Park CB, Tsuda H. Implications of the hyperinsulinaemia–diabetes–cancer link for preventive efforts. *Eur J Cancer Prev* 1998; **7**: 89–107.

38 Istvan J, Murray R, Voelker H. The relationship between patterns of alcohol consumption and body weight. Lung Health Study Research Group. *Int J Epidemiol* 1995; **24**: 543–6.

39 Bruning PF, Bonfrer JM, van Noord PA *et al.* Insulin resistance and breast-cancer risk. *Int J Cancer* 1992; **52**: 511–6.

40 Kazer RR. Insulin resistance, insulin-like growth factor I and breast cancer: a hypothesis. *Int J Cancer* 1995; **62**: 403–6.

41 Kaaks R. Nutrition, hormones, and breast cancer: is insulin the missing link? *Cancer Causes Control* 1996; **7**: 605–25.

42 Singh P, Rubin N. Insulin-like growth factors and binding proteins in colon cancer. *Gastroenterology* 1993; **105**: 1218–37.

43 Michalopoulos GK, DeFrances MC. Liver regeneration. *Science* 1997; **276**: 60–6.

44 Leffert HL, Koch KS, Moran T *et al.* Hormonal control of rat liver regeneration. *Gastroenterology* 1979; **76**: 1470–82.

45 McGowan JA, Strain AJ, Bucher NL. DNA synthesis in primary cultures of adult rat hepatocytes in a defined medium: effects of epidermal growth factor, insulin, glucagon, and cyclic-AMP. *J Cell Physiol* 1981; **108**: 353–63.

46 Macaulay VM. Insulin-like growth factors and cancer. *Br J Cancer* 1992; **65**: 311–20.

47 Bertrand F, Atfi A, Cadoret A *et al.* A role for nuclear factor κB in the antiapoptotic function of insulin. *J Biol Chem* 1998; **273**: 2931–8.

48 Bertrand F, Desbois-Mouthon C, Cadoret A *et al.* Insulin antiapoptotic signalling involves insulin activation of the nuclear factor κB-dependent survival genes encoding tumor necrosis factor receptor-associated factor 2 and manganese-superoxide dismutase. *J Biol Chem* 1999; **274**: 30596–602.

49 Lagopoulos L, Sunahara GI, Wurzner H *et al.* The effects of alternating dietary restriction and ad libitum feeding of mice on the development of diethylnitrosamine-induced liver tumours and its correlation to insulinaemia. *Carcinogenesis* 1991; **12**: 311–5.

50 Dombrowski F, Bannasch P, Pfeifer U. Hepatocellular neoplasms induced by low-number pancreatic islet transplants in streptozotocin diabetic rats. *Am J Pathol* 1997; **150**: 1071–87.

51 Nishiyama M, Wands JR. Cloning and increased expression of an insulin receptor substrate-1-like gene in human hepatocellular carcinoma. *Biochem Biophys Res Commun* 1992; **183**: 280–5.

52 Ito T, Sasaki Y, Wands JR. Overexpression of human insulin receptor substrate 1 induces cellular transformation with activation of mitogen-activated protein kinases. *Mol Cell Biol* 1996; **16**: 943–51.

53 Tanaka S, Wands JR. A carboxy-terminal truncated insulin receptor substrate-1 dominant negative protein reverses the human hepatocellular carcinoma malignant phenotype. *J Clin Invest* 1996; **98**: 2100–8.

54 Bach LA, Rechler MM. Insulin-like growth factors and diabetes. *Diabetes Metab Res Rev* 1992; **8**: 229–57.

55 Davies MJ, Rayman G, Gray IP *et al.* Insulin deficiency and increased plasma concentration of intact and 32/33 split proinsulin in subjects with impaired glucose tolerance. *Diabet Med* 1993; **10**: 313–20.

56 Daughaday WH. The possible autocrine–paracrine and endocrine roles of insulin-like growth factors of human tumors. *Endocrinology* 1990; **127**: 1–4.

57 Scharf JG, Dombrowski F, Ramadori G. The IGF axis and hepatocarcinogenesis. *Mol Pathol* 2001; **54**: 138–44.

58 Koch KS, Shapiro P, Skelly H *et al.* Rat hepatocyte proliferation is stimulated by insulin-like peptides in defined medium. *Biochem Biophys Res Commun* 1982; **109**: 1054–60.

59 Dunn SE, Kari FW, French J *et al.* Dietary restriction reduces insulin-like growth factor I levels, which modulates apoptosis, cell proliferation, and tumor progression in p53-deficient mice. *Cancer Res* 1997; **57**: 4667–72.

60 Sell C, Baserga R, Rubin R. Insulin-like growth factor I (IGF-I) and the IGF-I receptor prevent etoposide-induced apoptosis. *Cancer Res* 1995; **55**: 303–6.

61 Rogler CE, Yang D, Rossetti L *et al.* Altered body composition and increased frequency of diverse malignancies in insulin-like growth factor-II transgenic mice. *J Biol Chem* 1994; **269**: 13779–84.

62 Lin SB, Hsieh SH, Hsu HL *et al.* Antisense oligodeoxynucleotides of IGF-II selectively inhibit growth of human hepatoma cells overproducing IGF-II. *J Biochem (Tokyo)* 1997; **122**: 717–22.

63 Rubin R, Baserga R. Insulin-like growth factor-I receptor: its role in cell proliferation, apoptosis, and tumorigenicity. *Lab Invest* 1995; **73**: 311–31.

64 Baserga R. The insulin-like growth factor I receptor: a key to tumor growth? *Cancer Res* 1995; **55**: 249–52.

65 Miura M, Surmacz E, Burgaud JL *et al.* Different effects on mitogenesis and transformation of a mutation at tyrosine 1251 of the insulin-like growth factor I receptor. *J Biol Chem* 1995; **270**: 22639–44.

66 Resnicoff M, Burgaud JL, Rotman HL *et al.* Correlation between apoptosis, tumorigenesis, and levels of insulin-like growth factor I receptors. *Cancer Res* 1995; **55**: 3739–41.

67 Yang S, Lin HZ, Hwang J *et al.* Hepatic hyperplasia in non-cirrhotic fatty livers: is obesity-related hepatic steatosis a premalignant condition? *Cancer Res* 2001; **61**: 5016–23.

68 Heston W, Vlhakis G. Genetic obesity and neoplasia. *J Natl Cancer Inst* 1962; **29**: 197–209.

69 Yang S, Zhu H, Li Y *et al.* Mitochondrial adaptations to obesity-related oxidant stress. *Arch Biochem Biophys* 2000; **378**: 259–68.

70 Weltman MD, Farrell GC, Liddle C. Increased hepatocyte CYP2E1 expression in a rat nutritional model of hepatic steatosis with inflammation. *Gastroenterology* 1996; **111**: 1645–53.

71 Leclercq IA, Farrell GC, Field J *et al.* CYP2E1 and CYP4A as microsomal catalysts of lipid peroxides in murine non-alcoholic steatohepatitis. *J Clin Invest* 2000; **105**: 1067–75.

72 Weltman MD, Farrell GC, Hall P *et al.* Hepatic cytochrome P450 2E1 is increased in patients with non-alcoholic steatohepatitis. *Hepatology* 1998; **27**: 128–33.

73 Sanyal AJ, Campbell-Sargent C, Mirshahi F *et al.* Non-alcoholic steatohepatitis: association of insulin resistance

and mitochondrial abnormalities. *Gastroenterology* 2001; **120**: 1183–92.

74 Martinez-Chantar ML, Corrales FJ, Martinez-Cruz LA *et al.* Spontaneous oxidative stress and liver tumors in mice lacking methionine adenosyltransferase 1A. *FASEB J* 2002; **16**: 1292–4.

75 Lu SC, Alvarez L, Huang ZZ *et al.* Methionine adenosyltransferase 1A knockout mice are predisposed to liver injury and exhibit increased expression of genes involved in proliferation. *Proc Natl Acad Sci USA* 2001; **98**: 5560–5.

76 Cai J, Mao Z, Hwang JJ *et al.* Differential expression of methionine adenosyltransferase genes influences the rate of growth of human hepatocellular carcinoma cells. *Cancer Res* 1998; **58**: 1444–50.

77 Martinez-Chantar ML, Garcia-Trevijano ER, Latasa MU *et al.* Methionine adenosyltransferase II β subunit gene expression provides a proliferative advantage in human hepatoma. *Gastroenterology* 2003; **124**: 940–8.

78 Ockner RK, Kaikaus RM, Bass NM. Fatty-acid metabolism and the pathogenesis of hepatocellular carcinoma: review and hypothesis. *Hepatology* 1993; **18**: 669–76.

79 Gonzalez FJ, Peters JM, Cattley RC. Mechanism of action of the non-genotoxic peroxisome proliferators: role of the peroxisome proliferator-activator receptor α. *J Natl Cancer Inst* 1998; **90**: 1702–9.

80 Peters JM, Cattley RC, Gonzalez FJ. Role of PPARα in the mechanism of action of the non-genotoxic carcinogen and peroxisome proliferator Wy-14,463. *Carcinogenesis* 1997; **18**: 2029–33.

81 Hashimoto T, Fujita T, Usuda N *et al.* Peroxisomal and mitochondrial fatty acid β-oxidation in mice nullizygous for both peroxisome proliferator-activated receptor α and peroxisomal fatty acyl-CoA oxidase: genotype correlation with fatty liver phenotype. *J Biol Chem* 1999; **274**: 19228–36.

82 Bass NM. Three for the price of one knockout: a mouse model of a congenital peroxisomal disorder, steatohepatitis and hepatocarcinogenesis. *Hepatology* 1999; **29**: 606–8.

83 Fan CY, Pan J, Usuda N *et al.* Steatohepatitis, spontaneous peroxisome proliferation and liver tumors in mice lacking peroxisomal fatty acyl-CoA oxidase: implications for peroxisome proliferator-activated receptor α natural ligand metabolism. *J Biol Chem* 1998; **273**: 15639–45.

84 Holden PR, Tugwood JD. Peroxisome proliferator-activated receptor α: role in rodent liver cancer and species differences. *J Mol Endocrinol* 1999; **22**: 1–8.

23 Does NASH or NAFLD contribute to comorbidity of other liver diseases?

Andrew D. Clouston & Elizabeth E. Powell

Key learning points

1 Although steatosis without steatohepatitis is not progressive in its pure form, it can exacerbate a second liver disease, such as chronic hepatitis C, or alcoholic liver disease, to promote and accelerate fibrosis.
2 Increased body mass index and viral genotype contribute to steatosis in chronic hepatitis C. Weight loss and increased exercise in these patients can lead to a reduction in steatosis and, in some, reduced stellate cell activation and fibrosis score.
3 Many patients with non-alcoholic fatty liver disease (NAFLD) and non-alcoholic steatohepatatis (NASH) have elevated serum ferritin with or without increased hepatic iron stores, but the role of increased liver iron in disease progression remains unclear.

Abstract

The current epidemic of obesity in Western populations has led to the increasingly common finding of steatosis in liver biopsies. Whereas steatosis without true steatohepatitis is generally benign as an isolated finding, in the presence of a second chronic liver disease it may exacerbate the liver damage and promote and accelerate the development of fibrosis. There is now clear evidence that steatosis is a cofactor for progressive fibrosis in chronic hepatitis C virus (HCV) infection. This steatosis is multifactorial and, although viral factors have a role in genotype 3, increased body mass index (BMI) is closely correlated with the degree of steatosis in many patients. Weight loss in these patients can ameliorate not only the steatosis but also fibrosis in some cases. The role of coexistent non-alcoholic fatty liver disease (NAFLD) in other liver diseases is less clear, but it may be an important cofactor in alcoholic liver disease and some cases of drug-induced liver disease. The inter-action of NAFLD and increased hepatic iron is not clear-cut and is discussed.

Introduction

NAFLD is an increasingly common histological finding in liver biopsies, probably related to the marked increase in obesity that has occurred over the past 20 years. Because there is no specific diagnostic laboratory test for NAFLD, the diagnosis is based on a characteristic constellation of histological features in patients with obesity, visceral adiposity, type 2 diabetes or insulin resistance. In the past, the strict definition of NAFLD required the exclusion of patients consuming potentially hepatotoxic amounts of alcohol (more than 20 g/day in women and more than 40 g/day in men) and patients with other serologically identifiable liver disease. However, this definition requires revision in view of the increasing recognition of patients with overlapping clinical and histological features of NAFLD and other chronic liver diseases.

NAFLD encompasses a spectrum of histological changes, from steatosis through steatohepatitis to fibrosis and cirrhosis (see Chapter 2) [1]. Although the minimum histological criteria for NAFLD and non-alcoholic steatohepatitis (NASH) have varied in different studies, recent work suggests that four patterns of injury can be seen [2]. The first two, steatosis and steatosis with lymphocytic infiltrates, are relatively benign. Steatosis with hepatocellular ballooning, neutrophilic infiltrates and/or Mallory's hyaline, now regarded as classic NASH, shows a greater likelihood of developing progressive fibrosis, as does steatosis accompanied by sinusoidal fibrosis. Thus, patients with NAFLD can be stratified for the risk of progressive fibrosis according to histology. In a recent analysis of 3581 consecutive liver biopsies, histological evidence of steatohepatitis was found in 12% [3]. Using strict histological criteria to diagnose steatohepatitis, including perisinusoidal fibrosis, these authors found that steatohepatitis coexisted with another chronic liver disease in 4–5% of all liver biopsies. Coexistent steatohepatitis was present in 5.5% of all biopsies from patients with chronic HCV infection and 4.0% of other forms of chronic liver disease. Similar analyses have not been published for the more common NAFLD.

The histological features of steatohepatitis are distinct and usually allow for discrimination from coexistent disease processes. The types of inflammation and fibrosis usually do not overlap with the predominantly portal-based findings of other chronic liver diseases. In particular, the pattern of fibrosis in progressive forms of NAFLD is one of the identifying characteristics of this disorder [1]. Collagen deposition is initially observed in the perivenular and perisinusoidal spaces in acinar zone 3. In the early stages, the changes are subtle and may only be recognized with specific stains for collagen. In some areas, the perisinusoidal collagen appears to invest single cells in a 'pericellular' or 'chicken-wire' pattern, similar to that described in alcoholic liver disease (ALD). In non-alcoholic liver injury, this pattern of fibrosis distinguishes NAFLD from other forms of metabolic, necroinflammatory and cholestatic chronic liver diseases in which fibrosis initially occurs in the portal tracts [4].

It is not uncommon to identify more than one disease process concurrently affecting the liver. Some examples of dual pathology include chronic HCV and ALD,

haemochromatosis and HCV infection, and haemochromatosis and ALD. In these cases, the coexistence of more than one disease process is thought to have a role in the progression of liver disease. Similarly, data are now emerging to suggest that NAFLD, coexisting with other types of chronic liver disease, may act synergistically to accelerate the progression of chronic liver injury. Thus, the necroinflammatory injury of two distinct processes simultaneously affecting the liver may increase the progression of fibrosis. When present without hepatocyte injury or fibrosis, simple steatosis in non-alcoholic patients has been shown to have a benign non-progressive natural history [2,5]. In the pathogenesis of true NASH, a second 'hit' must occur in addition to steatosis. This is generally some form of oxidative stress, postulated to result from inflammation, gut-derived endotoxin, micronutrient deficiency or drug-induced inhibition of β-oxidation of fatty acids (Fig. 23.1). However, this second 'hit' may not be necessary in patients with another chronic liver disease. In this setting, steatosis may serve as a substrate for or induce metabolic pathways that result in necroinflammation and progressive fibrosis [6]. This has important therapeutic implications, as a reduction in steatosis may minimize liver injury and decrease the progression of fibrosis in a number of chronic liver diseases (Fig. 23.1).

In the following sections we discuss the role of coexistent NAFLD in chronic HCV and the effect of treating the underlying diseases that are the risk factors for steatosis in each individual patient. In addition, we discuss the possibility that NAFLD contributes to alcohol and drug toxicity, and address the role of NAFLD in iron overload, and the role of iron overload in NASH.

NAFLD/NASH and chronic hepatitis C virus infection

Steatosis in chronic HCV infection is associated with viral genotype 3 and increased body mass index

Steatosis is a very common histological finding in patients with chronic hepatitis C, occurring in more than 50% of liver biopsy samples. Both viral and host factors have been demonstrated to have a role in its development. In support of a direct cytopathic effect of the virus, some transgenic cell lines and animal models expressing HCV proteins accumulate intracellular lipids

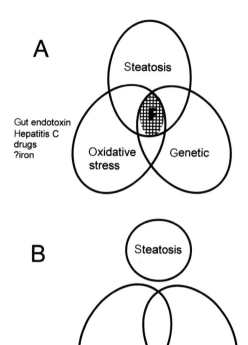

Gut endotoxin
Hepatitis C
drugs
?iron

Inflammatory (TNF-α, CTLA-4)
Profibrotic (TGF-β, AT)
antioxidant (MnSOD)
insulin resistance (?multiple)

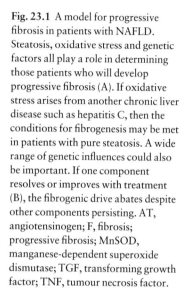

Fig. 23.1 A model for progressive fibrosis in patients with NAFLD. Steatosis, oxidative stress and genetic factors all play a role in determining those patients who will develop progressive fibrosis (A). If oxidative stress arises from another chronic liver disease such as hepatitis C, then the conditions for fibrogenesis may be met in patients with pure steatosis. A wide range of genetic influences could also be important. If one component resolves or improves with treatment (B), the fibrogenic drive abates despite other components persisting. AT, angiotensinogen; F, fibrosis; progressive fibrosis; MnSOD, manganese-dependent superoxide dismutase; TGF, transforming growth factor; TNF, tumour necrosis factor.

[7,8]. The specific mechanism remains uncertain, but may be brought about by viral proteins interfering with mitochondrial function and impairing fatty acid oxidation or to interference with pathways of lipid metabolism. The HCV core protein has recently been shown to reduce the activity of microsomal triglyceride transfer protein, a factor involved in the assembly and secretion of very-low-density lipoprotein [9]. Interestingly, all of these *in vitro* models of steatosis have used HCV genotype 1-derived constructs. This contrasts with clinical studies conducted in patients with chronic HCV infection, which link the presence of steatosis to HCV genotype 3 [10]. Patients infected with genotype 3 have a higher prevalence of steatosis and more severe steatosis than those infected with other genotypes, and there is a correlation between the level of viraemia and the grade of steatosis [10,11]. Following successful antiviral treatment with a sustained viral response, patients infected with viral genotype 3 had a significant reduction in steatosis [12]. In contrast, patients with HCV genotype 1 had no change in hepatic steatosis after antiviral treatment, irrespective of the treatment

response. The mechanism responsible for this viral genotype 3-specific association with more severe steatosis remains unclear.

Viral proteins may be important but may not be sufficient to result in steatosis. Host factors, in particular an increased BMI, are important cofactors in the development of steatosis [11,13–22]. In many patients, particularly those infected with viral genotype 1, steatosis appears to be a result of the coexistence of obesity-related fatty liver with HCV infection. In these patients, the steatosis is associated with both perisinusoidal fibrosis, a characteristic feature of NAFLD, and increased BMI [23]. The concurrence of these disorders probably reflects the frequency with which both conditions occur in the population in 'industrialized' developing countries.

In our series of 148 consecutive patients with chronic HCV infection, steatosis was present in 61% [13]. Steatosis was mild in 41% and moderate or severe in 20%. This is similar to other histopathological studies of chronic HCV infection, which have reported fatty change in 30–70% of patients. In our study we found a very significant association between increasing BMI and grade of steatosis. The mean BMI (± standard deviation [SD]) of patients with no steatosis was 23.9 (± 4.3) kg/m², which is within the acceptable weight range for men and women. The mean BMI of patients with mild steatosis and patients with moderate or severe steatosis were within the overweight range: 26.5 (± 5.1) kg/m² and 28.4 (± 4.9) kg/m² for men and women, respectively. Of the 64 patients with an acceptable weight (BMI up to 25.5 kg/m²), four had grade 3 steatosis and three had grade 2 steatosis. Of the 23 obese patients (BMI over 30 kg/m²), only three patients had no steatosis and 10 had grade 1 steatosis. Diabetes was an infrequent finding in this group of patients (N = 4) and therefore its impact could not be evaluated. There was no statistically significant relationship, either crudely or adjusted, between grade of steatosis and alcohol intake or viral load. After adjusting for age, sex and alcohol consumption using multiple ordinal logistical regression, the effect of BMI on grade of steatosis remained significant (P = 0.0002).

Interestingly, in our group of patients with viral genotype 3, patients without steatosis were leaner (mean BMI 24 ± 3.3 kg/m²) than those with steatosis (BMI 27 ± 4.9 kg/m²) [24]. However, in contrast to patients with viral genotype 1, there was no significant relationship between grade of steatosis in patients with genotype 3 and increasing BMI. We conclude that in patients infected with HCV genotype 1, increasing BMI has a role in the pathogenesis of steatosis. In patients with genotype 3, steatosis may be caused by a cytopathic effect of the virus; however, we suspect that host body fat also contributes as a cofactor. This suggests a permissive rather than a direct role for increased BMI in genotype 3, and suggests that efforts to restore a lean BMI are relevant in patients infected with either genotype.

Steatosis accelerates the development of fibrosis in chronic HCV infection

The clinical importance of steatosis in patients with chronic HCV infection is because of the accelerated progression of fibrosis. A number of studies have demonstrated a significant relationship between steatosis and fibrosis, suggesting that in chronic HCV steatosis has a role in disease progression (Table 23.1) [11,13–22]. We have previously shown that in patients with chronic

Table 23.1 Studies evaluating the role of steatosis in chronic hepatitis C virus (HCV) infection and its association with host and viral factors and fibrosis.

| Reference | No. of patients | Steatosis (% patients) | Association of steatosis with | | | | | |
| | | | Host factors | | | Viral factors | | |
			BMI	Alcohol	DM	Genotype	Viral load	Fibrosis
Castera, 2003 [22]	96	54	Yes	No	NA	Yes, 3a	No	Yes
Serfaty, 2002 [21]	142	42	Yes	No	No	Yes, 3a	NA	Yes
Westin, 2002 [20]	98	42	Yes	No	NA	Yes, 3a	NA	Yes
Ong, 2001 [19]	170	53	Yes	No	No	NA	NA	Yes
Hwang, 2001 [18]	106	52	Yes	NA	NA	No	No	Yes
Adinolfi, 2001 [11]	180	48	Yes, genotype 1	NA	NA	Yes, 3a	Yes, 3a	Yes
Rubbia-Brandt, 2000 [10]	101	41	NA	NA	NA	Yes, 3a	Yes	Yes
Hourigan, 1999 [13]	148	61	Yes	No	No	Yes, 3a	No	Yes
Giannini, 1999 [17]	172	70	NA	NA	NA	No	NA	Yes
Czaja, 1998 [16]	60	52	Yes	NA	Yes	NA	NA	NA
Wong, 1996 [15]	200	38	NA	NA	NA	NA	NA	Yes
Fiore, 1996 [14]	121	60	Yes	No	No	NA	NA	Yes

NA = not assessed.

HCV infection, higher grades of steatosis were predictive of more severe levels of fibrosis ($P = 0.01$) [13]. In another study, patients with grades 3 and 4 steatosis had a significantly greater amount of fibrosis and a progression rate of fibrosis twice as high as those with grade 0–2 steatosis [11]. Similarly, patients infected with genotype 3, who showed the highest prevalence of steatosis, had a degree of fibrosis comparable with those infected with genotype 1 despite a significantly shorter duration of disease [11]. In a more recent study, worsening of steatosis was shown to be an independent factor associated with progression of fibrosis in paired liver biopsies from patients with untreated chronic HCV [22].

The mechanisms by which steatosis contributes to progression of this chronic viral infection remain uncertain. The majority of these patients do not exhibit the classic features of steatohepatitis with ballooning degeneration or Mallory's hyaline. However, many of the patients have zone 3 perisinusoidal fibrosis with a chicken-wire appearance, similar to that seen in steatohepatitis (Plate 12, facing p. 22) [23]. In our cohort of patients with steatosis and chronic HCV infection, we found a statistically significant relationship between perisinusoidal fibrosis and age ($r_s = 0.33$; $P = 0.003$) and grade of steatosis ($r_s = 0.35$; $P = 0.001$). Mean BMI was higher in patients with focal (28.4 ± 4.7 kg/m^2) or extensive (29.6 ± 5.9 kg/m^2) perisinusoidal fibrosis than in those patients with no perisinusoidal fibrosis (25.5 ± 3.7 kg/m^2). These findings suggest that in HCV infection, host factors, particularly adiposity, contribute to both steatosis and acinar fibrosis.

In patients with hepatic steatosis, the coexistence of HCV infection may provide an additional source of oxidative stress. A number of studies have shown that HCV proteins overexpressed in cultured cells and transgenic mice are associated with increased production of reactive oxygen species (ROS) and mitochondrial injury [25]. Any additional increase in the production of ROS may further deplete glutathione or other antioxidant pathways and result in oxidative stress. The fatty liver appears to be more vulnerable to cellular injury from ROS [26]. Chavin *et al.* [27] have demonstrated a relationship between obesity and hepatic energy homoeostasis that may help explain the vulnerability of a steatotic liver. Lipids or products of lipid metabolism have been shown to alter the expression of various mitochondrial membrane proteins. Some of these induced proteins (such as antiapoptotic factors)

are beneficial. Induction of other regulatory proteins may deplete hepatocytes of adenosine triphosphate (ATP) and make them more vulnerable to necrosis. Hepatocytes from genetically obese mice upregulate the expression of uncoupling protein-2, a mitochondrial protein that uncouples oxidative phosphorylation from mitochondrial respiration, decreasing the efficiency of mitochondrial ATP synthesis [27]. The addition of new insults on a background of increased uncoupling protein-2 expression may result in marked ATP depletion and further hepatocyte necrosis. However, most of these findings in animal models have not been systematically evaluated or confirmed in humans, and the mechanisms of liver injury associated with human fatty liver disease remain speculative.

Effect of weight reduction in patients with steatosis and chronic HCV infection

Since steatosis is associated with an accelerated development of hepatic fibrosis, there is currently interest in whether reducing the steatosis can slow the progression of chronic HCV infection. This would be of particular importance for patients who are nonresponders to current antiviral therapy.

We examined the effect of a 12-week dietary intervention on liver biochemistry and metabolic parameters in 19 subjects with steatosis and chronic HCV infection [28]. The patients were seen weekly by a dietitian during the intervention and monthly during a 6-month weight maintenance period. They followed an individualized calorie-controlled diet and increased their daily exercise for a goal of 0.5 kg/week weight loss. Paired liver biopsies were performed in 10 subjects, prior to and 3–6 months following the intervention, to determine the effect of weight loss on liver histology. There was a mean weight loss of 5.9 ± 3.2 kg and a mean reduction in waist circumference of 9.0 ± 5.0 cm. In 16 of the 19 patients, serum ALT levels fell progressively with weight loss. Mean fasting insulin fell from 16 ± 7 mmol/L to 11 ± 4 mmol/L ($P < 0.002$). Nine of the 10 patients with paired liver biopsies had a reduction in steatosis irrespective of viral genotype (Plate 13 A,B). The patient who did not show an improvement in steatosis had the smallest amount of weight loss, less than 2.5% of body weight. In the subjects with a reduction in steatosis, the median modified Knodell fibrosis score decreased from 3 to 1 ($P = 0.04$) and activated stellate cells significantly decreased in sinusoids and portal tracts ($P < 0.004$). Stellate cell activation (detected by α smooth muscle actin staining) showed a wide variation in the pretreatment group, ranging from 2–81 cells/mm^2 in acini and 168–1273 cells/mm^2 in the portal tracts. This wide variation may account for our failure to find a correlation between steatosis, perisinusoidal fibrosis and activated stellate cell density in an earlier study [23]. Although the range of stellate cell densities remained relatively wide after weight reduction, the mean values decreased from 32 (± 28 SD) to 3 (± 16) in the acini, and from 333 (± 322) to 149 (± 200) in the portal tracts and septa. The latter reduction is intriguing and suggests that steatosis has a distant effect on portal myofibroblasts, through pathways that remain unexplored. These results suggest that weight reduction has a role in minimizing liver injury and may provide an important adjunct treatment strategy for patients with steatosis and chronic HCV infection.

Obesity and alcoholic liver disease

Increased body mass index is a risk factor for fibrosis in alcoholic liver disease

Excess body weight has also been identified as a risk factor for the progression of fibrosis in ALD. In a study of 268 patients with an alcohol consumption of 110 ± 4 g/day for 24 ± 0.8 years, BMI and fasting blood glucose were independent risk factors for hepatic fibrosis [29]. These authors previously reported a study of 1604 patients drinking more than 50 g/day alcohol, in which excess body weight (BMI > 25 in women and > 27 in men) for at least 10 years was an independent risk factor for steatosis, acute alcoholic hepatitis and cirrhosis [30]. Patients who were overweight for at least 10 years were 2.15 times more likely to have cirrhosis than non-overweight patients, after adjustment for age, sex, daily alcohol consumption and total duration of alcohol abuse. Similarly, an earlier study of 152 recently abstinent alcoholics also demonstrated a significant relationship between increased body weight and the severity of histological changes [31].

Concurrent steatosis and alcohol consumption increases hepatic fibrosis in chronic HCV infection

In patients with chronic HCV infection, at least two recent studies have shown a synergistic interaction between steatosis (associated with increased BMI or viral genotype 3) and a relatively low alcohol consumption and the severity of hepatic fibrosis [21,11]. Serfaty *et al.* [21] found that in 142 untreated patients with chronic HCV infection, the median progression rate of fibrosis was twice as high among drinkers with steatosis than among drinkers without steatosis or non-drinkers with or without steatosis ($P = 0.02$). In an earlier study, Adinolfi *et al.* [11] examined the impact of a low alcohol intake (15–20 g/day) on the progression of hepatic fibrosis in patients with chronic HCV (viral genotype 1) infection in relation to the presence or absence of steatosis. The fibrosis score in the subgroup with steatosis and alcohol intake was significantly higher than that observed in patients with steatosis and no alcohol intake (2.82 ± 0.19 versus 2.05 ± 0.20, respectively; $P < 0.02$).

Mechanisms by which an increased body mass index contributes to fibrosis in alcoholic liver disease

The mechanisms by which increased weight contributes to ALD remain to be clarified. The histological features of obesity-related fatty liver disease and ALD are very similar and cannot be readily differentiated. In alcoholic patients, obesity may increase the development and severity of steatosis. The degree of fatty infiltration seen on liver biopsy is a risk factor for fibrogenesis in alcoholic patients [32]. The increased delivery of free fatty acids to the liver in obesity may result in a greater induction of cytochrome P450 2E1 (CYP2E1) resulting in increased formation of ROS and lipid peroxidation [33]. CYP2E1 is highly inducible by ethanol, and is also upregulated in obesity and by a high-fat low-carbohydrate diet [34]. As a key microsomal oxidase involved in fatty acid oxidation, it generates pro-oxidant species that produce cellular injury when antioxidant pathways are depleted [35].

An additional factor that may contribute to liver injury in obese alcoholics is an alteration in hepatic macrophage function. In a study of 36 alcoholics, a positive correlation was found between production of the pro-inflammatory cytokine interleukin 1β (IL-1β) by stimulated monocytes and BMI, percentage body fat, abdominal circumference and total histological score (derived from the sum of fat, necrosis, fibrosis and inflammation) [36]. The liver has a very large population of resident macrophages (Kupffer cells) derived from circulating monocytes. In ALD, elevated circulating endotoxin leads to the activation of Kupffer cells, resulting in the synthesis and secretion of pro-inflammatory cytokines, prostaglandins and other factors [37]. These molecules promote an inflammatory response, which may result in peroxidative damage to cellular membranes. Altered Kupffer cell function and cytokine production has also been shown to contribute to the pathogenesis of liver injury in animal models of NAFLD [38].

These studies suggest that excess body weight in alcoholic patients can potentiate the metabolic effects of ethanol. This is important because weight reduction and dietary fat restriction may have a role in minimizing liver injury in patients with ALD. A prospective study in a large group of alcoholic patients is warranted to address this issue and may provide further insights into the pathogenesis of fatty liver disease.

Hepatic iron storage and NAFLD

The relationship between NAFLD and hepatic iron storage remains unclear. Two questions have been raised in the literature. First, can NAFLD (or more specifically the insulin resistance syndrome) be associated with an increased level of hepatic iron in the absence of HFE mutations and, secondly, is iron a cofactor in exacerbating NASH? Abnormalities of serum iron studies, usually expressing as hyperferritinaemia [39], are common in patients with steatosis and NASH and have been described in up to 60% of cases. The trans-ferrin saturation is variably elevated [39–41], but usually it is within normal limits [41–43]. When HFE mutations have been assessed, an increased frequency of the major C282Y and H63D mutations have been demonstrated in most series, with up to two-thirds or more of patients carrying one of the mutant alleles (Table 23.2).

Insulin resistance-associated iron overload

The abnormal iron studies that can be seen in NASH do not necessarily correlate with the presence of stainable iron, and conversely siderosis of grade 2+ or greater can occur without HFE mutation. With respect to this latter group, it has been postulated that insulin resistance itself may somehow lead to iron loading, a phenomenon termed insulin resistance-associated hepatic iron overload (IR-HIO) [41]. This form of iron overload has been suggested recently to be up to 10 times more common than genetic haemochromatosis [44]. Mendler et al. [41] found that patients with normal transferrin saturation, elevated serum ferritin and siderosis on liver biopsy almost always (94%) demonstrated the insulin resistance syndrome, although only 52% actually showed NAFLD on biopsy. In support of this, treatment of insulin resistance by strict dietary and antidiabetic control was shown to lead to a reduction in serum iron indices as well as hepatic iron stores in some patients [45], although this has not been confirmed [44]. The pattern of iron deposition in patients with this metabolically induced iron loading differs

Table 23.2 Studies evaluating the role of iron in disease progression in patients with NALFD and NASH.

Reference	Number of patients	NASH or NAFLD (% patients)	Increased liver iron (≥2) (% patients)	HFE mutation (%)		Correlation HFE mutation and fibrosis	Correlation iron and fibrosis
				C282Y	Any		
Bacon, 1994 [48]	33	100	29	NA	NA	NA	No
George, 1998 [39]	51	100	41	31	53	Yes	Yes
Bonkovsky, 1999 [40]	57	100	NS	20	69	Yes	No
Younossi, 1999 [49]	65	100	NS	NA	NA	NA	No
Angulo, 1999 [47]	144	100	NS	NA	NA	NA	No
Mendler, 1999 [41]	161	52	100	20	70	No	No
Fargion, 2001 [42]	40	78	45	45	65	No	No
Chitturi, 2002 [43]	93	100	10	22	39	No	No

NA, not assessed; NAFLD, non-alcoholic fatty liver disease; NASH, non-alcoholic steatohepatitis; NS, not stated.

from typical genetic haemochromatosis [46], showing milder deposition with a mixed distribution in both hepatocytes and sinusoidal (Kupffer) cells. The mechanism responsible for iron loading remains unclear.

Iron as a cofactor in NASH progression

The coexistence of increased iron stores and NAFLD is of potential importance because iron is a source of oxidative stress and can be a cofactor for disease progression in ALD and chronic HCV infection. The role of iron as a cofactor has been studied in NAFLD/NASH, but the results are not clear-cut. In two studies (Table 23.2), the presence of at least one copy of the C282Y allele was associated with increased hepatic iron and with more advanced hepatic fibrosis [39,40]. Using multivariate analysis, George et al. [39] showed that the effect was caused by increased hepatic iron concentration induced by the gene mutation. However, the second study found that although the presence of an HFE mutation was linked to increased fibrosis, there was no statistical association between the iron concentration or histological iron score and fibrosis. Other groups have been unable to confirm the iron–fibrosis association in NASH, and most of the studies addressing the role of iron have concluded that increased hepatic iron content shows no significant association with the degree of fibrosis in these patients (Table 23.2) [41–43,47–49].

Interpretation of these studies is complicated for several reasons. The definition of NASH varies, and many include cases of steatosis with lymphocytic infiltrates (but without ballooning degeneration, neutrophil polymorphs or Mallory bodies) in the NASH group. These cases probably should be regarded as type 2 NAFLD rather than true NASH. The assay for tissue iron can give artificially low levels in steatotic liver because of cellular swelling by fat, which could lower the tissue iron concentration in patients who have more severe fatty liver disease. Finally, referral bias to centres specializing in iron storage diseases could also be a confounding factor [43]. It is also worth noting that although the study by George et al. [39] found an association between C282Y, increased hepatic iron and fibrosis, analysis of their patients by gender showed that females had significantly less iron deposition than males. However, they had significantly greater BMI and liver fibrosis, suggesting that iron has, at best, a secondary role in the progression of liver injury.

Venesection as a therapeutic option

Because the nature of the interaction between NAFLD and increased hepatic iron remains clouded, it is not possible to offer clear recommendations on management. Preliminary data in small groups of patients, however, suggest that venesection could result in improvement of liver enzyme abnormalities and reduced inflammatory activity in the liver [50]. Venesection has also been advocated for IR-HIO and is successful at iron mobilization, but in this instance may not be associated with any significant change in the liver enzymes [44]. Interestingly, venesection was shown to improve peripheral insulin resistance in a group of patients with high-ferritin type 2 diabetes [51], but the mechanism remains unclear. The role of iron depletion therefore warrants prospective study in a large group of patients who must be carefully defined histologically as to the type of NAFLD, but until such studies are carried out venesection in NAFLD should be regarded as experimental.

NASH and liver transplantation

Orthotopic liver transplantation (OLT) potentially introduces several extra problems for patients with NAFLD/NASH. These include the complications of corticosteroids, and other immunosuppressive agents that could lead to a further increase in insulin resistance [52], low-grade antigraft responses contributing to inflammatory oxidative stress, and possibly enhanced fibrogenesis mediated by immunosuppressives causing enhancement of the TGF-β pathway. NASH has not been a common biopsy diagnosis after transplantation, and in a recent series it accounted for only 1% of diagnoses 1 year post-OLT [53]. However, there are three main clinically relevant questions:

1 Does NASH recur in the allograft?
2 If it does recur, is the progression faster (as it seems to be in some patients with recurrent hepatitis C)?
3 Is pure steatosis as benign in the context of liver transplantation as it is in the native liver?

Recurrence of NASH after liver transplantation

Recurrence of NASH has been documented in small numbers of patients in a number of studies; overall, however, it appears that recurrence is frequent when NASH is documented in the explanted liver. An early report of eight patients transplanted for NASH described the subsequent development of NAFLD in six recipients (75%) and NASH in three (38%) [54]. The two patients who did not develop NAFLD had lost weight postoperatively. Others have similar findings, with the frequent development of NAFLD in 60–75% of patients, and also classical NASH in 33–66% of patients [55–57].

Because steatosis can disappear in end-stage liver disease [58], it has been suggested that some cases of cryptogenic cirrhosis result from 'burnt-out' NASH [58,59]. In support of this, NAFLD/NASH can develop after OLT for cryptogenic cirrhosis, although this occurs less frequently than in patients with histological evidence of NASH at the time of transplantation. In 114 patients combined from three recent series [52,60,61], 47% had NAFLD diagnosed in a post-OLT biopsy but NASH developed in only 7–16% [52,61,62].

Natural history of NASH after transplantation

Assessment of outcomes is hampered again by small numbers and limited duration of follow-up. Although some have suggested that the risk of progressive liver disease is low [52], other reports describe the development of fibrosis and cirrhosis in up to 33% of cases [54,56,61]. Importantly, in a minority of patients the disease progresses more rapidly compared with the native liver. Cirrhosis and graft failure have occasionally been seen after post-OLT intervals of only 20–27 months [55,61]. The risk factors for rapid progression and the optimal management remain unknown.

Although Ong et al. [61] found that four patients who developed pure steatosis after transplantation for cryptogenic cirrhosis had a benign course similar to steatosis in the native liver, others have noted that steatosis can be followed by the later development of classical NASH and bridging fibrosis [52,54]. It remains unclear just how frequently pure steatosis can convert to progressive disease. However, in the absence of clear data it seems prudent to recommend that follow-up of patients who have risk factors for NASH and pure steatosis on graft biopsy (without classical NASH) should be more careful in the post-OLT setting.

NAFLD in the donor liver

When steatosis is present in the donor liver at the time of OLT it can have an adverse impact [63]. Grafts with severe macrovesicular steatosis have a high risk of primary graft non-function and the use of such donor organs is contraindicated. Ischaemia and/or reperfusion injury to vulnerable steatotic hepatocytes results in the release of free lipid into the sinusoids, activation of the coagulation cascade and heightened free radical formation [64], causing haemorrhagic necrosis in the graft. Obesity, increased donor age and alcohol have been shown to have a role in the genesis of fatty donor liver (reviewed in [64]). The use of donor liver with mild to moderate steatosis is not contraindicated, but ideally such grafts should be considered for use when donor and recipient risk factors are minimized (short ischaemic time, good recipient condition and non-emergency transplant). Microvesicular steatosis has not been found to cause primary graft non-function [63,65] and it is possible that in some cases the lesion described by the pathologist as microvesicular steatosis may, in some cases, represent reversible, pre-terminal mitochondrial swelling.

NASH and other liver diseases

The coexistence of NASH and a second liver disease other than those already described does not appear to be a common problem. Brunt et al. [3] analysed 3581 liver biopsies and found histological evidence of strictly defined NASH in almost 12%. In 93 of 419 biopsies with NASH (22%) there was evidence of a second liver disease, but this was usually hepatitis C; only 13 biopsies had evidence of NASH and a second non-HCV chronic liver disease. The coexistant diseases included primary biliary cirrhosis, α-1 antitrypsin deficiency, haemochromatosis, chronic hepatitis B and drug-induced hepatitis. Despite the rarity of NASH as an identifiable cofactor in other chronic liver diseases, its recognition is important since weight loss could theoretically be of therapeutic benefit. Moreover, as Brunt's analysis was restricted only to NASH with at least perivenular fibrosis; a much larger number of patients are likely to have co-existing NAFLD types 1 and 2, and a second liver disease. As discussed earlier, the benign nature of pure steatosis and steatosis with lymphocytic infiltrates cannot be assumed in the presence of a second form of chronic liver disease. In our own unpublished series of over 200 consecutive liver biopsies, moderate or severe steatosis was identified in 20%.

The potential relationship between NASH and α_1-antitrypsin deficiency is worth noting. Heterozygous phenotypes, including MS and MZ, have been found at significantly higher frequencies in patients with NASH [56,57]. Czaja [66] found that 20% of patients with NASH have a variant phenotype and this was significantly higher than the frequency in patients with chronic hepatitis C. It has also been noted that of 30 patients with end-stage NASH who were assessed at the Mayo Clinic for OLT, five had the MZ phenotype [56]. Just as other liver diseases have been reported to be at an increased risk of progression in the presence of heterozygosity for α_1-antitrypsin deficiency, the coexistence of NASH and the MZ phenotype could identify a subgroup of patients who are more prone to develop progressive fibrosis. Since α_1-antitrypsin serum levels are routinely tested, without recourse to allelic analysis for heterozygosity, it is likely that this state is currently under-recognized in NASH patients.

The effect of drug-induced hepatitis and pre-existing NASH has not been studied in a systematic way. In methotrexate-induced liver injury, obesity and diabetes have been identified as risk factors for fibrosis. A study of 24 patients by Langman *et al.* [67] found that some patients receiving methotrexate who developed progressive fibrosis had histological NASH as well as risk factors for this disease, such as obesity or diabetes. On the other hand, other patients without risk factors for NASH, but with a higher mean cumulative dose, developed similar histological changes, suggesting that methotrexate may be sufficient to cause steatohepatitis with fibrosis. Anecdotally we have seen several cases of drug-induced hepatitis and NASH occurring simultaneously. In one, a patient with cirrhosis had histological evidence of both (non-alcoholic) steatohepatitis and chronic hepatitis, the latter resulting from nitrofurantoin toxicity. Treatment with drug withdrawal as well as weight loss resulted in reversal of the steatohepatitis and marked symptomatic improvement despite the persistence of cirrhosis. In the second case, an obese patient receiving tamoxifen was diagnosed with NASH and bridging fibrosis. Withdrawal of this drug, a documented cause of NASH, failed to result in any improvement in liver enzymes and histology over several months, but the subsequent institution of a weight-loss programme under the supervision of a dietician led to improvement in liver function and symptoms. Others have suggested an interaction between tamoxifen and additional factors such as obesity involved in the development of NAFLD [68]. NASH is likely to be multifactorial in these cases, and the presence of two exacerbating causes could be a factor in the advanced fibrosis seen on biopsy.

Conclusions

In patients with NASH, progressive fibrosis is multifactorial and is related to steatosis, oxidative injury and genetic factors. Treatment of any one of these three may abrogate injury.

Although NAFLD without true steatohepatitis is generally a benign condition, the presence of a second liver disease may provide a synergistic combination of steatosis, cellular adaptation and oxidative damage that exacerbates any liver damage. Indeed, steatosis is now well recognized as a factor that accelerates the development of fibrosis in chronic HCV infection. Increased BMI and viral genotype contribute to the pathogenesis of steatosis in these infected patients. Similarly, obesity and its attendant insulin resistance are potential additive factors in the progression of alcoholic liver disease. This suggests that both alcoholic and non-alcoholic steatohepatitis may exacerbate the other and they could be more usefully grouped as a single non-prejudicial entity, steatohepatitis. If this becomes the case, all contributing causes could then be attributed a potential role and be treated as necessary. Although less common, a similar argument holds for drug-induced liver diseases.

The abnormal ferritin in many patients with insulin resistance, NAFLD and NASH is reflected in mildly increased hepatic iron stores (insulin resistance-associated hepatic iron overload). There may be an increased frequency of *HFE* mutation, but the evidence for a role of increased liver iron in disease progression is not proven.

The finding that patients with cryptogenic cirrhosis have risk factors for NASH now suggests that end-stage disease may be a greater problem than previously recognized.

Among OLT recipients, those transplanted for NASH or cryptogenic cirrhosis are at increased risk to develop NAFLD and NASH in the allograft. Pure steatosis can evolve into steatohepatitis and progressive fibrosis after OLT, and a minority of patients will have a rapidly progressive course.

These findings indicate that NAFLD/NASH must be taken into account even when it is not the primary cause of chronic liver disease, for it will be present with ever-increasing frequency in coming years. The challenge of future studies is to dissect, understand and ultimately control the critical pathogenetic pathways that drive the synergistic effect of steatosis on disordered cellular homoeostasis and fibrogenesis and to quantify its effects in a variety of diseases. In patients with chronic HCV infection, weight reduction improves steatosis and, in some patients, may reduce fibrosis and stellate cell activation. The degree to which weight loss and treatment of the insulin resistance syndrome can minimize liver injury in patients with other forms of chronic liver disease remains to be determined.

References

1 Brunt EM. Non-alcoholic steatohepatitis: definition and pathology. *Semin Liver Dis* 2001; **21**: 3–16.

2 Matteoni CA, Younossi ZM, Gramlich T *et al.* Non-alcoholic fatty liver disease: a spectrum of clinical and pathological severity. *Gastroenterology* 1999; **116**: 1413–9.

3 Brunt EM, Ramrakhiani S, Cordes BG *et al.* Concurrence of histologic features of steatohepatitis with other forms of chronic liver disease. *Mod Pathol* 2003; **16**: 49–56.

4 Ishak KG. Chronic hepatitis: morphology and nomenclature. *Mod Pathol* 1994; **7**: 690–713.

5 Teli MR, James OF, Burt AD *et al.* The natural history of non-alcoholic fatty liver: a follow-up study. *Hepatology* 1995; **22**: 1714–9.

6 Day CP, James OFW. Hepatic steatosis: innocent bystander or guilty party? *Hepatology* 1998; **27**: 1463–6.

7 Moriya K, Yotsuyanagi H, Shintani Y *et al.* Hepatitis C virus core protein induces hepatic steatosis in transgenic mice. *J Gen Virol* 1997; **78**: 1527–31.

8 Lerat H, Honda M, Beard MR *et al.* Steatosis and liver cancer in transgenic mice expressing the structural and nonstructural proteins of hepatitis C virus. *Gastroenterology* 2002; **122**: 352–65.

9 Perlemuter G, Sabile A, Letteron P *et al.* Hepatitis C virus core protein inhibits microsomal triglyceride transfer protein activity and very low density lipoprotein secretion: a model of viral-related steatosis. *FASEB J* 2002; **16**: 185–94.

10 Rubbia-Brandt L, Quadri R, Abid K *et al.* Hepatocyte steatosis is a cytopathic effect of hepatitis C virus genotype 3. *J Hepatol* 2000; **33**: 106–15.

11 Adinolfi LE, Gambardella M, Andreana A *et al.* Steatosis accelerates the progression of liver damage of chronic hepatitis C patients and correlates with specific HCV genotype and visceral obesity. *Hepatology* 2001; **33**: 1358–64.

12 Kumar D, Farrell GC, Fung C, George J. Hepatitis C virus genotype 3 is cytopathic to hepatocytes: reversal of hepatic steatosis after sustained therapeutic response. *Hepatology* 2002; **36**: 1266–72.

13 Hourigan LF, Macdonald GA, Purdie D *et al.* Fibrosis in chronic hepatitis C correlates significantly with body mass index and steatosis. *Hepatology* 1999; **29**: 1215–9.

14 Fiore G, Fera G, Napoli N *et al.* Liver steatosis and chronic hepatitis C: a spurious association? *Eur J Gastroenterol Hepatol* 1996; **8**: 125–9.

15 Wong VS, Wight DG, Palmer CR, Alexander GJ. Fibrosis and other histological features in chronic hepatitis C virus infection: a statistical model. *J Clin Pathol* 1996; **49**: 465–9.

16 Czaja AJ, Carpenter HA, Santrach PJ, Moore SB. Host- and disease-specific factors affecting steatosis in chronic hepatitis C. *J Hepatol* 1998; **29**: 198–206.

17 Giannini E, Ceppa P, Botta F *et al.* Steatosis and bile duct damage in chronic hepatitis C: distribution and relationships in a group of northern Italian patients. *Liver* 1999; **19**: 432–7.

18 Hwang SJ, Luo JC, Chu CW *et al.* Hepatic steatosis in chronic hepatitis C virus infection: prevalence and clinical correlation. *J Gastroenterol Hepatol* 2001; **16**: 190–5.

19 Ong JP, Younossi ZM, Speer C, *et al.* Chronic hepatitis C and superimposed non-alcoholic fatty liver disease. *Liver* 2001; **21**: 266–71.

20 Westin J, Nordlinder H, Lagging M, Norkrans G, Wejstal R. Steatosis accelerates fibrosis development over time in hepatitis C virus genotype 3 infected patients. *J Hepatol* 2002; **37**: 837–42.

21 Serfaty L, Poujol-Robert A, Carbonell N *et al.* Effect of the interaction between steatosis and alcohol intake on liver fibrosis progression in chronic hepatitis C. *Am J Gastroenterol* 2002; **97**: 1807–12.

22 Castera L, Hezode C, Roudot-Thoraval F *et al.* Worsening of steatosis is an independent factor of fibrosis progression in untreated patients with chronic hepatitis C and paired liver biopsies. *Gut* 2003; **52**: 288–92.

23 Clouston AD, Jonsson JR, Purdie DM *et al.* Steatosis and chronic hepatitis C: analysis of fibrosis and stellate cell activation. *J Hepatol* 2001; **34**: 314–20.

24 Jonsson JR, Edwards-Smith CJ, Purdie D *et al.* Body composition and hepatic steatosis as precursors of fibrosis in chronic hepatitis C patients [Reply]. *Hepatology* 1999; **30**: 1531–2.

25 Okuda M, Li K, Beard MR *et al.* Mitochondrial injury, oxidative stress, and antioxidant gene expression are induced by hepatitis C virus core protein. *Gastroenterology* 2002; **122**: 366–75.

26 Day CP, James OFW. Steatohepatitis: a tale of two 'hits'? *Gastroenterology* 1998; **114**: 842–5.

27 Chavin KD, Yang S, Lin HZ et al. Obesity induces expression of uncoupling protein-2 in hepatocytes and promotes liver ATP depletion. *J Biol Chem* 1999; **274**: 5692–700.

28 Hickman IJ, Clouston AD, Macdonald GA et al. The effect of weight reduction on liver histology and biochemistry in patients with chronic hepatitis C. *Gut* 2002; **51**: 89–94.

29 Raynard B, Balian A, Fallik D et al. Risk factors of fibrosis in alcohol-induced liver disease. *Hepatology* 2002; **35**: 635–8.

30 Naveau S, Giraud V, Borotto E et al. Excess weight risk factor for alcoholic liver disease. *Hepatology* 1997; **25**: 108–11.

31 Iturriaga H, Bunout D, Hirsch S, Ugarte G. Overweight as a risk factor or a predictive sign of histological liver damage in alcoholics. *Am J Clin Nutr* 1988; **47**: 235–8.

32 Reeves HL, Burt AD, Wood S, Day CP. Hepatic stellate cell activation occurs in the absence of hepatitis in alcoholic liver disease and correlates with the severity of steatosis. *J Hepatol* 1996; **25**: 677–83.

33 de la Maza MP, Hirsch S, Petermann M et al. Changes in microsomal activity in alcoholism and obesity. *Alcohol Clin Exp Res* 2000; **24**: 605–10.

34 Mezey E. Dietary fat and alcoholic liver disease. *Hepatology* 1998; **28**: 901–5.

35 Robertson G, Leclercq I, Farrell GC. Non-alcoholic steatosis and steatohepatitis. II. Cytochrome P450 enzymes and oxidative stress. *Am J Physiol Gastrointest Liver Physiol* 2001; **281**: G1135–9.

36 Bunout D, Munoz C, Lopez M et al. Interleukin 1 and tumor necrosis factor in obese alcoholics compared with normal-weight patients. *Am J Clin Nutr* 1996; **63**: 373–6.

37 Casini A. Alcohol-induced fatty liver and inflammation: where do Kupffer cells act? *J Hepatol* 2000; **32**: 1026–30.

38 Diehl AM IV. Non-alcoholic fatty liver disease abnormalities in macrophage function and cytokines. *Am J Physiol Gastrointest Liver Physiol* 2002; **282**: G1–5

39 George DK, Goldwurm S, MacDonald GA et al. Increased hepatic iron concentration in non-alcoholic steatohepatitis is associated with increased fibrosis. *Gastroenterology* 1998; **114**: 311–8.

40 Bonkovsky HL, Jawaid Q, Tortorelli K et al. Non-alcoholic steatohepatitis and iron: increased prevalence of mutations of the *HFE* gene in non-alcoholic steatohepatitis. *J Hepatol* 1999; **31**: 421–9.

41 Mendler MH, Turlin B, Moirand R et al. Insulin resistance-associated hepatic iron overload. *Gastroenterology* 1999; **117**: 1155–63.

42 Fargion S, Mattioli M, Fracanzani AL et al. Hyperferritinemia, iron overload, and multiple metabolic alterations identify patients at risk for nonalcoholic steatohepatitis. *Am J Gastroenterol* 2001; **96**: 2448–55.

43 Chitturi S, Weltman M, Farrell GC et al. HFE mutations, hepatic iron, and fibrosis: ethnic-specific association of NASH with C282Y but not with fibrotic severity. *Hepatology* 2002; **36**: 142–9.

44 Guillygomarc'h A, Mendler MH, Moirand R et al. Venesection therapy of insulin resistance-associated hepatic iron overload. *J Hepatol* 2001; **35**: 344–9.

45 Vigano M, Vergani A, Trombini P, Paleari F, Piperno A. Insulin resistance influence iron metabolism and hepatic steatosis in type II diabetes. *Gastroenterology* 2000; **118**: 986–7.

46 Turlin B, Mendler MH, Moirand R et al. Histologic features of the liver in insulin resistance-associated iron overload: a study of 139 patients. *Am J Clin Pathol* 2001; **116**: 263–70.

47 Angulo P, Keach JC, Batts KP, Lindor KD. Independent predictors of liver fibrosis in patients with non-alcoholic steatohepatitis. *Hepatology* 1999; **30**: 1356–62.

48 Bacon BR, Farahvash MJ, Janney CG, Neuschwander-Tetri BA. Non-alcoholic steatohepatitis: an expanded clinical entity. *Gastroenterology* 1994; **107**: 1103–9.

49 Younossi ZM, Gramlich T, Bacon BR et al. Hepatic iron and non-alcoholic fatty liver disease. *Hepatology* 1999; **30**: 847–50.

50 Nitecki J, Jackson FW, Allen ML, Farr VL, Jackson FW. Effect of phlebotomy on non-alcoholic steatohepatitis. *Gastroenterology* 2000; **118**: A1474.

51 Fernandez-Real JM, Penarroja G, Castro A et al. Blood letting in high-ferritin type 2 diabetes: effects on insulin sensitivity and β-cell function. *Diabetes* 2002; **51**: 1000–4.

52 Contos MJ, Cales W, Sterling RK et al. Development of non-alcoholic fatty liver disease after orthotopic liver transplantation for cryptogenic cirrhosis. *Liver Transpl* 2001; **7**: 363–73.

53 Berenguer M, Rayon JM, Prieto M et al. Are post-transplantation protocol liver biopsies useful in the long term? *Liver Transpl* 2001; **7**: 790–6.

54 Kim WR, Poterucha JJ, Porayko MK et al. Recurrence of non-alcoholic steatohepatitis following liver transplantation. *Transplantation* 1996; **62**: 1802–5.

55 Molloy RM, Komorowski R, Varma RR. Recurrent non-alcoholic steatohepatitis and cirrhosis after liver transplantation. *Liver Transpl Surg* 1997; **3**: 177–8.

56 Charlton M, Kasparova P, Weston S et al. Frequency of non-alcoholic steatohepatitis as a cause of advanced liver disease. *Liver Transpl* 2001; **7**: 608–14.

57 Chinnakotla S, Schafer D, Radio SJ et al. Is non-alcoholic steatohepatitis a systemic disease? Evidence from liver transplantation. *Hepatology* 2001; **34** (Part 2): 361A.

58 Caldwell SH, Oelsner DH, Iezzoni JC et al. Cryptogenic cirrhosis: clinical characterization and risk factors for underlying disease. *Hepatology* 1999; **29**: 664–9.

59 Poonawala A, Nair SP, Thuluvath PJ. Prevalence of obesity and diabetes in patients with cryptogenic cirrhosis: a case–control study. *Hepatology* 2000; **32**(Part 1): 689–92.

60 Amaro R, Montalbano M, Acosta RC *et al.* Non-alcoholic fatty liver disease (NAFLD) after orthotopic liver transplantation (OLT) in patients with cryptogenic cirrhosis (CC) and non-alcoholic steatohepatitis (NASH). *Gastroenterology* 2001; **120**: A118.

61 Ong J, Younossi ZM, Reddy V *et al.* Cryptogenic cirrhosis and post-transplantation non-alcoholic fatty liver disease. *Liver Transpl* 2001; **7**: 797–801.

62 Charlton MR, Kondo M, Roberts SK *et al.* Liver transplantation for cryptogenic cirrhosis. *Liver Transpl Surg* 1997; **3**: 359–64.

63 Cheng YF, Chen CL, Lai CY *et al.* Assessment of donor fatty livers for liver transplantation. *Transplantation* 2001; **71**: 1221–5.

64 Urena MAG, Moreno Gonzalez E, Romero CJ, Ruiz-Delgado FC, Moreno Sanz C. An approach to the rational use of steatotic donor livers in liver transplantation. *Hepatogastroenterology* 1999; **46**: 1164–73.

65 Fishbein TM, Fiel MI, Emre S *et al.* Use of livers with microvesicular fat safely expands the donor pool. *Transplantation* 1997; **64**: 248–51.

66 Czaja AJ. Frequency and significance of phenotypes for alpha1-antitrypsin deficiency in type 1 autoimmune hepatitis. *Dig Dis Sci* 1998; **43**: 1725–31.

67 Langman G, Hall PM, Todd G. Role of non-alcoholic steatohepatitis in methotrexate-induced liver injury. *J Gastroenterol Hepatol* 2001; **16**: 1395–401.

68 Chitturi S, Farrell GC. Etiopathogenesis of non-alcoholic steatohepatitis. *Semin Liver Dis* 2001; **21**: 27–41.

24 Recent advances

Richard Kirsch, Pauline de la M. Hall, Jacob George, Arthur J. McCullough & Geoffrey C. Farrell

Introduction

The purpose of this chapter is to highlight significant conceptual advances in the field of NAFLD/NASH that have occurred in the last 12 months, and hence does not seek to be a comprehensive review of all papers in the field. In many instances, work that was submitted in abstract form has now been published as definitive papers, thus allowing for a more detailed discussion than was possible in the preceding chapters. In other instances, new reports – both published papers and abstracts – particularly those relating to management, methods for evaluating liver pathology, as well as animal models of NAFLD, have become available. The topics discussed will largely follow the order of chapters in the book.

Pathology of NAFLD

Gramlich *et al.* [1] investigated the clinical and pathological features in patients with NAFLD that are associated with the development of fibrosis. Of the 132 NAFLD patients studied, 21% had advanced fibrosis (septal/bridging fibrosis or cirrhosis), 20% had sinusoidal fibrosis, 17% had perivenular fibrosis and 27% had periportal/portal-type fibrosis. A large number of histological and clinical parameters were studied but only ballooning degeneration and Mallory bodies were found to be independent predictors of perivenular and sinusoidal fibrosis. Serum aspartate aminotransferase : alanine aminotransferase (AST : ALT) ratio and ballooning degeneration were independent predictors of periportal/portal-type fibrosis. This study highlights the importance of ongoing liver injury, in the form of ballooning degeneration and Mallory bodies, in the development of fibrosis in NAFLD.

Megamitochondria with crystalline inclusions (MMC) are well documented in hepatocytes of patients with NASH (see Chapters 2 and 11). Le *et al.* [2] investigated the zonal distribution of MMC by transmission electron microscopy and examined their relationship to stage of disease [2]. The study included liver biopsy specimens from 31 patients, 29 with NASH and two with cryptogenic cirrhosis thought to represent 'burnt out' NASH. MMC were equally and randomly distributed throughout all zones, and showed no variation in number with respect to fibrosis stage. They also showed no apparent relationship with the presence and number of ballooned hepatocytes, or with markers of oxidative stress. The exact biochemical nature and biological function of MMC is yet to be elucidated.

A novel, semi-quantitative, numerical grading system for NASH has recently been proposed by Mendler *et al.* [3] in which an activity score (AS) is obtained by adding the scores (0–3) assigned to four histologic parameters: lobular necroinflammation, Mallory bodies, hepatocyte ballooning and perisinusoidal fibrosis. Portal fibrosis (PF) is graded separately (0–6). The combination of AS and PF is used for grading NASH severity as follows: Grade 1 (PF: 0–2 and AS: 0–4), Grade 2 (PF: 3 or AS: 5–7) and Grade 3 (PF: 4–6 or AS: 8–12). The authors report satisfactory inter- and intraobserver reproducibility of this system. Advanced grade was found to correlate with diabetes mellitus, elevated alkaline phosphatase and low platelets in a small cohort of 25 patients with NAFLD. Further studies are needed to evaluate the clinical utility and reproducibility of this novel scoring system compared with existing grading systems [3].

The pathology of NASH has been the subject of recent reviews with a special focus on the various pathological lesions encountered in NASH [4–8]. Challenging areas in NASH diagnosis, including NAFLD/NASH in children and NASH-related cirrhosis are discussed [4]. The role of and controversy surrounding liver biopsies in NAFLD/NASH are likewise addressed [6–8].

Pathogenesis of NAFLD/NASH

The pathogenesis of NAFLD/NASH in humans as discussed in Chapter 7, and the role of animal models as discussed in Chapter 8, have been the subject of several recent reviews [9,10] and an editorial [11].

Human studies

The role of oxidative stress

Videla et al. [12] investigated oxidative stress-related parameters in livers of 31 patients with NAFLD (15 with simple steatosis, 16 with NASH) compared with 12 controls. Patients with steatosis showed a fourfold increase in hepatic protein carbonyl content and reduced glutathione content, superoxide dismutase (SOD) activity and ferric reducing ability of plasma (FRAP) by 57%, 48% and 21% respectively compared to controls). Patients with steatohepatitis showed decreased glutathione content (27%), SOD activity (64%), catalase activity (48%) and FRAP (33%) compared with controls. Protein carbonyl content was comparable with controls. In contrast to livers with simple steatosis, livers with steatohepatitis showed significantly increased levels of microsomal p-nitrophenol hydroxylation (52%) and CYP2E1 content (142%) compared with controls. These findings confirm the presence of oxidative stress in NAFLD and provide further evidence that oxidative stress is increased with transition from steatosis to steatohepatitis (see Chapter 7).

Weight loss and cytochrome P4502E1 (CYP2E1) activity

Emery et al. [13] investigated the effect of weight loss on CYP2E1 activity in morbidly obese patients. The study included 16 morbidly obese patients with NAFLD undergoing gastroplasty for weight reduction, and 16 normal weight controls. Hepatic CYP2E1 activity,

determined by chlorzoxazone (CLZ) clearance, was evaluated pre-operatively and postoperatively (at 6 weeks and 1 year) in the morbidly obese patients. Total and unbound CLZ clearance (Cl_u/F) was elevated approximately threefold compared with controls. The Cl_u/F was significantly higher in patients with steatosis involving > 50% of hepatocytes compared with those in which steatosis was present in ≤ 50% of hepatocytes. At postoperative week 6, the median body mass index (BMI) decreased by 11%, total CLZ clearance by 16% and Cl_u/F by 18%. At 1 year median BMI decreased by 33%, total CLZ clearance by 46% and Cl_u/F by 35%. Those subjects with a year-1 BMI < 30 kg/m^2 had a median Cl_u/F that was 63% lower than the median recorded for all other subjects. In summary, this study demonstrates an association between morbid obesity and upregulation of hepatic CYP2E1 activity. It also provides further evidence to suggest that the latter may be related to, or caused by, the hepatic pathology that results from morbid obesity.

Leptin and adiponectin

A study by Chalasani et al. [14] investigated the relationship between serum leptin levels and NASH. Serum leptin levels were measured in 26 patients with NASH and 20 well-matched controls; values were then correlated with anthropometric, biochemical, metabolic and histological data. In addition, hepatic leptin and leptin receptor messenger RNA (mRNA) expression were measured in liver biopsy specimens in subsets of patients with NASH ($n = 5$) and simple steatosis ($n = 5$). There was no statistically significant difference in serum leptin levels between patients with NASH and their controls. Serum leptin levels did not correlate significantly with liver histology, serum ALT, fasting insulin levels or insulin resistance. Leptin mRNA was not detected in the cell lysate of liver biopsy specimens of subjects with NASH or steatosis. Patients with NASH and simple steatosis did not differ statistically with respect to serum leptin levels and hepatic leptin receptor mRNA expression.

Adiponectin has recently been shown to have anti-lipogenic and anti-inflammatory effects. A recent study by Hui et al. [15] examined the levels of the adipokines leptin and adiponectin, as well as activation of the tumour necrosis factor (TNF) system, in 109 subjects with NAFLD, including 80 with NASH and 29 with simple steatosis in comparison with a control cohort (matched according to age, gender and BMI) with normal liver enzymes. By multivariate analysis, reduced adiponectin level, increased TNF and increased soluble TNF receptor 2 levels occurred in subjects with NASH compared with controls. This was independent of the increased insulin resistance (assessed by the homoeostasis model assessment [HOMA]) in NASH subjects. Further, when compared with simple steatosis, NASH was associated with lower adiponectin levels and higher insulin resistance but not with differences in TNF-α or TNF-α receptor 2 levels. In addition, low serum adiponectin levels were independently associated with increased grades of hepatic inflammation. These results indicate that adipokines such as leptin and adiponectin have a critical role in the pathogenesis of hepatic steatosis and inflammation in NASH, where as TNF-α may not be relevant to the transition from steatosis to steatohepatitis. There is also a need for thorough assessments of metabolic and hormonal factors in NAFLD/NASH.

Weiss et al. [16], in a study of 439 obese children and adolescents, found similar results. There was a higher than expected prevalence of the metabolic syndrome (odds ratio, 1.12; 95% confidence interval, 1.16–2.08). The features of the metabolic syndrome worsened with increasing obesity, and were strongly correlated with increasing insulin resistance and decreasing levels of adiponectin.

Ghrelin

A novel peptide, ghrelin (which enhances appetite and promotes energy sparing, thus leading to weight gain), has recently been reported to be reduced in patients with NAFLD and to show a strong negative correlation with insulin resistance [17]. The reasons for the low levels of ghrelin in the setting of NAFLD and insulin resistance are not entirely clear. However, it has been speculated that reduced levels may somehow be teleologically aimed at preventing an increase in body mass. The significance (if any) of ghrelin in the pathogenesis of NAFLD/NASH remains to be determined.

Vascular injury

A study by Wanless and Shiota [18] has drawn attention to the role of hepatic venular obstruction in the pathogenesis and progression of NASH. Needle liver biopsies from 36 patients with NASH (and larger liver samples from three additional patients: one with NASH, one with lipopeliosis and one with alcoholic liver disease) were carefully examined and graded for steatosis, hepatocellular injury (ballooning), obstruction of small hepatic veins and stage of fibrosis. Based on data obtained in this study and on previous observations [19], a four-step model for the pathogenesis and progression of NASH was proposed:

1 Hepatic steatosis
2 Necrosis of steatotic hepatocytes
3 Release of bulk lipid into the interstitial space resulting in both direct and inflammatory damage to hepatic veins
4 Obliteration of hepatic veins with resulting parenchymal collapse and fibrosis.

Animal studies

Nutritional models of NASH
Starkel et al. [20] compared two dietary models of NAFLD, one of uncomplicated steatosis (5% orotic acid [OA] diet) and the other of steatohepatitis (lipogenic methionine- and choline-deficient [MCD] diet), with respect to inflammation, oxidative stress and stellate cell activation. Only MCD-fed animals showed evidence of inflammation, stellate cell activation, collagen deposition and upregulation of transforming growth factor-β1 (TGF-β1) and Kruppel-like factor 6 (KLF6) mRNA expression. Lipid peroxidation was increased in the MCD model in contrast to only minor changes in the OA model. Both groups showed increased uncoupling protein-2 (UCP-2) and interleukin-6 (IL-6) mRNA expression. CYP2E1 (expression and activity) was increased in the OA group but decreased in the MCD group. This study indicates that in the setting of experimental hepatic steatosis, lipid peroxidation is associated with inflammation, stellate cell activation and TGF-β1 expression, perhaps through upregulation of KLF6. These findings differ from some other studies (see Chapter 12).

Lieber et al. [21] have developed another nutritional model that reproduces many of the key features of human NAFLD. In this model, rats fed a high-fat liquid diet (71% of energy from fat, 11% from carbohydrates and 18% from protein) for 3 weeks developed panlobular steatosis, patchy mononuclear inflammation, increased plasma insulin concentrations, mitochondrial abnormalities, increased hepatic TNF-α (protein and mRNA), collagen type I and α(I) procollagen mRNA, increased CYP2E1 activity and mRNA levels and increased 4-hydroxynonenol levels; the latter indicates oxidative stress. Unlike most cases of human NAFLD, animals fed the high-fat diet did not show a significant increase in body weight or serum ALT levels compared with control animals fed a standard diet. Most of these features were attenuated by dietary restriction. Like most other animal models of NASH, and at variance with the strict histopathological criteria for the diagnosis of NASH (see Chapter 2), the inflammatory infiltrate was composed predominantly of mononuclear cells with no specific reference to neutrophils. The key clinicopathological correlate of disease outcome in NAFLD is the development of progressive hepatic fibrosis and cirrhosis. It will therefore be of interest to see whether longer term feeding of the diet results in significant weight gain, elevation of ALT levels and, most importantly, fibrosis. Although no one particular animal model is likely to reproduce all the important clinical, pathogenetic and pathological features of human NASH, this new experimental model is a significant addition to our armamentarium of models pivotal to advancing our understanding of NASH pathogenesis and outcomes.

The new Lieber *et al.* [22] model was further used to evaluate the effect of acarbose, an α-glucosidase inhibitor that is useful in the prevention of type 2 diabetes, on experimental NAFLD/NASH. Acarbose attenuated hepatic steatosis, inflammation, TNF-α mRNA and protein levels, CYP2E1 mRNA levels and collagen protein in rats fed a high fat diet for 3 weeks. Clinical studies are indicated to determine whether these beneficial effects of acarbose are applicable to human NAFLD.

Another recent novel observation is that hepatocyte expression of the Th1 cytokine, *osteopontin* (OPN) is upregulated in mice fed an MCD diet [23]. OPN protein expression was markedly increased on day 1 of the MCD diet, preceding the elevation of serum ALT (day 3), increased expression of TNF-α (day 3 to 2 weeks), hepatic steatosis (1 week), inflammation (2 weeks), oxidative stress (8 weeks) and fibrosis (8 weeks). MCD diet induced elevation in serum ALT levels, hepatic inflammation and fibrosis were markedly reduced in OPN–/– mice compared with OPN+/+ mice. This study suggests a possible role for OPN in signalling the onset of liver injury and fibrosis in experimental NAFLD.

Transgenic models for NAFLD/NASH

A study by Laurent *et al.* [24] involving genetically obese (*ob/ob*) mice has highlighted the important role of *superoxide anions* in murine steatohepatitis and suggests a potentially beneficial effect for antioxidant molecules. The production of reactive oxygen species (ROS) by liver mitochondria was measured in the presence and absence of antioxidant molecules, N-acetyl cysteine (NAC) and the superoxide dismutase mimics, ambroxol, manganese [III] tetrakis (5,10,15,20 benzoic acid) (MnTBAP), and copper [II] diisopropyl salicylate (CuDIPS). Liver mitochondria isolated from *ob/ob* mice were found to generate higher levels of $O_2^{\cdot-}$ than those of lean littermates. *Ex vivo* generation of $O_2^{\cdot-}$ was decreased in the presence of all three SOD mimics and was associated with complete inhibition of lipid peroxidation. *In vivo*, the SOD mimics, MnTBAP and this CuDIPS resulted in a significant decrease in body weight, serum ALT levels and hepatic steatosis but neither ambroxol nor NAC exerted significant effects. This study provides support for a role for superoxide anions in liver injury in NAFLD; if borne out by human studies there could be a possible role for nonpeptidyl mimics of SOD in the treatment of NASH.

Figge *et al.* [25] reported that mice overexpressing *Abcb11*, a gene that encodes for the liver bile salt export pump, are resistant to developing steatosis when fed a lithogenic diet (high cholesterol/fat/cholic acid). These animals showed markedly reduced hepatic steatosis compared with wildtype controls. This study raises the interesting possibility that regulation of *Abcb11* could play a part in the pathogenesis of NAFLD and may provide another target for therapy.

AlbCrePten^flox/flox^ mice, which have a hepatocyte-specific null mutation of the tumour suppressor gene *Pten*, develop a phenotype similar to that of NASH in humans [26]. In this model, adipocyte-specific genes and also genes involved in lipogenesis and β-oxidation were induced. These mice had massive hepatomegaly and steatohepatitis that was rather more pronounced in males than in females. An important finding was the presence of adenomas in 100% of the mice, and of hepatocellular carcinomas (HCCs) in 66%. Thus, it can be concluded that *Pten* is an important regulator not only of lipogenesis, but also of tumorigenesis in the liver.

The *db/db* mouse has a phenotype that is leptin receptor deficient, obese, diabetic, insulin resistant and has NALFD type 1 (P. Hall and R. Kirsch, unpublished observations). This transgenic model of NAFLD may be a useful model for the investigation of the effects of 'second hits'.

In a study using *ob/ob* mice, Xu *et al.* [27] administered adiponectin and showed attenuation of hepatomegaly, steatosis and serum ALT elevation. Kamada *et al.* [28] likewise showed that adiponectin lessened carbon tetrachloride-induced hepatic fibrosis in wildtype mice. In the latter study, the expression of TGF-β1 was greatly increased in adiponectin-knockout mice, leading the authors to speculate that adiponectin could be used to prevent fibrosis in obesity-associated liver injury where adiponectin levels are decreased [15]. These and other animal studies of NAFLD pathogenesis are likely to increase our understanding of the human disease and could indicate potential for novel therapeutic strategies.

Clinical features and diagnosis

Liver enzymes

It is well recognized that NAFLD/NASH can exist without elevation of serum ALT levels. A retrospective study investigated the clinical and pathological spectrum of liver disease in a subset of NAFLD/NASH patients who had normal serum ALT levels ($n = 51$) and compared these results with those seen in NAFLD/NASH patients with elevated serum ALT ($n = 50$) [29]. The entire histological spectrum of NAFLD was seen in patients with normal serum ALT levels. Furthermore, the pathology did not differ significantly from that seen in patients with elevated ALT levels. Most importantly, a low to normal serum ALT level was no guarantee for the absence of underlying steatohepatitis or advanced fibrosis [29].

C-reactive protein

A study by Hui *et al.* [30] evaluated the utility of high-sensitivity human serum C-reactive protein (hsCRP) in differentiating steatosis from steatohepatitis. Seventy-five patients with biopsy-proven NASH and 33 patients with simple steatosis were compared with respect to hsCRP levels. No relationship was demonstrated between hsCRP levels and the two conditions (mean hsCRP for NASH was 2.68 ± 2.1 mg/L versus 2.23 ± 1.68 mg/L for simple steatosis). Further, hsCRP levels did not correlate with grades of hepatic steatosis,

necroinflammation or fibrosis. However, this study was confounded by the fact that 29% of patients were taking 3-hydroxy-3-methylglutaryl coenzyme A (HMG-CoA) reductase inhibitors that are known to reduce hsCRP levels. While a larger multicentre study might have the statistical power to detect subtle differences between the two groups, the findings from this study suggest a limited clinical utility for hsCRP in distinguishing between patients with NASH and simple steatosis.

Autoantibodies in NAFLD

A study by Loria *et al.* [31] investigated the prevalence of non-organ-specific autoantibodies (NOSA), which include antinuclear antibodies (ANA) and smooth muscle antibodies (SMA) and antimitochondrial antibody (AMA), in 84 Italian patients with 'NAFLD' diagnosed on ultrasound (less than one-third of the patients were subjected to liver biopsy). The overall prevalence of NOSA was 36% (ANA 21%, SMA 4.8%, AMA 2.4%, ANA and SMA 7.1%), higher than the reported rate in the general Italian population of 6%. A subset of patients with high-titre ANA (> 1 : 100) were found to have greater degrees of insulin resistance than ANA-negative patients. However, larger studies are needed to confirm these findings in patients with biopsy-proven NAFLD and the relationship, if any, between circulating auto-antibodies and the severity of liver pathology in NAFLD.

Endocrine disturbances

Hypothalamic and pituitary dysfunction has been shown by Adams *et al.* [32] to be associated with progressive NAFLD in a subset of patients. Their study described 21 patients who had NAFLD in association with hypopituitarism, hypothalamic obesity or craniopharyngioma. The 21 patients were identified from a total of 879 patients with hypothalamic or pituitary dysfunction (a prevalence of 2.3%) at a single institution over a period of 12 years. The diagnosis was based on raised transaminases, liver ultrasound and/or liver biopsy. On average, the patients were diagnosed with NAFLD approximately 6 years after the diagnosis of hypothalamic or pituitary dysfunction. Most of the patients had developed elevated glucose levels, dyslipidaemia and excessive weight gain by the time of NAFLD diagnosis.

Of the 10 patients undergoing liver biopsy, six had cirrhosis, two had NASH with fibrosis and two had simple steatosis. Two patients required liver transplantation and two died from liver-related causes. The reported prevalence of NAFLD of 2.3% (no higher than the prevalence in the general population) in this study probably represents an underestimate as these patients were initially selected on the basis of liver enzyme tests, which were performed only once on many of the patients. In addition, normal liver enzymes do not completely exclude the presence of NAFLD (see earlier). Larger prospective studies are required to gauge the true prevalence of NAFLD in patients with hypothalamic or pituitary dysfunction. None the less, the recognition in this study of a subset of patients with hypothalamic or pituitary dysfunction who develop progressive NAFLD may have important implications for the management and surveillance of individuals with these disorders.

Drugs and NAFLD

A number of drugs cause steatohepatitis but this is usually considered to be drug-induced liver disease rather than NAFLD. However, a recent study of the side-effects of valproate suggests an increased risk of NAFLD in patients treated with this drug, perhaps related to insulin resistance [33]. An ultrasound study showed the features of fatty liver in 14 out of 23 epileptic patients treated with valproate (61%) and in only five of 22 persons treated with carbamazepine (23%). Compared with carbamazepine-treated patients, those treated with valproate showed higher BMIs, serum triglycerides, fasting glucose and insulin levels as well as insulin resistance as measured by the HOMA-IR index.

This report raises the question as to whether NAFLD is a consequence of valproate therapy or, alternatively, whether obese insulin-resistant subjects are more likely to be treated with valproate than with carbamazepine. Larger studies, preferably with liver biopsies, are required to address these questions.

Alcohol and NAFLD/NASH

The quantity of alcohol intake that precludes a diagnosis of NAFLD/NASH continues to be the subject of controversy and inconsistency in the literature. It is recognized that clinical histories are not always accurate in excluding 'significant' alcohol intake and rarely is a history of total lifetime alcohol intake (TLAI) obtained. This is despite the fact that a lifetime threshold for liver disease of 100 kg (equivalent to 30 g/day for 10 years) may exist [34,35]. Hayashi et al. [36] subjected 23 patients with biopsy-proven NAFLD to a carefully structured questionnaire aimed at determining daily alcohol intake and TLAI. A prior physician-obtained alcohol history from all patients had determined the daily intake to be less than 20 g/day. While the majority of patients in the study (87%) were found to have TLAIs of less than 100 kg, three patients (13%) had significantly higher intakes (all above 300 kg). Two of these patients had daily intakes of over 20 g/day. In addition, a fourth patient had a TLAI of just below 100 kg. Although this is a small study, it raises several important issues. First, a significant proportion of patients diagnosed with NAFLD may in fact have alcohol-induced fatty liver disease. In this regard, the relevance of TLAI intake in NAFLD warrants further research, particularly in patients with other risk factors for NAFLD in whom alcohol may serve as the toxic factor or 'second hit'. The results of a recent study on the effects of 'low-dose' alcohol in a rodent nutritional model add support to the suggestion that alcohol may be one of the 'second hits' that trigger steatohepatitis [37]. Secondly, the study by Hayashi et al. [36] suggests an important role for a standardized and reproducible questionnaire in subjects considered to have 'pure' metabolic forms of liver disease. This report also highlights the need for consensus on 'acceptable' levels of alcohol intake in persons recruited into NAFLD studies. Despite the above cogent concerns on alcohol intake in relation to the conduct of *clinical* studies of NAFLD pathogenesis, it should be noted that in office practice, the combination of alcohol intake and insulin resistance worsens liver injury irrespective of the semantics of the diagnosis, namely NAFLD or NAFLD/alcoholic liver disease.

Steatosis and hepatitis C

A number of recent reports have focused on the close relationship between hepatitis C virus (HCV), steatosis and insulin resistance [38–41]. In patients with HCV, fatty liver is strongly associated with features of the metabolic syndrome and is a risk factor for advanced fibrosis; the latter has been shown to be related to weight, presence of diabetes and the degree of hepatocyte ballooning [38]. A review by Lonardo et al. [39] highlights the many new advances in this field and focuses specifically on the mechanisms and signficance of steatosis in chronic HCV infection. The discussion below draws attention to some of the most recent advances.

HCV and insulin resistance

Hui et al. [40] investigated the relationship between liver pathology and insulin resistance in 260 patients with chronic HCV infection. Insulin resistance, as measured by the HOMA-IR, fasting insulin and C-peptide levels were compared in a subset of 121 HCV infected patients and 137 controls matched for age, BMI and waist : hip ratio. Higher levels of insulin resistance were demonstrated in HCV-infected patients compared with controls, irrespective of the severity of the liver disease. This effect was genotype specific, with genotype 3 infection being associated with significantly lower HOMA-IR than other genotypes. This is an interesting finding in view of the more extensive steatosis reported in genotype 3-infected patients compared with other genotypes. This is consistent with the proposal that steatosis in genotype 3 infection is mediated by viral factors rather than by insulin resistance [42–44]. Moreover, although obesity has a role in the development of steatosis in patients infected with genotypes 1, and possibly 2a/c, it is not required in patients infected with genotype 3a [42]. A second important finding was that insulin resistance was an independent predictor of the degree of fibrosis in chronic HCV infection. Thus insulin resistance may contribute to fibrogenesis in this condition [39]. More recently, this has been applied to the development of a fibrosis probability index to determine, using non-invasive parameters, the fibrosis stage in persons with chronic HCV infection [44].

Hepatitis C genotype 3 and steatosis

The relationship between HCV genotype 3 infection and the well-known risk factors for steatosis (including BMI and serum lipid levels) were examined in a retrospective study by Sharma et al. [45]. They studied 293 consecutive HCV patients (218 with genotype 1, 43 with genotype 2 and 32 with genotype 3). HCV genotype 3 patients were younger, had lower serum cholesterol levels and a higher prevalence of moderate to severe steatosis compared with non-genotype 3 patients. This study adds further support for the strong association between HCV genotype 3 infection and steatosis, and also confirms that in genotype 3-infected patients the steatosis is aetiologically distinct and not related to the usual factors predisposing NAFLD.

Steatosis and apolipoprotein B in hepatitis C

Petit et al. [46] reported a strong correlation between steatosis and apolipoprotein B (ApoB) levels in chronic HCV infection, consistent with another recent study [47]. The authors suggest a potential role for impaired metabolism of ApoB in the pathogenesis of chronic HCV infection and speculate that this might occur via the direct action of HCV core protein on microsomal triglyceride transfer protein (MTP) function.

Potential mechanisms for hepatic fibrogenesis in persons with chronic hepatitis C and steatosis

The mechanisms by which steatosis might contribute to liver injury and fibrosis in HCV infection were addressed by Walsh et al. [48]. They examined the relationship between liver cell apoptosis and disease severity in 125 patients with chronic HCV infection. Increasing grades of steatosis were associated with increased levels of apoptosis, decreased Bcl-2 mRNA levels and an increased pro-apoptotic ratio (Bax : Bcl-2). In the presence of steatosis, increasing apoptosis was associated with stellate cell activation and fibrosis. Such an association was not present in livers that were not steatotic, supporting the notion that steatotic livers are more susceptible to injury. Further studies are needed to elucidate the molecular pathways mediating the proapoptotic effect of steatosis and to determine whether hepatocyte apoptosis directly promotes fibrogenesis.

Iron and NAFLD/NASH

Bugianesi et al.[49] evaluated the relative contributions of iron burden, HFE mutations and insulin resistance to fibrosis in NAFLD. This prospective study included 263 patients with NAFLD in whom the diagnosis was based on liver ultrasound and/or liver biopsy. Peripheral iron overload was present in 7.4%, hepatic iron overload in 9% and hyperferritinaemia in 21% of patients. The presence of *HFE* mutations was similar to that seen in the general population and the mutations were not associated with iron overload. Serum ferritin levels and insulin resistance were independent risk factors for the development of hepatic fibrosis. Hepatic iron burden and *HFE* mutations were not significantly associated with liver fibrosis. These findings are in keeping with most recent studies, which have failed to demonstrate a significant association between hepatic iron burden, *HFE* mutations and liver fibrosis (see Chapter 23). Hyperferritinaemia, which was an independent predictor of fibrosis in this study, has been observed in association with diabetes, hypertension (in males) and hyperlipidaemia, and has been suggested to be a marker for the insulin resistance syndrome. The demonstration that insulin resistance is an independent risk factor for hepatic fibrosis adds to the evidence for an association between insulin resistance and the severity of liver pathology. It remains to be determined whether insulin resistance has a direct role in contributing to liver damage in the setting of steatosis and, if so, what are the relevant mechanisms. Nevertheless, it has been speculated that insulin resistance may act as both first and 'second hits' in the development and progression of NAFLD, indicating the potential limitations of this older concept (see Chapters 1, 8 and 12).

Non-invasive predictors of hepatic fibrosis

Liver biopsy continues to be the only reliable method for diagnosing, grading and staging NAFLD/NASH and for monitoring therapy. The search for non-invasive markers for hepatic fibrosis therefore continues. Laine *et al.* [50] reported, in a prospective study of 173 patients (both drinkers and non-drinkers) with clinical features of the metabolic syndrome, that no patients with a serum hyaluronate level < 35 µg/L had significant hepatic fibrosis (i.e. Metavir score > F2). They developed 'a simple algorithim, including serum hyaluronate and serum carbohydrate-deficient transferrin/transferrin ratio' for use in patients with the metabolic syndrome and raised ALT. No instance of

severe hepatic fibrosis (Metavir score > F2) was found when this ratio was > 0.9, irrespective of present or past alcohol consumption. The authors report a 100% predictive value for this algorithm. The results of further larger studies are awaited with interest.

Hepatocellular carcinoma in NAFLD

Regimbeau *et al.* [51] investigated the prevalence of risk factors for NAFLD in a cohort of 210 patients undergoing resection for HCC on a background of chronic liver disease. A subset of 18 patients (8.6%), who had no identifiable cause for liver disease, was further investigated for risk factors for NAFLD. Compared with matched patients with alcohol- and chronic viral hepatitis-related HCC, the prevalence of obesity was 50% (versus 17% and 14%, respectively) and diabetes 56% (versus 17% and 11%, respectively). The prevalence of hepatic steatosis (involving > 20% of hepatocytes) was significantly higher in patients with cryptogenic liver disease (61%) compared with patients with alcohol abuse (17%) or chronic viral hepatitis (19%). Well-differentiated tumours were significantly more common in patients with cryptogenic liver disease (89%) than in alcohol-related (64%) or chronic viral hepatitis-related (55%) HCC. This report indicates that obesity and diabetes mellitus could be important risk factors for HCC seen in association with cryptogenic chronic liver disease. It remains to be determined whether HCC in these patients is primarily related to obesity and diabetes mellitus or secondary to NAFLD/NASH. The recent report of the development of HCCs in 100% of *AlbCrePten^{flox/flox}* mice (discussed earlier) adds further support to the concept that disturbances of lipogenesis and hepatocyte lipid homoeostasis could be risk factors for hepatocarcinogenesis [26].

Natural history

The impact of patient subgroups and histological subtypes of NAFLD on the development of advanced fibrotic liver disease has been emphasized in three recent papers.

Dam-Larsen *et al.* [52] performed a large cohort study of 109 Danish patients with type 1 (steatosis alone)

NAFLD and 106 patients with alcoholic steatosis followed for a median of 17 and 9.2 years, respectively. While only one (1%) NAFLD patient progressed to cirrhosis, 22 (21%) of the patients with alcoholic steatosis did so. Another study [53] compared sequential liver biopsies (mean of 5.7 years between biopsies) obtained in 22 patients with NAFLD, of whom 19 had NASH. The results demonstrated that the histopathological course of these patients was variable. One-third progressed to fibrosis and 10% had a rapid progression to advanced fibrosis. These combined data confirm previous reports that the development of fibrosis or cirrhosis in NAFLD is related to the histopathology found in the index biopsy. Further, cirrhosis develops much more frequently in alcoholic steatosis than in non-alcoholic steatosis.

A report from Younossi *et al.* [54] investigated the impact of type 2 diabetes in the development of cirrhosis and liver-related death in NAFLD patients; 44 with and 88 without diabetes. Cirrhosis (25% versus 10.2%) and liver-related death (18.2% versus 2.3%) occurred more frequently in the diabetic group.

Hepatic steatosis in living donor livers

The effect of donor weight reduction on hepatic steatosis

There is a consensus that livers showing 'total steatosis' of > 30% of hepatocytes should not be used for living donor transplantation; this has led to the exclusion of many potential donors. This growing problem led Hwang *et al.* [55] to encourage nine potential living donors who had excessive hepatic steatosis and/or were overweight to lose ~ 9% of their body weight. None of the initial liver biopsies showed features of NASH; seven showed NAFLD type 2 while the remaining two showed steatosis and mild portal inflammation. The nine volunteers lost $5.9 \pm 2\%$ of initial body weight during a 2–6 month period. The BMI reduced from 25 ± 3.8 to 24 ± 3.4 and hepatic steatosis, especially microvesicular steatosis, decreased significantly from $49 \pm 26\%$ to $20 \pm 16\%$ after weight loss. All nine became donors, and all recipients survived. This study confirms the role of weight loss alone as an effective means for reducing hepatic steatosis and thereby increasing the potential pool of living liver transplant donors.

Management of NAFLD/NASH

Clinical studies

Drug trials continue but there is still no proven pharmacological treatment for NAFLD/NASH that alters long-term outcomes. Management is mainly aimed at controlling predisposing conditions such as obesity, diabetes mellitus and dyslipidaemia. Several pharmacological therapies have shown promise in small short-term pilot studies; agents have included insulin-sensitizing medications, lipid-lowering agents, antioxidants and the naturally occurring bile acid, ursodeoxycholic acid. Few of these agents have been subjected to large randomized and placebo controlled long-term study. The most recent reports are highlighted below.

Weight reduction

A number of recent studies have confirmed that weight loss, by whatever means, including diet alone [55,56], medication such as oristat [57] or bariatric surgery such as gastric banding [58] or gastroplasty [13], is accompanied by a decrease in hepatic steatosis. Whether this weight loss and the associated reduction in hepatic steatosis will be maintained and translate into better long-term outcomes awaits further study.

Xydakis *et al.* [56] report a marked improvement in glucose, insulin and triglycerides in 40 obese individuals following 4–6 kg weight loss, but no changes in adiponectin or TNF-α). They concluded that an increase in plasma adiponectin levels and a decrease in TNF-α are not necessary for the improvement in insulin sensitivity that occurs in association with weight loss.

Harrison *et al.* [57] reported three obese patients with biopsy-proven NASH who showed significant weight loss, and clinical and histopathological improvement following treatment for 6–12 months with orlistat.

Dixon *et al.* [58] examined the effect of weight loss on NAFLD/NASH and hepatic fibrosis. Their study included 36 obese patients (BMI > 35 kg/m^2; 11 males, 25 females) who were subjected to two liver biopsies, the first at the time of laparoscopic adjustable gastric band placement and the second after weight loss (mean 26 ± 10 months, range 9–51 months after band placement). Gastric banding resulted in a mean weight reduction of 34 ± 17 kg and a marked improvement in liver histology, including a reduction in the severity of steatosis, necroinflammation and fibrosis (82% of patients showed resolution or lessening in the severity of NASH) ($P < 0.001$ for all). Initial liver biopsies revealed NASH in 23 patients and simple steatosis in 12, while only four follow-up biopsies fulfilled the histological criteria for a diagnosis of NASH. Only three patients had fibrosis scores of 2 or more compared with 18 of the initial biopsies ($P < 0.001$).

Patients with the metabolic syndrome ($n = 23$) showed more pronounced liver injury before surgery as well as greater improvement in liver pathology following weight loss. The mean duration of the study was 25 months after surgery. Most of the patients not only lost weight, but maintained this weight loss. This differs from weight loss associated with low-carbohydrate diets, which tends to be followed by some weight gain.

This important study highlights the major benefits of gastric banding surgery, in selected severely obese subjects, for both weight loss and for the lessening of liver injury.

Lipid-lowering medications

Rallidis and Drakoulis [59] treated five patients with biopsy-proven NASH and liver enzyme abnormalities with the HMG CoA reductase inhibitor *pravastatin* (20 mg/day for 6 months). Excluded from the study were those with diabetes, obesity or elevated aminotransferases to more than three times the upper limit of normal. Treatment significantly reduced cholesterol levels but not serum triglyceride. Liver enzymes normalized in all five patients after treatment. Histologically, treatment resulted in a variable improvement in the grade of inflammatory activity but not in the fibrosis score using the Brunt criteria. Three patients showed an improvement in the extent of inflammation and one a reduction in steatosis. These results indicate a possible beneficial effect of pravastatin in a subset of patients with NASH, but larger studies are needed to confirm these preliminary observations.

Merat *et al.* [60] evaluated the use of *probucol*, a lipid-lowering agent with strong antioxidant properties in a double-blind, randomized placebo-controlled study including 27 patients with biopsy-proven NASH (treatment group $n = 18$, placebo group $n = 9$). The treatment group received 500 mg/day probucol for 6 months and showed a significant decrease in serum ALT levels compared with the control group. Both serum AST and ALT levels normalized in nine of the treatment group (50%) but in none of the control group. Probucil has subsequently been withdrawn from clinical use in the US.

Insulin-sensitizing agents

The aim of a study by Neuschwander-Tetri *et al.* [61] was to determine whether improving insulin sensitivity with *rosiglitazone* lessened the severity of liver injury in 30 adult patients with biopsy-proven NASH. All patients were overweight (BMI > 25 kg/m^2), and 23% of them were severely obese (BMI > 35 kg/m^2); 50% had impaired glucose tolerance or diabetes. The patients received rosiglitazone, 4 mg twice daily, for 48 weeks. All patients had a pretreatment liver biopsy that was initially diagnosed as NASH but on subsequent blinded evaluation only 22 of these biopsies met the published criteria for NASH. Twenty-six patients had post-treatment biopsies; those that met the histological criteria for a diagnosis of NASH before treatment showed a significant reduction in the amount of hepatocellular ballooning and zone 3 perisinusoidal fibrosis. Significantly, improved insulin sensitivity and lower mean serum ALT levels (104 U/C initially, 42 U/L at the end of treatment) were seen in the 25 patients who completed 48 weeks of treatment. However, weight gain occurred in 67% of patients; the median weight increase was 7.3%, and by 6 months after completion of treatment liver enzyme levels had increased to near pretreatment levels.

Similar results were obtained by Promrat *et al.* [62], who evaluated the role of the insulin-sensitizing agent *pioglitazone* in 18 non-diabetic patients with biopsy-proven NASH. Patients received 30 mg/day pioglitazone for 48 weeks, with tests for insulin resistance, body fat composition, serum ALT levels and liver biopsies being performed before and after treatment. At 48 weeks, 72% of patients showed normalization of serum ALT levels. Hepatic fat content and size (determined by magnetic resonance imaging) decreased, and glucose and free fatty acid sensitivity to insulin improved uniformly. Liver biopsies showed a significant reduction in steatosis, inflammation, cellular injury, Mallory bodies and fibrosis after treatment (all $P < 0.05$). Although pioglitazone was well tolerated, patients experienced slight weight gain (average 4%) and an increase in total body adiposity. While this pilot study suggests that pioglitozone can lead to biochemical and histological improvement in NASH, larger and longer term studies with the relevant controls are required to determine whether pioglitazone is truly beneficial in NASH, both with respect to histological and clinical outcomes, and with respect to long-term safety.

The weight gain that was observed in both these studies of insulin-sensitizing agents [61,62] indicate potential limitations of the otherwise promising peroxisome proliferator-activated receptor-γ (PPARγ) agonist in the treatment of NASH.

Antioxidants

Harrison *et al.* [63] investigated the effects of a combination of vitamins E and C on liver enzymes and liver histology in 45 NASH patients. In a double-blind, randomized, placebo controlled trial, patients received either combination vitamin E and C (1000 IU and 1000 mg, respectively) or placebo daily for 6 months. There was a statistically significant reduction in the fibrosis score (by Brunt criteria) in those receiving vitamins compared with pretreatment values. However, the vitamin group did not show statistically significant improvement when compared with the placebo group, and in fact some patients in the placebo group showed an apparent reduction in their fibrosis scores. Six months of vitamin E and C administration did not alter the necroinflammatory activity or serum ALT levels.

Ursodeoxycholic acid

A randomized, double-blind, placebo controlled trial involving more than 100 patients with NASH found that treatment with ursodeoxycholic acid (UDCA) for 2 years had no detectable effect on disease course [64]. While this negative trial most likely reflects a true lack of efficacy of UCDA on NASH outcomes, a recent editorial by Clark and Brancati [65] addressed some of the methodological considerations of the trial that could have conspired to mask a true beneficial effect of UCDA; these are of relevance to the design of future therapeutic trials in NAFLD/NASH). These included:

1 Small study size, resulting in a 'statistically underpowered' trial.

2 The possibility that the primary outcomes, namely liver enzymes and histology, were not sufficiently sensitive to detect subtle differences in a relatively small sample size.

3 Temporal fluctuation in liver biochemistry and histology (well described in patients with NASH) may, in combination with key eligibility criteria, have biased the study towards a negative result.

4 Aspects of study design may have influenced the outcome: e.g. whether or not the dosage of UCDA was optimal, whether or not the study was of sufficient duration, whether or not the correct preparation was used, and whether or not compliance was ensured.

This editorial highlights several important points. First, there is an urgent need for a histological grading scheme for NAFLD/NASH that is 'valid, precise and standardizable across research sites'. Such a scheme could generate quantitative or semi-quantitative data that improves the statistical power of relatively small trials. It is of note that several of the recent clinical studies involving scoring of liver injury have used modification of the scoring system proposed and modified by Brunt [4]; in particular, a separate score is given for portal fibrosis in some studies [3,55]. Secondly, the variability associated with widely used NASH markers such as ALT, AST and steatosis should be accurately determined and carefully accounted for in study design and statistical analysis. Thirdly, it should be appreciated that the clinical study of NASH poses significant challenges, not least with respect to patient recruitment and retention which result, in part, from the relatively low profile of NALFD/NASH in primary care settings, and the requirement for an invasive procedure for diagnosis and surveillance.

Animal studies

Dietary modification

A recent study in *ob/ob mice* reports the amelioration of hepatic steatosis following a diet high in carbohydrate, supplemented with polyunsaturated fatty acids (PUFAs)—either eicosapentaenoic acid or tuna fish oil for 7 days [66]. PUFAs are negative regulators of hepatic lipogenesis; such negative downstream regulation is thought to be mediated by repression of sterol regulatory element-binding protein-1 (SREBP-1). PUFAs both downregulate SREBP-1 and therefore triglyceride synthesis, and activate PPARα. The clinical value of a diet rich in PUFAs in the treatment of NAFLD/NASH is now worthy of study.

Lipid-lowering medications

A study in mice reported that *pitavastatin*, a 3-hydroxy-3-methylglutaryl-coenzyme A reductase inhibitor, is capable of restoring impaired fatty acid β-oxidation with amelioration of severe hepatic steatosis in aromatase-deficient mice defective in instrinsic oestrogen synthesis [67]. This effect is mediated via the PPARα signalling pathway.

Insulin-sensitizing agents
Pioglitazone has also been reported to improve hepatic steatosis and to prevent liver fibrosis in rats fed a choline-deficient diet [68]. Pioglitazone reduced the expression of tissue inhibitors of metalloproteinases (MMP), TIMP-1 and TIMP-2 mRNA, without changing mRNA expression of the matrix metalloproteinase MMP-13. *In vitro*, pioglitazone prevented the activation of hepatic stellate cells resulting in reduced expression of type 1 procollagen, MMP-2, TIMP-1 and TIMP-2 mRNA and increased MMP-13 mRNA expression. These effects were thought to be mediated by the action of pioglitazone acting as a PPARγ ligand.

PPARα
The PPARα Wy-14,643 has been shown to reverse steatosis, necroinflammation and fibrosis in the MCD mouse model for NAFLD [69]. This effect is probably via a reduction in fibrogenic stimuli, such as lipid peroxides, that activate collagen-producing hepatic stellate cells.

The value of these various therapies used in animal models, as treatment for human NAFLD remains to be determined.

Conclusions

Publications in the last 12 months have been dominated by those providing further insights into the importance of insulin resistance in NAFLD/NASH, pathophysiological mechanisms and comorbidity brought about by other types of liver injury, especially HCV infection.

New animal models have provided insights into pathogenic mechanisms and provide an opportunity to test novel hypotheses and potential therapeutic agents.

Regrettably, in most of the new studies employing either medical or surgical management, where improvement was assessed by comparison of scores in pre- and post-treatment liver biopsies, the investigators use their own modified scoring systems, making comparisons between studies difficult. Thus, there is an urgent need for an internationally accepted scoring system to be used in future therapeutic trials.

Despite many reports on the benefits of weight loss and a plethora of studies on pharmacological agents, the challenge for the future is to demonstrate alterations in the natural history of NAFLD/NASH and disease outcomes.

References

1 Gramlich T, Kleiner DE, McCullough AJ *et al*. Pathologic features associated with fibrosis in nonalcoholic fatty liver disease. *Hum Pathol* 2004; **35**: 196–9.
2 Le TH, Caldwell SH, Redick JA *et al*. The zonal distribution of megamitochondria with crystalline inclusions in nonalcoholic steatohepatitis. *Hepatology* 2004; **39**: 1423–9.
3 Mendler MH, Kanel G, Govidarajan S. Proposal for a histological scoring and grading system for nonalcoholic liver disease. *Liver Int* 2005; **25**: (in press).
4 Brunt EM. Nonalcoholic steatohepatitis. *Semin Liver Dis* 2004; **24**: 3–20.
5 Clouston AD, Powell EE. Nonalcoholic fatty liver disease: is all the fat bad? *Intern Med J* 2004; **34**: 187–91.
6 Friedman LS. Controversies in liver biopsy: who, where, when, how, why? *Curr Gastroenterol Rep* 2004; 630–6.
7 Laurin J. Motion: all patients with NASH need to have a liver biopsy—arguments against the motion. *Can J Gastroenterol* 2002; **16**: 722–6.
8 Wong F. The role of liver biopsy in the management of patients with liver disease. *Can J Gastroenterol* 2003; **17**: 651–6.
9 Lieber CS. New concepts of the pathogenesis of alcoholic liver disease lead to novel treatments. *Curr Gastroenterol Rep* 2004; **6**: 60–5.
10 Lieber CS. CYP2E1: from ASH to NASH. *Hepatol Res* 2004; **28**: 1–11.
11 Nanji AA. Another animal model for nonalcoholic steatohepatitis: how close to the human condition? *Am J Clin Nutr* 2004; **79**: 350–1.
12 Videla LA, Rodrigo R, Orellana M *et al*. Oxidative stress-related parameters in the liver of non-alcoholic fatty liver disease. *Clin Sci (Lond)* 2004; **106**: 261–8.
13 Emery MG, Fisher JM, Chein JY *et al*. CYP2E1 activity before and after weight loss in morbidly obese subjects with non-alcoholic fatty liver disease. *Hepatology* 2003; **38**: 428–35.
14 Chalasani N, Crabb DW, Cummings OW *et al*. Does leptin play a role in the pathogenesis of human nonalcoholic steatohepatitis? *Am J Gastroenterol* 2003; **98**: 2771–6.
15 Hui JM, Hodge A, Farrell GC *et al*. Beyond insulin resistance in NASH: TNF or adiponectin. *Hepatology* 2004; **40**: 46–54.

16 Weiss R, Dziura J, Burget TS *et al.* Obesity and the metabolic syndrome in children and adolescents. *N Engl J Med* 2004; **350**: 2362–74.

17 Marchesini G, Pagotto U, Bugianesi E *et al.* Low ghrelin concentrations in nonalcoholic fatty liver disease are related to insulin resistance. *J Clin Endocrinol Metab* 2003; **88**: 5674–9.

18 Wanless IR, Shiota K. The pathogenesis of nonalcoholic steatohepatitis and other fatty liver diseases: a four-step model including the role of lipid release and hepatic venular obstruction in the progression to cirrhosis. *Semin Liver Dis* 2004; **24**: 99–106.

19 Wanless IR, Nakashima E, Sherman M. Regression of human cirrhosis: morphologic features and genesis of incomplete septal cirrhosis. *Arch Pathol Lab Med* 2000; **124**: 1599–607.

20 Starkel P, Sempoux C, Leclercq I *et al.* Oxidative stress, KLF6 and transforming growth factor-β up-regulation differentiate non-alcoholic steatohepatitis progressing to fibrosis from uncomplicated steatosis in rats. *J Hepatol* 2003; **39**: 53846.

21 Lieber CS, Leo MA, Mak KM *et al.* Model of non-alcoholic steatohepatitis. *Am J Clin Nutr* 2004; **79**: 502–9.

22 Lieber CS, Leo MA, Mak KM *et al.* Acarbose attenuates experimental non-alcoholic steatohepatitis. *Biochem Biophys Res Commun* 2004; **315**: 699–703.

23 Sahai A, Malladi P, Melin-Aldana H, Green RM, Whitington PF. Upregulation of osteopontin is involved in the development of nonalcoholic steatohepatitis in a dietary murine model. *Am J Physiol Gastrointest Liver Physiol* 2004; **287**: G264–73.

24 Laurent A, Nicco C, Tran Van Nhieu J *et al.* Pivotal role of superoxide anion and beneficial effect of antioxidant molecules in murine steatohepatitis. *Hepatology* 2004; **39**: 1277–85.

25 Figge A, Lammert F, Paigen BJ *et al.* Hepatic overexpression of murine *Abcb11* increases hepatobiliary lipid secretion and reduces hepatic steatosis. *Biol Chem* 2004; **279**: 2790–9.

26 Horie Y, Suzuki A, Kataoka E *et al.* Hepatocyte-specific *Pten* deficiency results in steatohepatitis and hepatocellular carcinomas. *J Clin Invest* 2004; **113**: 1774–83.

27 Xu A, Wang Y, Keshaw H, Lam KS, Cooper GJ. The fat-derived hormone adiponectin alleviates alcoholic and non-alcoholic fatty liver diseases in mice. *J Clin Invest* 2003; **112**: 91–100.

28 Kamada Y, Tamura S, Kiso S *et al.* Enhanced carbon tetrachloride-induced liver fibrosis in mice lacking adiponectin. *Gastroenterology* 2003; **125**: 1796–807.

29 Mofrad P, Contos MJ, Haque M *et al.* Clinical and histologic spectrum of nonalcoholic fatty liver disease associated with normal ALT values. *Hepatology* 2003; **37**: 1286–92.

30 Hui J, Farrell GC, Kench JG, George J. High sensitivity CRP protein values do not reliably predict the severity of histological change in NAFLD (Letter). *Hepatology* 2004; **39**: 1458–9.

31 Loria P, Lonardo A, Leonardi F *et al.* Non-organ-specific autoantibodies in nonalcoholic fatty liver disease: prevalence and correlates. *Dig Dis Sci* 2003; **48**: 2173–81.

32 Adams LA, Feldstein A, Lindor KD, Angulo P. Nonalcoholic fatty liver disease among patients with hypothalamic and pituitary dysfunction. *Hepatology* 2004; **39**: 909–14.

33 Luef GJ, Waldmann M, Sturm W *et al.* Valproate therapy and nonalcoholic fatty liver disease. *Ann Neurol* 2004; **55**: 72009–32.

34 Bellentani S, Tiribelli C. The spectrum of liver disease in the general population: lesson from the Dionysos study. *J Hepatol* 2001; **35**: 531–7.

35 Bellentani S, Saccoccio G, Costa G *et al.* Drinking habits as cofactors of risk for alcohol induced liver damage. The Dionysos Study Group. *Gut* 1997; **41**: 845–50.

36 Hayashi PH, Harrison SA, Torgerson S *et al.* Cognitive lifetime drinking history in nonalcoholic fatty liver disease: some cases may be alcohol related. *J Gastroenterol* 2003; **9039**: 76–81.

37 Clarkson VC, Hall P, Shephard E, Kirsch R, Marais D. Ethanol feeding increases CYP2E11 activity in the methionine choline deficient mouse model for NASH (Abstract). *Liver Int* 2004; **24** (Suppl. 4): 18.

38 Sanyal AJ, Contos MJ, Sterling RK *et al.* Nonalcoholic fatty liver disease in patients with hepatitis C is associated with features of the metabolic syndrome. *Am J Gastroenterol* 2003; **98**: 2064–71.

39 Lonardo A, Adinolfi LE, Loria P *et al.* Steatosis and hepatitis C virus: mechanisms and significance for hepatic and extrahepatic disease. *Gastroenterology* 2004; **126**: 586–97.

40 Hui J, Sud A, Farrell GC *et al.* Insulin resistance is associated with chronic hepatitis C and virus infection fibrosis progression. *Gastroenterology* 2003; **125**: 1695–704.

41 Monto A, Alonzo J, Watson JJ, Grunfeld C, Wright TL. Steatosis in chronic hepatitis C: relative contributions of obesity, diabetes mellitus and alcohol. *Hepatology* 2002; **36**: 729–36.

42 Hui JM, Hench J, Farrell GC *et al.* Genotype specific mechanisms for hepatic steatosis in chronic hepatitis C infection. *J Gastroenterol Hepatol* 2002; **17**: 873–81.

43 Adinolfi LE, Gambardella M, Andreana A *et al.* Steatosis accelerates the progression of liver damage of chronic hepatitis C patients and correlates with specific HCV genotype and visceral obesity. *Hepatology* 2001; **33**: 1358–64.

44 Sud A, Hui JM, Farrell GC *et al.* Improved prediction of fibrosis in chronic hepatitis C using measures of insulin resistance in a probability index. *Hepatology* 2004; **39**: 1239–47.

45 Sharma P, Balan V, Hernandez J *et al.* Hepatic steatosis in hepatitis C virus genotype 3 infection: does it correlate with body mass index, fibrosis, and HCV risk factors? *Dig Dis Sci* 2004; **49**: 25–9.

46 Petit JM, Benichou M, Duvillard L *et al.* Hepatitis C virus-associated hypobetalipoproteinemia is correlated with plasma viral load, steatosis, and liver fibrosis. *Am J Gastroenterol* 2003; **98**: 1150–4.

47 Serfaty L, Andreani T, Giral P *et al.* Hepatitis C virus induced hypobetalipoproteinemia: a possible mechanism for steatosis in chronic hepatitis C. *J Hepatol* 2001; **34**: 428–34.

48 Walsh J, Vanags DM, Clouston AD *et al.* Steatosis and liver cell apoptosis in chronic hepatitisC: a mechanism for increased liver injury. *Hepatology* 2004; **39**: 1230–8.

49 Bugianesi E, Manzini P, D'Antico S *et al.* Relative contribution of iron burden, *HFE* mutations, and insulin resistance to fibrosis in nonalcoholic fatty liver. *Hepatology* 2004; **39**: 179–87.

50 Laine F, Bendavid C, Moirand R *et al.* Prediction of liver fibrosis in patients with features of the metabolic syndrome regardless of alcohol consumption. *Hepatology* 2004; **39**: 1639–46.

51 Regimbeau JM, Colombat M, Mognol P *et al.* Obesity and diabetes as a risk factor for hepatocellular carcinoma. *Liver Transpl* 2004; **10** (Suppl. 1): 69–73.

52 Dam-Larsen S, Frank Mann M, Andersen IB *et al.* Long-term prognosis of fatty liver: risk of chronic liver disease and death. *Gut* 2004; **53**: 750–5.

53 Harrison SA, Torgerson S, Hayashi PH. The natural history of non-alcoholic fatty liver disease: a clinical histopathological study. *Am J Gastroenterol* 2003; **98**: 2042–7.

54 Younossi ZM, Gramlich T, Matteoni CA, Bopari N, McCullough AJ. Non-alcoholic fatty liver disease in patients with type 2 diabetes. *Clin Gastroenterol Hepatol* 2004; **2**: 262–5.

55 Hwang S, Lee S-G, Jang S-J *et al.* The effect of donor weight reduction on hepatic steatosis for living donor liver transplantation. *Liver Transpl* 2004; **10**: 721–5.

56 Xydakis AM, Case CC, Jones PH *et al.* Adiponectin, inflammation, and the expression of the metabolic syndrome in obese individuals: the impact of rapid weight loss through caloric restriction. *J Clin Endocrinol Metab* 2004; **89**: 2697–703.

57 Harrison SA, Ramrakhiani S, Brunt EM *et al.* Orlistat in the treatment of NASH: a case series. *Am J Gastroenterol* 2003; **98**: 926–30.

58 Dixon JB, Bhathal PS, Hughes NR, O'Brien PE. Nonalcoholic fatty liver disease: improvement in liver histological analysis with weight loss. *Hepatology* 2004; **39**: 1647–54.

59 Rallidis LS, Drakoulis C. Pravastatin in patients with non-alcoholic steatohepatitis: results of a pilot study. *Atherosclerosis* 2004; **174**: 193–6.

60 Merat S, Malekzadeh R, Sohrabi MR *et al.* Probucol in the treatment of non-alcoholic steatohepatitis: a double-blind randomized controlled study. *J Hepatol* 2003; **38**: 414–8.

61 Neuschwander-Tetri BA, Brunt EM, Wehmeier KR, Oliver D, Bacon BR. Improved nonalcoholic steatohepatitis after 48 weeks of treatment with the PPAR-γ ligand rosiglitazone. *Hepatology* 2003; **38**: 100817.

62 Promrat K, Lutchman G, Uwaifo GI *et al.* A pilot study of pioglitazone treatment for nonalcoholic steatohepatitis. *Hepatology* 2004; **39**: 18896.

63 Harrison SA, Torgerson S, Hayashi P, Ward J, Schenker S. Vitamin E and vitamin C treatment improves fibrosis in patients with nonalcoholic steatohepatitis. *Am J Gastroenterol* 2003; **98**: 2485–90.

64 Lindor KD, Kowdley KV, Heathcote EJ *et al.* Ursodeoxycholic acid for treatment of nonalcoholic steatohepatitis: results of a randomized trial. *Hepatology* 2004; **39**: 770–8.

65 Clark JM, Brancati FL. Negative trials in nonalcoholic steatohepatitis: why they happen and what they teach us. *Hepatology* 2004; **39**: 602–3.

66 Sekiya M, Yahagi N, Matsuzaki T *et al.* Polyunsaturated fatty acids ameliorate hepatic steatosis in obese mice by SREBP-1 suppression. *Hepatology* 2003; **38**: 1529–39.

67 Egawa T, Toda K, Nemoto Y *et al.* Pitavastatin ameliorates severe hepatic steatosis in aromatase-deficient (Ar–/–) mice. *Lipids* 2003; **38**: 19–23.

68 Kawaguchi K, Sakaida I, Tsuchiya M *et al.* Pioglitazone prevents hepatic steatosis, fibrosis and enzyme-altered lesions rat liver cirrhosis induced by a choline-deficient L-amino acid-deficient diet. *Biochem Biophys Res Commun* 2004; **315**: 187–95.

69 Ip E, Farrell G, Hall P, Robertson G, Leclercq I. Administration of the potent PPARα antagonist Wy-14,643, reverses nutritional fibrosis and steatohepatitis in mice. *Hepatology* 2004; **39**: 1286–96.

Index